# Pediatric Drugs and Nursing Implications

**Ruth McGillis Bindler, RNC, MS**
Associate Professor
Intercollegiate Center for Nursing Education
Spokane, Washington

**Linda Berner Howry, RN, MS**
Former Assistant Professor
Intercollegiate Center for Nursing Education
Spokane, Washington

## APPLETON & LANGE
Norwalk, Connecticut/San Mateo, California

0-8385-7819-5

Notice: Our knowledge in clinical sciences is constantly changing. As new information becomes available, changes in treatment and in the use of drugs become necessary. The authors and the publisher of this volume have taken care to make certain that the doses of drugs and schedules of treatment are correct and compatible with the standards generally accepted at the time of publication. The reader is advised to consult carefully the instruction and information material included in the package insert of each drug or therapeutic agent before administration. This advice is especially important when using new or infrequently used drugs.

91 92 93 94 95 / 10 9 8 7 6 5 4 3 2

Prentice Hall International (UK) Limited, *London*
Prentice Hall of Australia Pty. Limited, *Sydney*
Prentice Hall of Canada Inc., *Toronto*
Prentice Hall Hispanoamericana, S.A., *Mexico*
Prentice Hall of India Private Limited, *New Delhi*
Prentice Hall of Japan, Inc., *Tokyo*
Prentice Hall of Southeast Asia Pte. Ltd., *Singapore*
Editora Prentice Hall do Brasil, Ltda., *Rio de Janeiro*
Prentice Hall, *Englewood Cliffs, New Jersey*

**Library of Congress Cataloging-in-Publication Data**
Bindler, Ruth McGillis.
    Pediatric drugs and nursing implications / Ruth McGillis Bindler, Linda Berner Howry.
        p.      cm.
    ISBN 0-8385-7819-5
    1. Drugs—Administration. 2. Pediatric pharmacology.
3. Pediatric nursing. I. Howry, Linda Berner. II. Title.
    [DNLM: 1. Drug Therapy—in infancy & childhood. WS 366
B612pb]
RJ560.B57    1989
DNLM/DLC                                                    89-18333
for Library of Congress                                         CIP

Acquisitions Editor: Marion Kalstein-Welch
For information about our audio products, write us at:
Newbridge Book Clubs, 3000 Cindel Drive, Delran, NJ  08370

PRINTED IN THE UNITED STATES OF AMERICA

*To our husbands and children*

# Consultants and Reviewers

We wish to thank the professionals who have given their time and shared their expertise to review sections of this book and offer us valuable consultantship service. Their contributions add to the pertinence and applicability of the content.

**Madge Brasch, RN, BSN**
Pediatric Oncology Nurse
Deaconess Hospital
Spokane, Washington

**T.R. Garcia, BS Pharm, MD**
Community Pediatrics
Pediatric Consultant for Corpus Christi Independent
  School District
Corpus Christi, Texas

**Karen Groth, RN, MS**
Instructor
Intercollegiate Center for Nursing Education
Spokane, Washington

**Joanne K.H. Howard, RN, PhD**
Assistant Professor
Intercollegiate Center for Nursing Education
Spokane, Washington

**Victor Lee, PharmD**
Pharmacy Manager
Long's Half Moon Bay Pharmacy
Moss Beach, CA

**Shirley Lockwood, RN, BSN**
Assistant Unit Manager—Pediatric Intensive Care Unit
Deaconess Hospital
Spokane, Washington

**Jan Nottingham, RN, MN**
Assistant Professor
Gonzaga University
Spokane, Washington

**Richard Orth, DO**
Private Family Practice
Estacada, Oregon

**R. Stanley Robinson, MD**
Ophthalmologist
Rockwood Clinic
Spokane, Washington

**Patricia Ruzyla-Smith, RN, MS**
Instructor
Intercollegiate Center for Nursing Education
Spokane, Washington

**Fred San Miguel, BS Pharm, MBA**
Director of Pharmacy Services
Riverside Hospital Pharmacy
Corpus Christi, Texas

**Craig Stucky, MD**
Pediatrician
Rockwood Clinic
Spokane, Washington

**Jo Trilling, RN, MN**
Instructor
Intercollegiate Center for Nursing Education
Spokane, Washington

**Brad White, BPh**
Pharmacist
Deaconess Hospital
Spokane, Washington

# Contents

# Preface

"Physicians and other health care professionals are increasingly aware that children require special treatment. Children are different . . ." (Ross Laboratories, 1978).

There is certainly a plethora of books available that discuss drugs and application of pharmacological knowledge to nursing, although few of these volumes are totally devoted to the discussion of such information in relation to children. Children, however, need to be viewed separately from adults in application of phamacokinetic principles. Their immaturity of body organs and systems create unique responses to medications. Absorption of medications may differ due to gastrointestinal, peripheral, and transport system variations. Metabolic activity may be quite different in children with some drugs metabolized rapidly, others slowly, and others traveling metabolic pathways different than those followed in adults. Excretion of certain drugs can also be influenced by the child's liver and kidney maturity and differing body fluid status.

A volume that focuses solely on children and on the uniqueness of prematures, neonates, and older children is needed. Childhood dosages are different because it is often inaccurate to extrapolate appropriate dosages from those established for adults. Such dosages are often difficult to find because they may be used clinically but not published in many drug references. We have attempted to gather these doses from the various publications and professionals using them, indicating in the *Routes and Dosages* section when dosages provided are suggested or provided by clinicians. It is recognized that these dosages may therefore differ somewhat from those that other clinicians use, but these dosages can be used as general guidelines. This illustrates the need for continued assessment and observation of children's responses to drugs, establishment of research projects, and dissemination of dosages used and responses achieved in children. Generally children who are above 16 years of age may be given adult dosages and other drug references may be used.

This volume also focuses all other parts of the drug reference format on children. For example, the *Absorption and Fate* section states pharmacokinetic norms in children if they are known, *Side Effects* focus on those most common in children, and *Nursing Implications* deal with drug forms used in children and suggest nursing actions related to children.

This childhood focus is a unique feature of this volume. The book is also comprehensive; drugs used commonly or in specific situations in children are included, even if they have not been approved by the

Food and Drug Administration for use in the pediatric population. It is frequently difficult for practicing nurses to obtain information about drugs commonly used in children simply because the drugs have not been tested formally in this population. Thus the comprehensive inclusion of drugs will offer invaluable assistance to those in practice who need data about drugs in the pediatric age group. Although the book is intended mainly for nurses and nursing students and centers on the information they use in practice, it is expected that others such as physicians, pharmacists, and physicians' assisants will find this to be a beneficial reference.

In addition to the drug monographs in this text, Part I includes information in clear outline format that deals with pharmacokinetics in children, administration of medications to the pediatric population, and developmental approaches to children. This data, in addition to sample medication calculation problems, will likely be most helpful to nursing students and beginning nurses in pediatrics.

Some terminology used in the text may need clarification. Recognizing that a number of licensed professionals prescribe medications (i.e., physicians, nurse practitioners, physicians' assistants), we frequently refer to this variety of individuals as *the prescriber*. Because the book may be used by many persons who provide care for children, the term *health care provider* is frequently seen, although at other times the word *nurse* is used when such care is nearly always provided by a nurse. The words *medication* and *drug* are used synonymously throughout the text.

In summary, we believe that this drug reference will provide essential information for a number of health care providers and we wish them success in their interactions with children.

A book of this magnitude could not be written without the help of countless people. Our families weathered the time commitment of writing and we thank them for their support. The professionals who reviewed sections of the book are listed separately. Yvonne Tso is the pharmacist with whom we wrote two former books and, although we missed her on this project, many of her contributions can be found interwoven here. We appreciate the typing assistance of Linda Jones and Joe Schafer and the computer assistance of David Solis. We especially wish to thank our editors, Marion Kalstein-Welch and Amanda D. Egan for their assistance and support in making this project a reality.

# PART I
## Administration
## of Pediatric Medications

# Physiological Considerations

## I. PHARMACOKINETIC PRINCIPLES

A. Pharmacokinetics
   1. Pharmacokinetics is the study of the processes of absorption, distribution, and excretion of drugs. These processes involve a constantly dynamic interaction between the drugs and the human body.
   2. Because of the unique characteristics of a child, pediatric pharmacokinetics is a distinct field. The child may tolerate drugs differently depending on age.

B. Key Terms
   1. The *therapeutic level* or *index* is the concentration of a drug that is needed to elicit the desired clinical response without causing toxic effects.
   2. *Serum concentration* is the level of drug present in the serum, as measured by a blood sample, in the laboratory. This may be helpful in establishing the dosage needed to create the therapeutic level, and to avoid toxic effects. Serum concentration levels are not available for all drugs due to the limitation in assay techniques and the inability to predict pharmacological response from the levels of some drugs. In the latter case, clinical response rather than serum levels is used to establish therapeutic dosages.
   3. *Trough level* is the lowest concentration of the drug reached between dosages (Fig. I–1).
   4. *Peak level* is the highest concentration of the drug reached after administration of dosages (Fig. I–2).
   5. The *steady-state concentration* is reached when the drug's distribution is in equilibrium in the body. The amount of drug taken into the body equals the amount excreted. This is attained after repetitive dosing and is dependent on the half-life of the drug. A longer half-life requires a longer time to reach the steady state (Fig. I–3).
   6. The *half-life* of a drug is the time required for 50 percent of a dose to be excreted. It is used to determine frequency of drug dosages. To avoid accumulation and toxic effects, drugs are given at intervals close to their half-lives.
   7. The *loading dose* is a large dose used with some drugs to begin therapy and shorten the time it takes for the body to reach the steady-state concentration. The loading dose is sometimes referred to as a bolus, or in the case of digitalis, a digitalizing dose. Once the loading dose is given, the patient is given a smaller *maintenance dose* on a scheduled basis.

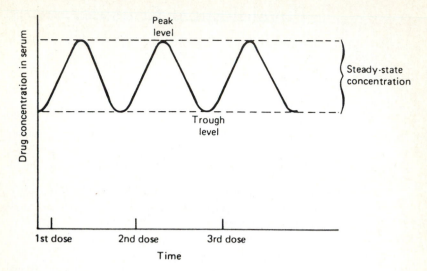

Figure I–1. Peak and trough levels of a drug in serum when steady-state concentration is achieved.

## II. PEDIATRIC VARIATIONS
   **A.** Height, Weight, Body Surface Area
   **1.** Height increases about 3 1/2 times between birth and adulthood.
   **2.** Weight increases about 20 times between birth and adulthood.
   **3.** Body surface area, measured by the relationship of height and weight, increases about 7 times between birth and adulthood.
   **4.** Body surface area, measured in square meters, is a good reflection of many physiological processes significant in metabolizing, transporting, and eliminating drugs, such as metabolic rate, extracellular fluid and total fluid volumes, cardiac output, and glomerular filtration rate. See nomogram for computation of body surface area in square meters (Fig. I–4).
   **5.** Body surface area or weight are generally used to calculate pediatric dosages of medications, as pediatric dosages are usually stated in terms of mg/kg or $mg/m^2$.
   **B.** Muscle Mass
   **1.** Muscle comprises 25 percent of body weight in infancy; 40 percent in adulthood (Table I–1).
   **2.** Infants and young children have little muscle tissue available for injection and may have erratic blood flow to muscle tissue, thus decreasing medication absorption.
   **C.** Fat
   **1.** Fat comprises 16 percent of an infant's body weight, 23 percent of a 1-year-old's, 8 to 12 percent of a preschooler, and 15 percent of an adult (Table I–1).

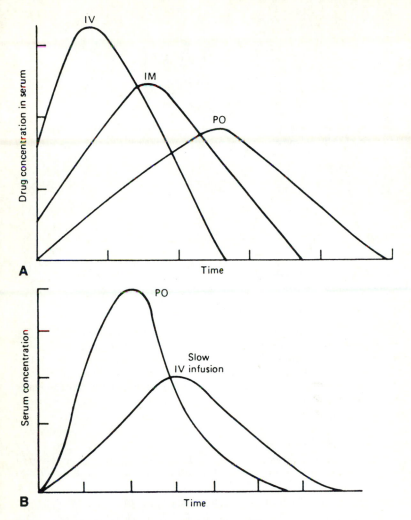

**Figure I-2. A** Peak serum levels following different routes of administration. **B** Differences in peak serum concentrations after oral administration and during slow IV infusion.

2. Blood levels of lipid-soluble drugs are dependent on the amount of fat tissue in the body, as the fat must get saturated with these drugs before blood levels begin to increase (e.g., diazepam, barbiturates).

3. The variable fat percentages observed throughout childhood as well as between individual children may lead to a need for differing mg/kg dosages to achieve therapeutic blood levels.

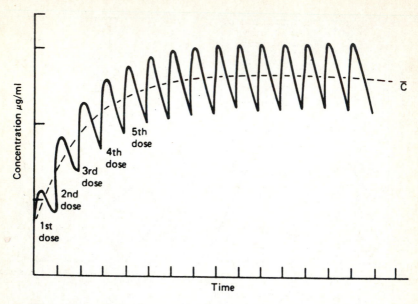

$\bar{C}$ Average steady-state concentration in serum

**Figure I–3.** Achievement of steady-state concentration after repetitive dosing. When the fixed dose of a drug is given repeatedly at intervals approximating the half-life of the drug, a steady-state concentration results after about five half-lives of the drug; hence, the longer the half-life of a drug, the longer the time required for steady-state concentration to occur. If a loading dose is used, the process is shortened considerably (*dotted line*).

**D.** Body Fluid

    **1.** Eighty-five percent of the body weight in prematures is fluid; 80 percent in term infants; 60 percent in 2-year olds and throughout childhood (Fig. I–5).

    **2.** Forty-five percent of body weight in infancy is extracellular fluid; 35 percent is intracellular. Fifteen percent of body weight in the adult is extracellular; 40 percent is intracellular.

    **3.** Greater mg/kg dosages of aqueous- (water) soluble drugs are needed in young children, as their total body fluid levels, especially extracellular (circulating) volumes, are greater (e.g., sulfisoxazole).

    **4.** The greater proportion of extracellular fluid in young children makes them more prone to dehydration. Dehydration states can alter needed dosages and response to medications.

**E.** Skin

    **1.** Variations in children include:

        **a.** large body surface area and, therefore, more skin surface

        **b.** thin dermis, epidermis (especially stratum corneum or outer layer of epidermis)

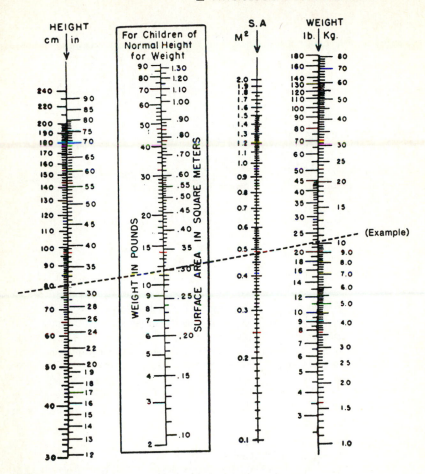

**Figure I–4.** The surface area is indicated at the intersection of a straight line connecting the height and weight column with the surface area column; if the patient is of roughly average size, it is determined by the weight alone (*enclosed area*). (*From Shirkey HC: Drug therapy. In Vaughan VC, McKay, RJ, Behrman RE (eds): Nelson Textbook of Pediatrics, 13 ed. Philadelphia, WB Saunders, 1987*)

     **c.** relatively inactive sebaceous glands before puberty

   **2.** Variations result in tendency to absorb topical medications through the skin, creating systemic effects (e.g., hexachlorophene, boric acids, steroids).

   **3.** Skin of young children, especially infants, is prone to irritation and allergy. Diaper rash, hives, eczema, contact dermatitis are not uncommon.

**F.** Eye

   **1.** Eye medications, especially those in solution form, create systemic effects when they pass through the nasolacrimal duct, be-

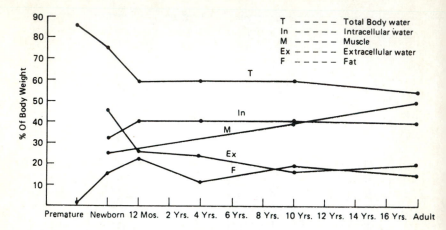

Figure I-5. Percentage of body weight composed of water, muscle, and fat.

come absorbed through the nasal mucous membranes, or get swallowed and absorbed from the gastrointestinal tract. Ointments are often used in children rather than solutions to minimize this effect (e.g., atropine).

  2. It may be difficult to administer eye medications to young children. Caution and correct techniques are advised.

  3. Oxygen used therapeutically in newborns may lead to retrolental fibroplasia that causes blindness. Premature infants administered high levels of oxygen over prolonged periods are most at risk of this complication.

G. Gastrointestinal System

  1. Variations in children include:

    a. gastric emptying time is prolonged (6 to 8 hours) in newborns as compared with children in the second year (2 hours)

**TABLE I-1. PERCENTAGE OF BODY WEIGHT MADE UP OF WATER, MUSCLE, AND FAT.**

|  | Muscle | Fat | Total body water | Extracellular water | Intracellular water |
|---|---|---|---|---|---|
| Premature | * | 1 | 86 | * | * |
| Birth | 25 | 16 | 70–80 | 45–47 | 32–35 |
| 12 months | * | 22–24 | 58–60 | 25–27 | 41 |
| 4 years | * | 12 | 60 | 24 | 41 |
| 10–11 years | 40 | 18–20 | 60 | 17 | 41 |
| Adult | 50 | 15 | 50–60 | 15 | 40 |

*not determined

    **b.** peristalsis is irregular in infants

    **c.** the gastrointestinal tract is long in proportion to the body size

    **d.** some substances needed for active transport of certain drugs are not yet produced in infants

    **e.** the gastric pH of newborn infants is acidic (1 to 3) and gradually nears the more adult pH of 0.9 to 1.5 by about 4 months

    **f.** infants eat every 2 to 4 hours, therefore, food is in their stomachs much of the time; food and digestive enzymes may interfere with drug absorption

  **2.** Variations result in slower, more erratic absorption of oral medications, especially in newborns and infants in the first half year of life. Acidic drugs, such as the penicillins, may be more readily absorbed in newborns and very young infants due to their lower gastric pH. In contrast basic drugs, such as diazepam and theophylline, may have delayed absorption.

  **3.** Sublingual administration to children younger than adolescence is generally avoided due to their inability to carry out this route of administration correctly.

**H.** Liver

  **1.** Enzyme systems are less well developed in infants and young children. Enzymes used for drug binding are, therefore, at lower levels (Table I–2).

  **2.** The neonate has some substances that compete with medications for plasma protein binding sites, such as maternal hormones and free and fatty acids.

  **3.** Proportionately smaller doses of some drugs that bind to plasma proteins are, therefore, needed, such as phenytoin and salicylate.

  **4.** The lower levels of many liver enzymes also decrease biotransformation rates of many drugs. Toxic effects of such drugs may be reached more readily, for example, chloramphenicol leads to the "gray baby" syndrome.

  **5.** Monitoring for side and toxic effects and sometimes blood levels is particularly important in infants and young children.

**TABLE I–2. SERUM PROTEIN VALUES AT VARIOUS AGES.**

|  | Premature | Neonate | Infant | 5–15 years |
|---|---|---|---|---|
| Total serum protein (g/100 ml) | 4.5–6.0 | 5.0–6.9 | 5.0–6.6 | 6.5–8.0 |
| Albumin | 2.5–3.5 | 3.0–4.5 | 3.8–5.0 | 4.5–6.0 |
| Globulin | 1.0–2.2 | 1.3–2.4 | 1.4–2.4 | 2.0–3.0 |
| Gamma globulin | 0.5–0.9 | 0.8–1.0 | 0.3–0.6 | 0.9–1.3 |
| Fibrinogen | 0.4 | 0.2–0.4 | 0.2–0.4 | 0.2–0.4 |

*(Lowrey GH: Growth and Development of Children, 7 ed. Copyright 1978 by Year Book Medical Publishers, Chicago)*

**I.** Respiratory System

    **1.** Variations in children include:

        **a.** a proportionately small lung size and high metabolic rate

        **b.** alveoli of newborn are immature and not fully functional

        **c.** the upper respiratory passages (e.g., nose, trachea, bronchi, eustachian tube) are shorter and narrower in infants and young children

        **d.** infants breathe almost totally through the nose to facilitate breathing while nursing

        **e.** the lower respiratory passages (bronchioles, alveoli) are shorter and narrower in infants and young children

        **f.** the immune system is immature in young children

    **2.** Variations result in:

        **a.** more rapid respiratory rates in young children (Table I–3).

        **b.** more frequent respiratory infections

        **c.** inability of the infant to breathe and nurse simultaneously when nasal passages are full from a respiratory infection

        **d.** middle ear infection (otitis media) frequently follows upper respiratory infection

**J.** Cardiovascular System

    **1.** Poorly developed peripheral circulation in the infant may cause intramuscular and subcutaneous injections to be absorbed slowly or erratically. Vasoconstriction due to a cold environment can further decrease or slow the absorption (Table I–4).

    **2.** Intravenous and oral routes are more often used in young children due to greater predictability of drug action by these routes.

    **3.** Proportionately large amounts of circulating extracellular fluid creates the need for relatively high doses of water-soluble drugs.

**K.** Neurological System

    **1.** The blood-brain barrier is not mature in the first 2 years of life;

**TABLE I–3. RESPIRATORY RATES.**

| Age | Average respiratory rates (breaths/min) |
| --- | --- |
| Premature | 40–90 |
| Newborn | 30–80 |
| 1 year | 20–40 |
| 2 years | 20–30 |
| 3 years | 20–30 |
| 5 years | 20–25 |
| 10 years | 17–22 |
| 15 years | 15–20 |
| 20 years | 15–20 |

*(Lowrey GH: Growth and Development of Children, 8 ed. Copyright 1978, by Year Book Medical Publishers, Chicago)*

**TABLE I–4. PULSE RATES AND BLOOD PRESSURES.**

| Age | Average pulse rates at rest (beats/min) |
| --- | --- |
| Birth | 140 |
| 1–6 months | 130 |
| 6–12 months | 115 |
| 1–2 years | 110 |
| 2–4 years | 105 |
| 4–6 years | 100 |
| 6–10 years | 95 |
| 10–14 years | 85 |
| 14–18 years | 82 |

| Age | Average blood pressure (mmHg) |
| --- | --- |
| Newborn | 78/42 |
| 1 month | 86/54 |
| 6 months | 90/60 |
| 1 year | 96/65 |
| 2 years | 99/65 |
| 4 years | 99/65 |
| 6 years | 100/60 |
| 8 years | 105/60 |
| 10 years | 110/60 |
| 12 years | 115/60 |
| 14 years | 118/60 |
| 16 years | 120/65 |

*(Lowrey, GH. Growth and Development of Children. 8 ed. 1986, Yearbook Medical Publication, Chicago)*

therefore, encephalopathy is more commonly seen as a toxic drug effect.

2. Central nervous system stimulants and depressants more often cause unpredictable results in children.

L. Renal System (Tables I–5 and I–6)
   1. Variations in children include:
      a. glomerular filtration rates are 30 to 50 percent that of adults in the young infant; mature rates are reached in the first half year of life
      b. tubular secretion is less in the infant due to a smaller number of tubular cells, shorter tubules, less blood flow, and less active transport systems; mature rates are reached by 7 months of age
      c. urinary pH of the newborn is more acidic and remains the

**TABLE I–5. DAILY WATER REQUIREMENTS AT VARIOUS AGES.**

| Age | Average body weight (kg) | Total water requirements per 24 hr (ml) | Water requirements per kg per 24 hr (ml) |
|---|---|---|---|
| 3 days | 3.0 | 250–300 | 80–100 |
| 10 days | 3.2 | 400–500 | 125–150 |
| 3 months | 5.4 | 750–850 | 140–160 |
| 6 months | 7.3 | 950–1100 | 130–155 |
| 9 months | 8.6 | 1100–1250 | 125–145 |
| 1 years ´ | 9.5 | 1150–1300 | 120–135 |
| 2 years | 11.8 | 1350–1500 | 115–125 |
| 4 years | 16.2 | 1600–1800 | 100–110 |
| 6 years | 20.0 | 1800–2000 | 90–100 |
| 10 years | 28.7 | 2000–2500 | 70–85 |
| 14 years | 45.0 | 2200–2700 | 50–60 |
| 18 years | 54.0 | 2200–2700 | 40–50 |

*(Vaughan VC, McKay RJ, Behrman RE: Nelson Textbook of Pediatrics, 13 ed. Philadelphia, WB Saunders, 1987)*

**TABLE I–6. GUIDELINES FOR MAXIMAL AMOUNTS OF SOLUTIONS TO BE INJECTED INTO MUSCLE TISSUES.**

| Muscle Group | Birth to 1½ years (ml) | 1½ to 3 years (ml) | 3 to 6 years (ml) | 6 to 15 years (ml) | 15 years to adulthood (ml) |
|---|---|---|---|---|---|
| Deltoid | Not recommended | Not recommended unless other sites are not available 0.5 | 0.5 | 0.5 | 1 |
| Gluteus maximus | Not recommended | Not recommended unless other sites are not available 1 | 1.5 | 1.5–2 | 2–2.5 |
| Ventrogluteal | Not recommended | Not recommended unless other sites are not available 1 | 1.5 | 1.5–2 | 2–2.5 |
| Vastus lateralis | 0.5–1 | 1 | 1.5 | 1.5–2 | 2–2.5 |

same over 24 hours of the day (older children and adults have a more basic urine during the daytime and a more acidic urine at night)

    **d.** little ability to concentrate or dilute urine

  **2.** Variations result in:

    **a.** longer half-life in infants for drugs excreted by glomerular filtration (e.g., kanamycin, streptomycin, gentamicin, digoxin)

    **b.** longer half-life in infants for drugs excreted by tubular secretion (e.g., penicillins)

    **c.** increased reabsorption of acidic drugs in the infant (e.g., sulfisoxazole)

    **d.** increased incidence of dehydration and overhydration

    **e.** oliguria or anuria necessitates close observation for drug toxic effects as well as decreased dosages of drugs excreted by the kidneys

**M.** Immune system

  **1.** The immune system is immature due to low exposure to and slow response to infections. Greater number of infections (particularly respiratory and gastrointestinal) are seen.

  **2.** Allergies, for example, of skin and respiratory system, are common.

  **3.** Allergy to medication should be carefully described and recorded.

## III. PRINCIPLES OF PEDIATRIC DOSAGES

**A.** Solutions

  **1.** Intravenous flow rates are most frequently calculated in microdrops in pediatrics. For all companies, 60 microdrops equals 1 ml of solution. Note the number of drops required to administer 1 ml of IV fluid using tubing manufactured by different companies.

| Company | Number of drops (gtt/1 ml) |
|---|---|
| Travenol | 10 drops (gtt) |
| Abbot | 15 drops (ggt) |
| McGaw | 15 drops (gtt) |
| Cutter | 20 drops (gtt) |
| All companies | 60 microdrops (*m*gtt) − 1 milliliter (ml) |

To calculate flow rate:

$$\text{Drops/min} = \frac{\text{Total volume ordered} \times \text{gtt/ml}}{\text{Total infusion time (min)}}$$

For example if 250 ml of fluid were to be administered by microdrip over 3 hours, the drops/minute would be calculated as follows:

$$\text{Ex: drops/min} = \frac{250 \times 60}{180} = 83 \text{ drops/minute}$$

$$\text{drops/min} = \frac{15,000}{180}$$

$$\text{drops/min} = 83.3$$

The IV flow rate in this example would be adjusted to administer 83 drops per minute.

**B.** Methods of Measurement

    **1.** Metric system. The basic units are a gram for measuring the weight of solids, a liter for measuring the volume of liquids, and a meter for measuring length. Prefixes indicate the division or multiplication by ten of the basic unit as follows:

```
  deci- = 0.1 of the basic unit
 centi- = 0.01 of the basic unit
  milli- = 0.001 of the basic unit
 micro- = 0.00001 of the basic unit = 0.001 of milli-
  nano- = 0.000000001 of the basic unit
  deka- = 10 of or times the basic unit
 hecto- = 100 of or times the basic unit
  kilo- = 1000 of or times the basic unit
```

Metric system

**Weight**

    μg or mcg = microgram

        mg = milligram

g or gm or G = gram

       kg = kilogram

**Volume**

    ml = milliliter

  L or l. = liter

cc or c.c. = cubic centimeter

**Length**

  m = meter

Commonly used metric equivalents

**Weight**

1 milligram (mg) = 1000 micrograms (μg or mcg)

1 milligram (mg) = 0.001 gram (g, gm, or G)

1 gram = 1000 milligrams (mg)

1 kilogram (kg) = 1000 grams (g, gm, or G)

**Volume**

1 milliliter (ml) = 1 cubic centimeter (cc)
1 liter (L) or (l) = 1000 milliliters (ml) = 1000 cubic centimeters (cc)

2. Apothecary system. Measures of weight in this system are grain, dram, ounce, and pound. Volume is measured by minim, fluidram, fluidounce, pint, and quart. Symbols are frequently used. The quantity or weight or volume follows the symbol and is indicated by Roman numbers. Thus:

$$15 \text{ grains} = \text{gr xv or gr } \overline{\text{xv}}$$
$$2 \text{ drams} = \text{℥ ii or ℥ ii}$$

Apothecaries' system

**Weight**

gr = grain
dr or ℥ = dram
oz or ℥ = ounce
lb = pound

**Volume**

m or ℳ = minim
fl dr or f℥ = fluidram
fl oz or f℥ = fluidounce
O or pt = pint
qt = quart

Commonly used apothecary equivalents

**Weight**

1 dram (dr or ℥ ) = 60 grains (gr)
1 ounce (oz or ℥ ) = 8 drams (dr or ℥ ) = 480 grains (gr)
1 pound (lb) = 12 ounces (oz or ℥ ) = 5760 grains (gr)

**Volume**

1 fluidram (fl dr or f℥) = 60 minims (m or ℳ)
1 fluidounce (fl oz or f℥) = 8 fluidrams (fl dr or f℥) = 480 minims (m or ℳ)
1 pint (O or pt) = 16 fluid ounces (fl oz or f℥)
1 quart (qt) = 2 pints (O or pt) = 32 fluid ounces (fl oz or f℥)

3. Household system. Volume measurements used include the teaspoon, tablespoon, cup, and glass. There is great variation in volume measured by household implements, therefore, their use to administer medications should be discouraged.

Household system

gtt = drop

$$t \text{ or tsp} = \text{teaspoon}$$
$$T \text{ or tbsp} = \text{tablespoon}$$
$$c = \text{cup}$$

Commonly used household equivalents

**Volume**
1 teaspoon (t or tsp) = 5 cubic centimeters (cc)
1 tablespoon (T or tbsp) = 3 teaspoons (t or tsp)
1 cup (c) = 6 fluidounces (fl oz or f℥) = 180 cubic centimeters (cc)
1 glass = 8 fluidounces (fl oz or f℥) = 240 cubic centimeters (cc)

    **4.** Transfer between systems is also a nursing responsibility.
Equivalents for transfer among metric, apothecaries', and household systems

|  | **Metric** | **Apothecaries'** | **Household** |
|---|---|---|---|
| Weight | 1 milligram (mg) | 1/60–1/65 grain (gr) | |
| | 60–65 milligrams (mg) | 1 grain (gr) | |
| | 1 gram (g) | 15/16 grains (gr) | |
| | 30 grams (g) | 1 ounce (oz) | |
| | 1 kilogram (kg) | 2.2 pounds (lb) | |
| Volume | 0.06 milliliter (ml) | 1 minim (♏) | |
| | 1 milliliter (ml) or 1 cubic centimeter (cc) | 15–16 minims (♏) | |
| | 4–5 milliliters (ml) | 1 fluidram (fl dr) | 1 teaspoon (tsp) |
| | 15 milliliters (ml) | 4 fluidrams (fl dr) | 1 tablespoon (tbsp) |
| | 30 milliliters (ml) | 1 fluidounce (fl oz) | |
| | 180 milliliters (ml) | 6 fluidounces (fl oz) | 1 cup (c) |
| | 240 milliliters (ml) | 8 fluidounces (fl oz) | 1 glass |
| | 473.2 or 500 milliliters (ml) | 1 pint (pt) | |
| | 1000 milliliters (ml) or 1 liter or 1000 cubic centimeters (cc) | 1 quart (qt) | |

The above are approximate equivalents of weights and volumes among metric, apothecaries', and household systems that are useful in giving medications. It is important to remember that these are approximate and not exact equivalents. Some loss of accuracy occurs whenever one system of measure is converted to another.

    **C.** Dosage Calculation
        **1.** A certain number of milligrams of a drug is specified for each kilogram of body weight. This is commonly written as mg/kg.

2. A certain number of milligrams of a drug is specified for each square meter of body surface area. This is commonly written as mg/m$^2$.
3. When pediatric dosages are not available, rules for calculation of pediatric dosages from adult dosages are sometimes used. They include:

    **a.** surface area rule

$$\text{Child's approximate dose} = \frac{\text{Surface area of child (square meters)}}{1.7} \times \text{Adult dose}$$

**b.** Fried's rule for children under 1 year

$$\text{Infant dose} = \frac{\text{Age of child (months)}}{150} \times \text{Adult dose}$$

**c.** Clark's rule

$$\text{Child's approximate dose} = \frac{\text{Weight of child (pounds)}}{150} \times \text{Adult dose}$$

**d.** Young's rule

$$\text{Child's approximate dose} = \frac{\text{Age of child (years)}}{\text{Age} + 12 \text{ years}} \times \text{Adult dose}$$

**D.** Guidelines for Medication Administration

Before giving any medication to a child, ask yourself these questions:

1. How will the drug be absorbed, metabolized, and excreted?
2. How will the child's illness and developmental physiology influence the absorption, metabolism, and excretion of the drug?
3. Is the child taking other drugs that will interact or compete with this drug for utilization and excretion?
4. What dose should be given?
5. What are the child's pulse, temperature, respiratory rate, blood pressure, skin color and condition, fluid status, and behavior? (Document in the medical record.)

After giving any medication to a child, ask these questions:

1. What time, route, amount, and site (for injections) were used for medication administration? (Document in the medical record.)

2. What pertinent physical findings are available, such as changes in condition, lack of expected findings, side effects, or unusual effects of the drug? (Document in the medical record.)
3. Would it be useful to obtain blood levels of the drug in establishing the therapeutic dose?
4. How can results of this therapy be shared with other health professionals?

## IV. PROBLEMS IN PEDIATRIC DOSING

A. Lack of approved drugs for use in children results from:
   1. difficulty in controlling experimental conditions to test drugs adequately with children.
   2. risk of side effects and long-term effects leading to ethical considerations.
   3. high experimental costs.
   4. unusual, unique response to some drugs that is sometimes observed in children (e.g., chloramphenicol causes toxic effects in newborns).
B. This lack of approved drugs for use in children results in:
   1. depriving children of some drugs that may be useful for them.
   2. use of drugs in children when there are no clearly established dosages for various age groups. In this book, under the dosage section, a dosage established by clinicians is sometimes given rather than one recommended by drug companies. This indicates that the drug is used in pediatrics even though the manufacturer has not been licensed to label the drug as safe and effective in children and to provide pediatric dosages.
C. The child has been referred to as a "therapeutic orphan" due to the lack of information about pharmacokinetics of many drugs in pediatric bodies.

# Developmental Considerations

**I. CHILD DEVELOPMENT**
- **A.** Areas of Development
  - **1.** Psychosocial development influences the child's interaction with the person giving a medication.
  - **2.** Cognitive development determines the child's understanding of the need for a medication. It is important to assess the child's intellectual understanding of medications to plan effective interactions and teaching.
  - **3.** Physical growth characteristics may influence the child's medication experience.

**II. METHODS OF COMMUNICATING WITH CHILDREN ABOUT MEDICATIONS**
- **A.** Drawings
  - **1.** Body line drawings can be used as assessment tools (Fig. I–6) to determine the child's understanding of anatomy or medication effects. The health-care provider gives the child an appropriate picture and asks the child questions such as "What is in the chest? Draw it on the picture," or "Where does this medicine go when you swallow it?"
  - **2.** Children often display feelings about medication administration in drawings. The child may draw spontaneously or can be encouraged to do so, such as "Will you draw a picture of a little girl in the hospital like you?" Open-ended statements are used to encourage children to explain their drawings.
  - **3.** The nurse can use body line drawings to teach the child about the body and the effects of medicines.
- **B.** Stories
  - **1.** Pictures of children in health-care settings or receiving medicine can be shown and a child asked to make up a story about what is happening in a particular picture. Anxiety may be displayed in this fantasy experience that is not evident in direct conversation.
  - **2.** The nurse can tell stories to convey necessary information, a technique that works particularly well with preschoolers. For example, "Susie was a 4-year-old girl who had to get a shot every week for an allergy. She was very afraid about the shots and wondered why she had to get them. Then the nurse told Susie all about what the shots would do. Do you know what she told Susie? She told her that . . ."
  - **3.** Books written for various age groups are available to explain health conditions or procedures as well as the medications required for treatment. The nurse can read these stories to the child to enhance understanding.

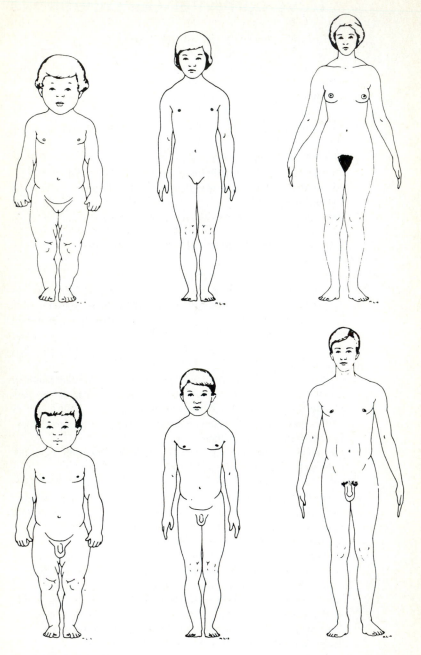

**Figure I-6.** Line drawings can be used to teach the child about the effects of medication on the body.

**C.** Toy Boxes
  **1.** The health care provider who wishes to discover which events about a child's medication experience are important to him can easily compile a toy box or small suitcase that can be provided to the child. The care provider should tell the child that she has come to visit him for 20 minutes (or whatever time is allotted) and has brought a box of toys. The child is told he is free to play with anything in the box while the care provider is present, but that the box will be packed up and taken when she leaves. Much information can be elicited regarding the feelings of the child by observing the items chosen for play, the content of the dramatic play in which the child engages, and the behavior manifested by the child during the play session.
  **2.** Playing with items used to administer medications can help the child feel more in control and less fearful of such equipment. The child must be closely and individually supervised if allowed to use needles or other potentially dangerous equipment in play with dolls.

**D.** Puppets
  **1.** Puppets are another effective tool used to impart information. The child believes in the identity of the puppet, forgets that the adult is actually playing the part of the character portrayed, and listens attentively to what is being discussed.

**E.** Music
  **1.** Music may be used to soothe and calm children. This may be particularly effective with infants after uncomfortable procedures or with toddlers and preschoolers at sleep time. If children listen to tapes at home, they can be brought to the hospital as an important link to provide security.

**F.** Discussion
  **1.** The older school-age child and the adolescent often respond best to clear explanations regarding their medications. They may also like to meet other children with the same condition. An adolescent coping with the disfiguring effects of antineoplastic drugs may gain much from a relationship with a similar adolescent who adjusted successfully to the same situation. The nurse should introduce such children to each other to encourage helpful relationships.
  **2.** Feedback is needed to determine if explanations are understood.

**G.** Audio-visual Media
  **1.** Audio-visual aids, such as pictures and key words, assist in capturing attention and increasing clarity during teaching sessions.
  **2.** A number of videotapes are available for children of various ages to provide information on certain health conditions.

# Techniques of Administration

## I. GENERAL PRINCIPLES

**A.** Information is built on general knowledge and methods of giving medication to adults. Therefore, if administrative techniques are similar to those for adults they will not be discussed.

**B.** A child needs well-planned, careful administration of medication to prevent physical and psychosocial trauma.

  **1.** Consideration of the child's physiologic variations, growth and development, and diseased condition is imperative for understanding and accuracy in pediatric drug administration.

  **2.** The care provider must possess knowledge of each drug's therapeutic effect on the child's body.

  **3.** After accurate calculation of drug dose and individual assessment of the child, and discussion with the parent about how the child takes medication, the care provider is ready to begin drug administration.

**C.** Good hand washing technique should always be used before preparing and giving medications to the child.

**D.** Identify correct drug, dose, and child with every medication given.

  **1.** Always check dosage prescribed against safe dosage ranges. Nurses are liable legally for any drug they administer.

  **2.** Identify each child carefully to avoid giving a medication to the wrong child. In the hospital check identification bands and in the office or outpatient setting have the parent or child identify himself.

## II. ORAL ADMINISTRATION

**A.** Liquid Preparations

  **1.** The child under 5 years of age usually experiences difficulty in swallowing tablets and capsules; thus, most medications for pediatric use are also available in the form of elixirs, syrups, or suspensions.

  **2.** Liquid preparations contain the active drug (dissolved or suspended in a liquid base) and a flavoring agent to disguise the drug's taste. Syrups and elixirs contain drugs in a homogeneous solution and are clear in appearance. Syrups are sugar based (some contain asparaginase) and elixirs contain differing percentages of alcohol. Suspensions are not homogeneous solutions; the active drug is suspended in a liquid base, giving the solution a cloudy appearance.

  **3.** Liquid medications are supplied in a unit dose of drug; for example, milligram or microgram per cubic centimeter or milliliter of fluid (e.g., 5 mg/0.5 ml). Medication is usually prescribed in the unit drug dosage for administration in the medical setting (e.g., 125 mg every 6 hours) and in the household measurement for administration by parents (e.g., 1 tsp every 6 hours).

**4.** In 1903, the American Medical Association defined the standard teaspoon to contain 5 cc or ml. Research has demonstrated that the average household teaspoon may hold between 2.5 ml and 7.8 ml, thus only calibrated devices (e.g., plastic medicine cups, spoonlike devices, droppers, or syringes) should be used.

   **a.** A medication dose that computes to less than 5 cc or to an uneven number, such as 7 cc, needs to be measured with a calibrated dropper or syringe to ensure accuracy of the dose. Some medications come with scored droppers and these should only be used to measure and give this particular medication.

**5.** Tasting a very small amount of the medication before giving it to the child can assist the care provider to describe the taste of the drug. Some medications that smell good may taste quite unpleasant; odor is not a reliable index of the taste.

**6.** Check expiration date of liquid medications before each dosage.

**B.** Tablets and Capsules

   **1.** Tablets and capsules are often available in doses appropriate for the child. Before deciding on this route of administration, carefully assess the individual child's ability to swallow this form of medication.

   **2.** If medication is only available in a tablet or capsule form and the child is unable to swallow it, the tablet may have to be crushed or the powder, "spansules," or liquid removed from the capsule for administration.

   **a.** Factors to consider when crushing a tablet.

   *1.* Is the dose required accurately measurable from the form of drug available? If not, can a particular tablet or capsule be accurately divided in half? Tablets are extremely difficult to divide into thirds or fourths and this practice should be avoided. If a very small dose is required, the pharmacy may be able to put the drug into solution so that the correct dose can be administered. This is especially important when the drug has a narrow therapeutic index.

   *2.* Enteric-coated tablets have a special coating so that the tablet will be dissolved in the duodenum and not destroyed by stomach acidity. Do not crush because the drug would then be dissolved in the stomach resulting in undesirable effects. Certain liquids, such as milk, may also destroy the enteric coating of a tablet, for example, the bisacodyl tablet (Dulcolax).

   *3.* Sustained-release tablets are formulated with the drug embedded inside the tablet in such a manner that gradual release of the drug in the gastrointestinal tract is achieved. Crushing these tablets causes improper release of the drug.

*4.* If the child cannot swallow the desired medication and it cannot be crushed, notify the prescriber so that a decision to change the medication's route or form can be made.

**b.** Crushed tablets and contents taken from capsules usually have a bitter or unpleasant taste, therefore, they need to be mixed with something to disguise their flavor.

*1.* When choosing a vehicle, consider if the drug will alter the food's taste; essential foods or fluids (e.g., orange juice) should be avoided, in case the child develops an aversion. Some commonly used vehicles are jelly, honey, chocolate syrup, apple sauce, and fruit-flavored drinks.

*a.* Apple sauce is primarily used in young infants because it is a nonessential food; it is one of the first foods given to infants, and allergic reaction to it is rare. Honey is not recommended in the child under 12 months of age, because there is evidence that some honey contains *Clostridium botulinum* spores and causes infants to develop botulism. Data demonstrates that the use of honey is not unsafe for the older child with normal intestinal microflora and immunities.

*b.* Jelly and honey have a very high sugar content and should be avoided in a child whose sugar intake is restricted. Good oral care after intake of medication in these sweet foods helps prevent dental caries.

*c.* Elixirs have alcohol content and may cause choking.

*d.* Medication should be placed in the smallest amount of liquid or food possible to assure that the child will take the entire amount.

**c.** With chewable tablets, chewing affects the disintegration of these tablets and is important in assuring proper absorption of the drug from the gastrointestinal tract.

*1.* The child loosing deciduous teeth needs to take care not to inadvertently dislodge and swallow a loose tooth while chewing the tablet.

**d.** Most capsules can be safely separated, although the powder or liquid contents may be unpalatable and may need to be placed in a disguising vehicle. Capsules that contain sustained-release particles can be safely opened for administration because the coating on each particle will control its release in the gastrointestinal tract. The child, however, should be instructed not to chew the particles, which would destroy the protective coating.

**e.** Gelatin capsule containers can be used to disguise the taste of bitter tablets for the child who can safely swallow a capsule. The crushed or safely divided tablet may be placed in the empty capsule.

**C.** Positioning the Child and Administering Medication

    **1.** The most important point in positioning the child for oral medication administration is to prevent aspiration of the drug. The child must be placed in an upright position and should never lie flat. The medication should be given in small amounts (0.2 to 0.5 ml) to prevent choking.

        **a.** Prematures. Assess for sucking reflex; if weak child may need to receive oral medications by nasogastric or gastrostomy tube. Assess for tube placement and patency before instillation. Follow agency procedure. Be sure to flush the tube of medication after instillation to assure that the dosage is delivered into the infant's stomach. If giving orally, take great care to prevent aspiration.

        **b.** Infants

            *1.* The infant should be positioned or held comfortably with the head elevated to 45 degrees and the extremities restrained as necessary.

            *2.* An infant under 3 to 4 months of age with a normal sucking and rooting reflex, will usually suck medication from a nipple, dropper, or syringe. He will take the medication more readily if hungry. If a nipple is placed in his mouth, the medication can be poured in small amounts directly into the nipple. The infant of this age does not have a good sense of taste, therefore, he will usually take the medication without difficulty. Support the child's head and back.

            *3.* An infant under 5 or 6 months of age will push anything solid out of his mouth and off his tongue because of the normal tongue movements used in sucking. This may interfere with giving crushed tablets disguised in solid food. The medication may need to be mixed in a liquid rather than a solid and administered by syringe instead of by a teaspoon. This child has good grasp, therefore, hands may need to be restrained while giving.

            *4.* An infant of 6 to 12 months can spit out whatever he does not want in his mouth. An oral syringe or medicine cup may work more effectively than a nipple. The plastic medicine cup can be bent slightly so that it fits into the infant's mouth and can deliver the medication in small amounts. A dropper, syringe, or medication spoon can also be used. The oral syringe or injectable syringe without a needle works effectively when it is placed across the tongue and directed toward the side of the mouth rather than the throat. This prevents aspiration or eliciting of the cough reflex. The child cannot spit out the medication because the syringe is across the tongue. This method works best with a child who will not take the medication from a cup. If the infant will not swallow the medication, the throat may be lightly stroked in a downward motion. This technique may be used effectively with infants or older children who have difficulty swallowing.

**c.** Toddlers

*1.* The approach to use with the toddler directly affects the medication experience in a positive or a negative manner. Be positive and approach him on his developmental level. If the child will drink the medication from a cup or hollow-handled medication spoon, use this method. Either have the child hold the cup and drink from it or have the care provider give the medication in small amounts. If the child refuses to take the medication in this manner, it can be given in a syringe. Seat the child across your lap facing the hand that will be used to give the medication. Put the child's arm that is nearer to your body along your side and under your arm. Grasp the child's free arm in the hand not giving the medication. To control the child's head place it against your shoulder. Use your free hand to give the medication. The medication can be given by the syringe method as described for the infant. Prevent aspiration.

**d.** Preschoolers

*1.* Most preschoolers will take oral medications without much difficulty. This child can reason; with the use of appropriate developmental approaches, he will usually take the medication. If he will not, the technique described for the toddler may be used. The use of play enables the preschooler to vent his fears and frustrations.

**e.** School-Age Child

*1.* This child takes medication well. The child sometimes procrastinates in taking medication. This can be effectively dealt with by imposing time limits.

**f.** Child Who Refuses Medication

*1.* A child from any age group may refuse to take oral medications because of a negative experience with medications or his desire to be independent. Work with this child to alleviate this negative experience first and then to gain his cooperation. Try to involve the parents or significant others to see if they can get the child to take the medication.

*2.* Sometimes a child will spit out medication. The best way to prevent this is to place the syringe across the tongue. If the child refuses to swallow, stroke his throat as described in the infant section. If the child spits out all the medication, repeat it immediately. If he spits out more than half but not all of the dose administered, repeat half of the dose. If the child spits out less than half the dose, if it is difficult to estimate how much has been spit, or if the care provider has any questions about repeating the medication, the prescriber should be consulted.

**D.** Special Considerations

    **1.** A child who is unable to retain oral medication because of vomiting needs careful evaluation by the prescriber. The medication treatment may need to be reassessed and another route of administration selected (rectal, IM, or IV). It is important to note that drug dose may vary among these different routes. For example, the oral dose may need to be higher to achieve the same therapeutic blood level maintained by IV administration. Consult drug dosage references when routes of administration are changed.

    **2.** The child who is taking daily medication for chronic illness requires careful evaluation of his medication needs if he is receiving nothing by mouth (NPO) or is vomiting. If the child is taking vitamins or laxatives daily, these can usually be omitted for 24 to 48 hours without negative effects. Cardiac medications and anticonvulsants are examples of drugs that usually need to be administered by another route if the child is NPO more than 12 hours.

**III. RECTAL ADMINISTRATION**

  **A.** Rectal medications usually are not the most desirable route of drug administration in the child because of erratic and unpredictable absorption from the colon. Fecal matter present in the rectal area may cause part or all of the drug not to be absorbed. The rectal route occasionally becomes the method of choice if a child is vomiting or is NPO. This route, however, may be contraindicated in the child prone to rectal abscesses (e.g., a child being treated with certain antineoplastic agents).

    **1.** Suppositories

      **a.** Suppositories are the most frequent form of drug used rectally in the child. The drug is usually combined in a base of glycerin or lanolin that melts at body temperature.

      **b.** Splitting or quartering of a suppository is difficult and does not guarantee that the child will receive the proper dose, therefore, it is best to give suppositories only as manufactured, especially with drugs with a narrow therapeutic index.

      **c.** Generally the normal full-term infant's rectum will accommodate the insertion of an adult's fifth digit. This finger should be used to insert suppositories in infants and toddlers.

     **d.** Insert suppository in infants and toddlers with an adult's fifth digit. The child's rectum is those over 3 years can usually accommodate the insertion of an adult's index finger into the rectum.

     **e.** Because a child dislikes having a suppository inserted, proper restraint is necessary. The preschool child can become extremely upset by this procedure because of his age-related fear of body entry. It becomes particularly important to give adequate explanations to the child over 2 years of age and to use developmental approaches to decrease the child's fears.

  **2.** Positioning the child and administering suppositories

     **a.** Follow manufacturer's recommendations for need to lubricate the suppository before inserting it. When indicated, a water-soluble lubricating jelly can be used.

     **b.** The child is usually placed in the Sim's position or a knee–chest position for rectal administration.

     **c.** The suppository is inserted gently into the rectum and is pushed past the internal sphincter toward the child's umbilicus. The child may be instructed to breath deeply or to pant like a puppy to distract him from the procedure. This also helps to discourage defecation. The buttocks should be held together firmly for 5 to 10 minutes after drug administration or until the child loses the urge to defecate.

     **d.** If the child has a stool within 10 to 30 minutes after the insertion of the suppository, it should be examined for the presence of the suppository. If the suppository was not given for its laxative action and all of it is expelled with the stool, the prescriber should be contacted.

     **e.** Chart the expulsion of the suppository and the subsequent course of action in the child's medication record.

  **3.** Drug administration by enema

     **a.** Occasionally drugs are administered by an enema. Follow agency procedure for the administration of an enema to a child.

     **b.** The child, especially during infancy, is very susceptible to fluid overload and electrolyte imbalances; thus the vehicle and the amount of solution for the enema should be carefully evaluated.

**IV. OPHTHALMIC ADMINISTRATION**

  **A.** Special Considerations

    **1.** Sterile technique is essential when instilling medication into the child's eyes to prevent the introduction of pathogens into this delicate organ. The child should have an individually dispensed container of ophthalmic medication, and care must be taken even with individual medications to prevent contamination. If contaminated, the solution or ointment should be discarded.

**B.** Some factors that affect the absorption of a medication from the eye are child cooperation, gravity, blinking, and lid closure.

1. The young child greatly fears having anything placed in the eyes and even in infancy the child is able to close the eyelids tightly so that the care provider has difficulty opening them. When the child is old enough to comprehend the procedure, an explanation of ophthalmic instillation may help gain cooperation. Play also assists in dissipating fear and anxiety caused by eye instillations.

2. Most ophthalmic preparations come in liquid or ointment form. Solutions at room temperature are less irritating and decrease blinking.

3. Crying during the instillation of eye drops causes the solution to have little or no contact with the eye and the drug's therapeutic value may be lost. Thus, the child's cooperation greatly affects the therapy.

4. Positioning of the child for administration of either liquid or ointment ophthalmic medication is the same. Hyperextend the child's neck over an adult's lap or put pillows under the shoulders. The child's head will then be lower than the body and gravity will help to disperse the medication over the cornea.

5. Proper restraint of the child is necessary to prevent injury to the eye. More than one individual may be required to accomplish this task, especially when dealing with an infant or a toddler. A mummy restraint can be used so that the child's extremities will not impede the instillation. Some individuals prefer to place the child's arms alongside his head to stabilize the drug during instillation. Either of these methods is effective as long as head control is achieved.

6. Because fear appears to be increased when the child actually sees the dropper coming toward his eye, he may respond more positively if the care provider suggests that he close his eyes while she retracts the lower lid for instillation. A demonstration of how the eyelid will be retracted can further understanding and lessen fear. Having him close his eyes prevents him from looking at the dropper as it approaches. It also naturally deviates the cornea upward, preventing discomfort that could result in blinking or head movement. When the child blinks, the outflow of the medication from the eye increases, thereby decreasing the therapeutic value of the medication.

7. Stabilize the hand used for instilling medication by resting it on the child's forehead. Retract the lower lid to form a sac; apply medicine without touching the conjunctiva. To ensure sterility and to prevent blinking or ocular injury, do not allow the dropper to touch the child's eyelashes or the eye itself.

8. After instillation, keep the child in position for 1 to 3 minutes so that the medicine will have maximal contact with eye. The

child should close his eyes gently and keep them closed for several minutes to allow the medication greater contact time with the ocular area.

9. To minimize systemic absorption of eyedrops immediately after instillation; apply finger to periphery of nasolicrimal sac using light pressure for 1 to 2 minutes. Blot any excess medication with clean tissue.

10. If the ointment has been used previously, the care provider can prepare the ointment for instillation by squeezing a small amount of medication onto a sterile gauze pad and discarding it before instillation. This clears the end of tube that may have been inadvertently contaminated during previous instillation or storage.

11. Technique for administration of ophthalmic ointment is similar to that of placement of ophthalmic drugs. Squeeze a small line of ointment into the saclike areas along conjunctiva. To stop ointment flow, rotate the tube with a twisting motion. Close lid margin and have the child remain for several minutes in a hyperextended position with the eyes closed. Ointments usually blur vision for several minutes after instillation.

## V. OTIC ADMINISTRATION

A. Medication comes in a liquid form to be placed in the external ear canal by dropper. Because the external auditory canal is not sterile, the ear is not treated in a sterile manner. If, however, the eardrum is ruptured and draining, the ear canal should be treated with sterile technique. Separately dispensed ear medication should be used for each individual child.

B. Place the child on his side with the affected ear exposed. Two people may be needed to restrain a young child to prevent him from turning his head during instillation. An older child needs an explanation to gain his cooperation.

C. Sometimes a child's ears may need to be cleansed of cerumen if there is a large amount present in the outer ear canal. The prescriber may use otic drops designed for this purpose or may order gentle water irrigation of the ear. If the ear is draining, only the outer aspect of the ear should be cleansed, with care to prevent fluid from entering the canal. Drainage from the ear is usually quite irritating to the skin. It should be cleansed frequently and the outer ear should be closely observed for skin breakdown.

D. In a child under 3 years of age, structures surrounding the ear canal area are cartilaginous and straight. To separate the walls of the canal effectively for drop instillation with this child, pull the pinna gently down and back.

E. In a child over 3 years of age, the ear canal has more ossification and the canal angles slightly. To instill drops in this child, pull the pinna up and back. Direct drops toward the ear canal rather than toward the eardrum. Drops directly hitting the eardrum may produce pain; if they are cold, they may induce nausea or vertigo.

Drops should be at room temperature or body temperature when administered.

**F.** Immediately after instillation of the ear drops, massage the anterior ear gently to ease entry of the drops into the ear. The child should remain on his side a few minutes so the drops can permeate to the tympanic membrane.

**G.** Cotton pledgets are occasionally used to prevent medication from escaping from the ear canal. They are also used if the ear canal is draining. A child should be instructed not to play with his ears or with the pledgets.

## VI. NASAL ADMINISTRATION

**A.** Instillation of medication into the nares is a clean but not a sterile procedure. The nares drain into the back of the mouth and throat, and instillation of medication may produce sensations of difficulty in breathing, tickling, or bad taste. Oil-based drops should be avoided because this solution may be aspirated into the lungs and produce aspiration pneumonia.

**B.** A child often reacts negatively to the experience of having drops placed in his nares. The infant, who breathes primarily through his nose, will squirm and attempt to get away, whereas the older child may violently protest. Proper restraint of the child is imperative to accomplish nasal instillation and to prevent injury.

**C.** A small infant may be placed in the care provider's lap with his head hyperextended over his knees. If his extremities are bound, his head can be controlled effectively.

**D.** An older child's head can be hyperextended by placing pillows under his shoulders. It may be necessary for two individuals to restrain a child.

**E.** After instillation of drops, the child should remain in the instillation position for several minutes to facilitate the action of the drops. The child should be closely observed for choking or vomiting during or after nasal drop instillation.

**F.** The young infant who has a respiratory ailment may receive saline nose drops before feedings to clear his nasal passages and aid his breathing during feeding. Outer nares may need to be cleansed first if mucus has crusted over the nares.

## VII. AEROSOL THERAPY

**A.** A croup or mist tent is one of the most common aerosol therapies used with the child who is experiencing respiratory difficulties and it is designed to deliver continuous mist particles to thin tracheobronchial secretions. The child is placed in this tentlike structure, which consists of a tubular frame covered with plastic sheeting, with a mechanical device designed to deliver a cool wet mist. The dense aerosol mist may be increased in these tent structures by use of an ultrasonic nebulizer. The standard tent maintains water–mist concentrations of 44 to 75 mg/l. A Virateck small particle aerosol generator is used to deliver medication (such as ribavirin) into the tent. The primary responsibilities of the care provider during this therapy are to maintain mist level and to observe its effects on the child's respiratory effort. The child must be encouraged to remain in the tent and needs to be kept dry and warm.

**B.** Intermittent positive pressure breathing (IPPB) treatments are usually given by a respiratory therapist or by specially trained nurses. The care provider delivering treatment must be knowledgeable about the machine's operation. The prescriber will order the medication dose, amount of pressure to be exerted during therapy, duration of the treatment, and number of treatments in a 24-hour period.

   **1.** The infant and the young child are usually frightened by the IPPB machine itself, whereas an older child may fear being unable to breathe during the treatment. Many of the aerosol medications have an unpleasant smell and the child may be overwhelmed by the combination of machines and medication. The child who can comprehend directions needs careful instructions to increase understanding of the treatment.

   **2.** With an infant and a young child, a facial mask is used to deliver the IPPB treatment, therefore, both the nose and the mouth are covered.

      **a.** If a mouth piece is used and the child is having difficulty triggering the machine, nose plugs may aid in complete breathing into the machine and thus make the treatment effective.

      **b.** The young child will usually respond more positively if held during IPPB treatment.

   **3.** To prevent contamination, each child should have an individual mask or mouth piece and tubing for the machine. These pieces of equipment should be cleansed according to agency policy after each treatment.

**C.** Side effects experienced with administration of aerosol medications are the same as if the drug were taken systemically.

**D.** Hand-held nebulizers are usually used with an older child for intermittent aerosol treatment in the home environment. There are several types of hand-held devices that operate by use of a hand bulb, as well as aerosol types packed under pressure and propelled by Freon.

   **1.** With each type of aerosol drug, manufacturer's directions for use and prescriber's directions for administration should be followed. General directions include shaking the inhaler before each administration, tightly closing the lips around the inhaler, inhaling with a slow deep breath, and holding the breath as long as possible to ensure maximum effect of the drug.

      **a.** The child and the parents need careful instruction in the use of nebulizer. They must understand that it offers symptomatic relief, is not a curative device, and should be used only as directed.

    **2.** Cleansing of nebulizer after each dose as directed by the manu-facturer prevents the growth of bacteria in the nebulizer.

**VIII. TOPICAL AGENT ADMINISTRATION**

    **A.** Careful assessment of the skin area and charting of observations before topical agent treatment is necessary. This provides a point of reference for progress of healing or development of undesirable effects.

    **B.** The care provider must be aware of the ingredients present in the topical drug being applied. If undesirable reactions to compounds occur, then careful assessment must be made to identify which ingredient is causing the reaction.

    **C.** Topical agents are applied to a clean skin surface. Cleansing of the involved skin area is accomplished from inner to outer aspects using a clean technique.

        **1.** If the skin is broken, sterile technique should be used. The exception to this may be the diaper area, where clean rather than sterile technique is usually employed.

        **2.** Lotions are usually applied with sterile applicators onto the skin; they need frequent reapplication because of drying and flaking of residues.

        **3.** Ointments are usually rubbed on with gloved hands or are applied with sterile applicators. Thin-coat applications are pre-ferred unless otherwise directed.

        **4.** After the medication is applied to the skin, careful assessment of the area is once again necessary. Any new skin irritation, breakdown, or rashes should be noted, reported to the pre-scriber immediately, and use stopped until further direction.

    **D.** The child usually does not understand the necessity to refrain from scratching an infected area even with repeated reminders and ex-planations.

        **1.** The child's hands may need to be restrained or wrapped with clean cotton mittens, especially when the child is sleeping.

        **2.** All nails, including toenails, should be kept short and clean to prevent introduction of bacteria to the affected site.

        **3.** Drugs to relieve itching may be necessary.

        **4.** Toys must be carefully selected for the child to prevent trauma or infection. Fuzzy stuffed toys are usually not recommended, especially if the child's skin is broken or draining. Washable cotton or plastic toys are a better choice.

**IX. VAGINAL ADMINISTRATION**

    **A.** Vaginal medication is rarely used with the young female child or infant; adolescent girls more commonly receive this form of medi-cation.

        **1.** When a toddler or a preschool child receives vaginal medica-tion, great care must be taken to reduce psychologic trauma. Because these age groups have great fear of body entry, it is necessary to assess their developmental level carefully.

2. A school-age child and adolescent usually understands explanations of the vaginal administration process. This age child, however, needs sensitive assessment of the understanding of the vaginal area and its functions. Because the vagina is a sexual organ, it is important to ascertain what the beliefs are about sexuality, family values, and what cultural influences affect the beliefs. It is also important to assess parental views.

3. Vaginal medications commonly come in suppositories, creams, or irrigation form. These medications are instilled as they are for the adult woman. Because the vaginal opening is small, good visualization of area is necessary to prevent trauma. The medication should be inserted gently to reduce fear and possible discomfort. Adolescents usually can be instructed to administer their own vaginal medication.

4. Applicators should be cleansed after each administration, and separate applicators should be used with each child receiving vaginal drugs.

## X. PARENTERAL MEDICATION ADMINISTRATION

A. Care providers must be sensitive to the needs of the child and should administer injections in a manner that will decrease the physical as well as the psychosocial trauma.

1. Syringes should be prepared out of visual range of the child, to prevent anxiety created by viewing a needle. Needles may seem to get larger and more frightening if the child has to look directly at them for an extended time.

   a. Occasionally, an older child may wish to look at the needle just before the injection.

2. Structured play with needles and syringes has been found to lessen anxiety associated with injections.

3. Best results occur if play is performed several hours in advance of the injection or after an injection, rather than at the time of injection.

4. It is important to assist every child receiving an injection in relieving feelings through appropriate developmental approaches.

B. Reconstitution of Injectable Medications

1. Follow drug manufacturer's recommendations for the amount and types of solutions to reconstitute.

   a. When a newborn and premature infant require extremely small doses of medication, further dilution of the drug may be needed. The pharmacist can provide the necessary dilution information. Do not reconstitute medications for this age group using solutions containing benzyl alcohol because of the potential risk of causing fatal toxicity.

2. Store injectable medications according to the manufacturer's recommendations to ensure stability of the drug.

3. Refrigerated injectables should be stored in the refrigerator used

only for medications. The vials should not be stored on the refrigerator doors because frequent opening of the doors may cause significant temperature variations. The measles vaccine is one medication affected by temperature changes, which results in loss of its therapeutic value.

4. Injectable drugs must be properly labeled as to when they were opened or reconstituted with the total amount of solution in which the drug is dissolved, the solution strength, date and time it was prepared, and initials or name of individual who prepared the solution. The labels of reconstituting solutions, such as sterile water or normal saline, indicate whether preservatives are present in solution. Solutions that do not have preservatives should be used immediately. Solutions with preservatives (e.g., bacteriostatic water) should be discarded after 7 days, or immediately if contaminated. Expiration dates of all injectables should be checked before each injection preparation.

5. Mathematic calculations of drug dose should be checked by each person giving an injectable medication, even if the pharmacist has made the calculation. This ensures accuracy and prevents errors.

6. After injections are given, it is imperative to chart medication correctly and according to agency policy, always including site in which the injection was administered. This is not only a legal requirement but also assists the care provider who gives the next injection in rotating injection sites, thereby reducing tissue irritation.

C. Subcutaneous Injections
   1. Subcutaneous injections are placed in subcutaneous fat layers of a child's body and the child's fat deposits differ from those of adults. Preferred sites are anterior thighs, buttocks, upper arms, and abdomen.
      a. The subcutaneous layer can be picked up to isolate the site and avoid injecting a muscle; this is especially helpful if the child is thin and has very little subcutaneous tissue. The injection is given as for an adult.
      b. Restrain the child as necessary.

D. Intramuscular Injections
   1. Giving IM injections to a child requires understanding of anatomy and physiology, careful site selection, and adequate restraint of the child.
   2. The total volume of solution that may be injected into an injection site for each dose must be carefully assessed. Factors to be considered are size of the muscle, tissue integrity, and the child's age and development. Table I–7 shows maximal amounts of solutions to be injected into muscle tissues.
   3. Assess amount of subcutaneous fat over the injection site.

**TABLE I–7. GUIDELINES FOR MAXIMAL AMOUNTS OF SOLUTIONS TO BE INJECTED INTO MUSCLE TISSUES.**

| Muscle Group | Birth to 1½ years (cc) | 1½ to 3 years (cc) | 3 to 6 years (cc) | 6 to 15 years (cc) | 15 years to adulthood (cc) |
|---|---|---|---|---|---|
| Deltoid | Not recommended | Not recommended unless other sites are not available 0.5 | 0.5 | 0.5 | 1 |
| Gluteus maximus | Not recommended | Not recommended unless other sites are not available 1 | 1.5 | 1.5–2 | 2–2.5 |
| Ventrogluteal | Not recommended | Not recommended unless other sites are not available 1 | 1.5 | 1.5–2 | 2–2.5 |
| Vastus lateralis | 0.5–1 | 1 | 1.5 | 1.5–2 | 2–2.5 |

This determines the appropriate needle length for delivery of medication into a muscle mass. Most 1- to 1 1/2-inch needles, gauge 20, 21, or 22, are appropriate for the child. Use the smallest gauge needle to deliver a drug into the muscle mass.

4. Physiologically, the gluteus maximus muscle mass is not well developed until the child has walked for at least 1 full year. The sciatic nerve is large and runs through the medial portion of the muscle mass. The gluteus maximus is not the site of choice in a child before 2 or 2 1/2 years of age. Always approach this site with great care with every child because of the location of the sciatic nerve and identify the greater trochanter and posterior iliac spine and form an imaginary line injecting superior and laterally to this line. The authors recommend that the gluteus maximus never be used for an injection site in a child who has not walked for 1 year and that in the child under 4 to 6 years this site be used only if other sites are contraindicated (Fig. I–7).

5. The vastus lateralis muscle is the preferred site for injection because it is the largest muscle mass in a child under 3 years and is free of major nerves and vessels. The injection site is the medial outer aspect in the center one-third portion of the

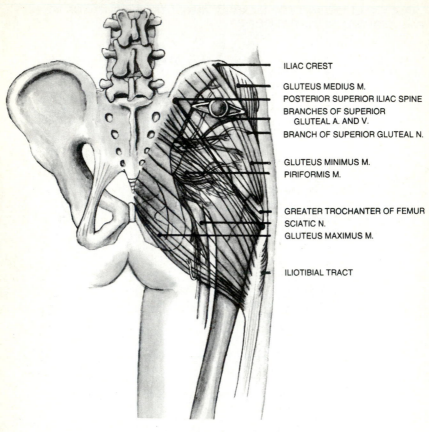

ILIAC CREST

GLUTEUS MEDIUS M.
POSTERIOR SUPERIOR ILIAC SPINE
BRANCHES OF SUPERIOR
    GLUTEAL A. AND V.
BRANCH OF SUPERIOR GLUTEAL N.

GLUTEUS MINIMUS M.
PIRIFORMIS M.

GREATER TROCHANTER OF FEMUR
SCIATIC N.
GLUTEUS MAXIMUS M.

ILIOTIBIAL TRACT

Figure I-7. Dorsogluteal.

thigh. This muscle can be isolated for injections by pinching up the muscle mass. Insert the needle at right angle, directing it toward the knee (Fig. I-8).

6. The ventrogluteal site is also relatively free of major nerves and vessels. This makes it an ideal site in a child over the age of 3 who has been walking for some years. Place the child on his side and have the child flex his top leg at the knee to relax the muscle site. Locate the greater trochanter and place the heal of the hand on this landmark, while pointing fingers toward the child's head and place the index finger over the anterior superior ilac tubercle and with the middle finger spread to the iliac crest forming a "V" with the fingers. Make the injection into the center of the triangle formed with the fingers placing the needle at a right angle but slightly canted toward the iliac crest. This site must be correctly identified to prevent injection into the bone or hip joint (Fig. I-9).

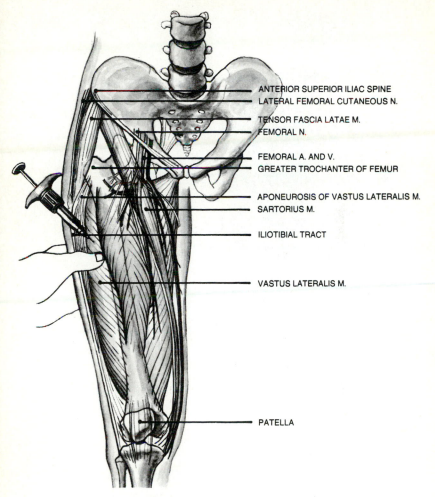

ANTERIOR SUPERIOR ILIAC SPINE
LATERAL FEMORAL CUTANEOUS N.

TENSOR FASCIA LATAE M.
FEMORAL N.

FEMORAL A. AND V.
GREATER TROCHANTER OF FEMUR

APONEUROSIS OF VASTUS LATERALIS M.
SARTORIUS M.

ILIOTIBIAL TRACT

VASTUS LATERALIS M.

PATELLA

**Figure I–8.** Vastus lateralis.

7. The deltoid muscle is rarely used in children under 4 or 5 years of age because of the small muscle mass. It is used for immunizations in the child over 1 1/2 years of age, because of the small amount of solution to be injected. This site also requires proper identification owing to the position of the nerves. Find the acromion process and give the injection into the upper one third of the muscle located about two fingers length below the acromion. Give the injection at right angle with the needle slightly canted toward the shoulder (Fig. I–10).

8. Because the child often moves during an injection, be sure to have a firm grip on the lower portion of syringe (to ensure

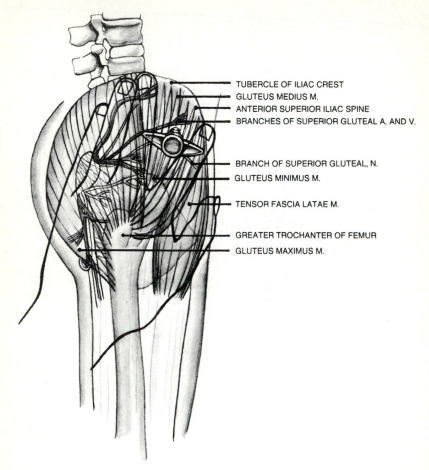

TUBERCLE OF ILIAC CREST
GLUTEUS MEDIUS M.
ANTERIOR SUPERIOR ILIAC SPINE
BRANCHES OF SUPERIOR GLUTEAL A. AND V.

BRANCH OF SUPERIOR GLUTEAL, N.
GLUTEUS MINIMUS M.

TENSOR FASCIA LATAE M.

GREATER TROCHANTER OF FEMUR
GLUTEUS MAXIMUS M.

**Figure I–9.** Ventrogluteal.

that the drug is injected at the site of aspiration) and have a second needle available in case the first one becomes contaminated.

9. A child may need some distraction during injection to facilitate relaxation of the muscle and thus permit ready needle entry. This can be accomplished by having the child pant, count, or wiggle or point toes during the injection. Use developmental approaches to assist in gaining the child's cooperation and in allaying fears.

10. Remember that overusage, frequent injections, or large volumes of drugs injected into IM sites can cause muscle wasting and atrophy.

E. A child must be securely restrained to avoid giving the injection in the wrong site or having the needle become dislodged or broken.

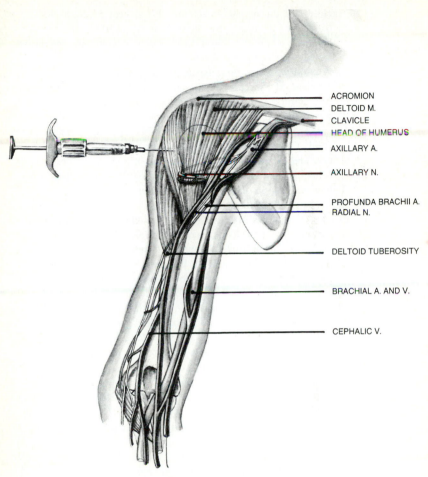

ACROMION
DELTOID M.
CLAVICLE
HEAD OF HUMERUS
AXILLARY A.

AXILLARY N.

PROFUNDA BRACHII A.
RADIAL N.

DELTOID TUBEROSITY

BRACHIAL A. AND V.

CEPHALIC V.

**Figure I–10.** Deltoid.

1. A child under 6 months can easily be restrained by one person. A health care provider can position herself horizontally above the infant, facing the legs, and use her body or arms as a gentle but effective restraint. Then she can select the exact site, pick up the muscle with one hand, and inject with the other.

2. When an infant can turn over or is particularly strong, a second person may be needed during an injection. The second person should restrain the infant's arms and the leg not being injected. The professional giving the injection then has more control over the needle and syringe and over the site being injected.

3. It is always best to have two adults present for injection administration to toddlers and preschoolers.

4. The care provider may need someone to help hold a school-age

child still during the injection. This is best accomplished by a parent or at times, by another health worker. On the other hand, a school-age child may prefer only having the professional who is giving the injection present.

5. A child who is combative may need more than two adults for restraint. If the child wants parents to help restrain, they must be carefully assessed for their ability to support and restrain their child during an injection. Some parents are invaluable and can assist not only by restraining but also by comforting the child. Other parents become upset by the thought of an injection and their anxiety only increases the child's. These parents need the care provider's understanding and assistance to learn how to support the child during future injections.

F. Intravenous Medication

1. The IV route is often preferred over the IM route for administration of certain drugs, such as antibiotics, to the child, especially with prematures, infants, and toddlers. With the IV route, therapeutic blood levels of the drug are achieved quickly because of direct access into the systemic circulation.

G. Insertion and Regulation of Intravenous Line

1. Maintenance of pediatric IV drug therapy poses many problems owing to the child's psychologic makeup and cognitive level. Recognition of the child's level of development and individual needs can assist the care provider in reducing scare and trauma of IV therapy.

2. Adverse reactions can be seen in a matter of seconds to minutes. Knowledge of each drug's therapeutic actions, calculation of dosage, and close monitoring of the child are imperative.

3. Veins of a child are small and fragile, requiring skilled insertions.

    a. Most individuals who start IVs on pediatric clients prefer to insert them in a treatment room rather than at child's beside, so the child does not view the bed as a place of punishment.

4. Method for starting an IV infusion will not be discussed in this book because the technique is similar to the technique used for adults. The child's veins are smaller and need small-gauge needles and in the infant, scalp veins are also used as infusion sites.

5. A young child requires restraint by one or more adults while an IV is started.

6. Intravenous lines must be securely anchored. Assess the child for tape allergies so that hypoallergenic tape can be used when necessary. Stabilize the IV site for freedom of the child's movement and to prevent IV infiltration.

    a. Paper cups or plastic medicine cups can be cut, padded, and placed over the infusion site to prevent the needle from being dislodged. These cups allow visualization of the needle site. Similar IV protective devices are also available commercially.

**b.** Parents need explanations about their child's limitations with IV therapy to prevent them from inadvertently dislodging the IV or stopping the flow.

**c.** Instruction given to the child aids in comprehension of the reason for an IV treatment and thus promotes cooperation with treatment.

**7.** The IV fluid and medication need close monitoring in the child because fluid overload can occur easily.

**a.** A younger child is most susceptible to fluid overloads. Most institutions regulate maximal volumes that may be used with various age groups. (See Table I–7)

**b.** Careful regulation of rate of fluid infusion also prevents fluid overload. The IV drip rate should be monitored every 15 to 30 minutes. Hourly IV infusion rates and amounts should be recorded on an IV flow chart.

**c.** A safeguard for pediatric clients is a measured volume chamber. Most of these measured chambers also have microdrip drop mechanisms. When using these chamber devices, no more than twice the amount of solution a child is to receive in an hour should be placed into the chamber at any one time. This prevents fluid overload.

**d.** Frequent checking of IV helps detect flow stoppage due to a change in the child's position, kinks in tubing, or other causes.

**e.** Medication infused by constant drip also requires close monitoring of IV site for potential infiltration, skin breakdown, or phlebitis. Infiltrations can occur suddenly and are usually noted by symptoms of edema at the needle site, changes in skin color or temperature, or complaints of pain at the needle site.

**f.** Most institutions recommend that IV tubing be changed every 24 to 48 hours.

**8.** The IV medications can be placed in the entire bottle of solution for infusion over an extended time, piggyback, or administered by IV push. With every drug given, the care provider must know the drug's dose range, side effects, interaction, and compatibility with the IV solution and the drug's safe infusion rate. Piggyback bottles can be inserted into a heparin lock or into an infusing IV.

**a.** If the drug is placed in a measured chamber, the chamber should be flagged in some manner to inform other care providers that no more fluid should be placed in the chamber until the drug has been completely infused.

**b.** Parents and the child need to be instructed not to tamper with either the fluid levels in the measured chamber or the IV infusion rate.

9. Immediately before injecting the drug, the site should be checked for signs of infusion intactness.
10. When drugs are given by constant infusion, it is important to keep the flow rate on schedule. Constant infusion pumps deliver the solution into the vein at a constant and controlled rate. Small volumes of solution (2 to 3 ml/hour) can be infused while keeping the infusion patent.
    a. Infusion pumps are not infallible and need to be observed for dry chambers, air in the tubing, and improper pump rates.
    b. Battery-powered infusion pumps allow the child greater freedom of movement.
    c. Patient control analgesia (PCA) pumps are used to deliver pain relievers as the patient needs them and are currently in usage for older children and adolescents.
    d. Drugs given by IV push method should not be injected quickly but should follow the manufacturer's maximal rate of drug infusion.
11. The heparin lock is a needle or catheter that is placed into the vein with a specially designed cap. A heparin solution is placed into the cap to maintain needle patency.
    a. Heparin locks are maintained as they are for adults. The heparinized solution most hospitals use for pediatric flush is 50 to 100 U/ml.
    b. The child must be cautioned not to tamper with the heparin lock, as immediate hemorrhage could result.
H. Hyperalimentation Infusions
    1. Hyperalimentation infusions require skillful monitoring and maintenance. The physician inserts the catheter surgically, under sterile conditions, into the subclavian vein, the jugular vein, or the umbilical vein of newborns or prematures. The site is then covered with a sterile dressing that is changed every 24 to 48 hours under sterile conditions according to the agency policy.
        a. The child must be instructed not to touch or play with the catheter dressing and the young child may need to be restrained to prevent contamination of the site.
        b. The hyperalimentation infusion rate is usually maintained with an infusion pump. Extreme care in recording infusion rate and volume of fluid infused is imperative as well as strict input and output measurements and daily weighings to detect fluid imbalances.
        c. Special tubing and filters designed for hyperalimentation administration are used; tubing and filters are changed down to the catheter site every 24 to 48 hours, depending on agency policy.
        d. Medication should not be administered through the hyperalimentation fluid, or blood be drawn through this central line.

The pharmacist must be consulted before any drugs are added to this fluid. If drugs are given intravenously, they are usually administered through another IV infusion site or through a heparin lock.

 **e.** Hyperalimentation fluid is prepared in the pharmacy under laminar flow hoods to prevent contamination. It is ideally made no more than 8 hours in advance of the infusion time; a bottle should be considered safe for infusion for only 24 hours after preparation. Most hyperalimentation fluids should be refrigerated in the medication refrigerator until usage, but should be allowed to come to room temperature before infusion.

 **f.** Before each new bottle of hyperalimentation fluid is hung, carefully check against the prescriber's orders for the contents of the solution.

 **g.** If hyperalimentation fluid begins to leak from the tubing, the tubing should be changed immediately; tape should not be placed over the tubing.

 **h.** The catheter site and the patient should be carefully observed for any signs of infection during hyperalimentation therapy.

**I.** Lipid Emulsions

 **1.** Lipid emulsions are usually infused through a central venous line. These emulsions have a milky appearance because of the suspended fat globules in the solution.

  **a.** Appearance of this solution may frighten a child and the parents, therefore, explanations are necessary.

  **b.** Lipid emulsions are refrigerated and then brought to room temperature by standing for 30 minutes before infusion.

  **c.** Nothing should ever be added to the emulsion mixture, and it should be checked for consistency, texture, and color.

  **d.** Rates of infusion need to be carefully checked with the physician and pharmacist before infusion.

  **e.** Observe for signs of adverse reaction, especially in the first 30 minutes. The infusion rate should not exceed 1 ml/minute.

  **f.** The child receiving this infusion should be monitored constantly during the infusion and should be observed for delayed symptoms after the infusion.

**XI. CONCLUSION**

 **A.** Drug administration with the child requires knowledge of the child's individual needs, developmental level, and cognitive understanding and is based on good administration principles and techniques.

 **B.** Time taken for adequate individual child assessment will enable the care provider to plan and approach the child in a manner that will decrease anxiety usually associated with medication administration.

# PART II
# Pediatric Medications

# Guide to Drug Reference Format

**Name:** The generic name is in capital bold face letters and common trade names are listed alphabetically in parenthesis.

**Pronunciation:** Stated in parenthesis.

**Combination Products:** Products that contain the drug in combination with other medications are listed.

**Classification:** Class(es) to which the drug belongs is stated.

**Available Preparations:** Dose and types of preparations are listed with oral forms first, then parenteral, and last, those given by other routes.

**Action and Use:** The drug's pharmacological actions in the body are stated. Most common pediatric uses are listed, beginning with those approved, followed by uses not currently approved by the Food and Drug Administration.

**Routes and Dosages:** Routes of administration are listed with oral first, then parenteral, and last, other routes such as inhalation, rectal, and ophthalmic. Pediatric dosages for each route are stated. If dosages differ for various uses, the specific use and dosage are listed. When dosages vary for different pediatric age groups, this is noted. The manufacturers have not tested some drugs adequately in children and, therefore, have not made pediatric dosage recommendations. Some drugs are used in clinical practice: the doses established in that area are listed as clinician established. It is possible that variations may exist between these dosages and those observed in your specific health care facility.

**Absorption and Fate:** Areas included, when information is available and pertinent, are absorption and distribution in the body, amount of binding to plasma proteins, metabolic route, and method of excretion. Time to onset of action, peak action, time to peak level, duration of action, half-life, and therapeutic level by each route are described.

**Contraindications and Precautions:** Pregnancy category is stated (see Appendix for description of each category). Information pertinent to children is listed next. Contraindications are stated, followed by precautions.

**Side Effects:** Side effects are listed in the following categories: Central Nervous System (CNS), Cardiovascular (CV), Gastrointestinal (GI), Respiratory, Hepatic, Genitourinary (GU), Skin, Hemic, Endocrine, Musculoskeletal,

Sensory, and Other. In general, the most common side effects are listed first in each category, followed by those less often reported. It is sometimes impossible to list in specific order of occurrence as data from various studies and references may conflict or may not be definite. Life-threatening side effects are listed in **boldface**.

**Nursing Implications:** This section is organized to assist the practicing nurse to use the nursing process with clients. Under *Assess*, information that should be collected or reviewed before giving the drug is stated. Next, under *Administer*, general information useful when giving the drug is stated first. Then information to assist with PO routes are noted, followed by parenteral routes, and then other routes. For example, instructions on mixing, time of potency after mixing, time for administration, compatibilities, and use of infusion devices are included for IV medications when pertinent. The *Monitor* section states observations to be made of patients during and/or after drug administration. In *Patient Teaching*, a summary of important information to be shared with the child and/or parents is listed. Some teaching which pertains to all drugs is not included (Examples: Keep drugs out of reach of children; do not share drugs with family members or others.)

**Drug Interactions:** Important interactions of the drug with other medications are stated. In some situations the drug alters the effect of other medications or in other cases some medications change the effect of the drug being discussed. If this drug is contraindicated with certain medications, this is noted. Although major interactions are noted, this is not intended as a complete drug interaction handbook. Some drugs that might interact but are not commonly given to children have been omitted. Especially for children, readers are referred to drug interaction texts for a complete listing of interactions on numerous or uncommon medications.

**Food Interactions:** Interactions of the drug with foods are included when known.

**Laboratory Test Interferences:** The effects of the drug on laboratory test findings are included. These may reflect a change created by the drug (for example, decreased potassium with a drug causing hypokalemia), or may be a false reading due to interference with the method used for laboratory analysis.

**Storage Requirements:** The temperature for storage is stated in both centigrade and fahrenheit. If the drug must be kept in dark, tightly closed, or must not be frozen, this is noted.

# ☐ ACETAMINOPHEN

(a-seat-a-min'o-fen)

(Acephen, Aceta, Actamin, Anacin-3, Anuphen, Apacet, Banesin, Bromo-Seltzer, Conacetol, Dapa, Datril, Dolanex, Genapap, Genebs, Halenol, Liquiprin, Meda Cap, Meda Tab, Myapap, Neopap, Oraphen-PD, Panadol, Panex, Pedric, Phenaphen, Suppap, Tapanol, Tempra, Tenol, Ty-Caplets, Tylenol, Valadol, Valorin)

**Combination Products:** Numerous products, for example, Aceta with codeine, Codaminophen, Excedrin, Trigesic, Vanquish.

**Classification:** analgesic, antipyretic

## Available Preparations:

- 120, 325, 500, 650-mg tablets
- 80-mg chewable tablets
- 160, 325, 500-mg film-coated tablets
- 500-mg capsules
- 120 mg/5 ml, 160 mg/5 ml, 167 mg/5 ml, 325 mg/5 ml elixir
- 100 mg/ml elixir
- 160 mg/5 ml oral solution
- 48, 100 mg/ml oral solution
- 120, 125, 325, 650-mg rectal suppositories

Also available in numerous combination products, such as in combination with codeine, pseudoephedrine, aspirin and caffeine, phenylopropanolamine, and propoxyphene.

**Action and Use:** May interfere with prostaglandin synthesis in the nervous system. Acts on the hypothalmus to cause antipyresis and the CNS to provide analgesia. May have mild antiinflammatory effect but likely this is not therapeutic. Used in treatment of fever and mild to moderate pain.

## Routes and Dosages:
*PO:*

- under 3 months: 40 mg
- 4–11 months: 80 mg
- 1–2 years: 120 mg
- 2–3 years: 160 mg
- 4–5 years: 240 mg
- 6–8 years: 320 mg
- 9–10 years: 400 mg
- 11 years: 480 mg
- over 11 years: 325–650 mg; not to exceed 4 g/day for short-term therapy or 2.6 g/day for long-term therapy.

Doses above may be repeated q4–6 h PRN, not to exceed 5 doses/day and not to exceed 5 days of treatment without medical advice.

Alternative dosing: 10–12 mg/kg q4h.
**PR:** PO doses above may be used for PR doses for children over 2 years.

**Absorption and Fate:** Rapidly and well absorbed after PO administration; decreased absorption when given with carbohydrate. Distributed widely in body tissues and only partially (25%) bound to plasma proteins. Metabolized by the liver and excreted in the urine as metabolized and unchanged drug. Peak serum levels reached in 30 to 120 minutes with peak effect observed in 1 to 3 hours. Duration of action, 3 to 4 hours, and half-life, 1 to 4 hours.

**Contraindications and Precautions:** Pregnancy category B. Present in breast milk but not known to be harmful to infants. Contraindicated in those with previous allergy to the drug. Repeated use not recommended for those with cardiac, lung, hepatic, or renal dysfunction. Preparations with sulfite not to be given to those with sulfite allergy; preparations with aspartame (Children's Anacin-3 and Children's Tylenol) not to be given to children with phenylketonuria. Cautious use in children especially those under 3 years, in patients with hepatic dysfunction, anemia, or renal dysfunction.

**Side Effects:**
**CNS:** mental confusion, lethargy, behavior changes, seizures; all symptoms of accompanying hepatic damage. **GI:** nausea, vomiting, diarrhea, anorexia. **Hepatic:** liver damage with abnormal liver function tests within 2 to 4 days of overdose. **GU:** hematuria, renal damage and dysfunction more common in those with renal disease. **Skin:** rash, urticaria as symptoms of rare anaphylaxis. **Hemic:** bleeding, ecchymosis, anemia, thrombocytopenia, leukopenia, pancytopenia; all more common with long-term use. **Other:** anaphylaxis with respiratory and skin symptoms.

**Nursing Implications:**
**Assess:** Hepatic and renal function are noted.
**Administer:** May be crushed and given with fluid; avoid carbohydrate that can decrease drug absorption.
**Monitor:** Periodic renal and hepatic studies may be done with the patient on long-term therapy.
**Patient Teaching:** Do not give with other OTC drugs unless directed by health-care provider. Consult physician for dosage in child younger than 2 to 3 years, if fever or illness persist over 3 days, or if relief not obtained. Limit children to 5 doses/day. This is a frequent drug that is accidentally ingested.

**Drug Interactions:** Increased risk of liver damage in persons who are alcoholic or are taking other hepatotoxic drugs. Persons on chronic barbiturates may have decreased acetaminophen action. Increased anticoagulant effect of coumarin with chronic acetaminophen use. Nephrotic side effects more common if chronic use is combined with chronic aspirin use. Potential for hypothermia when given with phenothiazines.

**Food Interactions:** Decreased absorption with high carbohydrate meal.

**Laboratory Test Interferences:** False-positive 5-hydroxyindoleacetic acid. False decrease in serum glucose. False increase in urine glucose and serum uric acid. Interferes with bentiromide test for pancreatic function.

**Storage Requirements:** Store tightly covered at 15 to 30°C (59–86°F).

---

## □ ACETYLCYSTEINE                                   (a-se-til-sis'tay-een)

(Airbron, Mucomyst, Mucosol)

**Classification:** mucolytic

**Available Preparations:** 100 mg/ml, 200 mg/ml for oral, intratracheal inhalation; oral solution

**Action and Use:** Decreases the viscosity of purulent and nonpurulent respiratory secretions apparently through reduction of disulfide linkages of mucoproteins. Enables the removal of mucous secretions through coughing, postural drainage, or mechanical means. Used in treatment of cystic fibrosis, bronchitis, pneumonia, tuberculosis, mucus obstruction atelectasis, emphysema, preparation for bronchial studies. Treatment of acetaminophen overdosage to prevent hepatotoxicity probably through maintaining or restoring glutathione levels.

**Routes and Dosage:**
*PO:* Acetaminophen Overdosage: initially 140 mg/kg; then in 4 hours, 70 mg/kg/dose and every 4 hours for total of 17 doses
*Inhalation:*
- Nebulization: 3 to 5 ml of 20% solution or 6 to 10 ml of 10% solution 3 to 4 times per day
- Closed Tent or Croupette: 300 ml of the 10 or 20% solution for single continuous treatment
- Intratracheal: 1 to 2 ml of 10 to 20% solution every 1 to 4 hours.

**Absorption and Fate:** After inhalation; onset of action within 1 minute, peak effect 5 to 10 minutes. Deacetylated in liver to cysteine.

**Contraindications and Precautions:** Pregnancy category B. Use caution during lactation. Contraindicated if hypersensitivity to drug. Use caution in asthma, severe respiratory insufficiency, conditions predispose to GI hemorrhage.

**Side Effects:**
*CNS:* drowsiness. *GI:* nausea, vomiting, stomatitis. *Resp:* rhinorrhea, **bronchospasm** (more common with asthmatics), hemoptysis. *Skin:* generalized urticaria. *Other:* fever, chills.

## Nursing Implications:

**Assess:** Cough: type, characteristic, frequency, amount and type of mucous secretions. Note rate and characteristics of respirations. Ingestion: may be difficult to assess how much acetaminophen was taken, serum level should be drawn 4 hours after reported ingestion to ensure peak level of drug has been reached. Treatment with acetylcysteine can start before results of serum levels. Drug should be given immediately if 24 hours or less has elapsed since ingestion.

**Administer: PO:** Drug most effective if given within 10 to 12 hours of overdosage. A 20% solution dilute to 5% solution or 1:3 ratio using cola, soft drinks, or citrus fruit drinks. Use within 1 hour of dilution. Drug has offensive odor of rotten eggs; reduce odor by placing diluted solution in glass with plastic top or lid and giving through straw. Drug odor becomes less noticeable with continued usage. Dosage vomited in 1 hour should be repeated. If child is unable to drink fluid, may give drug diluted with water through duodenal intubation. Dilute drug due to its irritating or sclerosing tendencies.

**Inhalation:** Do not use with hand-held nebulizer; particle size too large and output usually too small. Drug reacts with iron, copper, nickel, and rubber, therefore, use glass or plastic nebulizer. Nebulized drug should be inhaled directly from face mask or tent, mouth piece, oxygen tent, croupette, or head tent. Do not use with heated (hot-pot) nebulizer. Compressed air provides pressure for drug nebulization, however, oxygen can be used; nebulize with caution in those who have carbon dioxide retention. Before giving inhalation have child clear airway by coughing. Follow agency procedure for use of nebulizer. In continuous nebulization, solution evaporates impeding drug delivery and nebulization. When 3/4 of initial solution dispensed, add an equal volume of sterile water.

**Monitor:** This drug is just part therapy, supportive therapy is necessary in acetaminophen overdosage. Monitor renal and cardiac function. Liver function tests and prothrombin time should be obtained daily for 96 hours or until plasma tests indicate hepatotoxicity is not evident. Monitor for drug side effects and if generalized urticaria occurs discontinue drug. After drug inhalation therapy, there may be an increase in volume of bronchial secretions that may necessitate mechanical suction. Facial stickiness may occur after using face mask, which can be removed by washing with water. Nebulizing equipment must be cleaned immediately after each use because residues can clog device or corrode metal. Assess respiratory status.

**Patient Teaching:** A teaching plan should be developed for the family by the nurse and the respiratory therapist. Child should have regular medical evaluations and supervision.

**Drug Interactions:** Activated charcoal decreases effectiveness of this drug. Incompatible in same solution with amphotericin B, chlortetracycline HCl, erythromycin lactobionate, oxytetracycline HCl, ampicillin, tetracycline, iodized oil, trypsin, and hydrogen peroxide.

**Storage Requirements:** Store at 15 to 30°C (59 to 86°F). Stable for 96 hours after opening if stored in refrigerator.

# ☐ ACTIVATED CHARCOAL

(Absorba, Arm-a-char, Charcoaide, CharcoalantiDote, Charcocaps, Characodote, Charcotabs, Digestalin, Insta-Char, Liquid Antidose)

**Classification:** antidote, adsorbent

## Available Preparations:
- 0.625 g/5ml, 0.7 g/5ml, 1 g/5ml, 1.25 g/5ml oral suspensions
- 15, 30, 120, 240, 450-g powder for oral solution
- 325 g, 650-mg tablets
- 260-mg capsules

**Action and Use:** Inhibits GI absorption of wide variety of chemical compounds by means of adsorptive capacity of its total surface area. It is formed from residue from the destructive distillation of various organic materials. Because of the small particle size, it has the adsorptive power to form a complex with poisons in the GI tract and aids in their removal. Burnt toast is not a substitute for activated charcoal and has no adsorptive activity. Used in the treatment of poisoning or drug overdose or as a marker in testing GI function.

## Routes and Dosage:
**PO:** 5 to 10 times the amount of toxins ingested or 20 to 30 g/dose, initially

**Absorption and Fate:** Not absorbed from GI tract, excreted in feces.

**Contraindications and Precautions:** Pregnancy category C. Safety not established as antiflatulent in those under 3 years of age. Not effective for all poisonings as adsorbent of corrosives, mineral acids, solvents, petroleum distillates, iron, ethanol, methanol, or cyanide.

## Side Effects:
*GI:* nausea, black stools, constipation

## Nursing Implications:
*Assess:* Assess what child ingested, time of ingestion, how much ingested, did parents give anything for treatment. Assess level of consciousness and if any contraindication conditions are present; notify poison control center. Obtain vital signs and start flow chart.

*Administer: PO:* Powder most adsorbent form. To achieve significant binding of poison, administer charcoal within 30 minutes of poison ingestion; the longer the interval, the less effective it becomes. If giving ipecac it is best to give charcoal after emetic action; activated charcoal negates ipecac's effect. To mix powder (30 g/100 to 200 ml) stir constantly into tap water. To increase palatability add bentonite, sorbitol, concentrated fruit juice, corn syrup, or chocolate powder, and place in opaque glass with cover and use straw to administer. The appearance and consistency make it difficult for some children to consume. Some children may take it better if you let them suck on Popsicle or drink dilute fruit juice between swallows of drug to clear mouth of taste until medication is consumed. Child and parent must realize the importance of taking all of this medication. Do not mix with milk, milk products, or sherbet; it decreases charcoal's absorptive properties. May need to repeat dosage if child vomits shortly after administration.

*Monitor:* Assess child's response to medications and carefully observe for side effects of poison. Have gastric lavage and emergency equipment available. Do not use for more than 72 hours because it interferes with absorption of nutrients. Maintain hydration level for age group to prevent constipation.

*Patient Teaching:* Call poison control center before using. Explain how to give; how to monitor child's condition. Review how to prevent poisonings, what to do if incident occurs (e.g., determine what child took, try to assess how much consumed, time of ingestion, and if bringing child to emergency room bring container with them). Observe for constipation, stools will be black.

**Drug Interactions:** Activated charcoal neutralizes ipecac's emetic effect. This drug diminishes absorption of therapeutic agents if administered concurrently, give 3 to 4 hours after charcoal.

**Food Interactions:** Milk decreases adsorptive capacity of drug.

**Storage Requirements:** Store at 15 to 30°C (59 to 86°F), in tightly closed glass or metal containers.

---

## □ ACYCLOVIR, ACYCLOVIR SODIUM (Zovirax)                                    (ay-sye-kloe-ver)

**Classification:** antiinfective, antiviral

**Available Preparations:**
- 200 mg capsules
- 500 mg for parenteral administration
- 5% ointment for topical administration

**Action and Use:** Synthetic purine nucleoside analog whose action inhibits viral replication by interfering with DNA synthesis. Used in the treatment of cytomegalovirus infections, initial and recurrent mucocutaneous herpes simplex (HSV-1, HSV-2), in children who are and are not immunocompromised, and in treating nonimmunocompromised children with first episodes of genital herpes. Parenteral form has been given for varicella–zoster in immunocompromised children.

**Routes and Dosage:** (Dosage adjustment necessary with renal impairment)
**PO:** Safety of oral form has not been established in children. Some clinicians recommend 200 5 times/day for 5 days (genital lesions)
**IV:**
- neonates: 5 to 15 mg/kg or 250 mg/m$^2$ every 8 hours (dosage adjusted to maturity and renal function).
- under 12 years: 250 mg/m$^2$ every 8 hours
- over 12 years: 5 mg/kg every 8 hours

**Topical:** Information on usage in children is lacking; some clinicians recommend applying to affected area every 3 hours 6 times a day for 7 days

**Absorption and Fate:** Poor absorption from GI tract; percutaneous absorption minimal. Peak levels: PO, 1.5 to 2.5 hours, IV at end of infusion. Half-life: under 3 months, 3.8 to 4.1 hours; 1 to 2 years, 1.9 hours; 2 to 12 years, 2.2. to 2.8 hours; 12 to 17 years, 3.6 hours. Widely distributed to body fluids and tissues including CSF. Excreted principally in urine.

**Contraindications and Precautions:** Pregnancy category C and safety during lactation not established. Safe usage of oral form not established in children and limited information is available on IV or topical usage. Contraindicated if hypersensitivity to drug, herpes zoster immunosuppressed child. Use with caution in renal or hepatic disease, dehydration, neurologic abnormalities, electrolyte imbalance, hypoxia, previous neurologic reactions to cytotoxic drugs.

**Side Effects:**
**CNS:** headache, dizziness, fatigue, insomma, irritability, depression, IV: lethargy, obtundation, tremors, confusion, hallucinations agitation, **seizures, coma**.
**CV:** Hypotension, palpitations. **GI:** nausea, vomiting, diarrhea (oral).
**Hepatic:** transient rise in SGOT, SGPT, alkaline phosphatase. **GU:** hematuria, transient rise in serum creatinine. **Skin:** rash, urticaria, acne, accelerated hair loss. **Hemic: thrombocytosis, thrombocytopenia, leukopenia, lymphopenia**.
**Musculo-Skeletal:** arthralgia, pars planitis, muscle cramps, leg pain. **Other:** fever, sore throat, lymphadenopathy, superficial thrombophlebitis.

**Nursing Implications:**
**Assess:** Record appearance and number of lesions. Confirm diagnosis through laboratory cultures. Obtain baseline renal and liver studies.
**Administer:** Drug should be given at first symptoms of infection (tingling, burning, itching, or pain). This drug is not to be given SC, IM, ID, or ophthalmically. **IV: Do not give IV push**; causes crystals to form in renal tubules with ensuing renal damage. Reconstitute using 10 ml of sterile water (do not use bacteriostatic water containing benzyl alcohol in neonates). Do not use solutions containing parabens. This dilution is stable for 12 hours. Dilute to concentration of 7 mg/ml or less and infuse over at least 60 minutes. This solution is stable for 24 hours. Compatible with $D_5W$, $D_{10}W$, $D_5W/0.2\%NS$, $D_5W/0.5\%NS$, $D_5W/NS$, NS, LR. Incompatible with biological or colloidal fluids and avoid mixing with other drugs. **Topical:** Application should be

started as soon as possible after noting lesions. Strict medical asepsis (hand washing) should be used before and after contact with lesions. Cleanse with soap and water, dry thoroughly. Apply to cover lesion completely, gently rub in using gloves to protect individual applying ointment. Herpes virus has been reported to survive on fomites for 88 hours. If area is covered by clothing, it should be loose fitting to avoid irritation.

*Monitor:* Maintain adequate hydration during infusion and for 2 hours after. Monitor carefully for CNS symptoms and assess urinary function with I & O, and periodic renal function studies. If creatinine clearance decreases, dosage adjustments should be made as long as child is well hydrated and not in electrolyte imbalance. Avoid extravasation; it causes inflammation and phlebitis. Contact psyician if no improvement in 7 days after usage of ointment.

*Patient Teaching:* Proper application to avoid spreading virus to others; good hand washing techniques (liquid soap preferred). Child should have separate towels and washcloths, as well as undergarments. If itching is a problem, the area should not be scratched, it could cause secondary infections; contact physician. Do not use OTC creams and other preparations on lesions. Do not apply ointment more frequently than directed. Children who are sexually active need to understand how genital herpes is transmitted and avoid sexual activity during prodromal stage (several hours to days before appearance of lesion or until lesions are entirely healed). Healthy young children are unlikely to contract this disease except through incest or sexual assault. Parents and child must understand scope of this condition and what may precipitate attacks and how to handle this condition because drug does not cure disease. Follow-up health nurse consult may be helpful for aiding families in understanding the disease.

**Drug Interactions:** Probenecid and this drug may increase half-life and renal clearance of acyclovir. Cautiously use IV acyclovir in children who have previously experienced interferon- or cytotoxic-induced neurologic reactions or who are receiving methotrexate intrathecally.

**Storage Requirements:** Store at 15 to 30°C (59 to 86°F) in tight, light-resistant containers. Refrigeration of reconstituted solutions will cause precipitate to form, which will redissolve at room temperature without effecting potency.

---

## ☐ ALBUTEROL                                    (al-byoo'ter-ole)

(Proventil, Ventolin)

**Classification:** adrenergic, bronchodilator

**Available Preparations:**
- 2 mg/5 ml solution
- 2, 4-mg tablets
- 4-mg extended-release, film coated tablets
- 90 μg/metered spray aerosol, oral inhalation

- 0.083%, 0.5%, solution for nebulization

**Action and Use:** A synthetic sympathomimetic amine that appears to act on β-adrenergic receptors resulting in bronchodilation; it seems to have most effect on bronchial, uterine, and vascular muscles. Used for relief of reversible obstructive bronchospasms of asthma, bronchitis, and cystic fibrosis.

**Routes and Dosage:**
*PO:*
- 2 to 6 years: Initial: 0.1 mg/kg/day in 3 divided doses. (Maximum dosage 2 mg 3 times/day); if child fails to respond, gradually increase to 0.2 mg/kg/day in 3 divided doses. (Maximum dosage 4 mg 3 times/day)
- 6 to 12 years: 2 mg 3 to 4 times per day (may be increased to maximum of 24 mg/day)
- over 12 years: 2 to 4 mg 3 to 4 times per day; Extended-release tablets: 4 to 8 mg every 12 hours

*Inhalation:* Oral Inhalation:
- under 12 years: 1 to 2 inhalations (100 μg/inhalation) 4 times a day
- over 12 years: 1 to 2 inhalations (90 μg/inhalation) every 4 to 6 hours

Nebulizer: Manufacture does not recommend use of nebulization in those under 12 years, however, some clinicians use:
- under 5 years: 1.25 to 2.5 mg every 4 to 6 hours as necessary
- over 5 years: 2.5 to 5 mg every 4 to 6 hours as necessary
- over 12 years: 2.5 mg 3 to 4 times a day

**Absorption and Fate:** Well absorbed from GI tract. Onset of action: PO, 30 minutes; aerosol, 5 to 15 minutes; nebulization, 5 minutes. Peak effect: PO, 2 to 3 hours; aerosol, 0.5 to 2 hours; nebulization, 1 to 2 hours. Duration of action: PO, 4 to 6 hours; inhalation (both forms), 3 to 4 hours. Metabolized in liver and rapidly excreted in urine and feces.

**Contraindications and Precautions:** Pregnancy category C. Safe usage not established during lactation; tablets with those under 6 years, oral solution in those under 2 years, nebulization in those under 12 years. Contraindicated if hypersensitivity to drug or its ingredients. Use with caution in sensitivity to other sympathomimetic drugs, diabetes mellitus, hypertension, hyperthyroidism, cardiovascular disorders.

**Side Effects:**
*CNS:* (more common in those 2 to 5 years) excitement, nervousness, insomnia, hyperactivity; tremors, dizziness, headache. *CV:* tachycardia, palpitations, **hypertension**, hypotension, peripheral vasodilation. *Sensory:* irritation of nose and throat. *GI:* heartburn, nausea, vomiting, bad taste, increased appetite (common in 2 to 5 years). *Other:* muscle cramps, hypersensitivity (rare).

**Nursing Implications:**
*Assess:* Assess respiratory status and obtain baseline pulse.
*Administer: PO:* Can crush plain tablets, mix with small amounts of food or

fluids. Do not crush coated tablets. Side effects more common with oral form.
***Inhalations:*** Shake container well. See Part I for administration. If second inhalation is prescribed, manufacture recommends that 2 minutes elapse between doses. For administration by nebulization with IPPB apparatus, follow agency policy for operation. Follow package insert for solution dilution.
***Monitor:*** Monitor pulse (cardiovascular effects may occur); respiratory response to medication. Maintain hydration for weight. Should not use other sympathomimetic agents with this drug; it increases risk of cardiovascular symptoms.
***Patient Teaching:*** Teach proper usage and care of inhaler, it is beneficial to have child demonstrate inhaler usage. Inhaler should not be used more frequently than prescribed; if symptoms worsen, contact physician. If paradoxical bronchospasm occurs, discontinue immediately. Do not use other inhalers than those ordered by physician. Tolerance can develop with long-term therapy.

**Drug Interactions:** Avoid usage with other sympathomimetic amines because of additive effects. Effects of β-adrenergic blocking agents antagonize bronchodilation effects of this drug. May potentiate vascular effects of this drug when used with MAO inhibitors.

**Storage Requirements:** Store inhaler at 15 to 30°C (59 to 86°F) and do not puncture canister or place near heat or in open flame. Store nebulization solutions, extended-release tablets, and oral solutions at 2 to 30°C in light-resistant containers.

---

## □ ALLOPURINOL                                      (al-oh-pure'i-nole)

(Lopurin, Zyloprim)

**Classification:** antilithic, antigout agent

**Available Preparations:** 100, 300-mg tablets

**Action and Use:** Both allopurinol and its by-product oxypurinol inhibit xanthine oxidase, thereby interfering with production of uric acid. An increase in serum xanthine and hypoxanthine are observed. May inhibit hepatic microsomal enzymes. Used to lower serum and urinary uric acid levels in gout. Its main use in children is to lower uric acid concentration, which is observed in neoplastic disease, and particularly after chemotherapy and radiation therapy, which cause increased uric acid levels from cell breakdown. May be used to prevent future renal calculi in those with history of recurrent stones.

**Routes and Dosages:** PO, IV, and PR experimental
***PO:***
- under 6 years: 150 mg/day
- 6 to 10 years: 300 mg/day

■ adult dose: 600 to 800 mg/day for 2 to 3 days
*IV:* 100 to 200 mg/m²/day divided into 4 doses

**Absorption and Fate:** About 80 to 90% absorbed from GI tract. Distributed throughout body with lower amounts in brain. Not bound to plasma proteins. Metabolized to oxypurinol and excreted in original and metabolized form mainly in urine with smaller amounts in feces. Onset of action in 2 to 3 days with lowest uric acid levels reached in 1 to 3 weeks. Peak level of 2 to 3 μg/ml is reached in 1/2 to 2 hours after a 300-mg dose. The peak level of oxypurinol is 5 to 6.5 μg/ml and is reached in 4.5 to 5 hours. Duration of action 1 to 2 weeks after last dose. Half-life of allopurinol is 1 to 3 hours; oxypurinol, 18 to 30 hours.

**Contraindications and Precautions:** Pregnancy category C. Safe use in lactation not established. Not indicated for use in children except those with hyperuricemia of neoplasms, chemotherapy, or genetic purine metabolic disease. Contraindicated in acute gout, idiopathic hemochromatosis. Cautious use in hepatic or renal dysfunction, peptic ulcer, and bone marrow depression.

**Side Effects:**
*CNS:* drowsiness, peripheral neuropathy, neuritis, headache, vertigo, dizziness, depression, confusion, foot drop, optic neuritis. *GI:* nausea, vomiting, diarrhea, gastritis, abdominal pain, dyspepsia, aggravation of peptic ulcer. *Hepatic:* elevated alkaline phosphatase, SGOT, SGPT, urobilinogen; hepatomegaly, hepatitis, jaundice. *Skin:* pruritis, maculopapular rash, dermatitis, alopecia, ichthyosis, Stevens-Johnson syndrome; skin reactions may be delayed for up to 2 years after therapy. *Hemic:* leukocytosis, leukopenia, eosinophilia, thrombocytopenia, granulocytopenia, bone marrow suppression. *Sensory:* cataracts (rare), retinitis, iritis, conjunctivitis, amblyopia, tinnitus. *Other:* fever; hypersensitivity reaction with fever, chills, altered WBC count, arthralgia, rash, pruritis, nausea and vomiting.

**Nursing Implications:**
*Assess:* CBC, liver, and renal function tests must be done before initiating therapy
*Administer:* Given PO often after meals to decrease GI discomfort. Fluid intake increased to maintain about 2000 ml output daily.
*Monitor:* CBC, liver, and renal function tests are done regularly. Drug dosage must be reduced as creatinine clearance levels decrease. Uric acid levels will determine dosage of drug needed (normal uric acid, 6 to 7 mg/100 ml, but varies with laboratory). Observe for rash and report as this may indicate a hypersensitivity reaction that could be life threatening. Observe for and report weight loss and anorexia. Weigh daily. Measure I & O. Perform urinary pH; urine maintained at neutral or slightly alkaline level.
*Patient Teaching:* Increase fluid intake to prescribed levels. Drug alters mental alertness, therefore adjust activities accordingly; avoid driving as drowsiness may occur. Avoid exposure of eyes to sunlight or ultraviolet light. Report painful urination, skin rash. Children usually are not on long-term therapy.

**Drug Interactions:** Inhibits metabolism of azothioprine and mercaptourine, therefore, doses of those drugs must be reduced. Increases myelosuppression with cyclophosphamide. Inhibits metabolism of dicumarol. Increases rashes when given with ampicillin or amoxicillin and concomitant administration may be avoided. Diuretics increase serum urate and allopurinol hypersensitivity. Possible thrombocytopenia with co-trimoxazole. Increased hepatic and renal reactions with chlorpropamide.

**Laboratory Test Interferences:** Elevated serum alkaline phosphatase, transaminase, SGOT, SGPT. Decreased urinary urobilinogen, serum hematocrit, hemoglobin, WBCs.

**Storage Requirements:** Store tightly closed at 15 to 30°C (59 to 86°F).

---

## □ ALUMINUM CARBONATE

(Basaljel)

**Classification:** antacid, antilithic

**Available Preparations:**
- 400 mg/5 ml oral suspension
- 500 mg tablets
- 500 mg capsules

**Action and Use:** Neutralizes gastric acids by increasing pH; lowers esophageal sphincter pressure. Used in relief of symptoms of peptic ulcer, gastritis, hyperacidity, and hiatal hernia. Because of adsorbent capacity (aluminum binding to phosphate), it is given to prevent development of renal calculi. Sodium content 2.3 mg/5 ml, 2.8 mg/capsule, and 2.1 mg/tablet.

**Routes and Dosage:**
*PO:* Peptic Ulcer: 5 to 15 ml/dose every 3 to 6 hours or 1 to 3 hours after meals and at bedtime. Dosage variable, depends on indication and reaction of child.

**Absorption and Fate:** Onset action slow. Duration determined by gastric emptying time and presence of food. Binds with phosphate ions in intestine to form insoluble aluminum phosphate, which is excreted unabsorbed.

**Contraindications and Precautions:** Pregnancy category C. Can be used during lactation. Not for use with children unless prescribed by physician. Contraindicated in hypersensitivity to this drug or aluminum products. Use caution in renal failure, dehydration, decreased GI motility, and sodium restrictions.

## Side Effects:
*GI:* constipation, anorexia, intestinal obstruction, fecal impaction. ***Other:*** hypophosphatemia, hypercalciuria, dementia (from aluminum toxicity).

## Nursing Implications:
***Assess:*** Assess serum phosphate level.

***Administer: PO:*** Shake suspension well. Give with small amount of water or fruit juice. If given for urinary calculi, give with as much juice or fluids as child will take.

***Monitor:*** Monitor stool consistency and pattern; notify physician if constipation occurs. Assess for hypophosphatemia, anorexia, malaise, muscle weakness (especially if in renal failure). Monitor serum phosphate levels. Maintain fluid intake for age level. For renal calculi, increase fluid intake, acid ash diet, strain urine, and record I & O.

***Patient Teaching:*** Take only as scheduled, in prescribed amount and do not increase dosage. Observe for constipation and maintain fluid intake for age group. Do not take OTC without consulting pharmacist or physician.

**Drug Interactions:** This drug interferes with absorption of tetracyclines, space doses 1 to 2 hours apart.

**Food Interactions:** Avoid phosphate foods: eggs, dairy products, fruits, carbonated beverages.

**Storage Requirements:** Store at 15 to 30°C (59 to 86°F) and protect from freezing.

---

## □ ALUMINUM HYDROXIDE

(ALternaGEL, Alu-Cap, Al-U-Creme, Alugel, Aluminett, Alu-Tab, Amphojel, Dialume)

**Combination Products:** Aluminum hydroxide is used with other drugs for OTC medications such as: Gaviscon, Maalox, Di-Gel, Gelusil, Mylanta, and others.

**Classification:** antacid, antilithic

## Available Preparations:
- 320 mg/5 ml, 400 mg/5 ml, 600 mg/5 ml oral suspension
- 300, 600-mg tablets
- 600-mg film-coated tablets
- 500-mg chewable tablets
- 475, 500-mg capsules

**Action and Use:** Neutralizes gastric acids by increasing pH; lowers esophageal sphincter pressure. Used in relief of symptoms of peptic ulcer, gastritis, hyperacidity, and hiatal hernia. Because of adsorbent capacity (aluminum binding to phosphate), it is given to prevent development of renal calculi. Sodium content varies with brand and formulation, check with pharmacist.

## Routes and Dosage:

*PO:* Peptic Ulcer: 5 to 15 ml/dose every 3 to 6 hours or 1 to 3 hours after meals and at bedtime
Prophylaxis GI Bleeding:
- infants: 2 to 5-ml/dose every 1 to 2 hours
- children: 5 to 15 ml/dose every 1 to 2 hours
Maintain gastric pH below 5. Dosage variable, depends on indication and reaction of child.

*Hyperphosphatemia:* 50–150 mg/kg/day every 4 to 6 hours.

**Absorption and Fate:** Onset of action slow. Duration determined by gastric emptying time and presence of food. Binds with phosphate ions in intestine to form insoluble aluminum phosphate, which is excreted unabsorbed.

**Contraindications and Precautions:** Pregnancy category C. Can be used during lactation. Not for use with children unless prescribed by physician. Contraindicated in hypersensitivity to this drug or aluminum products. Use caution in renal failure, dehydration, decreased GI motility, and sodium restrictions.

## Side Effects:

*GI:* constipation, anorexia, intestinal obstruction, fecal impaction. *Other:* hypophosphatemia, hypercalciuria, dementia (from aluminum toxicity)

## Nursing Implications:

*Administer: PO:* Shake suspension well and give with small amount of water or milk. Masticate chewable tablet well for maximum absorption. If given by nasogastric tube, check for patency and proper tube placement. After dosage, flush tube with enough water to clear tube and ensure medication is in stomach. If given for urinary calculi, give with as much juice or fluids as child will take.

*Monitor:* Monitor stool consistency and pattern; notify physician if constipation occurs. Assess for hypophosphatemia, anorexia, malaise, muscle weakness (especially if in renal failure). Monitor serum phosphate levels. Maintain fluid intake for age level. For renal calculi, increase fluid intake, acid ash diet, strain urine, and record I & O.

*Patient Teaching:* Take only as scheduled, in prescribed amount and do not increase dosage. Observe for constipation and maintain fluid intake for age group. Do not take OTC without consulting pharmacist or physician.

**Drug Interactions:** This drug interferes with absorption of tetracyclines, digoxin, phenytoin, isoniazid, iron, or chlorpromazine; space doses 2 to 3 hours apart.

**Food Interactions:** Avoid phosphate foods: eggs, dairy products, fruits, carbonated beverages.

**Storage Requirements:** Store at 15 to 30°C (59 to 86°F) and protect from freezing.

---

## □ AMANTADINE HYDROCHLORIDE

(a-man′ta-deen)

(Symmetrel)

**Classification:** antiinfective, antiviral

**Available Preparations:**
- 50 mg/5 ml oral solution
- 100-mg capsules

**Action and Use:** Exact mechanism of action unknown but appears to inhibit influenza A virus from penetrating respiratory epithelia cells and reducing possibility of viral replication. Only active against strains of influenza A virus. Prevention of disease is achieved only if drug is in tissues before exposure to virus. Symptoms of influenza may be less severe if drug is administered 24 to 48 hours from onset of symptoms.

**Routes and Dosage:** (Adjustment necessary with renal impairment)
*PO:*
- over 1 to 9 years: 4.4–8.8 mg/kg/day divided doses 2 times a day. (Maximum dosage 150 mg/day)
- 10 to 12 years: 4.4 mg/kg/day in divided doses 2 times a day (maximum dosage 200 mg/day).
- adults: 200 mg/day

**Absorption and Fate:** Well absorbed from GI tract. Peak levels, 1 to 4 hours. Half-life, 9 to 37 hours. Distributed to saliva, nasal secretions. 90% excreted in urine.

**Contraindications and Precautions:** Pregnancy category C. Use with caution during lactation. Contraindicated in those under 1 year, hypersensitivity to drug, herpes zoster-immunosuppressed child. Use caution in renal impairment, hepatic or cardiovascular disease, eczematoid dermatitis, epilepsy history, uncontrolled psychosis or psychoneurosis, orthostatic hypotension.

**Side Effects:**
*CNS:* dizziness, insomnia, irritability, problems in concentration, depression, anxiety, ataxia, confusion, headache, hallucinations, **psychosis**, weakness,

slurred speech, tremor, **seizures**. *CV:* orthostatic hypotension, peripheral edema, **congestive heart failure**. *GI:* nausea, anorexia, constipation, dry mouth, vomiting. *GU:* urinary retention. *Skin:* rash, urticaria, livedo reticularis with prolonged therapy. *Hemic:* leukopenia, neutropenia (rare). *Other:* dyspnea, visual disturbances.

## Nursing Implications:

*Assess:* Assess for exposure to influenza A virus.

*Administer: PO:* Drug should be given before or as soon as possible after child has contacted influenza A virus and should be continued for 10 days after known exposure. For treatment of symptoms, give 24 to 48 hours after onset and continue for 5 days after symptoms disappear. Can give with food or milk. Using divided daily doses may decrease CNS symptoms. Tablet can be crushed or capsule taken apart, mixed with small amount of food or fluid.

*Monitor:* Monitor carefully for drug side effects and symptoms of influenza. If insomnia occurs, take last dose several hours before bedtime.

*Patient Teaching:* Take for duration determined by physician. Orthostatic hypotension may occur; instruct not to stand or change positions quickly.

**Drug Interactions:** Use of alcohol with this drug may increase CNS effects. Use with caution with other CNS stimulants because of potential increase in these effects. Amantadine and anticholinergic drugs may cause increased CNS symptoms of hallucinations and confusion.

**Storage Requirements:** Store at 15 to 30°C (59 to 86°F) in light-resistant containers.

---

## ☐ AMIKACIN                                          (am-i-kay′sin)

(Amikin)

**Classification:** aminoglycoside

**Available Preparations:** 50 mg, 250 mg/ml for parenteral administration

**Action and Use:** Inhibits protein synthesis by binding irreversibly to bacterial ribosomes. Active against wide range of both gm+ and gm− bacteria, such as staphylococci, enterococci, *Escherichia coli, Proteus, Klebsiella, Enterobacter, Serratia,* and *Pseudomonas.* May be active against some of the *Pseudomonas; Proteus,* and *Serratia* strains are resistant to gentamicin and tobramycin. Used to treat infections of bone, burns, urinary tract, and infections such as otitis media, septicemias, meningitis.

## Routes and Dosage:

*IM and IV:* Loading dose for neonates is 10 mg/kg then:
- birth to 7 days (<2000g): 7.5 mg/kg every 12 hours

- 7 days (or 72000g) to 1 year: 7.5 mg/kg every 8 hours
- 1 year and older: 15 mg/kg/day every 8 hours or 7.5 mg/kg every 12 hours. (Maximum dosage not to exceed 15 mg/kg/day or 1.5 mg/day)

**Note:** Dosages based on normal renal function. Limit treatment to 7 to 10 days.

**Absorption and Fate:** IM absorption rapid and complete. Distributed mainly to extracellular fluids. CSF concentrations may reach 50% if meninges inflamed. Peak level: IM, about 1 hour; IV, end of infusion or in 30 minutes. Half-life: 2 to 2.5 hours; neonates, 4 to 8 hours. Protein binding low; 82 to 98% excreted unchanged in urine.

**Contraindications and Precautions:** Pregnancy category D. Safety during lactation not established. Use caution in premature infants and neonates due to renal immaturity. Contraindicated if hypersensitivity to this drug or other aminoglycosides or renal failure. Use caution in renal function impairment, botulism, hypocalcemia, dehydration, or eighth cranial nerve impairment.

**Side Effects:**
*CNS:* **neurotoxicity**: numbness, tingling, muscle twitching, seizures; **neuromuscular blockade** with muscle weakness, respiratory depression, lethargy, headache. *GI:* nausea, vomiting, loss of appetite. *GU:* **nephrotoxicity**, blood or casts in urine, oliguria, increased thirst, proteinuria, increased BUN and serum creatine, decreased urine creatinine clearance and specific gravity, renal failure. *Skin:* skin rash, drug fever. *Hemic:* eosinophilia, anemia. *Sensory:* **ototoxicity**: eighth cranial nerve damage, hearing loss, loss of balance, vertigo, tinnitus; cochlear damage, high frequency hearing loss only detected at first by audiometric testing

**Nursing Implications:**
*Assess:* Obtain cultures and sensitivity before treatment, but can start treatment before results. Obtain baseline weights, BUN, creatinine levels, and hearing tests before therapy.
*Administer:* Solution should be colorless to very pale yellow. Do not use if dark yellow color or has particulate matter. *IV:* Do not give IV push. Minimum dilution is 25 mg/10 ml. Dilute in maximum amount of solution possible, usually using amount of solution to be infused over 1 hour; give over 30 to 60 minutes. Infants infusion should be 1 to 2 hours. Compatible with $D_5W$, $D_5W$/ 0.2% NS, $D_5W$/ 0.45% NS, $D_5W$/NS, $D_{10}W$, NS, LR, Normosol M/$D_5W$, Normosol R/$D_5W$, Ionosol, Mannitol 20%. Do not premix with other medications. Flush line with normal saline or 5% dextrose in water. Stable for 24 hours at room temperature in concentrations of 0.25 and 5.0 mg/ml if mixed in above listed solutions.
*Monitor:* Observe signs of respiratory depression during IV infusion. Peak blood levels drawn 1 hour after IM dosage and 30 minutes to 1 hour after infusion ends. Desirable peak concentrations should be 15 to 30 µg/ml and maximum trough concentrations should not be above 5 to 10 µg/ml. Measurements above these levels associated with increased incidence of toxicity. Main-

tain daily hydration level for child's age group. If no response in 3 to 5 days, therapy should be discontinued. Monitor child's hearing levels daily (can use ticking watch). Renal function assessed by I & O, daily weights, urine specific gravity, urinalysis, creatinine levels, and BUN. Report side effects immediately to physician. Observe for superinfections. If therapy continues past 10 days, obtain daily renal function tests and weekly audiograms.

**Drug Interactions:** Increased chance for ototoxicity when used with other aminoglycosides or capreomycin. Amphotericin B, salicylates, bacitracin (parenteral), bumetanide (parenteral), carmustine, cephalothin, cisplatin, cyclosporine, ethacrynic acid, furosemide, paromomycin, streptozocin, and vancomycin in combination with amikacin may cause ototoxicity and nephrotoxicity. Masked symptoms of ototoxicity occur when used with dimenhydrinate. Neuromuscular blockade may occur with halogenated hydrocarbon inhalation anesthetic, citrate-anticoagulated blood transfusion, and neuromuscular blocking agents used with amikacin. Neonates have decreased renal clearance with amikacin and indomethacin. Nephrotoxicity and neuromuscular blockade may be increased with use of this drug with methoxyflurane or polymyxins. Amikacin causes increased respiratory depressant effects with opioid and analgesics. Inactivated by penicillin, carbicillin, and ticarcillin.

**Laboratory Test Interference:** LDH increased; serum sodium decreased.

**Storage Requirements:** Store at 15 to 30°C (59 to 86°F). Stable at room temperature for 2 years. IV dilutions retain potency for 24 hours at room temperature.

---

□ **AMINOPHYLLINE OR**           (am-in-off'i-lin)
**THEOPHYLLINE**
**ETHYLENEDIAMINE**

(Aminophyllin, Corophyllin, Lixaminol, Phyllocontin, Somophyllin-DF, Truphylline)

**Classification:** bronchodilator, xanthine

**Available Preparations:**
- 105 mg/5 ml oral solution
- 100, 200-mg tablets
- 100, 200-mg enteric-coated tablets
- 225-mg extended-release tablets
- 25 mg/ml for parenteral administration
- 1 mg/ml, 2 mg/ml in 45% sodium chloride for parenteral administration
- 60 mg/ml rectal solution
- 250, 500-mg rectal suppositories

**Action and Use:** An ethylenediamine compound with theophylline. An enzyme inhibitor of phosphodieterase that results in increased concentrations of cyclic AMP causing relaxation of bronchial smooth muscles. Used for the symptomatic relief of bronchial asthma, reversible bronchospasm of chronic bronchitis and emphysema. Also used in treatment of Cheyne-Stokes respiration apnea and bradycardia in prematures. This drug has about 79% anhydrous theophylline.

## Routes and Dosage:
*PO:*
- 1 to 9 years: 20 mg/kg/day in equally divided doses every 6 hours
- 9 to 16 years: 16 mg/kg/day in equally divided doses every 6 hours
- over 16 years (adult): 12 mg/kg/day in equally divided doses every 6 hours

*IV:* Neonatal Apnea: Loading dosage, 4 to 6 mg/kg for 1 dose only **(each 1 mg/kg dose raises serum theophylline levels 2 µg/ml)**
Maintenance:
- prematures at birth gestational age up to postnatal age of 40 weeks: 1 mg/kg divided dose every 12 hours
- term neonates at birth or 40 weeks postconception up to 4 weeks postnatal: 1-2 mg/kg every 8 hours
- 4 to 8 weeks postnatal: 1 to 3 mg/kg every 8 hours

Bronchospasm: Loading dosage, 6 mg/kg for 1 dose only
Maintenance:
- neonates up to 24 days: 1.25 mg/kg every 12 hours
- neonates over 24 days: 1.9 mg/kg every 12 hours
- 6 to 52 weeks: $\dfrac{0.008 \text{ (age in weeks)} + 0.21}{0.8}$ = mg/kg/hour
- 1 to 9 years: 1 mg/kg/hour
- 9 to 12 years: 0.9 mg/kg/hour
- 12 to 16 years (nonsmoker): 0.6 mg/kg/hour
- 12 to 16 years (smoker): 0.9 mg/kg/hour

**Dosage is individualized and should be based on serum concentrations.**
*Rectal:* Enema dosages rarely used; contact your pharmacist for dosage

**Absorption and Fate:** Peak level: PO: liquid, 1 hour; plain tablets, 2 hours; enteric-coated tablets, 5 hours; extended-release tablets, 4 to 7 hours; IV: within 30 to 60 minutes. Mean half-life: neonates and prematures, 30+ hours; over 6 months, 3.7 ± 1.1 hours. Half-life decreased by smoking and fever; half-life increased by alcoholism, decreased hepatic or renal function, congestive heart failure, and with some antibiotics. Therapeutic level: neonatal apnea, 5 to 15 µg/ml; bronchspasm, 10 to 20 µg/ml. Excreted in urine.

**Contraindications and Precautions:** Pregnancy category C. Distributed in breast milk and can cause irritability in nursing infants. Contraindicated by IM route (causes severe pain at injection site), enteric-coated tablets in those under 12 years, suppositories due to erratic absorption, and if hypersensitivity to drug or xanthines (caffeine), preexisting cardiac arrhythmias. Use caution in children, peptic ulcer, hyperthyroidism, glaucoma, diabetes mellitus, hepatic disease, hypertension, cor pulmonale, compromised cardiac, or circulatory function.

## Side Effects:

*CNS:* headaches, restlessness, dizziness, irritability, insomnia, muscle twitching, **seizures**. *CV:* palpitations, **sinus tachycardia**, extrasystoles, flushing, marked hypotension, **circulatory failure, cardiac arrest**. *GI:* nausea, vomiting, bitter aftertaste, epigastric pain, anorexia, diarrhea. *Resp:* tachypnea. *GU:* albuminuria. *Skin:* urticaria, exfoliative dermatitis. *Other:* hyperglycemia, inappropriate ADH; Local, redness, pain at IV site.

## Nursing Implications:

*Assess:* Assess respiratory status and vital signs. Obtain weight; dosage based on lean body mass, drug not distributed to fatty tissues. If child on any form of theophylline, ask when last dosage was given and may be necessary to obtain drug level before starting this drug. If neonates heart rate above 180/min; withhold drug; consult physician.

*Administer: PO:* Food delays the absorption of this drug, but if GI irritation occurs it can be taken with food. Lowering dosage may be necessary if GI irritation occurs. Dosages individualized. Oral dosage can also be given by nasogastric tube. Plain tablets can be crushed and mixed with small amounts of food or fluids. Extended-release or enteric-coated tablets should not be crushed or chewed. *IV:* Exposure of parenteral form to air liberates theophylline causing it to crystallize; do not use if this occurs. Make sure you have IV form before use and verify theophylline content. Drug is commercially diluted to 25 mg/ml. Intermittent infusion: usually dilute equal volume of $D_5W$ (preferred), but compatible with $D_5W/0.2\%NS$, $D_5W/0.5\%NS$, $D_5W/NS$, $D_{10}W$, NS, LR, Ionosol products. **Administering faster than 25 mg/minute may result in circulatory failure or excessive serum concentrations of drug.** Administration rate is usually over 25 to 30 minutes. Continuous infusion is diluted with at least an equal volume of compatible IV fluid and is usually infused at rate of 0.9 to 1.5 mg/kg/hour. Do not use continuous infusions for neonates. Incompatible with acid solutions, alkali labile drugs (penicillin G, isoproterenol, thiamine), vitamin B complex, vitamin B with C, insulin, phenytoin, methylprednisolone, and many others. Check with pharmacist before mixing with any drug.

*Monitor:* Carefully monitor respiratory status. Theophylline preparations have low therapeutic index. Thus, optimum serums levels between 10 and 20 μg/ml should be maintained. Toxic symptoms are more likely to occur when serum drug level is over 20 μg/ml. Monitor drug levels frequently. With an intermittent infusions, monitor for theophylline level in 4 to 6 hours of last IV dosage. Assess vital signs and I & O during IV infusion. Monitor IV site for pain and inflammation.

*Patient Teaching:* Report any CNS, cardiac, or GI side effects to physician. Monitor respiratory response. Maintain hydration level and weight level. Do not use any OTC drug that may contain ephedrine, which can cause excessive

CNS symptoms. Take drug as directed and take at same time of day every day to maintain blood levels of drug. Drug is meant for control of asthma only under physician's supervision.

**Drug Interactions:** Phenytoin and barbiturates decrease this drug's serum levels. This drug decreases therapeutic effectiveness of lithium and furosemide. Beta-adrenergic blockers (especially propranolol and nadolol) may induce bronchospasms when used with this drug. Erythromycin, cimetidine, troleandomycin decrease the hepatic clearance of this drug. This drug may enhance the toxic potential of cardiac glycosides. Adrenergics used with this drug may increase CNS stimulation.

**Laboratory Test Interference:** Produces false-positive serum uric acids with Bittner or colorimetric method.

**Storage Requirements:** Store at 15 to 30°C (59 to 86°F); protect parenteral form from light and freezing.

---

## □ AMITRIPTYLLINE　(a-meh-trip'ti-leen)

(Amitril, Elavil, Emitrip, Endep, Enovil)

**Combination Products:** Etrafon, Limbitrol, Travil

**Classification:** tricyclic antidepressant

**Available Preparations:**
- 10, 25, 50, 75, 100, 150-mg film-coated tablets
- 10 mg/ml vials for parenteral use

Also available in tablets in combination with chlordiazepoxide and with perphenazine.

**Action and Use:** Likely inhibits the reuptake and metabolism of endogenous catecholamines in the CNS, thus potentiating effects of norepinephrine and serotonin. Used in treatment of mental depression. Uses in children not approved by the FDA include treatment of anorexia and bulimia, attention deficit disorder in children over 6 years, enuresis, and for pruritus in cold urticaria.

**Routes and Dosages:**
*PO:* Antidepressant:
- 6 to 12 years: 10 to 30 mg/day or 1 to 5 mg/kg/day divided into 2 to 3 doses
- adolescent: 10 mg tid and 20 mg at hs; not to exceed 100 mg/day
  Enuresis:

- under 6 years: 10 mg at hs
- over 6 years: 10 to 25 mg at hs

Dose for enuresis established by clinicians rather than manufacturer.
*IM*: dose not used in children.

**Absorption and Fate:** Rapidly absorbed from GI tract. Distributed in body tissues and crosses blood-brain barrier and placenta; present in breast milk. 96% bound to plasma proteins. Metabolized in the liver and excreted mainly in the urine. Peak level in 2 to 12 hours after administration but full effect may not occur for 2 to 3 weeks. Half-life is 10 to 50 hours with up to 93 hours for metabolites. Therapeutic level is 110 to 250 ng/ml.

**Contraindications and Precautions:** Pregnancy category C. Used in pregnancy only if clearly needed as teratogenesis in laboratory animals has occurred. The general class of tricyclic antidepressants is not recommended for children under 12 years; however, this drug is used in children over 6 years with enuresis or attention deficit disorder. Contraindicated after myocardial infarction, hypersensitivity to any tricyclic antidepressant, in those with un-treated glaucoma, and during lactation. Used with caution in children, adolescents, treated glaucoma, respiratory and cardiovascular disease, those with seizures, in asthmatics, cardiovascular problems, bipolar disorder, GI problems, hyperthyroidism, hepatic or renal dysfunction.

**Side Effects:**
*CNS:* drowsiness, lethargy, fatigue (common); agitation, sleep disturbance, confusion, anxiety, mood changes, worsening of psychosis, fine motor tremor, ataxia, dysphagia, dysarthria, incoordination; seizures particularly in those with seizure history when doses are increased in large increments. *CV:* EKG changes particularly in children with AV dissociation, prolonged PR intervals, widened QRS, postural hypotension, arrhythmia, thrombosis, congestive heart failure, hypertension, tachycardia, ventricular flutter and fibrillation, heart block. *GI:* anorexia, nausea, vomiting, diarrhea, GI distress, dry mouth, constipation. *Hepatic:* jaundice, hepatitis, altered liver function tests. *GU:* urinary retention, renal damage. *Skin:* allergic reaction with rash, erythema, petechiae, edema of face and tongue, photosensitivity. *Hemic:* agranulocytosis, eosinophilia, leukopenia and thrombocytopenia (rare). *Endocrine:* breast engorgement, testicular edema, increase or decrease in blood glucose.

**Nursing Implications:**
*Assess:* Careful history to identify cardiac, blood, and other diseases. Take baseline vital signs.
*Administer: PO:* May give with food to lessen GI irritation. If drug is given for depression, be sure it is taken. Only small amount of drug is dispensed for home use. Drug is withdrawn before surgery but should be tapered rather than quickly withdrawn.
*Monitor:* Monitor vital signs especially pulse and blood pressure. Measure regularly and observe food and fluid intake and bowel and bladder elimination.

Watch patient for side effects of drug, especially if a history of seizures, allergies, or cardiac disease is present. Record night wettings if used as treatment for enuresis and mood if used as treatment of depression. If sore throat or fever occur, CBC should be done as hemic side effects may be present. If jaundice occurs, liver function tests should be done. EKG may be done in those with cardiac problems. Serum level may be monitored.

*Patient Teaching:* Take drug as directed. Do not discontinue quickly or without prescriber instructions. Return for follow-up visits as recommended. Report excess fatigue, mood changes, weight change, enuresis episodes, do not drive cars. Adjust activities accordingly; Good oral care may help symptoms of dry mouth. Do not use OTC drugs without consulting prescriber. Instruct to change position slowly especially when rising.

**Drug Interactions:** Increased side effects of both drugs if used with monoamine oxidase inhibitors with hyperpyrexia, hypertension, tachycardia, seizures. Additive effects with other CNS depressant drugs, including alcohol. Potentiation of side effects with barbiturates. Increased blood levels with phenothiazines. Increased sympathetic activity with sympathomimetics. May decrease the activity of antihypertensives. Can increase activity of dicumarol and warfarin. Increases gastric emptying time, therefore, may slow absorption and cause inactivation of some drugs in the stomach.

**Laboratory Test Interferences:** May increase or decrease blood glucose. May elevate serum bilirubin, alkaline phosphatase, transaminase. Increases urinary catecholamines.

**Storage Requirements:**
Store in tightly closed container between 15 and 30°C (59 and 86°F). Do not freeze injection solution.

---

### ☐ AMOXICILLIN    (a-mox-i-sil'in)

(A-Cillin, Amoxican, Amoxil, Apo-Amoxi, Larotid, Moxilean, Novamoxin, Polymox, Sumox, Trimox, Utimox, Wymox)

**Classification:** antibiotic, aminopenicillin

**Available Preparations:**
- 50 mg/ml pediatric drops
- 125 mg/5 ml, 250 mg/5 ml suspension
- 125, 250-mg chewable tablets
- 250, 500-mg capsules

**Action and Use:** Bactericidal action inhibits cell-wall synthesis in bacteria, a broader spectrum of activities than penicillin G. Effective on some gram-positive and gram-negative organisms, such as *Haemophilus influenzae, E. coli, Proteus mirabilis, Neisseria gonorrhoeae*, meningococci, enterococci, and *Salmonella*. Used to treat infections of the ear, upper respiratory tract, GU system, skin and soft tissue, and prophylaxis for bacterial endocarditis.

## Routes and Dosage:
*PO:*

- under 20 kg: 20 to 40 mg/kg/day in equally divided doses every 8 hours
- over 20 kg: 250 to 500 mg every 8 hours

Dosage adjustment necessary for renal impairment

## Absorption and Fate: 74 to 92% absorbed from GI tract. Distributed to all body tissues but brain and spinal fluid, except when meninges are inflamed. 20% bound to plasma proteins. Peak level, 1 to 2 hours. Half-life, about 60 minutes. Therapeutic level, 0.01 to 10 μg/ml. About 50% excreted unchanged in urine.

## Contraindications and Precautions: Pregnancy category B. Use with caution during lactation. Contraindicated if hypersensitivity to drug, penicillins, or cephalosporins. Use with caution with allergies, asthma, family history of allergies, infectious mononucleosis, history of GI disease, or impaired renal function.

## Side Effects:
*GI:* diarrhea (less than ampicillin), nausea and vomiting (2%), epigastric pain, stomatitis, glossitis, black tongue, **pseudomembranous colitis** (rare). *Hepatic:* moderate rise in SGOT and SGPT. *GU:* superinfections primarily yeast, **interstitial nephritis. Skin:** erythematous, maculopapular, mildly pruritus rash (starts 3 to 14 days after therapy initiated, begins on trunk, spreads to entire body even soles, palms, and oral mucosa, most intense at pressure areas elbows and knees). *Hemic:* eosinophilia, **anemia, thrombocytopenia, thrombocytopenic purpura,** leukopenia, **agranulocytosis. Other:** hypersensitivity: urticarial rash, drug fever, **anaphylaxis** (rare).

## Nursing Implications:
*Assess:* Assess previous allergy to this drug, penicillins, cephalosporins, other drugs, asthma, or family history of allergies. Obtain culture and sensitivity before treatment, but can start treatment before results.
*Administer: PO:* Stable in gastric acids, give without regard to meals. Shake suspension well. Capsules may be taken apart or tablets crushed; mixed in small amount of food or fluid.

## Monitor: Monitor child for hypersensitivity (especially in first 20 minutes of first dosage), rash (onset and characteristics), and side effects. Watch for symptoms of superinfection; diarrhea (may indicate pseudomembranous colitis, which can occur while on drug or 4 days to 6 weeks after drug is discontinued). Assess renal, hepatic, and hematological functions with prolonged or

high-dose therapy or with premature and neonates. Maintain fluid intake for age group. Therapy course continued for 48 to 72 hours after negative bacterial cultures or symptoms subside. If given for β-**hemolytic streptococcal** infection, 10-day course needed to prevent risk of acute rheumatic fever or glomerulonephritis.

*Patient Teaching:* Take as prescribed for full course of therapy. Observe for side effects, especially diarrhea or rash; report to physician. Store suspension in refrigerator out of reach of children. Reconstituted suspension should be discarded after 14 days if refrigerated.

**Drug Interactions:** Erythromycin, tetracycline, chloromycetin, and acids decrease the effects of amoxicillin. Probenecid combined with amoxicillin decreases renal excretion of drug, thus prolonging serum levels.

**Laboratory Test Interferences:** False-positive urine glucose with Clinitest and Benedict's test.

**Storage Requirements:** Store at 15 to 30°C (59 to 86°F). Reconstituted suspensions stable; refrigerated for 14 days, room temperature for 7 days. Label with time and date at time of reconstitution.

---

# ☐ AMOXICILLIN AND CLAVULANATE POTASSIUM

(a-mox-i-sil'in)

(Augmentin, Clavulin)

**Classification:** antibiotic, aminopenicillin

## Available Preparations:
- 125 mg amoxicillin with 31.25 mg clavulanic acid /5ml, 250 mg amoxicillin with 62.5 mg clavulanic acid /5ml suspension
- 125 mg amoxicillin with 31.25 mg clavulanic acid, 250 mg amoxicillin with 62.5 mg clavulanic acid chewable tablets
- 250 or 500 mg amoxicillin with 125 mg clavulanic acid tablets

**Action and Use:** Bactericidal action inhibits cell-wall synthesis in bacteria, broader spectrum of activities than penicillin G.Clavulanic acid is β-lactamases inhibitor that causes synergistic effect expanding spectrum of activity of amoxicillin. Effective on some gm+ and gm− organisms, such as *Staphylococcus aureus*, *S. epidermis*, β-hemolytic streptococci, *Hemophilus influenzae, E. coli, Proteus mirabilis, Neisseria gonorrhoeae, N. meningitidis, Branhamella catarrhalis, Klebsiella*, meningococci, enterococci, *Salmonella*, and others. Used to treat infections of the ear, upper respiratory tract, GU system, skin, and soft tissue.

## Routes and Dosage:
*PO:*
- under 40 kg: 20 to 40 mg/kg/day in equally divided doses every 8 hours
- over 40 kg: 250 to 500 mg every 8 hours

Dosage adjustment necessary for renal impairment

**Absorption and Fate:** Well absorbed from GI tract, 17 to 30% bound to plasma proteins. Peak level, 1 to 2 hours. Half-life, about 1.3 hours. 28 to 50% metabolized by liver; about 50% amoxicillin excreted unchanged in urine and 25 to 45% clavulanate excreted in urine.

**Contraindications and Precautions:** Same as amoxicillin.

## Side Effects:
*CNS:* dizziness, headache. *GI:* diarrhea (more than amoxicillin), nausea and vomiting (40% with clavulanate doses of 250 mg), epigastric pain, stomatitis, glossitis, black tongue, **pseudomembranous colitis** (rare). *Hepatic:* moderate rise SGOT and SGPT. *GU:* superinfections primarily yeast, **interstitial nephritis**. *Skin:* erythematous, maculopapular, mildly pruritus rash (starts 3 to 14 days after therapy initiated, begins on trunk, spreads to entire body even soles, palms, and oral mucosa, most intense at pressure areas elbows and knees). *Hemic:* eosinophilia, **anemia, thrombocytopenia, thrombocytopenic purpura, leukopenia, agranulocytosis**. *Other:* hypersensitivity: urticarial rash, drug fever, **anaphylaxis** (rare).

## Nursing Implications:
*Assess:* Same as for amoxicillin.
*Administer: PO:* Give without regard to meals. If nausea occurs give with food to minimize GI distress. Suspension, refrigerate, and shake well. Capsules may be taken apart, tablets crushed; contents can be mixed with small amount of food or fluid. Both 250- and 500-mg tablets contain 125 mg clavulanic acid per tablet; thus do not use two 250-mg tablets in place of 500 mg, it doubles clavulanic dosage.
*Monitor:* Same as for amoxicillin.
*Patient Teaching:* Same as for amoxicillin.

**Drug Interactions:** Erythromycin, tetracycline, chloromycetin, and antacids decrease the effects of amoxicillin. Questionable interaction between disulfiram and this drug.

**Laboratory Test Interferences:** False-positive urine glucose with Clinitest and Benedict's test. May cause false-positive direct Coomb's, which will interfere with cross-matching determinations.

**Storage Requirements:** Store at 15 to 30°C (59 to 86°F). Reconstituted suspensions stable; refrigerated for 14 days, room temperature for 7 days. Label with time and date at time of reconstitution.

# ☐ AMPHOTERICIN B

(am-foe-ter'i-sin)

(Fungizone)

**Combination Products:** Amphotericin B with tetracycline hydrochloride (Mysteclin-F)

## Classification: antifungal

## Available Preparations:
- 50 mg for parenteral administration
- 3% lotion, cream, and ointment for topical administration

**Action and Use:** Interferes with functions of the membranes of fungal cells and increases their permeability allowing leakage of intracellular components and potassium. Active against all kinds of systemic mycoses and parenteral form is used for fungal infections that are progressive and potentially fatal.

## Routes and Dosage:
*IV:* Dosage highly individualized.
- Test Dose: 0.05 to 0.1 mg/kg, infused over 20 to 30 minutes
- Maintenance: 0.25 to 0.5 mg/kg/day over 2 to 6 hours
- Increment Increases: 0.25–0.5 mg/kg/day increasing every 1 to 2 days as tolerated.
- Maximum Daily Dosages: infants: 1 mg/kg/day
- Children and adults: 1.5 mg/kg/day

*Intrathecal (IT):* Intitial dose 0.025 mg then 0.1 to 0.5 mg every 48 to 72 hours

*Topical:* apply sparingly to affected area 2 to 4 times per day

**Absorption and Fate:** IV peak level about 1 hour. Distribution appears to be multicompartmental. Poor penetration CSF, only achieved in significant levels by IT administration. 90 to 95% bound to serum proteins and metabolic fate unknown. Half-life, 24 to 48 hours. Slowly excreted in urine 40% over a 7-day period; may be detected for 7 weeks after drug stopped.

**Contraindications and Precautions:** Pregnancy category B. Safe use during lactation not established. Contraindicated if hypersensitivity to drug unless this drug is only drug that will treat infection. Use caution with renal impairment.

## Side Effects:
*CNS:* headache (IT): peripheral nerve pain, paresthesia, vision changes, arachnoiditis. *GI:* aanorexia, weight loss, dyspepsia, epigastric pain, nausea, vomiting. *GU:* (80%) hypokalemia, hyposthenuria, azotemia, **renal tubular acidosis, nephrocalcinosis,** (large doses) **permanent renal impairment, anuria, oliguria.** *Skin:* (lotion) pruritus, exacerbation of preexisting candidal le-

sions; (cream) drying effect, topical causing erythema, burning contact dermatitis. **Hemic:** thrombocytopenia, leukopenia, agranulocytosis, eosinophilia, reversible normocytic, normochromic anemia. **Musculoskeletal:** muscle weakness, muscle and joint pain. **Other:** febrile reaction to IV, 1 to 2 hours after start infusion causing fever, chills; local: pain at infusions site, phlebitis, **thrombophlebitis**.

## Nursing Implications:

**Assess:** Positively identify organism by culture or histological tests before starting drug. Obtain baseline BUN, serum creatinine, liver function tests, hematological tests, and weight.

**Administer: IV:** Preparation of solution must be done under strict aseptic technique; no preservatives in antibiotic or in solutions for preparation. All vial entries should be made with sterile 20-gauge needle. Initially dilute 50 mg with 10 ml **sterile water for injection** without preservatives. Other solutions may cause precipitate. Shake until solution clears and do not use if it has precipitate or foreign matter. Further dilute solution with **5% dextrose only** to minimum of 0.1 mg/ml. Solution must have pH above 4.2 or coagulation can occur. Sterile buffer may be added using strict aseptic technique. An in-line membrane filter may be used with mean pore diameter larger than 1 μm. Test dose should be given to avoid an anaphylactic reaction. To reduce vein irritation, use scalp vein in distal veins, change IV sites frequently and by adding small amounts of heparin to infusion fluid (check with physician). Do not mix with other drugs. Infuse slowly over 2 to 12 hours, 6 hours usually well tolerated. Rapid infusion can cause cardiovascular collapse. Manufacturer recommends that infusion be protected from light while administering but exposure of 8 hours does not appear to effect potency appreciably; consult your pharmacist. **Topical:** Physician should specify how area should be cleaned before drug application. Use cream or lotion for intertriginous areas. Apply sparingly, rubbing into area. Do not use occlusive dressings.

**Monitor: IV:** Obtain vital signs including temperature every 30 minutes during infusion, then every hour if afebrile. Febrile reactions may occur 1 or 2 hours into therapy (shaking chills, fever, headache, nausea) and usually subside in 4 hours after drug infusion ends. Antihistamines, antipyretics, and antiemetics may aid in symptom relief. Monitor for cardiovascular collapse. Assess for renal function: I & O, daily weights, potassium, magnesium, BUN, serum creatinine, bilirubin, alkaline phosphatase, and SGOT daily until routine dosage of drug is established, then once or twice a week. Obtain CBC weekly. Discontinue drug if BUN exceeds 40 mg%, serum creatinine exceeds 3 mg%, or liver studies are abnormal. Report signs of hypokalemia. Therapy may be 6 to 12 weeks in duration or longer.

**Patient Teaching:** Teach proper application of topical forms of medication. If no improvement in 2 weeks, contact physician. Total therapy may take several months. May stain clothing; remove cream or lotions stains by hand washing with soap and warm water, and ointment with standard cleaning fluid. Do not apply other OTC over infected areas without consulting physician.

**Drug Interactions:** Drugs with nephrotoxic side effects, such as aminoglycosides, capreomycin, colistin, cisplatin, methoxyflurane, mechlorethamine, polymyxin B, and vancomycin, may increase this drug's nephrotoxicity. Corticosteroids, cardiac glycosides, or skeletal muscle relaxants may enhance potassium loss with this drug. If corticosteroids used to reduce adverse reactions, monitor cardiac function and electrolytes. Use with caution in antineoplastic drugs.

**Storage Requirements:** Store topical preparations at 15 to 30°C (59 to 86°F), protect from freezing. Store powder at 2 to 8°C; protect for light and moisture. Reconstituted vials stable for 1 week if refrigerated.

---

# ☐ AMPICILLIN

(Amcap, Amcill, Ampicin, Ampilean, Nova Ampicillin, Omnipen, Penbritin, Pfizerpen, Polycillin, Principen, SK-Ampicillin, Supen, Totacillin).

# ☐ AMPICILLIN SODIUM                                            (am-pi-sill'in)

(Omnipen-N, Polycillin-N, SK-Ampicillin-N, Totacillin-N)

**Classification:** antibiotic, aminopenicillin

## Available Preparations:
- 100 mg/ml pediatric drops
- 125, 250, 500 mg/5ml suspension
- 250, 500-mg tablets and capsules
- 125, 250, 500-mg, 1, 2-g for parenteral administration

**Action and Use:** Bactericidal action inhibits cell-wall synthesis in bacteria, broader spectrum of activities than penicillin G. Effective against some gram-positive and gram-negative organisms, such as *Haemophilus influenzae*, *Escherichia coli*, *Proteus*, *Meningococci*, *Salmonella*, and *Shigella*. Treats infections of ear, meninges, upper respiratory tract, GU tract, skin and soft tissue. Injectable ampicillin sodium contain 2.9 mEq sodium per gram of drug.

## Routes and Dosage:
*PO:* 50 to 100 mg/kg/day in equally divided doses every 6 hours. (Maximum dosage 2 to 4 g/day)
*IM, IV:*
- birth to 7 days: 50 to 100 mg/kg/day in equally divided doses every 12 hours
- 7 days to 1 month: 100 to 200 mg/kg/day in equally divided doses every 8 hours
- over 1 month: Mild to Moderate Infections: 50 to 100 mg/kg/day in equally divided doses every 6 hours. (Maximum dosage 2 to 4 g/day);

Severe Infections: 200 to 400 mg/kg/day in equally divided doses every 4 to 6 hours. (Maximum dosage 12 g/day)

**Absorption and Fate:** Distributed to body tissues, penetrating brain and CSF only when meninges are inflamed. 20 to 25% bound to plasma proteins. Peak levels: PO, 1 hour; IM, 1 hour; 5 minutes after IV bolus. Half-life about 60 minutes. Therapeutic level, 0.01 to 1μg/ml. Excreted unchanged in urine and bile. Severe renal dysfunction prolongs plasma levels.

**Contraindications and Precautions:** Pregnancy category B. Use with caution during lactation. Contraindicated if previous reactions to drug, penicillins, or cephalosporins. Use with caution in renal disease, liver or GI disease, hyperuricemias, lymphatic leukemia, prematures, infectious mononucleosis, asthma, allergies, or family history of allergies.

**Side Effects:**
*CNS:* **seizures** (usually seen in excess of 400 mg/kg/day). *GI:* diarrhea 20% oral, 3% IV, dose-related (under 36 months most prone), nausea, vomiting, epigastric pain, **pseudomembranous colitis** (rare), stomatitis, glossitis, black tongue *Hepatic:* moderate rise in SGOT. *GU:* superinfections primarily yeast, **interstitial nephritis**. *Skin:* erythematous, maculopapular, mildly pruritus rash (onset 3 to 14 days after first dosage; begins on trunk, spreads entire body even soles, palms, oral mucosa; most intense at pressure areas elbows and knees); (5 to 10%) usually rash nonimmunologic occurs; 90% lymphatic leukemia, 65 to 100% infectious mononucleosis. *Hemic:* eosinophilia, **anemia, thrombocytopenia, thrombocytopenic purpura, leukopenia, agranulocytosis**. *Other:* hypersensitivity: urticarial rash, drug fever, **anaphylaxis** (rare); local: IM, pain; IV, phlebitis (rare)

**Nursing Implications:**
*Assess:* Assess previous allergy to drug, penicillins, cephalosporins, other drugs, asthma, or family history of allergies. Obtain cultures and sensitivity before treatment, but can start treatment before results.
*Administer: PO:* Stable in gastric acids, drug absorption hampered by food. Give 1 hour before or 2 hours after meals. Suspension, refrigerate and shake well. *IM, IV:* Reconstituted solutions should be used in 1 hour of preparation. IM: Reconstitute according to package inserts with either sterile or bacteriostatic water for injection. Do not use bacteriostatic preparations containing benzyl alcohol with neonates. IV: Reconstitute with sterile water or bacteriostatic water for injection. Can give IV push; dilute solution to minimum of 1 g/10 ml infuse slowly. **Do not exceed 100 mg/minute, if rate exceeded may cause seizures.** Preferred route is intermittent infusion infused over 20 to 30 minutes, do not exceed 1 hour. Compatible with $D_5W/0.5\%$ NS, $D_5W/0.2\%$ NS, NS, LR. Do not premix with other drugs. Stability decreases in dextrose solutions.
*Monitor:* Observe IV site for vein irritation and extravasation. Monitor for hypersensitivity (especially in first 20 minutes of first dosage), rash (onset and characteristics), and side effects. Watch for symptoms of superinfection; diar-

rhea (may indicate pseudomembranous colitis, which can occur while on drug or 4 days to 6 weeks after drug is discontinued). Drug's sodium content may effect patient's sodium restrictions. Assess renal, hepatic, and hematological functions with prolonged or high-dose therapy or with premature and neonates. Maintain fluid intake for age group. Therapy course continued for 48 to 72 hours after negative bacterial cultures or symptoms subside. If given for β-**hemolytic streptococcal** infection, 10-day course needed to prevent risk of acute rheumatic fever or glomerulonephritis.

***Patient Teaching:*** Take as prescribed for full course of therapy. Observe for side effects especially diarrhea or rash; report to physician. Store suspension in refrigerator out of reach of children.

**Drug Interactions:** Erythromycin, tetracycline, and chloramphenicol decrease effects of ampicillin. Allopurinol may enhance development of ampicillin rash. It may interfere with effectiveness of oral contraceptives.

**Laboratory Test Interferences:** False-positive urine glucose with Clinitest and Benedict's test. False-positive direct Coomb's interferes with cross-matching procedures.

**Storage Requirements:** Store at 15 to 30°C (59 to 86°F). Reconstituted PO suspensions stable; refrigerated for 14 days, room temperature for 7 days. Label time and date at time of reconstitution. Reconstituted parenteral form stable for 1 hour at room temperature.

---

## □ ANTIHEMOPHILIC FACTOR

(an-tie-hee-moe-feel'ik)

(AHF, AHG, Factor VIII, HT Profilate, Humate-P, Koate-HS, Koate-HT, Monoclate, Profilate)

**Classification:** hemostatic

**Available Preparations:** vials for parenteral use

**Action and Use:** A concentrated preparation of clotting Factor VIII, which is prepared from multiple blood and plasma donors. Factor VIII is essential to convert prothrombin to thrombin in the body so normal clotting can occur. Used in treatment of hemophilia A (classic hemophilia) in which a genetic disease prevents normal Factor VIII production.

**Routes and Dosages:**
*IV:*
- Prophylaxis: under 50 kg: 250 units qd in AM; over 50 kg: 500 units qd in AM
- Joint Hemorrhage: 10 units/kg q8–12h

■ Muscle Hemorrhage: 8 to 10 units/kg q24 h for 2 to 3 days
■ Bleeding: 15 to 25 units/kg; then 8 to 15 units q 8–12h for 3 to 4 days
Dosages above are approximate and are individualized to specific patients based on results of blood studies. A plasma Factor VIII level of 10 to 80% of normal is needed based on items such as whether there is active bleeding or the patient is undergoing surgery.

**Absorption and Fate:** Rapid action and elimination with half-life of 4 to 24 hours, average 12 hours.

**Contraindications and Precautions:** Pregnancy category C. Does not usually cross the placenta. Not effective in von Willebrand disease. Monoclate brand is contraindicated in those with allergy to mouse. Used cautiously when given repeatedly to persons with blood types A, B, AB due to increasing potential for hemolysis.

**Side Effects:**
*CNS:* headache, flushing, paresthesia, lethargy, loss of consciousness, chills. *CV:* tachycardia, hypotension. *GI:* nausea, vomiting. *Skin:* urticaria, stinging at IV site. *Other:* jaundice, disturbed vision, allergic reactions, fever.

**Nursing Implications:**
*Assess:* Take baseline vital signs. Laboratory tests include Factor VIII activity, Factor VIII inhibitor, PTT, PT, hematocrit, direct Coomb's. Platelet count, bleeding time, and prothrombin time will be normal in persons with hemophilia A.
*Administer:* Warm diluent to room temperature of 20 to 30°C (68 to 86°F). Concentrate is reconstituted with provided diluent and rotated gently to dissolve. Keep at room temperature and administer within 3 hours. Flow rates are generally 2 ml/minute for 34 or more units/ml solution and 10 to 20 ml/3 minutes for less than 34 units/ml solution. Do not confuse concentrate with cryoprecipitate that is kept frozen and gently warmed in warm water, gently rotated, and administered by IV filter. Although concentrate is labeled with specific number of units contained, cryoprecipitate is not. Concentrate is prepared from multiple donors, therefore, risk of infection with hepatitis B or HIV is greater than with cryoprecipitate; cryoprecipitate is the preparation of choice for children under 4 years or those with newly diagnosed disease. Cryoprecipitate also contains von Willebrand factor and fibrinogen. Fresh-frozen plasma may also be used for treatment but is not used for routine or frequent administration as the resultant fluid load may be too high.
*Monitor:* Monitor vital signs, remaining alert for signs of allergy. Discontinue infusion if signs of anaphylaxis such as chest tightness, sweating, fever, urticaria, erythema occur. Routine blood coagulation studies and direct Coomb's test are performed. Patients on repeated infusions are at highest risk of hepatitis B and HIV infection and should be monitored routinely in health-care center to rule out infection.
*Patient Teaching:* Care of the hemophiliac must be taught to the parents and the child when old enough. Avoidance of contact sports and maintenance of a

safe environment are some preventive measures. Use of ice, elevation, and pressure for injuries is important. Families are taught to begin intravenous therapy and administer the Factor. Correct technique and preparation must be taught and monitored periodically. Many children can perform parts of therapy at about 8 years of age. Perform good oral care with soft bristle brush. Watch for signs of bleeding such as dark urine, dark stools, change in behavior or consciousness. Wear medical alert identification and inform all care providers, such as dentists, of the diagnosis. Teachers need to be prepared for emergency treatment of bleeding. New heat-treated preparations have lowered the risk of acquiring viral infections such as hepatitis B or HIV; a risk of transmission still does exist, however.

**Storage Requirements:** Store concentrate powder at 2 to 8°C (35 to 46° F). Some preparations may be stored at room temperature; read labels. Avoid freezing diluent.

---

# ☐ ASPARAGINASE  (a-spar'a-gi-nase)

(Elspar, L-Asparaginase)

**Classification:** antineoplastic, enzyme

**Available Preparations:** 10,000 IU vial for parenteral use

**Action and Use:** This enzyme is derived from *Escherichia coli*, catalyzes the breakdown of asparagine, an essential amino acid into aspartic acid and ammonia. This interferes with protein and DNA synthesis and it is active in $G_1$ phase of cell division. Used to induce remission in children with acute lymphocytic leukemia.

**Routes and Dosages:** IM, IV Highly individualized
*IM:* Acute lymphocytic leukemia: 6000 IU/m² on days 4, 7, 10, 13, 16, 19, 22, 25, and 28 of induction period or given 3 times weekly
*IV:* Sole therapy: 200 IU/kg IV for 28 days. In combination with prednisone and vincristine: 1000 IU/kg/day IV for 10 days starting day 22 of treatment period.

**Absorption and Fate:** Not absorbed from GI tract. Rapid absorption from IV administration with 80% of drug remaining in intravascular spaces. IM injections are approximately 1/2 equivalency of IV dose levels. Metabolic pathways unknown. Small amounts of the drug are excreted in the urine. Peak level is 14.5 IU/ml with 1000 IU/kg dose daily and 50 IU/ml with 5000 IU/kg dose daily in children; occurs 14 to 24 hours after IM injection; duration 23 to 33 days. Half-life, 8 to 30 hours after IV and 39 to 49 hours after IM; not related to dose, age, body surface, hepatic or renal function.

**Contraindications and Precautions:** Pregnancy category C. Not to be used in pregnancy unless benefits clearly outweigh risks. Unknown if drug is present in breast milk, therefore, use during lactation is discouraged. Contraindicated in those hypersensitive to the drug, patients with renal failure, pancreatitis, chicken pox, or herpes zoster infection. Cautious use with hepatic disease, diabetes, and infections.

## Side Effects:

*CNS:* EEG changes, depression, headache, irritability, somnolence, dizziness, hallucinations, seizures. *GI:* nausea, vomiting, anorexia, abdominal pain secondary to pancreatitis, mucosal ulcers. *Hepatic:* liver function impairment manifested by increased SGOT, SGPT, alkaline phosphatae, bilirubin, gamma globulin, and ammonia and decreased cholesterol, fibrinogen, albumin, and calcium. *GU:* azotemia, renal insufficiency, transient proteinuria, hyperuricemia. *Hemic:* prolonged thrombin, prothrombin, and partial prothrombin times; decrease in clotting Factors V, VII, VIII, and IX; decrease in platelets and plasminogen; lowered hematocrit and hemoglobin, and leukopenia; bone marrow effects (rare). *Endocrine:* hyperglycemia, transient diabetes mellitus. *Other:* impaired pancreatic function, hyperglycemia, diabetic ketoacidosis; allergic response manifested by rash, urticaria, arthralgia, and anaphylaxis with hypotension, facial edema, dyspnea, diaphoresis, asthma, altered level of consciousness, chills, fever. This allergic response may be manifested in 20 to 35% of patients and can be life threatening.

## Nursing Implications:

*Assess:* Obtain history of prior courses of asparaginase as this may increase the risk of hypersensitivity. Sensitivity testing should be performed before giving drug the first time and if last dose was a week or longer ago. About 2 IU of the drug are injected intradermally and patient is observed for 1 hour. Allergy is determined by presence of a wheal or erythema. Allergy may be treated with desensitization or the drug may be withheld. Even patients with negative skin tests may manifest allergy to the treatment dose.

*Administer:* This drug has potentially severe toxic effects and should be given only under the supervision of a physician with training and experience in cancer chemotherapy. The drug's potential for toxic effects in health-care personnel as well as patients necessitates careful handling during preparation and administration. Generally, during preparation of chemotherapy, latex gloves, a mask, and a solid front gown are worn, and a laminar flow hood is used. Gloves and gown may also be recommended for administration. Contaminated equipment, such as needles, syringes, vials, and unused medications, is disposed of properly. Clean up of spills is carefully performed and accidental contact by patient or personnel receives prompt flushing and cleaning. *IM:* Reconstitute vial with 2 ml saline and roll gently to dissolve. Limit injections to 2 ml per site. Rotate sites; given deep IM into large muscle mass (avoid deltoid). *IV:* Reconstitute vial with 5 ml saline or sterile water and roll gently to dissolve. Reconstituted solution stable 8 hours if refrigerated. Administer into tubing of freely running IV of saline or 5% dextrose over at least 30 minutes.

Have emergency drugs (such as adrenalin, benadryl and solucortef) and equipment available in case of anaphylaxis.

***Monitor:*** Observe 30 to 60 minutes after IM injection for signs of anaphylaxis; observe after each IM injection. SGOT, SGPT, and other liver function tests are done twice weekly. Serum coagulation factors, hematocrit, hemoglobin, serum amylase, blood glucose, calcium, uric acid levels, and CBC are regularly monitored. When giving IM injections to patient, monitor platelet counts carefully as platelet transfusion may be needed before injections. WBC count is most important in first few days of therapy when dangerous leukopenia may occur. Bone marrow aspiration may be done. Monitor food intake, I & O, weight. Observe for signs of GI ulcers, nausea, and vomiting. Weigh daily. Observe for changes in vital signs, chills, and other signs of infection. Watch for signs of bleeding and bruising.

***Patient Teaching:*** Avoid contact with persons with infections such as colds, influenza, and chicken pox. Report signs of infection such as fever, chills, sore throat, cough, and malaise. Increase fluid intake. Report weight changes and edema. Drug should only be given in hospital under monitored conditions.

**Drug Interactions:** Increased hyperglycemic effect if given with corticosteroids or vincristine. The hyperglycemic and neuropathic effects are less if asparaginase is given after, rather than before, or with these drugs. Blocks antineoplastic effect of methotrexate if given together. Can enhance hepatotoxicity of other hepatotoxic drugs. Suppresses immune response to immunizations. Live virus vaccines or oral polio vaccine must not be given to those in close contact with the patient on this drug due to the chance of infection with a virus; these vaccines are delayed at least 3 months after chemotherapy when the patient is in remission.

**Laboratory Test Interferences:** Reduces serum thyroxine-binding globulin, a thyroid function test. Levels are normal 4 weeks after last asparaginase dose. May increase SGOT, SGPT, alkaline phosphatase, bilirubin, gamma globulin, ammonia. May decrease serum cholesterol, fibrinogen, albumin, calcium.

**Storage Requirements:** Store vials at less than 8°C (46°F). Reconstituted solution should be stored at 2 to 8°C (35 to 46°F) and discarded after 8 hours. Do not use cloudy solutions.

---

## ☐ ASPIRIN
(as′pir-in)

(A.S.A., Alka-Seltzer, Ascriptin, Aspergum, Bufferin, Cama Inlay-Tab, Easprin, Ecotrin, Magnaprin, Maprin, Salagen, Speedrin)

**Combination Products:** Anacin, Darvon Compound, Empirin with Codeine, Talwin Compound, Vanquish, and others

**Classification:** nonsteroidal antiinflammatory, analgesic, antipyretic, salicylate

## Available Preparations:
- 324, 325, 500, 650-mg tablets
- 325, 500-mg film-coated tablets
- 324, 325, 500, 650-mg enteric-coated tablets
- 650, 800-mg extended-release tablets
- 65, 81-mg chewable tablets
- 227-mg chewing gum
- 60, 65, 120, 125, 130, 195, 200, 300, 325, 600, 650-mg, and 1.2 g rectal suppositories

Available in buffered preparations:
- 324, 325, 486, 500, 650-mg tablets
- 500-mg film-coated tablets
- 324, 500-mg tablets for oral solution

Also available in numerous combination products, i.e., with caffeine, codeine, propoxyphene, butalbital, acetaminophen, meprobamate, oxycodone, and pseudoephedrine.

**Action and Use:** Likely inhibits prostaglandin synthesis and release in the CNS and throughout body. This creates an analgesic effect as prostaglandins cause sensitization of pain receptors in the peripheral system; additional CNS effect may occur. Drug produces vasodilation by its action on the hypothalmus, thereby causing antipyresis. Its antiinflammatory effect may be due to interference with prostaglandin activity. The drug also decreases platelet aggregation and increases bleeding time. Used in treatment of mild to moderate pain, fever, and to decrease inflammation. Common uses in children include treatment of pain, juvenile rheumatoid arthritis, and rheumatic fever

## Routes and Dosages:
*PO, PR:* Analgesia and Antipyresis:
- 2 to 11 years: 1.5 g/m$^2$/day or 65 mg/kg/day in 4 to 6 doses; rectal dose not to exceed 2.5 g/m$^2$/day
- over 11 years: 325 to 650 mg q4h PRN; not to exceed 4 g/day

Alternatively:
- 2 to 3 years: 160 mg q4h PRN
- 4 to 5 years: 240 mgq4h PRN
- 6 to 8 years: 325 mg q4h PRN
- 9 to 10 years: 400 mg q4h PRN
- 11 years: 480 mg q4h PRN

Chewing Gum:
- 3 to 5 years: 227 mg PRN; not to exceed 681 mg/day
- 6 to 11 years: 227 to 454 mg PRN; not to exceed 1.82 g/day
- over 11 years: 454 mg PRN; not to exceed 3.63 g/day

Tablets for Oral Solution:
- 3 to 5 years: 162 mg q4–6h PRN; not to exceed 648 mg/day

- 6 to 11 years: 324 mg q4–6h PRN; not to exceed 1.3 g/day
- over 11 years: 648 mg q4–6h; not to exceed 2.59 g/day

Juvenile Rheumatoid Arthritis:

- 25 kg or less child: 60 to 90 mg/kg/day in divided doses
- over 25 kg child: 2.4 to 3.6 g/day in divided doses
- alternatively, an initial dose of 1.5 g/m²/day in divided doses, increased by 10 mg/kg/day each week PRN; not to exceed 100 mg/kg/day if child is over 25 kg or not to exceed 3 g/m²/day; maintenance dose generally 80 to 100 mg/kg/day

Rheumatic Fever:

- 90 to 130 mg/kg/day divided into 4 to 6 doses initially; decreased gradually

**Absorption and Fate:** Well absorbed from GI tract. Food may decrease speed but not likely amount of drug absorbed. Widely distributed into body tissues and poorly bound (33%) to plasma proteins. Metabolized in the GI tract and liver and excreted in the urine. Onset of action within 5 to 30 minutes with peak effect by 2 hours. Half-life, 15 to 20 minutes in serum with a much longer half-life (4 to 12 hours) in breast milk. Therapeutic level for analgesia and antipyresis is 25 to 50 μg/ml and for antiinflammatory effect 150 to 300 μg/ml.

**Contraindications and Precautions:** Pregnancy category D. Because the drug crosses the placenta and has been known to cause defects in laboratory animals, its use in first trimester is discouraged. If used in high or chronic doses in the last trimester, prostaglandin and platelet effects may result in prolonged pregnancy, increased maternal hemorrhage, increased fetal or newborn hemorrhage, and premature closure of ductus arteriosus; its use in the last trimester is thus discouraged. The drug is present in breast milk with a prolonged half-life, therefore, chronic or high dosage in the lactating mother is discouraged. Doses for children under 2 years must be established by clinicians. Contraindicated in treatment of chicken pox and influenza, in those with prior allergy to aspirin or salicylates or other nonsteroidal antiinflammatories, bleeding disorders, thrombocytopenia, for those on anticoagulants, in congestive heart failure. Aspirin chewing gum or gargle not to be used within 1 week of tonsillectomy. Aspirin products generally discontinued 1 week before surgery. Product with sulfite contraindicated in those with allergy to that substance. Cautious use in children with fever or dehydration, anemia, GI dysfunction, renal dysfunction, asthmatics, thyrotoxicosis; cautious use of tablets for oral solution in those for whom increased sodium intake could be problematic.

**Side Effects:**
*CNS:* dizziness, headache, tiredness, behavior changes. *GI:* nausea, vomiting, GI pain, black stools, diarrhea, GI bleeding, rectal irritation with PR form. *Respiratory:* tachypnea, labored or deep breathing, dyspnea as signs of overdose or allergic reaction. *Hepatic:* hepatotoxicity with chronic high doses.

*Hemic:* prolonged bleeding time, decreased prothrombin time; iron deficiency anemia in G-G-PD deficient patient. *Sensory:* tinnitus and hearing loss with chronic high dose; vision changes. *Other:* sweating, thirst.

## Nursing Implications:

*Assess:* Inquire about history of asthma or previous allergy to salicylates. Liver function tests are often performed before chronic high-dose therapy. Because child with fever and dehydration is more prone to toxic effects, physical assessment of the ill child should identify these conditions. The drug should not be given during influenza or chicken pox in children or adolescents due to an increased incidence of Reye syndrome in those treated with aspirin for those illnesses, therefore, those illnesses should be ruled out before therapy.

*Administer:* Check proper administration of product being used. Tablets for oral solution can be used for 10 hours after being dissolved in water if kept at room temperature or for 90 hours if at 5°C (40°F).

*Monitor:* If used for pain or fever, assessments of pain and fever must be made and recorded frequently in the 30 to 120 minutes after administration. For long-term therapy, hematocrit, liver function studies, renal function tests, and serum salicylate are routinely performed. Because hypoglycemia may occur in children on chronic dose, serum glucose may be monitored.

*Patient Teaching:* Do not give to children under 2 years unless directed by physician. Do not give if chicken pox or influenza are possible causes of illness. Regular tablets may be given with food to decrease GI upset. Chewable tablets may be chewed, dissolved, or crushed. Film-coated tablets must be swallowed whole. Extended-release tablets may be broken but not crushed. Tablets for oral solution are dissolved in 3 oz of water just before administration. Do not repeat doses any more often than 5 total doses per day. If fever or pain is not improved within 3 days or if relief is not obtained, contact health-care provider. Be aware of aspirin present in many OTC products. This is a common drug for accidental overdose. Call poison control center immediately for overdose. If chronic high dose is used, be alert for and report child with behavior changes, tiredness, hearing changes, fast or deep breathing. Return for scheduled health visits.

**Drug Interactions:** Increased renal side effects if used chronically with acetaminophen. Decreased salicylate level with adrenocorticosteroids. Increased risk of GI side effects with other GI toxic drugs such as other nonsteroidal antiinflammatories and alcohol. Increased ototoxicity with other ototoxic drugs; use with ototoxic drugs such as aminoglycosides, furosemide, and others generally contraindicated. Increased risk of bleeding with anticoagulants. Salicylate can increase serum levels and toxicity of methotrexate, verapamil, and nifedipine. Lowered blood glucose with drugs having hypoglycemic effect. Urinary acidifiers and alkalinizers will decrease and increase salicylate excretion, respectively. May displace valproic acid from protein binding sites, therefore, generally not given with this drug.

**Food Interactions:** Chronic aspirin use may decrease vitamin C, folate, and vitamin K levels and promote iron deficiency anemia.

**Laboratory Test Interferences:** Prolongs bleeding time for 4 to 7 days. Prolongs prothrombin time. Abnormal SGOT, SGPT, alkaline phosphatase. Decreased serum cholesterol, potassium, thyroxine, triiodothyronine, protein bound iodine. Decreased urine PSP. Alters serum uric acid and urine VMA. Increased $T_3$ resin uptake. False-negative urine glucose. Interferes with Gerhardt test for acetoacetic acid. Decreases urine phenosulfonphthalein excretion. False decreased urine 17-hydroxycorticosteroids by some methods. Interferes with plasma theophylline test.

**Storage Requirements:** Store tablets at 15 to 30°C (59 to 86°F) in tightly closed container. Store suppositories at 8 to 15°C (46 to 59°F).

---

# ☐ ATROPINE

(Atropair, Atropine-Care, Atropisol, Dey Dose, Isopto Atropine, I-Tropine, Ocu-Tropine)

**Combination Products:** Antrocol, Mydraped

**Classification:** anticholinergic, antimuscarinic, antispasmodic, mydriatic

**Action and Use:** Blocks vagal impulses to the myocardium and stimulates the cardioinhibitory center in the medulla, thereby increasing heart rate and cardiac output and shortening the PR interval. Vasodilates small blood vessels. Diminishes smooth muscle contractions of GI and GU tracts. Decreases salivation and secretions of respiratory and GI tracts. Lessens response of ciliary and iris sphincter muscles in the eye, causing mydriasis. Used to restore normal heart contraction during cardiac arrest or in surgery. Used as a preoperative medication to decrease secretions in bronchioles and mouth. Used for treatment of uveitis and refractions of eyes in children up to 6 years; not used in older children for refractions due to long duration of action. Used occasionally as a bronchodilator in those experiencing bronchospasm such as asthmatics.

## Available Preparations:
- 0.4, 0.6-mg tablets
- tablets and capsules and elixir with phenobarbital
  0.05, 0.1, 0.3, 0.4, 0.5, 0.8, 1-mg/ml vials for parenteral use
- injection vials with meperidine, morphine, or neostigmine
- 0.2, 0.5% inhalation solution for nebulization
- 0.5%, 1% ophthalmic ointment
- 0.5%, 1%, 2%, 3% ophthalmic solution
- 1% ophthalmic suspension with prednisolone 0.25%

**Absorption and Fate:** Well absorbed from upper intestine, or from parenteral or inhalation administration. Well distributed throughout body. Moderately protein bound. Metabolized in liver; drug and metabolites excreted mainly in urine. Effect on heart rate observed 2 to 4 minutes after IV administration; 30 minutes after IM; 60 minutes or more after PO. Duration is 4 to 6 hours. Onset of effect after inhalation is 15 minutes with peak levels in 1.5 to 4 hours. Inhibition of salivation begins 30 minutes after administration, peaks in 1 to 2 hours, and persists for 4 hours. Duration of ophthalmic action is up to 14 days.

## Routes and Dosages: PO, SC, IM, IV, Inhalation, Topical (eye)

***PO:*** Antimuscarinic: 0.01 mg/kg or 0.3 mg/m², not to exceed 0.4 mg every 4 to 6 hours

***SC:***
- Antimuscarinic: 0.01 mg/kg or 0.3 mg/m² q4–6h, not to exceed 0.4 mg; may repeat every 4 to 6 hours
- Preop: weight 3 kg or less: 0.1 mg; 7 to 9 kg: 0.2 mg; 12 to 16 kg: 0.3 mg; 20 to 27 kg: 0.4 mg; 32 kg: 0.5 mg; 41 kg: 0.6 mg

***IV:***
- Arrhythmia: 0.01 to 0.03 mg/kg
- Cardiac Arrest: 0.02 mg/kg with a minimum dose of 0.1 mg and maximum of 1 mg; repeat PRN q5min up to 1 mg for child and 2 mg for adolescent

***Inhalation:*** 0.05 mg/kg in saline 3 to 4 times/day or 15 to 25.8 kg:1 mg; 25.9 to 37.6 kg:1.5 mg; 37.7 to 63.2 kg:2.5 mg

***Ophthalmic:***
- Refraction: 1 to 2 drops solution (infant: 0.125%; 1 to 5 year: 0.25%; over 5 years with blue eyes: 0.25%; over 5 years with dark eyes: 0.5%) 2 times/day for 1 to 3 days or 0.3 cm of ointment (under 2 years with blue eyes: 0.5%; under 2 years with dark eyes: 1%; over 2 years: 1%) 3 times/day for 1 to 3 days
- Uveitis: 1 to 2 drops of 0.125 to 1% solution up to 3 times/day or 0.3 cm 1% ointment 3 times/day

## Contraindications and Precautions: Pregnancy category B. Can produce fetal tachycardia. Infants and young children are especially susceptible to toxic effects, therefore, the drug is used cautiously in those under 6 years. Contraindicated in those with hypersensitivity to products used in the solution (such as sulfite in atropine/meperidine combination drug). Contraindicated in closed-angle glaucoma, obstructive GI disease, tachycardia secondary to cardiac insufficiency or thyrotoxicosis, acute hemorrhage. Used cautiously in blonds and those with blue eyes as they are more susceptible to toxic effects, in Down syndrome children, those with brain damage or spastic paralysis, fever, hyperthyroidism, hepatic or renal dysfunction, hypertension, congestive heart failure, arrhythmia, coronary artery disease, ulcerative colitis, and obstructive uropathy.

## Side Effects:

***CNS:*** atropine psychosis, CNS stimulation, restlessness, combativeness, confusion, hallucination, weakness, dizziness, insomnia, headache, paradoxical excitement in children. ***CV:*** tachycardia, bradycardia with low doses or slow injection, palpitation. ***GI:*** loss of taste, nausea, vomiting, bloating, dry mouth, constipation, paralytic ileus. ***GU:*** urinary retention. ***Skin:*** hot, dry skin, rash, urticaria, dermatitis. ***Sensory:*** mydriasis, blurred vision, cyclopegia, photophobia, local irritation to eye with repeated topical application, increased ocular tension especially with closed-angle glaucoma

## Nursing Implications:

***Assess:*** Assess vital signs before giving

***Administer: PO:*** Give 30 minutes before meals and at bedtime. Use mouth washes, sips of water, oral care for complaints of thirst. ***IM:*** Used for preop medication. Compatible with many other preop medications, such as meperidine and morphine, for 15 minutes in same syringe. Have patient void before giving. ***IV:*** Form usually used in cardiac arrest; given slowly IV. Not compatible with sodium bicarbonate injection or epinephrine. ***Ophthalmic:*** ointment rather than solution is preferred in children to decrease chance of systemic effects (solution can roll down nasolacrimal duct and gets swallowed, thereby producing systemic effects). Apply ointment several hours before refraction to avoid inaccurate refractions.

***Monitor:*** Monitor vital signs frequently. Monitor I & O. Evaluate bowel sounds and elimination. Observe for abdominal distention. Monitor the person on ophthalmic dose for systemic effects.

***Patient Teaching:*** Use only as directed. Observe for and notify prescriber if side effects occur. Avoid antacids and antidiarrheals within 1 hour of dose. Take PO form 30 to 60 minutes before meals. Avoid strenuous exercise or hot weather. Get up slowly. Prepare for possibility of photophobia. Avoid driving and operating hazardous machinery. Inform physician if ophthalmic form causes eye pain, conjunctivitis, or other unusual symptoms.

## Drug Interactions:
May have increased effect when given with MAO inhibitors. Can increase the effect of nitrofurantoin. Increased intraocular pressure in other drugs with same effect. Delayed atropine excretion with urinary alkalizers such as antacids or sodium bicarbonate. Increased GI antimuscarinic effects with meclizine, methylphenidate, phenothiazines, and procainimide. Decreased absorption with antacids and antidiarrheals. Ventricular arrythmias possible with cyclopropane anesthesia. Decreased GI effect with guanethidine and reserpine. Increased constipation with narcotics.

## Laboratory Test Interferences:
Alters gastric acid secretion test; do not give atropine for 24 hours before test. Alters phenolsulfophthalein (PSP) excretion test results.

## Storage Requirements:
Keep in tightly covered, light-resistant container at room temperature at 15 to 30°C (59 to 86°F).

---

# □ AZLOCILLIN SODIUM                    (az-loe-sill'in)

(Azlin)

## Classification: penicillin, extended spectrum

**Available Preparations:** 2, 3, 4-g for parenteral administration

**Action and Use:** Semisynthetic derivative of ampicillin whose bactericidal action inhibits cell-wall synthesis in bacteria. Effective on some gm − and gm + organisms, but it is principally used to treat gm − aerobic bacilli, e.g., *Pseudomonas aeruginosa, Proteus mirabilis, Escherichia coli.* Treats infections of lower respiratory tract (especially cystic fibrosis), GU tract, skin, soft tissue, bone, joint, and bacterial septicemias. Sodium content 2.17 mEq sodium per gram.

**Routes and Dosage:**
*IV:* Manufacturer recommends this drug not be used in neonates, however, some clinicians recommend:
- premature neonates under 7 days: 50 mg/kg every 12 hours (IM,IV)
- term neonates under 7 days: 100 mg/kg every 12 hours (IM,IV)
- over 1 month: 75 mg/kg every 4 hours. (Maximum dosage 24 g/day)
Dosage alteration need in renal impairment

**Absorption and Fate:** Distributed: bone, bronchial secretions, wounds, vascularized tissues, CSF especially when meninges are inflamed. 20 to 46% bound to plasma proteins. Half-life, 55 to 70 minutes. Drug and metabolites excreted in urine with some excreted in bile.

**Contraindications and Precautions:** Pregnancy category B. Excreted in breast milk, use caution during lactation. Due to limited testing manufacturer does not recommend usage with neonates. Contraindicated if hypersensitivity to drug, penicillins, or cephalosporins. Use with caution if sensitivity to multiple allergens or other drugs.

**Side Effects:**
*CNS:* dizziness, giddiness, neuromuscular hyperirritability, **seizures**. *GI:* alteration in taste, nausea, vomiting, flatulence, loose stools, diarrhea, stomatitis, abnormal smell. *Hepatic:* elevation of SGOT, SGPT, LDH, alkaline phosphatase, serum bilirubin. *GU:* increased serum creatinine, BUN, hypernatremia, hypokalemia, decreased serum uric acid *Skin:* rash, urticaria, pruritus, arthralgia. *Hemic:* eosinophilia, **thrombocytopenia**, leukopenia, neutropenia, **decreased hemoglobin and hematocrit, increased prothrombin time and bleeding time.** *Other:* Hypersensitivity: drug fever, **anaphylaxis**; local: too rapid IV: transient chest discomfort, vein irritation, phlebitis, thrombophlebitis.

**Nursing Implications:**
*Assess:* Assess previous allergy to this drug, penicillins, cephalosporins, other drugs, or history of allergies. Obtain cultures and sensitivity before treatment, but can start treatment before results. Obtain baseline data on renal, hepatic, hematological, potassium levels if on long-term therapy.
*Administer:* Powder and solutions may darken upon storage but does not appear to effect potency. Refrigerated reconstituted solutions may cause precipitate to form; drug can be redissolved by raising solution temperature to 37°C in

warm water bath for 20 minutes, then agitating vigorously. *IV:* Reconstitute by adding 10 ml of sterile water, 0.9% sodium chloride, or 5% dextrose. Shake vigorously to dissolve. If necessary, can give solution (10 mg/ml) slow IV push over 5 minutes or more. Preferred route is intermittent infusion, minimum dilution of 3 g/50 ml infused over 30 minutes. Compatible with $D_5W$, $D_5W$/ 0.2% NS, $D_5W$/0.5%NS, LR. Do not premix with aminoglycosides, inactivate each other; infuse separately. Incompatible with amphotericin B, chloramphenicol, lincomycin, oxytetracycline, polymyxin B, promethazine, tetracycline, and vitamins B with C. Use of large vein with small-bore needle may reduce local IV reactions.

*Monitor:* Check for hypersensitivity (especially in first 20 minutes of first dosage). Observe IV site for vein irritation and extravasation and change site every 72 hours. Monitor child for hypersensitivity and side effects. Closely observe for symptoms of bleeding; monitor platelet dysfunction and bleeding time especially on long-term therapy. Monitor potassium levels, renal and hepatic function. Maintain hydration for age group. Course of therapy usually 7 to 10 days or 48 hours after symptoms subside.

**Drug Interactions:** Probenecid in combination with azlocillin inhibits renal excretion of antibiotic, thus prolonging serum levels. Anticoagulants given with this drug may increase risk of bleeding. Erythromycin, tetracycline, and chloromycetin may decrease effects of azlocillin.

**Laboratory Test Interferences:** Decreased serum uric acid. Gives a false-positive urine protein level; only reliable method is bromphenol blue test.

**Storage Requirements:** Store powder at 15 to 30°C (59 to 86°F). Storage of reconstituted solutions: consult package insert, stability depends on strength and dilution.

---

## □ BACITRACIN                                            (bass-i-tray'sin)

(Ak-Tracin, Baci-IM, BACI-RX, Baciguent, Medi-Quik, Neo-Thrycex, Ocu-Tracin, Ziba-Rx)

**Combination Products:** Ophthalmic: bacitracin, polymyxin B and neomycin sulfate (Ak-Spore, Neocidin, Neosporin, Neotal, Ocu-Spor-B, Ocusporin, Ocutricin, Triple Antibiotic, Tri-Thalmic); bacitracin and polymyxin B (Ak-Poly-Bac, Ocumycin, Polysporin)
Topical: bacitracin, polymyxin B and neomycin sulfate (Neo-Thrycex, Septa); bacitracin and polymyxin B (Bactine, Medi-Quik, Mycitracin)

**Classification:** antiinfective

**Available Preparations:**
- 10,000, 500,000 units for parenteral administration

- 500 units/g ophthalmic ointment
- 500 units/g topical ointment

**Action and Use:** Polypeptide obtained from cultures of *Bacillus subtilis*. Action may be either bacteriostatic or bactericidal depending on drug concentration and susceptibility of organism. Prevents incorporation of amino acids and nucleotides into cell wall during its synthesis. Also damages the bacterial plasma membrane. Active against many gm+ organisms including streptococci, staphylococci, *Corynebacteria*, and *Clostridia*. Used to treat staphylococci pneumonia and empyema in infants who can be closely monitored. Topical and ophthalmic formulations treat short-term, superficial, topical infections.

### Routes and Dosage:
*IM:*
- infants weighing under 2.5 kg: 900 U/kg/day in 2 or 3 divided doses
- infants weighing over 2.5 kg: 1000 U/kg/day in 2 or 3 divided doses

Do not exceed dosages and give no longer than 12 days
*Ophthalmic:* Instill small strip of 500 Units/g into conjunctival sac 1 to 2 times per day
*Topical:* Apply sparingly to clean wound 2 to 3 times per day

**Absorption and Fate:** Rapidly and completely absorbed from IM site. Not absorbed significantly from mucous membranes or intact or broken skin. Peak level IM, 1 to 2 hours. Distributed to body tissues and not highly bound to plasma proteins. 10 to 40% drug excreted slowly into urine.

**Contraindications and Precautions:** Pregnancy category C. Contraindicated in hypersensitivity to this drug, those who experienced renal dysfunction while on this drug with normal fluid intake, or renal disease or impairment. Use caution with neuromuscular disease. Sensitivity to neomycin may indicate sensitivity to this drug.

**Side Effects:** More likely seen with high dosages or impaired renal function. *CNS:* believed to inhibit neuromuscular transmission that can cause **neuromuscular blockade** with respiratory paralysis. *GI:* anorexia, nausea, vomiting, diarrhea. *GU:* **renal tubular and glomerular necrosis:** albuminuria, cylindruria, hematuria, increased blood drug level without increasing dose, **azotemia, oliguria, renal failure** (infants less prone than older children), rectal itching and burning. *Hemic:* eosinophilia, **bone marrow toxicities, blood dyscrasias**. *Other:* Hypersensitivity: fever, skin rashes, urticaria, **anaphylaxis**; Local: IM: pain, induration; Ophthalmic, Topical: rash, itching, swelling, **anaphylaxis**.

### Nursing Implications:
*Assess:* Assess previous allergy to this drug or any renal impairment. Obtain cultures and sensitivity before treatment, but can start treatment before results. Obtain baseline renal function data and urinalysis. Record and observe appearance of wound or eye.

*Administer: IM:* Reconstitute with sterile 0.9% sodium chloride containing 2% procaine hydrochloride for injection. Restrain child as necessary. Rotate and record sites; give deep into large muscle mass avoiding major nerves and vessels, aspirate before injection. Injection may be painful. *Ophthalmic:* See Part I for instillation of ointments. Clean exudate from eye before instillation. Do not touch ointment tip to eye or any of its adjacent structures. Do not use as prophylaxis for neonatal ophthalmia. *Topical:* Clean wound according to physician's directions. Apply cream sparingly. May be used with or without dressing.

*Monitor:* IM injection can cause pain; observe for induration. Do not give IV because severe thrombophlebitis occurs. Monitor for nephrotoxicity and neuromuscular blockade. Assess renal function by I & O, weights, serum drug levels, daily urinalysis, BUN, and serum creatinine. If symptoms of nephrotoxicity occur, discontinue drug and notify physician. Watch for symptoms of superinfections. Maintain fluid I & O for age group; urine pH should be kept at 6. If rash, itching, or swelling occurs with ophthalmic or topical preparations, discontinue medication.

*Patient Teaching:* Teach proper administration of drug.

**Drug Interactions:** Avoid giving with other nephrotoxic drugs, aminoglycosides, amphotericin B, capreomycin, methoxyflurane, polymyxin B sulfate, vancomycin, curariform muscle relaxants (ether, tubocurarine, succinylcholine, gallamine, decamethoniuma, and sodium citrate may enhance neuromuscular reactions of bacitracin).

**Storage Requirements:** Store sterile powder at 2 to 15°C and protected from direct sunlight. Aqueous solutions stable for 2 weeks at 2 to 8°C (36 to 59°F). Ophthalmic and topical ointments stored at room temperature.

---

## □ BECLOMETHASONE DIPROPIONATE  (be-kloe-meth'a-sone)

(Beclovent, Beconase, Beconase Nasal Inhaler, Vancenase, Vancenase Nasal Inhaler, Vanceril)

**Classification:** corticosteroid, glucocorticoid

**Available Preparations:**
- 42 µg/metered aerosol spray for oral inhalation
- 42 µg/metered aerosol spray for nasal inhalation
- 42 µg/metered dose nasal suspension for inhalation

**Action and Use:** A synthetic corticosteroid with glucocorticoid and weak mineralocorticoid activity used for inhalation. Treats steroid-dependent asthmatics when it is necessary to decrease systemic steroids to reduce adverse side effects. Intranasal form for symptomatic control of rhinitis is occasionally used in children over 12 years.

## Routes and Dosage:
**Nasal:** Rhinitis: Over 12 years: 42 μg delivered per metered spray; give 1 spray 2 to 4 times a day. (Maximum dose 168 to 336 μg/day)
**Inhalation:** Bronchial Asthma:
- 6 to 12 years: oral inhalation 1 or 2 sprays (42 to 84 μg) inhaled 3 to 4 times per day. (Maximum dosage 420 μg/day [10 sprays])
- over 12 years: oral inhalation 2 sprays (84 μg) inhaled 3 to 4 times per day. (Maximum dosage 840 μg/day [20 sprays])

## Absorption and Fate:
Readily absorbed by respiratory and GI tract. 87% bound to plasma proteins; principally metabolized in liver. Excretion primarily fecal.

## Contraindications and Precautions:
Pregnancy category C. Use with caution during lactation. Beclomethasone should not be used for oral inhalation under 6 years, nasal suspension under 6 years, nasal aerosol under 12 years. Contraindicated in hypersensitivity to drug or its ingredients (fluorocarbons), relief of acute bronchospasm, status asthmaticus. Use with caution in pulmonary tuberculosis, untreated fungal, bacterial, or viral infections, ocular herpes, recent nasal surgery or trauma, and nasal septic ulcers.

## Side Effects:
**GI:** nausea, dysphonia, dry or sore mouth, irritation of tongue, dysgeusia. **Resp:** throat and tracheal irritation, cough, **bronchospasm**, hoarseness, **wheezing**, epistaxis. **Skin:** rash, urticaria, angioedema (rare). **Other:** candidal infection of mouth, throat, and larynx, lacrimation, **suppression of HPA function** especially in overdosage.

## Nursing Implications:
**Assess:** Ability of child to follow usage directions of hand-held inhalers. If child is on systemic steroids obtain height and weight of child.
**Administer: Nasal:** Use only nasal preparation. Before usage clear nasal passages of mucus. Shake well, tilt head backward, insert into nostril, and hold other nostril closed. While spraying inhale through nose and exhale through mouth. If two sprays are ordered per nostril direct first spray toward lower nostril and other spray toward upper nostril to ensure coverage of entire nasal mucosa. After each usage remove cap and nosepiece from canister, rinse in warm water, and dry thoroughly. **Oral Inhalation:** Use only oral preparation. If inhaler for bronchodilation is prescribed, use 5 to 15 minutes before beclomethasone so these drugs will augment steroid's penetration into peripheral airways. To use aerosol inhaler, shake well, first exhale completely, place lips around oral mouthpiece with tongue below inhaler, tilt inhaler upward and head backward, then inhale with steady even breath while depressing the top of metal canister. Remove inhaler, hold breath as long as possible to allow particles of medication to reach into lungs. Exhale slowly through pursed lips or nose. If second inhalation is prescribed, wait about 1 minute between inhalations.

*Monitor:* Monitor for side effects. Therapeutic effects of drug are usually seen within 1 to 4 weeks. If child is on concurrent systemic corticosteroid therapy, do not withdraw drug rapidly as it may cause adrenal insufficiency or life-threatening asthma exacerbation. Withdrawal should be gradual and under physician's strict supervision; total recovery of HPA function may take 1 year. Withdrawal symptoms could include: lassitude, joint and muscular pain, depression, fatigue, hypotension, nausea, vomiting. Blood pressure and weight should be monitored during withdrawal. Report to physician any symptoms of infections or other allergic conditions. Fungal infections of oropharyngeal area are common, inspect this area for infection. Encourage good oral hygiene and have child rinse mouth with water or mouthwash immediately after drug usage. If infections occur, notify physician because antiinfective therapy or discontinuance of drug is necessary. The systemic side effects seen with other steroids are usually not seen with this drug, but regular heights and weights should be obtained to assess for growth and development.

*Patient Teaching:* Teach proper usage and care of inhaler and it is beneficial to have child demonstrate inhaler usage. Use inhaler only as prescribed, at regular intervals, and do not use during acute attack; it is not a bronchodilator. Rinsing mouth with water after usage; good oral hygiene and inspection of mouth for fungal infections is necessary. It is advisable to keep record of number of doses administered so that refill bottles can be obtained as it is difficult to assess the number of doses left in canister. Inform any emergency caretaker that the child is on this medication and child should be under supervised medical care while on this drug.

**Storage Requirements:** Store at 2 to 30°C (36 to 86°F), protect from flame or heat above 102°F. Do not puncture or discard into fire or incinerator.

---

# □ BETHANECHOL CHLORIDE          (be-than'e-kole)

(Duvoid, Myotonachol, Urabeth, Urecholine)

**Classification:** cholinergic, direct acting

## Available Preparations:
- 5, 10, 25, 50-mg tablets
- 5 mg/ml for parenteral administration

**Action and Use:** Has cholinergic properties. At therapeutic dose, its actions are primarily on GI tract and detrusor muscle of urinary bladder. Used in the treatment of postoperative urinary retention, gastric retention, adynamic ileus; has been used experimentally for gastroesophageal reflux.

## Routes and Dosage:
*PO:* 0.6 mg/kg/day in divided doses every 6 to 8 hours. Gastroesophageal Reflux: 2.9 mg/m²/dose every 8 hours
*SC:* 0.15 to 0.2 mg/kg/day in divided doses every 8 hours

**Absorption and Fate:** Poorly absorbed orally. Onset of action: PO, 30 minutes; SC, 5 to 15 minutes. Peak level: PO, 30 to 60 minutes; SC, 15 to 30 minutes. Duration of action: PO, 1 to 6 hours; SC, 2 hour. Metabolic fate and excretion unknown.

**Contraindications and Precautions:** Pregnancy category C and safety during lactation not established. Contraindicated IV or IM, in hypersensitivity to drug, hyperthyroidism, bronchial asthma, seizure disorders, cardiac disease or coronary artery disease, obstructive pulmonary disease, bradycardia, atrioventricular conduction defects, hypotension, hypertension, peptic ulcer, mechanical obstruction of GI or GU tract, recent surgery of GI or GU tract, spastic GI disturbances, decreased bladder wall or GI tract strength or integrity, peritonitis, or acute inflammatory conditions of the GI tract.

**Side Effects:** Rare after oral, more common with SQ.
*CNS:* malaise, headache. *CV:* transient slight fall in BP accompanied by minor reflex tachycardia. *GI:* abdominal cramps, excessive salivation, diarrhea, belching, borborygmi. *Resp:* **bronchial constriction, asthmatic attacks**. *GU:* urinary urgency, incontinence. *Sensory:* EENT: miosis, blurred vision, lacrimation. *Other:* flushing of face, increased sweating, substernal pain or pressure.

**Nursing Implications:**
*Assess:* Discontinue other cholinergics before giving. Obtain baseline vital signs (P, BP, and respirations).
*Administer: PO:* Give on empty stomach 1 hour before or 2 hours after meals to decrease nausea and vomiting. Tablets may be crushed, mixed with small amount of food or fluid. *SC:* **Make sure that injection is given into subcutaneous tissue, do not give IM or IV.** Aspirate before injection. If inadvertently given IV or IM, symptoms include hypotension, bradycardia, reflex tachycardia, severe abdominal pain, bloody diarrhea, **shock, cardiac arrest, circulatory collapse**. Have atropine sulfate readily available with dosage for individual child (0.001 mg/kg); can give IV, IM, SC.
*Monitor:* Observe child and monitor vital signs for at least 1 hour after injection. Monitor for side effects. If given for urinary retention have bedpan, urinal, or potty chair available. Monitor I & O. Orthostatic hypotension or dizziness possible; alter activities as necessary.
*Patient Teaching:* Note side effects and inform care provider if they occur.

**Drug Interactions:** Do not give with other cholinergic drugs or anticholinesterase inhibitors because of increased chance of additive and toxicity effects. Concurrent usage with ganglion blocking agents may cause a sharp fall in blood pressure and severe abdominal symptoms. Quinidine and procainamide antagonize cholinergic actions of this drug.

**Laboratory Test Interference:** Increases serum amylase and lipase as result of increased pancreatic secretions. May increase serum bilirubin, SGOT by increasing contractions in sphincter of Oddi.

**Storage Requirements:** Store at 15 to 30°C (59 to 86°F); avoid freezing.

---

## □ BLEOMYCIN                                      (blee-oh-mye'sin)

(Blenoxane)

**Classification:** antineoplastic, antibiotic

**Available Preparations:** 15 units vial for parenteral use

**Action and Use:** Inhibits DNA synthesis and to a lesser degree RNA and protein synthesis. Most active in $G_2$ and M phases of cell division. It is an antibiotic effective against gram-positive and gram-negative bacteria and fungi, but is not used as an antibacterial due to its toxicity. Used in lymphoma such as Hodgkin's disease, non-Hodgkin's lymphoma, in head and neck cancers, and in squamous cell carcinomas.

### Routes and Dosages:
*IV, IM, SC:* 0.25 to 0.5 units/kg or 10 to 20 units/m² once or twice weekly.
- Maintenance: 1 unit/day or 5 units/week. Test doses not to exceed 2 units are given IM for the first 2 doses to lymphoma patients due to possibility of anaphylaxis.
- Arterial Perfusion: 10 to 20 units/m²/day over 12 to 24 hours for 5 to 14 days has been used experimentally.
- Intrapleural: 60 to 120 units have been used experimentally.
Total cumulative lifetime dose of the drug not to exceed 400 units/m²

**Absorption and Fate:** Distributed in highest concentrations to skin, lungs, kidneys, peritoneum, and lymphatics. Low concentration in bone marrow. Metabolism in body unknown, although 60 to 70% is excreted as unchanged drug in the urine. Distribution half-life after IV is 24 minutes and terminal is 4 hours. In those under 3 years, distribution half-life is 54 minutes and terminal is 3 hours. With continuous IV terminal half-life is 2.3 hours.

**Contraindications and Precautions:** Pregnancy category D. Contraindicated with allergy to the drug and during infection with chicken pox or herpes zoster. Use with caution in those with lung disease, hepatic or renal dysfunction, infection, or previous chemotherapy or radiation, especially pulmonary radiation.

### Side Effects:
*GI:* stomatitis, mild nausea and vomiting. ***Respiratory:*** interstitial pneumoni-

tis is common and a serious toxic effect; may progress to fatal pulmonary fibrosis. *Skin:* urticaria, erythema, hyperkeratosis, hyperpigmentation, alopecia, and other skin reactions. *Hemic:* minimal myelosuppressive effect, mild leukopenia, thrombocytopenia, decreased hemoglobin. *Other:* anaphylaxis with hypotension, fever, chills, confusion, paresthesia, phlebitis at injection site; wheezing (most common in lymphoma patients).

## Nursing Implications:

*Assess:* Obtain history of prior treatment with antineoplastics and radiation. Assess respiratory status including chest x-ray and pulmonary function studies.

*Administer:* This drug has potentially serious side effects and should be given only under the supervision of a physician with training and experience in cancer chemotherapy. The drug's potential for toxic effects on health-care personnel as well as patients necessitates careful handling during preparation and administration. Generally, during preparation of antineoplastics, latex gloves, a mask, and a solid front gown are worn, and a laminar flow hood is used. Gloves and gown may also be recommended for administration. Contaminated equipment, such as needles, syringes, and unused medication, is disposed of properly. Clean-up of spills is carefully performed and accidental contact by patient or personnel receives prompt flushing and cleaning. *IM:* Add 1 to 5 ml of sterile water, saline, 5% dextrose, or bacteriostatic water to vial. For test dose, give 1 to 2 units and if no reaction within 2 to 4 hours, IV infusion will be started. Reconstituted solution stable for 24 hours at room temperature. *IV, intraarterial:* Add at least 5 ml of sterile water, saline, 5% dextrose, or bacteriostatic water to vial and administer slowly over 10 minutes. Be prepared for anaphylactic reaction with resuscitative drugs and equipment readily available.

*Monitor:* Watch for anaphylaxis manifested by hypotension, fever, chills, confusion, wheezing immediately and up to several hours after administration. Monitor respiratory function with frequent lung auscultation and chest x-ray every 1 to 2 weeks. Carbon dioxide pulmonary diffusion capacity may be helpful in monitoring for pulmonary toxicity. Pulmonary function tests, such as decreased vital capacity, may indicate pulmonary toxicity. Perform regularly WBC with differential count. Monitor renal and hepatic function with periodic BUN, SGPT, SGOT, bilirubin, creatinine, LDH, uric acid. Serum creatinine of 2.5 to 4 necessitates lowering dose to 1/4 normal; 4.0 to 6.0 necessitates lowering dose to 1/5 normal; 6.0 to 10 necessitates lowering dose to 1/10 to 1/20 normal.

*Patient Teaching:* Report respiratory symptoms such as cough, wheezing, dyspnea, fever, and chills within 3 to 6 hours after a dose. Perform good oral care and report pain or sores in mouth. Prepare patient for possibility of hyperpigmentation and mild nausea and vomiting.

**Drug Interactions:** Increased toxicity with other antineoplastics or radiation. May reduce plasma phenytoin levels. Concomitant oxygen therapy increases possibility of lung damage. Suppresses immune response to immunization. Live virus vaccines or oral polio vaccine must not be given, to those in close contact with the patient on this drug due to the chance of infection with a virus; these vaccines are delayed until at least 3 months after chemotherapy when the patient is in remission.

**Storage Requirements:** Store at 15 to 30° C (59 to 86°F). Reconstituted solutions are stable for 24 hours at room temperature.

---

## □ BROMPHENIRAMINE MALEATE
(brome-fen-ir'a-meen)

(Bromarest, Brombay, Bromphen, Chlorphed, Dehist, Dimetane, Dimetane-Ten, Dimetane Extentabs, Histaject Modified, Nasahist B, Rolabromophen Spentane, Veltane)

**Combination Products:** Brompheniramine maleate is combined with other drugs such as pseudoephedrine HCl, pseudoephedrine sulfate, phenylephrine HCl, and phenylpropanolamine HCl.

**Classification:** antihistamine

### Available Preparations:
- 2 mg/5 ml oral elixir
- 4-mg tablet
- 8, 12-mg extended-release tablets
- 10 mg/ml for parenteral administration

**Action and Use:** Propylamine derivative that competes with histamine for $H_1$-receptor sites of effector cells. By blocking histamine it decreases the allergic reactions. Used to relieve rhinitis and allergy symptoms. Parenteral form given to prevent allergic reactions to blood, plasma, and in anaphylactic reactions.

### Routes and Dosages:
*PO:*
- under 6 years: 0.5 mg/kg/day or 15 mg/m²/day in 3 to 4 equally divided doses (Maximum dosage 6 mg/day)
- 6 to 12 years: 2 to 4 mg 3 to 4 times/day or one 8 or 12 mg extended-release tablet every 12 hours (Maximum dosage 12 mg/day)
- over 12 years: 4 mg every 4 to 6 hours or one 8 or 12 mg extended-release tablet every 12 hours (Maximum dosage 24 mg/day)

*SC, IM, IV:* under 12 years: 0.5 mg/kg/24 hours or 15 mg/m²/day in 3 to 4 equally divided doses

**Absorption and Fate:** Absorbed well from GI tract. Peak level, 2 to 5 hours. Half-life, 25 hours. Duration of action, 4 to 25 hours. Excreted primarily in urine.

**Contraindications and Precautions:** Pregnancy category C. Use during lactation not recommended. Do not use in neonates, prematures, no extended-release tablets in children under 6 years; in those under 6 years, drug should only be given under physician directions. Contraindicated in hypersensitivity to drug, acute asthma attack. Use caution in cardiovascular or renal diseases; asthma, hypertension, increased intraocular pressure, bladder neck obstruction, urinary retention, hyperthyroidism, stenosed peptic ulcers.

**Side Effects:**

*CNS:* drowsiness, paradoxical excitement, dizziness, headaches, nervousness, insomnia, tremors, **seizures**. *CV:* palpitations, **hypotension**. *GI:* anorexia, nausea, vomiting, diarrhea, dry mouth and throat. *Hepatic:* mild increase SGOT, SGPT. *Resp:* increased thick secretions, **wheezing, chest tightness**. *GU:* urinary retention or frequency. *Skin:* rash, urticaria. *Other:* hypersensitivity; Local (IV): sweating, syncope.

**Nursing Implications:**

*Assess:* Obtain CBC before long-term therapy.

*Administer: PO:* May give with food or milk to reduce GI distress. Elixir contains 3% alcohol. Can crush tablet, mix with small amounts of food or fluid. Extended release tablets are not to be crushed or chewed. *SC, IM:* Give as undiluted injection. *IV:* 100 mg/ml is not recommended for IV usage. To reduce side effects, dilute each 10 ml with normal saline; but can be given undiluted. Infuse over at least 60 minutes or longer. Compatible with D$_5$W or NS. Incompatible with aminophylline, insulin, pentobarbital, iodipamide meglumine. Crystallization of drug will occur under 32°F, but warming to 86°F will cause redissolving of crystals. Because local reaction to IV—such as hypotension, sweating, syncope—may occur, keep child recumbent while infusing.

*Monitor:* Assess for side effects. Periodic CBC if on long-term therapy.

*Patient Teaching:* Give only under physician supervision in those under 6 years. Observe for side effects and maintain hydration. Assess relief of symptoms. If CNS symptoms occur, may require adjustment of behavior, e.g., skate boarding, bike riding, and other activities requiring mental alertness. Do not use alcohol or take other OTC drugs that may increase CNS symptoms while on this drug. Chewing sugarless gum or sucking sugarless candy may relieve dry mouth.

**Drug Interferences:** This drug may increase CNS depression of alcohol, other CNS drugs, and barbiturates. Use of this drug and MAO inhibitors may cause increased anticholinergic effects.

**Laboratory Test Interferences:** May suppress reactions to skin testing; discontinue drug 4 days before testing.

**Storage Requirements:** Store at 15 to 30°C (59 to 86°F), in tight containers. Elixir and parenteral form, protect from light and avoid freezing.

# ☐ CAFFEINE  (kaf-een')

(Caffedrine, Dexitac, NoDoz, Quick Pep, Tirend, Vivarin)

**Classification:** CNS stimulant, xanthine

## Available Preparations:
- 65, 100, 150, 200-mg tablets
- 200, 250-mg capsules
- 250 mg/ml vials for parenteral use
- powder

**Action and Use:** Increases intracellular AMP and antagonizes central adenosine receptors. Acts as a stimulant at all CNS levels. Has stronger CNS and skeletal muscle effects than other xanthines, such as theophylline, and weaker cortical effects than the amphetamines. Has positive inotropic effect on the heart with increased heart rate and cardiac output. Causes constriction of cerebral vessels and dilation of peripheral vessels. Stimulates voluntary skeletal muscle and gastric acid secretion. Used in treatment of drowsiness and vascular headaches. Parenteral form used in treatment of circulatory failure in emergencies, in respiratory depression for overdosage with CNS depressants. The major use in children is unapproved treatment of neonatal apnea. Other uses not approved by FDA are for diuresis in fluid retention such as in menstruation and for atopic dermatitis.

## Routes and Dosages:
***SC, IM, IV:*** CNS Stimulation: 8 mg/kg or 250 mg/m$^2$; not to exceed 500 mg
***PO, IM, IV:*** Neonatal Apnea: 5 to 10 mg/kg as loading dose; then 1 to 5 mg/kg/day; not to exceed 12 mg/kg/day in two doses
Doses established by clinicians rather than manufacturers.

**Absorption and Fate:** Rapidly absorbed in PO and parenteral forms. Rapidly distributed in body; crosses placenta and blood-brain barrier. 17% bound to plasma proteins. Metabolized in the liver and excreted in metabolized and unchanged form in the urine. Peak level reached in approximately 1 hour after PO form. Half-life in adults, 3.5 hours; may be considerably prolonged in neonates, to 100 hours. Therapeutic level for neonatal apnea 8 to 20 mg/L.

**Contraindications and Precautions:** Pregnancy category C. Crosses placenta and is present in breast milk. The parenteral preparation in sodium benzoate is not to be given to neonates as it may disrupt bilirubin binding to albumin and cause kernicterus. Contraindicated in those hypersensitive to caffeine and with cardiac arrhythmias, palpitations, and recent myocardial infarction. Use as mild CNS stimulant not recommended in children. Cautious use in peptic ulcer, hepatic dysfunction, hypertension, insomnia, and panic states.

## Side Effects:

**CNS:** insomnia, restlessness, nervousness, delirium (more common in children); dizziness, tremors, headache, confusion, irritability, seizures, anxiety, tinnitus. **CV:** increased pulse, arrhythmia. **GI:** abdominal distention and vomiting in neonates, nausea, diarrhea, gastric irritation, rectal irritation with suppositories. **GU:** bacteriuria, nephritis, frequency. **Other:** kernicterus in neonates.

## Nursing Implications:

**Assess:** Take baseline vital signs.

**Administer: IM, IV:** Analeptic use in respiratory and cardiac failure is discouraged. **IV:** Only citrated caffeine injection is to be used for neonatal apnea, as caffeine and sodium benzoate preparation may cause kernicterus. 10 g of powder are dissolved in 250 ml of sterile water for injection. Add 250 ml additional sterile water. Filtered into 10-ml vials and autoclaved. Solution contains 20 mg/ml. Given slowly.

**Monitor:** Take vital signs every few minutes during administration. Therapeutic levels monitored during neonatal apnea treatment; taken 24 hours after initial dose, then once or twice weekly; maintained at 8 to 20 mg/L.

**Drug Interactions:** Increases inotropic effects of β-blockers. Increased metabolism of barbituates and caffeine when given concomitantly. Decreased metabolism of cimetidine. Increased side effects with other xanthines such as aminophylline. Can inhibit calcium absorption. Increases excretion of lithium. Increased half-life of caffeine when given with disulfiram.

**Laboratory Test Interferences:** False-positive serum urate by Bittner method. Increased VMA, catecholamines, 5-hydroxyindoleacetic acid. Increased blood glucose.

**Storage Requirements:** Store at 15 to 30°C (59 to 86°F).

---

## □ CAPTOPRIL                                    (kap′toe-pril)

(Capoten)

**Combination Products:** capozide

**Classification:** angiotensin-converting enzyme inhibitor, antihypertensive

## Available Preparations:
- 12.5, 25, 37.5, 50, 100-mg tablets
- 25, 50-mg tablets with hydrochlorothiazide

## Routes and Dosages:
*PO:*
- newborn: 10 µg/kg BID or TID; adjust PRN
- children: 300 µg/kg TID; increase by 300 µg/kg in 8- to 24-hour intervals PRN
- children on diuretics or who have water or sodium depletion, or with renal dysfunction should initially receive 150 µg/kg TID

**Absorption and Fate:** Rapidly absorbed from GI tract; food impairs absorption. Distributed widely in body with exception of CNS. 25 to 30 % bound to plasma proteins. Metabolized and excreted in urine. Onset of action, 15 to 60 minutes and peak action in 1 to 2 hours. Duration, 2 to 6 hours or longer. Half-life, 2 hours with much longer half-life in those with renal dysfunction.

**Contraindications and Precautions:** Pregnancy category C. Small amount present in breast milk, therefore, lactation should be discontinued when taking the drug. Safety and use in children has not been established; use in children only if other antihypertensives are not effective. Cautious use in renal dysfunction, sodium or water depletion, collagen vascular disease, when given with diuretics, or during dialysis.

## Side Effects:
*CNS:* dizziness, fatigue, headache, paresthesia, insomnia (all rare). *CV:* hypotension, tachycardia, chest pain, palpitations, angina, congestive heart failure, Raynaud's syndrome. *GI:* altered taste acuity that improves within 2 to 3 months after drug therapy starts, nausea, vomiting, anorexia, diarrhea, constipation. *Respiratory:* cough, bronchospasm, dyspnea. *GU:* proteinuria, nephrotic syndrome, renal dysfunction especially in those with renal dysfunction. *Skin:* maculopapular and urticarial rash (common), photosensitivity, nail changes. *Hemic:* neutropenia, agranulocytosis, eosinophilia, pancytopenia. *Other:* hyperkalemia, serum sickness with rash, fever, arthralgia, jaundice (rare).

## Nursing Implications:
*Assess:* Take baseline vital signs, particularly blood pressure. Obtain history of renal dysfunction such as renal artery stenosis or glomerulopathy. Obtain kidney function tests. Obtain WBC count. Assess for presence of hypovolemia, sodium or potassium imbalance, other antihypertensives.

*Administer: PO:* Give 1 hour before meals. Tablet has slight sulfurous odor. If tablet cannot be swallowed, the tablet may be crushed and added to water, shaken vigorously, and administered within at least 30 minutes.

*Monitor:* Measure daily weight, I & O. Measure urine for protein. Renal function studies done regularly. WBC count done every 2 weeks for first 3 months and then periodically (neutrophil count under 1000/mm$^3$ usually necessitates stopping therapy). Excessive hypotension may occur 1 to 3 hours after first dose; patient should be kept supine for this period and blood pressure taken frequently. Serum electrolytes, especially potassium and sodium, are performed regularly. Monitor blood sugar of diabetic for hypoglycemia.

*Patient Teaching:* Report weight gain and edema. Change position slowly to avoid postural hypotension. Urine protein dipstick may be recommended. Take drug as directed 1 hour before meals. Do not take other drugs unless instructed by physician. Use caution during hot weather or exercise to avoid hypovolemia. Avoid salt substitutes and low salt milk, which may contain excess potassium. Report nausea, vomiting, and diarrhea.

**Drug Interactions:** Increased hypotensive effect with other antihypertensives and diuretics; diuretic may be withheld or sodium intake increased for 3 to 7 days before captopril therapy. Possible increased hypotensive effect with nitroglycerine; concomitant use discouraged. Decreased antihypertensive effect with nonsteroidal antiinflammatories. Increased hyperkalemia with potassium-sparing diuretics necessitates close serum potassium monitoring. Administration with antacids decreases absorption. Increased serum concentrations of captopril when given with probenecid. Possible increased insulin sensitivity leading to hypoglycemia in diabetics. Increased myelosuppression with drugs that suppress bone marrow.

**Laboratory Test Interferences:** False-positive urinary acetone. Increased BUN, creatinine, hepatic enzymes, potassium. Decreased serum sodium.

**Storage Requirements:** Store tightly covered at 15 to 30°C (59 to 86°F).

---

□ **CARBAMAZEPINE**                          (kar-ba-maz′e-peen)

(Epitol, Tegretol)

**Classification:** anticonvulsant

**Available Preparations:**
- 200-mg tablets
- 100-mg chewable tablets

**Action and Use:** Similar in action to phenytoin; inhibits polysynaptic flexor reflexes thereby interfering with seizure propagation. Also has sedative, antidepressant, muscle relaxing, and antidiuretic effects. Used in treatment of psychomotor, grand mal, and mixed seizures, particularly when other drugs are not effective. Provides pain relief from trigeminal neuralgia. Uses not approved by FDA include control of pain and symptoms of multiple sclerosis, hemifacial spasm, dystonia, antidiuretic effects in diabetes insipidus, and other uses primarily in adults.

**Routes and Dosages:**
*PO:*
- Seizures: under 6 years: 5 mg/kg/day; increasing to 10 mg/kg/day in 5 to 7 days PRN and to 20 mg/kg/day in another 5 to 7 days PRN.

Alternatively initial doses at this age may be 10 to 20 mg/day in divided doses. This dose established by clinicians, not manufacturers.

- 6 to 12 Years: 100 mg BID; increasing by 100 mg/day in weekly intervals PRN; not to exceed 1 g/day. Doses given 3 to 4 times daily if daily dosage is over 200 mg. Usual maintenance dose at this age is 400 to 800 mg/day.
- over 12 years: 200 mg BID; increasing up to 200 mg/day in weekly intervals PRN; not to exceed 1 g/day for 13 to 15 years and 1.2 g/day for those over 15 years. Doses given 3 to 4 times daily if daily dosage is over 400 mg. Usual maintenence dose at this age is 800 to 1200 mg/day.

**Absorption and Fate:** Absorbed slowly from GI tract. Widely distributed in body and 75 to 90% bound to plasma proteins. Metabolized mainly by the liver and excreted primarily in urine. Onset of anticonvulsant activity is from hours to months; peak level is reached in 2 to 8 hours. Half-life is 8 to 72 hours, with a range from 25 to 65 hours initially and 12 to 17 hours after repeated doses. Therapeutic level is 3 to 14 µg/ml.

**Contraindications and Precautions:** Pregnancy category C. The drug should be used in pregnancy only if it is essential in the woman's seizure management. Not recommended during lactation. Safety in children under 6 years has not been established. Contraindicated in liver disease, history of bone marrow suppression, AV heart block, blood disorders, hypersensitivity to the drug, in absence, atonic, or myoclonic seizures, and those with a hypersensitivity to any tricyclic antidepressant. Cautious use in those with cardiac damage, latent psychosis, hepatic or renal dysfunction, diabetes, glaucoma, hyponatremia, and urinary retention.

**Side Effects:**
*CNS:* ataxia and dizziness with plasma level 10 µg/ml or more; nystagmus with plasma level over 4 µg/ml; drowsiness, vertigo, diplopia, speech changes, involuntary movements; behavior changes (more common in children); weakness, headache, depression, trembling, hallucinations. *CV:* congestive failure, hypertension, hypotension, thrombophlebitis, arrhythmia, chest pain, changes in heart rate. *GI:* nausea, vomiting, diarrhea, GI pain, constipation, dry mouth, sore throat, mouth ulcers. *Respiratory:* dyspnea, pneumonia. *Hepatic:* jaundice, hepatitis, abnormal liver function tests. *GU:* frequency, retention, oliguria, renal failure; inappropriate antidiuretic hormone secretion. *Skin:* rash, urticaria, pigmentation changes especially with sunlight exposure, alopecia, worsening of systemic lupus erythematosis. *Hemic:* aplastic anemia, leukopenia, thrombocytopenia, eosinophilia, agranulocytosis, leukocytosis. *Other:* fever, aching joints, muscle cramps, ocular changes.

**Nursing Implications:**
*Assess:* This drug has life-threatening toxic effects, therefore, careful assessment is necessary. It is used in those children who have had serious side effects or no therapeutic response to other anticonvulsants. CBC, platelet, reticulocyte, and iron studies are done initially, and the drug is withheld if results are

abnormal. Liver function tests are performed before therapy begins. BUN, ECG, UA, liver function tests are done. EEG monitoring is done to identify those children with mixed seizure disorders who may have a worsening of seizures with use of this drug. Eye studies with slit lamp, tonometry, and fundoscopy are performed. History of other drugs, particularly tricyclic antidepressants, bone marrow suppression, liver or kidney disease are important.

*Administer:* Drug is given with food to facilitate its absorption.

*Monitor:* CBC, platelets, reticulocytes, and iron counts are done weekly for at least 3 months and then monthly. Drug is discontinued if RBC count is under 4 million/mm³, hematocrit is under 32%, hemoglobin is under 11 g/dl, WBC count is under 4000/mm³, reticulocyte count is under 20,000/mm³, platelet count is under 100,000/mm³, *or* serum iron is over 150 µg/dl. Inform prescriber of laboratory results and withhold drug if necessary. The child with bone marrow suppression side effect is monitored by bone marrow studies as the effect can be fatal. Liver function tests and renal studies including BUN and UA are routinely performed. Serum electrolytes are monitored. Serum carbamazepine levels are taken with 6 to 12 µg usually the desired optimal range. Regular eye studies including tonometry, fundoscopy are performed especially in those with intraocular pressure. Measure I & O during establishment of dosage. Report fluid retention.

*Patient Teaching:* Take drug as directed. Do not discontinue drug suddenly as this may precipitate seizure activity. Avoid driving and other hazardous activities as drowsiness, dizziness, and ataxia are common. Avoid sunlight exposure. Notify prescriber immediately if bleeding, bruising, fever, sore throat, or fatigue occur. See prescriber on a regular schedule. Wear bracelet stating person has seizures and is on anticonvulsant medication.

**Drug Interactions:** Carbamazepine can decrease serum concentration of phenytoin, phenobarbital, doxycycline, and warfarin. Breakthrough bleeding may occur when given with oral contraceptives; alternative birth control methods should be used. Increased serum levels of carbamazepine occur when given with verapamil or erythromycin, therefore, dosage must be adjusted downward. This drug should not be given with or for less than 14 days after a monoamine oxidase inhibitor.

**Laboratory Test Interferences:** Can increase BUN, SGOT, SGPT, bilirubin. May cause albuminuria and glycosuria. Decreases serum calcium and thyroid hormones. False-negative pregnancy tests.

**Storage Requirements:** Store tightly covered at 15 to 30°C (59 to 86°F).

---

# ☐ CARBENICILLIN DISODIUM                (kar-ben-i-sill′in)

(Geopen, Pyopen)

**Classification:** penicillin, extended spectrum

**Available Preparations:** 2, 5, 30 g for parenteral administration

**Action and Use:** Mechanism similar to other penicillins that inhibit cell-wall synthesis in bacteria. Can be inactivated by penicillinase-producing staphylococci, and is primarily used for *Proteus vulgaris, Providencia rettgeri, Morganella morganii, P. mirabilis, Escherichia coli, Enterobacter,* and *Pseudomonas aeruginosa* strains; may be useful in *Bacteroides* infection using large doses. Treats infections of GU tract, respiratory tract, intraabdominal, skin, soft tissue, and in septicemia and meningitis. Contains 4.7-6.5 mEq of sodium per gram of drug.

**Routes and Dosage:**
*IM, IV:* Loading Dose: neonates: 100 mg/kg initially, then;
- neonates <2000 g, under 7 days: 75 mg/kg every 8 hours (225 mg/kg/day)
- over 7 days: 100 mg/kg every 6 hours (400 mg/kg/day)
- neonates > 2000 g, under 3 days; 75 mg/kg every 8 hours (300 mg/kg/day)
- over 3 days: 100 mg/kg every 6 hours (400 mg/kg/day)
- over 1 month: UTI: 50 to 200 mg/kg every 4 to 6 hours
- over 1 month: Severe infections: 400 to 600 mg/kg/day every 4 to 6 hours. (Maximum dosage 40 g/day)

**Absorption and Fate:** Distributed in pleura, synovia, peritoneum, sputum, lymph, bile, meninges when inflamed. Peak level: IM in neonates, about 4 hours; IM children, 1 hour; IV, 5 minutes after infusion. Half-life about 1.1 hours in children and 2.7 hours in neonates. 60 to 90% excreted unchanged in urine.

**Contraindications and Precautions:** Pregnancy category B. Excreted in breast milk, use caution with lactation. Contraindicated if hypersensitivity to drug, penicillins, or cephalosporins. Use with caution in sensitivity to multiple allergens, other drugs, renal impairment, bleeding tendencies, or sodium restrictions.

**Side Effects:**
*CNS:* neuromuscular irritability, **seizures** (with high serum levels). *GI:* nausea. *Hepatic:* Elevation of SGOT and SGPT. *GU:* hemorrhagic cystitis with frequency and pain, **acute interstitial nephritis**. *Hemic:* **anemia, eosinophilia, thrombocytopenia, leukopenia, neutropenia, abnormal prothrombin time and clotting time** (with high doses). *Other:* Hypersensitivity: skin rashes, pruritus, urticaria, drug fever, **anaphylaxis**; hypernatremia, hypokalemia; Local: IV pain, vein irritation, phlebitis, and IM (painful).

**Nursing Implications:**
*Assess:* Assess previous allergy to drug, penicillins, cephalosporins, other drugs, or history of allergies. Obtain cultures and sensitivity before treatment, but can start treatment before results. Obtain baseline data on renal, hepatic, hematological, potassium levels if on long-term therapy.

*Administer: IM:* Reconstitute with 2 ml of either sterile or bacteriostatic water or 0.5% lidocaine without epinephrine for injection. Injection painful, may minimize pain by giving slowly (over 12 to 15 seconds). Do not use bacteriostatic preparations containing benzyl alcohol in neonates. *IV:* Reconstitute according to package inserts with sterile water. If necessary can give slow IV push over 5 or more minutes (200 mg/minute); neonates infuse over 15 minutes. **Rapid infusion may cause seizures.** Preferred route is intermittent infusion; minimum dilution of 1 g/7 ml infused over 15 to 30 minutes. Continuous infusion over 4 to 24 hours, do not use dilution of less than 10 mg/ml. Compatible with $D_5W$, $D_5W/0.2\%$ NS, $D_5W/0.5\%$ NS, NS, LR, amino acids 4%/$D2_{25}W$, 10% fat emulsion. Do not premix with aminoglycosides, avoid mixing with other drugs, infuse separately. Incompatible with amphotericin B, bleomycin, chloramphenicol, lincomycin, oxytetracycline, polymyxin B, promethazine, tetracycline, and vitamins B with C. Using large vein with small-bore needle may reduce local IV reactions.

*Monitor:* Check child for hypersensitivity (especially in first 20 minutes of first dosage). Observe IV site for vein irritation and extravasation and change site every 72 hours. Monitor child for side effects. Closely observe for symptoms of bleeding; monitor platelet dysfunction and bleeding time especially on long-term therapy. Monitor potassium and sodium levels, renal and hepatic function. Maintain fluid level for age group. Avoid prolonged use of drug because of overgrowth of nonsusceptible organisms.

**Drug Interactions:** Anticoagulants given with this drug may increase risk of bleeding. Erythromycin, tetracycline, and chloromycetin may decrease effects of carbenicillin. Synergistic effect may occur against certain organisms when given with acetohydroxamic acid.

**Laboratory Test Interferences:** Increased SGOT and SGPT.

**Storage Requirements:** Store at 15 to 30°C (59 to 86°F); reconstituted solutions for IM at room temperature for 24 hours, 72 hours if refrigerated, and IV solutions according to packags insert.

---

## □ CEFACLOR                                                (sef'a-klor)

(Ceclor)

**Classification:** cephalosporin, second generation

## Available Preparations:
- 125, 187, 250, 375 mg/5 ml suspension
- 250, 500-mg capsules

**Action and Use:** Semisynthetic cephalosporin that renders cell wall osmotically unstable through cell-wall synthesis. Less active than most second generation cephalosporins but effective against both gm + and gm − bacteria, such as staphylococci, group A β-hemolytic *Streptoccocus*, *S. pneumoniae*, *E. coli*, *Proteus mirabilis*, *Haemophilus influenza*, and *Klebsiella* species. Used to treat otitis media, respiratory, urinary tract and skin infections.

## Routes and Dosage:
*PO:* over 1 month: 20 to 40 mg/kg/day in divided doses every 8 to 12 hours. (Maximum dosage 1 g/day)

## Absorption and Fate:
Absorbed well from GI tract and excreted unchanged in urine. Peak level 1 to 1.5 hours. Half-life 30 to 60 minutes.

## Contraindications and Precautions:
Pregnancy category B. Crosses into breast milk; safe use during lactation not established. Not recommended in infants under 1 month. Contraindicated in hypersensitivity to cephalosporins. Use caution in bleeding disorders, ulcerative colitis, hepatic and renal function impairments, and sensitivity to penicillin.

## Side Effects:
*CNS:* headache, dizziness, somnolence. *GI:* diarrhea, nausea, vomiting, anorexia, GI cramps, heartburn, **pseudomembranous colitis** (rare). *GU:* increased BUN and serum creatinine, vaginitis. *Hemic:* increased serum AST (SGOT), ALT (SGPT), alkaline phosphatase. *Other:* Hypersensitivity: maculopapular rash, dermatitis, pruritus, fever.

## Nursing Implications:
*Assess:* Assess if previous allergy to penicillins or cephalosporins. Obtain cultures and sensitivity before treatment, but can start treatment before results. Baseline data for long-term therapy: BUN, creatinine, CBC, Hct, AST, ALT, and alkaline phosphatase.
*Administer: PO:* Suspension; refrigerate, shake well. Capsules may be taken apart and given with a small amount of food or fluid. May be given with food but food does decrease absorption time. Medication is expensive, use only for susceptible organisms.
*Monitor:* Observe for superinfections: black tongue, sore mouth, itching, loose stools, fever. Yogurt may maintain normal intestinal flora. Take for 10 days especially if given for **A β-hemolytic streptococcal infection**.
*Patient Teaching:* Take as scheduled and prescribed for full course of therapy. Observe for side effects. Store suspension in refrigerator. Reconstituted suspension should be discarded after 14 days if refrigerated.

## Laboratory Test Interference:
Gives false-positive for: direct Coombs' (may interfere with cross matching and other hematologic tests), and urine glucose by copper sulfate reduction (Clinitest, Benedict's reagent).

## Storage Requirements:
Store capsules at 15 to 30°C (59 to 86°F). Reconstituted suspension stable if refrigerated for 14 days; at room temperature for 7 days. Label suspension at time of reconstitution with date and time.

# □ CEFADROXIL                                    (sef-a-drox'ill)

(Duricef, Ultracef)

**Classification:** cephalosporin, first generation

## Available Preparations:
- 125, 250, 500 mg/5 ml suspensions
- 1-g tablets
- 500-mg capsules

**Action and Use:** Semisynthetic that renders cell wall osmotically unstable through cell-wall synthesis. Bactericidal action against A β-hemolytic *Streptococcus*, staphylococci, *Streptococcus*, *Escherichia coli*, *Proteus mirabilis*, and *Klebsiella*. Used to treat infections of the urinary tract, skin and adjacent structures and nasopharynx.

## Routes and Dosage:
*PO:* 30 mg/kg/day in divided doses every 12 hours

**Absorption and Fate:** Rapidly, completely absorbed from GI tract. Peak level, 1 to 2 hours. Half-life, 1.1 to 2 hours. 90% excreted unchanged in urine.

**Contraindications and Precautions:** Pregnancy category B. Use with caution during lactation. Contraindicated in hypersensitivity to this drug or cephalosporins. Use with caution if allergic to penicillins, allergy to other drugs, impaired renal function or history of GI disease, especially colitis.

## Side Effects:
*GI:* **pseudomembranous colitis,** nausea and vomiting. *GU:* pruritus, genital moniliasis, vaginitis. *Skin:* Hypersensitivity: rash, urticaria, angioedema. *Hemic:* transient neutropenia.

## Nursing Implications:
*Assess:* Assess if previous allergy to penicillins or cephalosporins. Obtain cultures and sensitivity before treatment, but can start treatment before results. Baseline data for long-term therapy: BUN, creatinine, CSC, Hct, AST, ALT, and alkaline phosphatase.
*Administer: PO:* Suspension; refrigerate and shake well. Capsules may be taken apart, given with a small amount of food or fluid. May be given with food or without food; if nausea occurs give with food or milk.
*Monitor:* Observe for superinfections: black tongue, sore mouth, itching, loose stools, fever. Yogurt (4 oz) daily may maintain normal intestinal flora. Take for 10 days especially if given for **A β-hemolytic streptococcal infection** to reduce incidence of rheumatic fever and glomerulonephritis.
*Patient Teaching:* Take as scheduled for full course of therapy. Observe for side effects. Store suspension in refrigerator out of reach of children. Reconstituted suspension should be discarded after 14 days if refrigerated.

**Laboratory Test Interference:** Gives false-positive: direct Coombs' (may interfere with cross-matching and other hematologic tests), and urine glucose by copper sulfate reduction (Clinitest, Benedict's reagent).

**Storage Requirements:** Store tablets and capsules at 15 to 30°C (59 to 86°F). Reconstituted suspension stable; refrigerated for 14 days, room temperature for 7 days. Label suspension at time of reconstitution with date and time.

---

□ **CEFAMANDOLE NAFATE**                    (sef-a-man'dole)

(Mandol)

**Classification:** cephalosporin, second generation

**Available Preparations:** 500 mg, 1, 2 g for parenteral administration

**Action and Use:** Inhibits mucopeptide synthesis in bacterial cell wall causing osmotic instability. Appears to have broader spectrum of activities than other cephalosporins against some gm− bacilli such as *Proteus, Enterobacter, Acinetobacter*, and *Haemophilus influenzae*.

**Routes and Dosage:**
*IM, IV:* Safe use in children under 1 month not established. However, some clinicians have recommended following dosage:
- birth to 1 week, <2000 g: 90 mg/kg/day in divided doses every 8 hours
- 1 to 4 weeks, >2000 g: 120 mg/kg/day in divided doses every 6 hours
- children over 1 month: 50 to 100 mg/kg/day in divided doses every 4 to 8 hours, depending on severity of infection. (Maximum dosage 12 g/day)

**Absorption and Fate:** Peak level: IM, 30 to 60 minutes; IV, end of infusion. Half-life, 1 to 1.5 hours. Bound to proteins; excreted unchanged in urine. Therapeutic level of 4 μg/ml for most gm+ species and 25 μg/ml for some *Enterobacter* and indole-positive *Proteus* species.

**Contraindications and Precautions:** Pregnancy category B. Excreted in breast milk, thus safety during lactation not established. Do not use in infants under 1 month old. Contraindicated if hypersensitive to drug or other cephalosporins. Use caution in sensitivity to penicillins, renal disease, or history of bleeding problems.

**Side Effects:**
*CNS:* headache, vertigo, paresthesia, weakness. *GI:* **pseudomembranous colitis**, nausea, vomiting, diarrhea, anorexia, abdominal cramps, thrush. *Hepatic:*

transient rise in SGOT, SGPT, and alkaline phosphatase levels. *GU:* elevated BUN, vaginitis, pruritus. *Hemic:* **thrombocytopenia** (rare), eosinophilia, hypoprothrombinemia, **bleeding**. *Other:* Hypersensitivity: maculopapular and erythematous rashes, urticaria, drug fever, dyspnea; Local: pain, induration, sterile abscesses, phlebitis and **thrombophlebitis** at IV site.

## Nursing Implications:

*Assess:* For previous allergy to cefamandole, cephalosporins, and penicillins. Obtain cultures and sensitivity before treatment, but can start treatment before results. Obtain baseline data on renal function.

*Administer:* Cefamandole powder discolors with exposure to light causing reconstituted solution to be light yellow to amber in color. Do not use if another color or has precipitate. *IM:* Reconstitute powder with 3 ml to 1 g of medication of either bacteriostatic or sterile water or 0.9% sodium chloride for injection. Powder can be difficult to dilute into solution; clumping of powder occurs when only surface of powder is hydrated. Invert vial, inject diluent above powder and quickly, vigorously shake vial. Less painful than cefoxitin; not given with lidocaine. After reconstitution, carbon dioxide develops inside vial during storage; pressure may be dissipated before withdrawal of contents, or it may be used to aid withdrawal if vial is inverted over the syringe needle and contents are allowed to flow into syringe. *IV:* Reconstitute with 10 ml sterile water, 0.9% sodium chloride, or 5% dextrose. Can be given IV push over 3 to 5 minutes. Intermittent infusion (perferred) with minimum dilution of 1 g/50 ml, infused over 30 to 60 minutes. Compatible with $D_5W$, $D_5W/NS$, $D_5W/0.5\%NS$, $D_5W/0.2\%NS$, $D_{10}/W$, NS, and others; check with pharmacists. Do not premix with other medications and infuse separately.

*Monitor:* Observe IV site for vein irritation, extravasation, and change site every 72 hours. Monitor child for hypersensitivity and side effects. Check for bruising and bleeding. Watch for symptoms of superinfection and diarrhea. Yogurt (4 oz) daily may maintain normal intestinal flora. If given for β-**hemolytic streptococcal infections**, 10-day therapy course needed to prevent risk of rheumatic fever and glomerulonephritis. Therapy course usually continued for 48 to 72 hours after symptoms subside.

## Drug Interactions: 
Cefamandole contains sodium bicarbonate making it incompatible in solutions containing magnesium or calcium ions. In combination with aminoglycosides, colistins, furosemides, probenecid, polymyxin B, sulfinpyrazone, vancomycin; nephrotoxicity may result. Aminoglycosides, chloramphenicol, and penicillins in combination with cefamandole may cause a synergistic effect with certain organisms. If combined with alcohol ingestion a disulfiram-like reaction may result. Alcohol should not be used for several day after ingestion of this drug.

## Laboratory Test Interferences: 
False-positive urine glucose by copper sulfate reductions (Clinitest or Benedict's reagent). Causes false-positive direct Coombs', which can interfere with cross-matching determinations.

## Storage Requirements: 
Store powder at 15 to 30°C (59 to 86°F), protect

from light. Reconstituted solution stable; room temperature for 24 hours, refrigerated for 96 hours.

---

# □ CEFAZOLIN SODIUM                                    (sef-a′zoe-lin)

(Ancef, Kefzol, Zolicef)

**Classification:** cephalosporin, first generation

**Available Preparations:** 250, 500 mg, 1, 5, and 10 g for parenteral administration

**Action and Use:** Semisynthetic that inhibits mucopeptide synthesis in bacterial cell wall; generally considered a broad-spectrum antibiotic active against most gm + bacteria (*Staphylococcus* and *Streptococcus*) and limited strains of gm − bacteria (e.g., *E coli, Haemophilus influenzae, Proteus, Klebsiella, Enterobacter*). Used to treat respiratory, biliary and GU tract, skin, bone and joint infections, as well as septicemias and endocarditis.

## Routes and Dosage:
*IM, IV:* Safe use in children under 1 month not established; however, some clinicians recommend:
- birth to 1 week: 40 mg/kg/day in equally divided doses every 12 hours;
- 1 to 4 weeks: 60 mg/kg/day in equally divided doses every 8 hours.
- over 1 month: 25 to 100 mg/kg/day in equal divided doses every 8 hours, 1.25 g/m²/day.

(Maximum dose 6 g-day)
Dosage adjustment necessary in renal function impairment

**Absorption and Fate:** Peak level: IM, 30 minutes; IV, 5 to 10 minutes after infusion. Half-life: 1.8 hours. Therapeutic level: 0.25 to 12.5 μg/ml. Bound to plasma proteins. Distributed in body fluids, tissues especially gallbladder, bile, and inflamed synovial membranes. Excreted unchanged into urine.

**Contraindications and Precautions:** Pregnancy category B. Use with caution during lactation. Contraindicated in hypersensitivity to this drug or cephalosporins. Use with caution if allergic to penicillins, allergy to other drugs, impaired renal function or history of GI disease, especially colitis.

## Side Effects:
*GI:* **pseudomembranous colitis**, anorexia, diarrhea, thrush, abdominal cramps, nausea and vomiting (rare). *GU:* transient rise BUN, SGOT, SGPT, and alkaline phosphatase without evidence of renal or hepatic involvement, pruritus, genital moniliasis, vaginitis. *Hemic:* transient neutropenia, leukopenia, **thrombocythemia**. *Other:* Hypersensitivity: drug fever, rash, pruritus,

**anaphylaxis**; Local: phlebitis at IV site (rare); pain, induration at IM site (rare).

## Nursing Implications:

*Assess:* For previous allergy to cefazolin, cephalosporins, and penicillins. Obtain cultures and sensitivity before treatment, but can start treatment before results. Obtain baseline data on renal function.

*Administer:* Reconstituted solution is pale to yellow color. Shake well, if solution has particulate matter discard. *IM:* Reconstitute powder according to package insert with sterile water. Injection usually not painful. *IV:* Reconstitute according to package inserts with sterile or bacteriostatic water, or 0.9% sodium chloride for bulk vials; single-dose vial, add sterile water. Can give slow IV push (75 to 100 mg/ml, varies with manufacturer, consult pharmacist) over 3 to 5 minutes. Intermittent infusion (preferred) with minimum dilution of 1 g/ 50 ml infused over 30 to 60 minutes. Compatible with $D_5W$, $D_5W/NS$, $D_5W/$ 0.5%NS, $D_5W/0.2\%NS$, $D_{10}/W$, NS, amino acid 4.25% dextrose 25%, normosol and lactated Ringer's. Do not premix with other medications and infuse separately.

*Monitor:* Observe IV site for vein irritation and extravasation; thrombophlebitis has occurred 36 to 48 hours after infusion. Monitor child for hypersensitivity and side effects. Watch for symptoms of superinfection and diarrhea (may indicate pseudomembranous colitis). Yogurt (4 oz) daily may maintain normal intestinal flora. If given for **A β-hemolytic streptococcal infections**, 10-day therapy course needed to prevent risk of rheumatic fever and glomerulonephritis. Therapy course usually continued for 48 to 72 hours after symptoms subside.

**Drug Interactions:** Probenecid in combination with cefazolin inhibits renal excretion of cephalosporin, thus prolonging serum levels. Aminoglycosides, chloramphenicol, and penicillins combined with cefazolin may cause synergistic effect with certain organisms.

**Laboratory Test Interferences:** False-positive urine glucose by copper sulfate reductions (Clinitest or Benedict's reagent). Causes false-positive direct Coombs' that can interfere with cross-matching determinations.

**Storage Requirements:** Store powder at 15 to 30°C (59 t 86°F), protect from light. Reconstituted solution stable; room temperature for 24 hours, 96 hours refrigerated. Store frozen preparation below −15°C, stable for 12 weeks.

---

# □ CEFOTAXIME SODIUM

(sef-oh-taks′eem)

(Claforan)

**Classification:** cephalosporin, third generation

**Available Preparations:** 1, 2, 10 g for parenteral administration

**Action and Use:** Semisynthetic cephalosporin that acts by inhibiting muco-peptide synthesis in bacterial cell wall causing osmotic instability. More active against wide range of gm − bacteria, such as *Citrobacter, Neisseria meningitidis, N. gonorrhoeae, Haemophilus influenzae, Shigella, Enterobacter aerogenes, Escherichia coli, Proteus mirabilis, Klebsiella*. Also active against some gram-positive strains (*e.g., Staphylococcus aureus, S. epidermidis, S. pyogenes, S. agalactiae, Streptococcus pneumoniae*). Used to treat infections of lower respiratory tract, skin, GU tract, bone, joint, and septicemias, gynecologic, CNS infections and gonococcal ophthalmic infections.

**Routes and Dosage:**
*IM, IV:*
- neonates, birth to 1 week: 50 to 100 mg/kg/day every 12 hours
- neonates, 1 to 4 weeks: 50 to 150 mg/kg/day every 8 hours
- infants 1 to 12 years, < 50 kg: 50 to 180 mg/kg/day in 4 to 6 equally divided doses
- children weighing over 50 kg: 1 to 2 g every 6 to 8 hours. (Maximum dose not to exceed 10 to 12 g daily)

Dosage adjustment needed for renal impairment

**Absorption and Fate:** Widely distributed to body fluids and tissues including CSF when meninges are inflamed. Peak levels: IM, 30 minutes; IV, 5 minutes after infusion. Half-life is 1 hour. Partially metabolized by the liver. Metabolites and drug excreted primarily in the urine by tubular secretion.

**Contraindications and Precautions:** Pregnancy category B. Use with caution during lactation. Contraindicated in hypersensitivity to this drug or cephalosporins. Use with caution in type I hypersensitivity to penicillins, allergy to other drugs, impaired renal function, or GI disease especially colitis.

**Side Effects:**
*CNS:* headache. *GI:* **pseudomembranous colitis**, diarrhea, nausea, vomiting. *Hepatic:* transient rise of SGPT, SGOT, serum LDH, serum alkaline phosphatase levels. *GU:* transient rise of BUN, moniliasis, vaginitis. *Skin:* maculopapular or erythematous rash, pruritus, fever. *Hemic:* **granulocytopenia**, transient eosinophilia, leukopenia, neutropenia, **thrombocytopenia**. *Other:* Hypersensitivity: **anaphylaxis**; Local: IV: site, inflammation; IM: pain, induration, tenderness at IM site (most frequent side effects).

**Nursing Implications:**
*Assess:* Assess if previous allergy to cefotaxime, penicillins, or cephalosporins. Obtain cultures and sensitivity before treatment, but can start treatment before results.
*Monitor:* Solution and powder tends to darken with exposure to light and heat. Color variance other than light yellow to amber may indicate loss in potency. *IM:* Reconstitute with either sterile or bacteriostatic water for injection. Injection painful. *IV:* Reconstitute according to package insert with sterile

bacteriostatic water, 0.9% sodium chloride, or 5% dextrose. Can give 1 g slow IV push over 3 to 5 minutes. Preferred route is intermittent infusion with minimum dilution of 1 g/50 ml infused over 30 to 60 minutes. Compatible with $D_5W$, $D_5W/NS$, $D_5W/0.5\%$ NS, $D_5W/0.2\%NS$, $D_{10}W$, NS, LR. Do not premix with other aminoglycosides aminophylline, sodium bicarbonate, or alkaline solutions. Use of large vein with small-bore needle may reduce local IV reactions.

***Monitor:*** Check IM site for induration. Observe IV site for vein irritation and extravasation, and change site every 72 hours. Monitor child for hypersensitivity and side effects. Watch for symptoms of superinfection or diarrhea (may indicate pseudomembranous colitis, which can occur 4 days to 6 weeks after drug discontinued). Yogurt (4 oz) daily may maintain normal intestinal flora. If given for **A β-hemolytic streptococcal infections**, 10-day therapy course needed to prevent risk of rheumatic fever and glomerulonephritis. Therapy course usually continued for 48 to 72 hours after symptoms subside.

**Drug Interactions:** Probenecid in combination with cefotaxime inhibits renal excretion of cephalosporin, thus prolonging serum levels. Aminoglycosides, chloramphenicol, and penicillins combined with cefotaxime may cause a synergistic effect with certain organisms.Concomitant administration aminoglycosides, potassium-depleting diuretics, and other cephalosporins may increase nephrotoxicity.

**Laboratory Test Interferences:** False-positive urine glucose by copper sulfate reductions (Clinitest or Benedict's reagent). Cause a false-positive direct Coombs' that can interfere with cross-matching determinations.

**Storage Requirements:** Store powder at 15 to 30°C (59 to 86°F), protect from heat and light. Reconstituted solution stable; 24 hours room temperature, 10 days if refrigerated. Reconstituted solutions with sterile water, 5% dextrose, and 0.9% sodium chloride are stable if frozen immediately in their original container for 13 weeks at −15°C.

---

## □ CEFOXITIN SODIUM                                    (se-fox'i-tin)

(Mefoxin)

**Classification:** cephalosporin, second generation

**Available Preparations:** 1, 2 g for parenteral administeration

**Action and Use:** Semisynthetic cephamycin that is pharmacologically related to cephalosporins. Active against both gram-positive bacteria (*Staphylococcus* and *Streptococcus*) and gm− bacteria (*Escherichia coli, Klebsiella, Proteus mirabilis*, indole-positive *Proteus, Haemophilus influenzae, Salmonella, Shigella, Providencia, Neisseria gonorrhoeae*, and some strains of *Serratia*).

Also active against *Bacteroides fragilis*. Treats infection caused by susceptible pathogens.

## Routes and Dosage:

*IM, IV:* Safe use in children under 3 months not established. However, some clinicians recommend 90–100 mg/kg/day in divided doses every 8 hours.
- over 3 months: 80 to 160 mg/kg/day in divided doses every 4 to 6 hours
  (Maximum dose should not exceed 160 mg/kg/day or 12 g/day)
- Perioperative Prophylaxis: over 3 months: 30 to 40 mg/kg 30 to 60 minutes preop, then same dosage every 6 hours for 24 hours.

**Absorption and Fate:** Peak level: IM, 1 hour; IV, end of infusion. Half-life is 0.8 hour. Widely distributed into body fluids (except cerebral spinal fluid) and tissues. Excreted in urine. Therapeutic levels: 8 to 16 μg/ml for most gram-positive and gram-negative bacteria; 16 to 32 μg/ml for bacteroides infection.

**Contraindications and Precautions:** Pregnancy category B. Excreted in breast milk; use caution during lactation. Do not use if infant under 3 months old. Contraindicated if hypersensitive to drug or other cephalosporins. Use caution in sensitivity to penicillins, allergy to other drugs, renal disease, or history of GI disease.

## Side Effects:

*CV:* hypotension. *GI:* **pseudomembranous colitis**, nausea, vomiting, diarrhea (rare). *GU:* elevated BUN, vaginitis, pruritus. *Hemic:* **eosinophilia**, transient leukopenia, granulocytopenia, **thrombocytopenia**, **anemia**. *Hepatic:* transient rise in SGOT, SGPT, serum LDH, and alkaline phosphatas levels. *Other:* Hypersensitivity: maculopapular and erythematous rashes, exfoliative dermatitis, urticaria, drug fever, **anaphylaxis** (rare); Local: IV: pain, tenderness, induration, phlebitis, **thrombophlebitis**.

## Nursing Implications:

*Assess:* For previous allergy to cefoxitin, cephalosporins, and penicillins. Obtain cultures and sensitivity before treatment, but can start treatment before results. Obtain baseline data on renal function; dosages are altered with renal impairment.

*Administer:* Powder and solutions may darken; this usually does not effect potency. Do not use if it has precipitate. Do not reconstitute with bacteriostatic water if used for infants; the benzyl alcohol preservative has been associated with toxicity (especially if large dosage used). *IM:* Reconstitute powder with either bacteriostatic or sterile water, 0.9% sodium chloride, 5% dextrose, or 0.5% or 1% lidocaine hydrochloride (without epinephrine) for injection. Lidocaine decreases pain at injection site. Shake vial well after addition of diluent and solution will clear upon standing. *IV:* Reconstitute with sterile water for injection. Can be given IV push over 3 to 5 minutes or by intermittent infusion (preferred). Minimum dilution is 1 g/50 ml. Infuse over 30 to 60 minutes. Compatible with $D_5W$, $D_5W/NS$, $D_5W/0.5\%NS$, $D_5W/0.2\%NS$, $D_{10}/W$, NS, LR and others; check with pharmacists. Do not premix with other aminoglycosides, cephalosporins, penicillins, or alkaline solutions in same Volutrol or bag; infuse separately.

*Monitor:* Observe IM site for induration and IV site for vein irritation, extravasation, and change site every 72 hours. Monitor child for hypersensitivity and side effects. Check for bruising and bleeding. Watch for symptoms of superinfection; yogurt (4 oz) daily may maintain normal intestinal flora. If given for **A β-hemolytic streptococcal infections**, 10-day therapy course prevents risk of rheumatic fever or glomerulonephritis. Therapy course usually continued for 48 to 72 hours after symptoms subside. Cefoxitin contains sodium that may effect sodium restrictions.

**Drug Interactions:** Cefoxitin contains sodium bicarbonate making incompatible in solutions containing magnesium or calcium ions. In combination with aminoglycosides, colistins, furosemides, probenecid, polymyxin B, sulfinpyrazone, vancomycin; nephrotoxicity may result. Aminoglycosides, chloramphenicol, and penicillins in combination with cefoxitin may cause a synergistic effect with certain organisms.

**Laboratory Test Interferences:** False-positive urine glucose by copper sulfate reductions (Clinitest or Benedict's reagent). Cause false-positive direct Coombs' that can interfere with cross-matching determinations. Jaffe creatinine reaction test may indicate falsely elevated serum or urine creatinine in concentrations 100 μg/ml 2 hours after cefoxitin dosage.

**Storage Requirements:** Store powder at 15 to 30°C (59 to 86°F), protect from temperatures above 50°C. Reconstituted solution stable; room temperature 24 hours, 1 week if refrigerated, frozen preparations 30 weeks at −20°C.

---

□ **CEFTAZIDIME**                                          (sef'tay-zi-deem)

(Fortaz, Tazicef, Tazidime)

**Classification:** cephalosporin, third generation

**Available Preparations:** 500 mg, 1, 2, 6 g for parenteral administration

**Action and Use:** Semisynthetic cephalosporin that acts by inhibiting mucopeptide synthesis in bacterial cell wall causing osmotic instability. More active against wide range of gm − bacteria, such as *Citrobacter, Neisseria meningitidis, N. gonorrhoeae, Haemophilus influenzae, Shigella, Enterobacter aerogenes, Escherichia coli, P. mirabilis,* and *Klebsiella.* More active than other cephalosporins against *Pseudomonas aeruginosa.* Also active against some gm + strains (*e.g., Staphylococcus aureus, S. epidermidis, Streptococcus pneumoniae*). Used to treat infections of lower respiratory tract, skin, intraabdominal area, GU tract, bone, joint, and septicemias, gynecologic, and meningitis.

## Routes and Dosage:
*IM, IV:*
- neonates up to 4 weeks: 30 mg/kg (IV) every 12 hours; however, some clinicians recommend neonates < 7 days (< 2000 g): 30–50 mg/kg (IV) every 12 hours, and neonates > 7 days (> 2000 g): 30 mg/kg (IV) every 8 hours
- infants 1 month to 12 years: 30 to 50 mg/kg every 8 hours
- 12 years and older: 1 g every 8 to 12 hours

Do not exceed 6 g/day

**Absorption and Fate:** Widely distributed to body fluids, tissues, including CSF when meninges are inflamed. Peak levels: IM, dosage 1 hour; IV, 0.5 minutes following infusion. Half-life: neonates, 2.2 to 4.7 hours; infants 2 to 12 months, 2 hours; children, 1.9 to 2 hours. Partially metabolized. 80 to 90% excreted unchanged in urine by glomerular filtration.

**Contraindications and Precautions:** Pregnancy category B. Use with caution during lactation. Contraindicated in hypersensitivity to this drug or cephalosporins. Us with caution if allergic to penicillins, allergy to other drugs, impaired renal function, or GI disease especially colitis.

## Side Effects:
*CNS:* headache, vertigo, paresthesia. *GI:* diarrhea, nausea, vomiting, abdominal pain, **pseudomembranous colitis**. *Hepatic:* transient rise of SGPT, SGOT, serum LDH, GGT, and serum alkaline phosphatase levels. *GU:* transient rise of BUN and serum creatinine, candidiasis, vaginitis. *Skin:* maculopapular or erythematous rash, pruritus, fever. *Hemic:* eosinophilia, transient leukopenia, neutropenia, **thrombocytopenia**, lymphocytosis. *Other:* Hypersensitivity: **anaphylaxis**; Local: inflammation and phlebitis at IV site and pain, induration and tenderness at IM site.

## Nursing Implications:
*Assess:* For previous allergy to ceftazidime, penicillins, or cephalosporins. Obtain cultures and sensitivity before treatment, but can start treatment before results.

*Administer:* Mixing powder and diluent generates carbon dioxide. To release pressure build-up, follow package insert instructions and when withdrawing fluid keep needle below fluid levels of inverted vial. *IM:* Reconstitute with either sterile or bacteriostatic water or 0.5 or 1% lidocaine hydrochloride for injection. Injection moderately painful lasting for 2 to 5 minutes and subsiding within 10 to 20 minutes. *IV:* Reconstitute with sterile water, 0.9% sodium chloride, or 5% dextrose. Can give slow IV push over 3 to 5 minutes. Consult with pharmacist for dilution ratios. Preferred route is intermittent infusion over 30 minutes. Compatible with $D_5W$, $D_5W/NS$, $D_5W/0.5\%$ NS, $D_5W/0.2\%NS$, $D_{10}W$, NS, LR. Less stable in sodium bicarbonate solutions. Do not premix with other aminoglycosides and other bacteriostatic agents. Use of large vein with small-bore needle may reduce local IV reactions.

*Monitor:* Check IM site for induration. Observe IV site for vein irritation and extravasation and change site every 72 hours. Monitor child for hypersensitivity and side effects. Watch for symptoms of superinfection or diarrhea (may indicate pseudomembranous colitis, which can occur 4 days to 6 weeks after drug discontinued). Yogurt (4 oz) daily may maintain normal intestinal flora. If given for **A β-hemolytic streptococcal infections**, 10-day therapy course needed to prevent risk of rheumatic fever and glomerulonephritis. Therapy course usually continued for 48 to 72 hours after symptoms subside.

**Drug Interactions:** Probenecid in combination with ceftazidime inhibits renal excretion of cephalosporin thus prolonging serum levels. Concomitant administration aminoglycosides, potassium-depleting diuretics, and other cephalosporins may increase nephrotoxicity.

**Laboratory Test Inferferences:** False-positive urine glucose by copper sulfate reductions (Clinitest or Benedict's reagent). Causes false-positive direct Coombs' that can interfere with cross-matching determinations.

**Storage Requirements:** Store powder at 15 to 30°C (59 to 86°F), protect from light. Reconstituted solution stable; room temperature for 18 hours, 7 days refrigerated. Reconstituted solutions with sterile water, 5% dextrose, and 0.9% sodium chloride are stable if frozen immediately in their original container for 3 months at −20°C.

---

□ **CEFTIZOXIME**          (sef-ti-zox'eem)
   **SODIUM**

(Cefizox)

**Classification:** cephalosporin, third generation

**Available Preparations:** 1, 2, 10 g for parenteral administration

**Action and Use:** Semisynthetic cephalosporin that acts by inhibiting mucopeptide synthesis in bacterial cell wall causing osmotic instability. More active against wide range of gm − bacteria, such as *Citrobacter, Neisseria meningitidis, N. gonorrhoeae, Haemophilus influenzae, Shigella, Enterobacter aerogenes, Escherichia coli, P. mirabilis, Klebsiella, Serratia,* and *Pseudomonas aeruginosa.* Also active against some gm + strains (*e.g., Staphylococcus aureus, S. epidermidis, Streptococcus pneumoniae*). Used to treat infections of lower respiratory tract, skin, intraabdominal area, GU tract, bone, joint, and septicemias, gynecologic, and meningitis.

**Routes and Dosage:**
*IM, IV:* Not recommended for neonates and infants under 6 months
- over 6 months: 150 to 200 mg/kg/day in divided doses every 6 to 8 hours

(Dosage should not exceed 12 g daily or 200 mg/kg)

**Absorption and Fate:** Widely distributed to body fluids, tissues, CSF especially when meninges ars inflamed. Peak levels: IM, 1 hour; IV, 10 minutes after infusion. Half-life: 1.7 hours. 30 % protein bound; excreted unchanged in urine.

**Contraindications and Precautions:** Pregnancy category B. Use with caution during lactation. Manufacturer does not recommend usage in children under 6 months. Contraindicated in hypersensitivity to this drug or cephalosporins. Use with caution if allergic to penicillins, in allergy to other drugs, impaired renal function, or GI disease especially colitis.

**Side Effects:**
*CNS:* headache, vertigo, tinnitus. *GI:* diarrhea, nausea, vomiting, **pseudomembranous colitis**. *Hepatic:* transient rise of SGOT, SGPT, serum creatine phosphokinase (may be related to IM injection of drug), serum alkaline phosphatase levels, bilirubin. *GU:* transient rise of BUN and serum creatinine, vaginitis (rarely). *Skin:* rash, pruritus, fever. *Hemic:* transient eosinophilia, anemia, leukopenia, neutropenia, thrombocytopenia. *Other:* Hypersensitivity: numbness (rarely), **anaphylaxis**; Local: IV: burning, cellulitis, phlebitis; IM: pain, induration, paresthesia, tenderness.

**Nursing Implications:**
*Assess:* Assess if previous allergy to ceftizoxime, penicillins, or cephalosporins. Obtain cultures and sensitivity before treatment, but can start treatment before results.
*Administer:* Clear to pale yellow upon reconstitution but darkening upon storage to amber, does not effect potency. *IM:* Reconstitute with either sterile water. Injection may burn. *IV:* Reconstitute with sterile water, 0.9% sodium chloride, or 5% dextrose according to package inserts. For IV push, give undiluted reconstitute slowly; IV push, 3 to 5 minutes. The preferred route is intermittent infusion over 30 minutes. For dilution levels and compatible fluids consult pharmacist. Do not premix with other drugs. Use of large vein with small-bore needle may reduce local IV reactions.
*Monitor:* See ceftazidime.

**Drug Interactions:** Probenecid in combination with ceftizoxime inhibits renal excretion of cephalosporin, thus prolonging serum levels. Concomitant administration aminoglycosides, potassium-depleting diuretics, and other cephalosporins may increase nephrotoxicity.

**Laboratory Test Interferences:** A false-positive direct Coombs' can interfere with cross-matching determinations.

**Storage Requirements:** Store powder at 15 to 30°C (59 to 86°F), protect from light. Reconstituted solution stable at room temperature for 8 hours and 48 days if refrigerated. Frozen preparations are stable for 18 months at −20°C.

## ☐ CEFTRIAXONE SODIUM

(sef-try-ax'one)

(Rocephin)

**Classification:** cephalosporin, third generation

**Available Preparations:** 250, 500 mg, 1, 2, 10 g for parenteral administration

**Action and Use:** Semisynthetic cephalosporin that acts by inhibiting mucopeptide synthesis in bacterial cell wall causing osmotic instability. More active against wide range of gm − bacteria, such as *Citrobacter, Neisseria meningitidis, N. gonorrhoeae, Haemophilus influenzae, Shigella, Enterobacter aerogenes, Escherichia coli, P. mirabilis, Klebsiella, Serratia,* and *Pseudomonas aeruginosa.* Also active against some gm+ strains (*e.g., Staphylococcus aureus, S. pyogenes, Streptococcus pneumoniae*). Used to treat infections of lower respiratory tract, skin, intraabdominal area, GU tract, bone, joint, and septicemias, uncomplicated gonorrhea, pelvic inflammatory disease, and meningitis.

**Routes and Dosage:**
*IM, IV:*
- neonates: 50 mg/kg/day as single dose
- infants, children: 50 to 75 mg/kg/day in equally divided doses every 12 hours. (Dosage not to exceed 2 g/day)
- over 12 years: 1 to 2 g daily or in equally divided doses every 12 hours. (Dosage not to exceed 4 g/day)

Meningitis:
- neonates to 12 years: Loading Dose: 75 to 100 mg/kg once, then 100 mg/kg/day in equally divided doses every 12 hours

Prophylaxis for infants of mothers with peripartum gonococcal infections:
- Single dose 50 mg/kg IM given or IV at birth (125 mg maximum dose)

**Absorption and Fate:** Widely distributed to body fluids, tissues, CSF especially when meninges are inflamed. Peak levels: IV, concentrations vary from about 30 to 60 minutes in infants to about 30 minutes in older children; IM, 2 hours. Half-life: 16.2 hours in neonates; 9.2 hours in infants under 1 month; 6 to 9 hours in older children. Primarily excreted unchanged in urine and 1/3 is excreted in feces.

**Contraindications and Precautions:** Pregnancy category B. Use with caution during lactation. Contraindicated in hypersensitivity to this drug or cephalosporins. Use with caution if allergic to penicillins, in allergy to other drugs, impaired renal or hepatic function, malnutrition, impaired vitamin K synthesis, or GI disease especially colitis.

## Side Effects:

*CNS:* headache, vertigo. *GI:* diarrhea, nausea, vomiting, dysgeusia, **pseudomembranous colitis**. *GU:* transient rise of BUN and serum creatinine, casts in urine, moniliasis or vaginitis. *Hemic:* eosinophilia, thrombocytosis, leukopenia, **anemia**, neutropenia, **thrombocytopenia, prolongation of prothrombin time** (rare). *Hepatic:* transient rise of SGOT, SGPT, and less frequently rise in serum alkaline phosphatase levels, bilirubin. *Skin:* rash, pruritus, fever. *Other:* Hypersensitivity: fever and chills, **anaphylaxis**; Local: **Phlebitis at IV site**; IM: pain, induration, tenderness at site.

## Nursing Implications:

*Assess:* Assess if previous allergy to ceftriaxone, penicillins, or cephalosporins. Obtain cultures and sensitivity before treatment, but can start treatment before results.

*Administer: IM:* Reconstitute with either sterile or bacteriostatic water, 0.9% sodium chloride, 5% dextrose, or 1% lidocaine hydrochloride (without epinephrine) for injection. Injection painful. Do not use bacteriostatic water with benzyl alcohol for reconstitution in neonates. *IV:* Reconstitute according to package insert with compatible IV fluid. Intermittent infusion is infused over 10 to 30 minutes in recommended concentrations of 10 to 40 mg/ml compatible with $D_5W$, $D_{10}W$, $D_5W/0.5\%$ NS, $D_5W/NS$, NS. Do not premix with other aminoglycosides and other bacteriostatic agents. Use of large vein with small-bore needle may reduce local IV reactions.

*Monitor:* Check IM site for induration. Observe IV site for vein irritation and extravasation, and change site every 72 hours. Monitor child for hypersensitivity and side effects. Watch for symptoms of superinfection or diarrhea (may indicate pseudomembranous colitis, which can occur 4 days to 6 weeks after drug discontinued). Yogurt (4 oz) daily may maintain normal intestinal flora. Watch for symptoms of bleeding due to possible prolonged bleeding time especially in malnutrition, children on anticoagulants, and other susceptible patients. If given for A β-**hemolytic streptococcal infections**, 10-day therapy course needed to prevent risk of rheumatic fever and glomerulonephritis. Therapy course usually is from 4 to 14 days.

**Drug Interactions:** Probenecid in combination with ceftriaxone inhibits renal excretion of cephalosporin thus prolonging serum levels. Concomitant administration aminoglycosides, potassium-depleting diuretics, and other cephalosporins may increase nephrotoxicity.

**Laboratory Test Interferences:** False-positive urine glucose by copper sulfate reductions (Clinitest or Bendict's reagent).

**Storage Requirements:** Store powder at 15 to 30°C (59 to 86°F), protect from light. Reconstituted solution stability is dependent on diluent used, check package inserts for this information.

# □ CEFUROXIME AXETIL, GLAXO

(se-fyoor-ox'eem)

(Ceftin, Zinnat)

**Classification:** cephalosporin, second generation

**Available Preparations:** 125, 250, 500-mg film-coated tablets

**Action and Use:** Ethyl ester of cefuroxime, a cephalosporin that acts by inhibiting mucopeptide synthesis in bacterial cell wall causing osmotic instability. More active against gram-negative bacteria, especially *Branhamella catarrhalis, Citrobacter* sp, *Enterobacter* sp, *Haemophilus influenzae*; including some that are resistant to other penicillins and cephalosporins. This is in part because of its resistance to hydrolysis of β-lactamases. Also active against some gram-positive strains. Used to treat pharyngitis, tonsillitis, otitis media, bronchitis, URI, skin, and soft tissue infections.

## Routes and Dosage:
*PO:*
- infants to 12 years: 125 mg every 12 hours

Otitis Media:
- under 2 years: 125 mg every 12 hours;
- over 2 years: 250 mg every 12 hours
- over 12 years: 250 mg twice a day; for severe infections dosage may be increased to 500 mg twice a day

**Absorption and Fate:** Rapidly absorbed from GI tract. Half-life, 1.2 hours. 50% bound to plasm proteins. Excreted unchanged in urine.

**Contraindications and Precautions:** Pregnancy category B. Excreted in breast milk; do not use during lactation. Contraindicated if hypersensitive to drug or other cephalosporins. Use caution if sensitivity to penicillins, allergy to other drugs, renal disease, or history of GI disease

## Side Effects:
*CNS:* headache, dizziness. *GI:* diarrhea, nausea, vomiting, **pseudomembranous colitis** (rare). *Hepatic:* transient rise in SGOT, SGPT, LDH. *GU:* vaginitis, pruritus. *Hemic:* eosinophilia, positive Coombs' test. *Other:* Hypersensitivity: rash, pruritus, urticaria, **severe bronchospasms** (rare).

## Nursing Implications:
*Assess:* For previous allergy to cefuroxime, cephalosporins, and penicillins. Obtain cultures and sensitivity before treatment, but can start treatment before results. Obtain baseline data on renal function.
*Administer: PO:* May be given without regard to meals but absorption is

increased when given with food. Tablet may be crushed and mixed with small amounts of food or fluid. It is best, however, if child can swallow tablet whole, due to fact tablet has a very bitter taste. Have child suck on ice or flavored ice treat before taking. Follow with fluids of child's choice to remove taste from mouth. Liquid form should be available in near future.

*Monitor:* Monitor child for hypersensitivity and side effects. Watch for symptoms of superinfection and diarrhea. Yogurt (4 oz) daily may maintain normal intestinal flora. If diarrhea occurs assess for pseudomembranous colitis. If given for **A β-hemolytic streptococcal infections**, 10-day therapy course needed to prevent risk of rheumatic fever and glomerulonephritis.

## Laboratory Test Interferences: 
False-positive urine glucose by copper sulfate reductions (Clinitest or Benedict's reagent). Causes false-positive direct Coombs' that can interfere with cross-matching determinations.

## Storage Requirements: 
Store powder at 15 to 30°C (59 to 86°F), protect from moisture.

---

# □ CEFUROXIME SODIUM

(se-fyoor-ox'eem)

(Kefurox, Zinacef)

**Classification:** cephalosporin, second generation

**Available Preparations:** 750 mg, 1.5, 7.5 g for parenteral administeration

**Action and Use:** Semisynthetic, methoxyamino group, cephalosporin that acts by inhibiting mucopeptide synthesis in bacterial cell wall causing osmotic instability. More active against gm− bacteria because of its resistance to hydrolysis of β-lactamases. Also active against some gm + strains. Used to treat infections of lower respiratory tract, skin, GU tract, bone, joint, and septicemias, meningitis. Used perioperatively for open heart surgical patients.

## Routes and Dosage:
*IM, IV:*
- Under 3 months: safe use not established, however, some clinicians recommend neonates receive 10 mg/kg every 12 hours
- over 3 months: 50 to 100 mg/kg/day in divided doses every 6 to 8 hours

Meningitis:
- 200 to 240 mg/kg/day in divided doses every 6 to 8 hours; until improvement then 100 mg/kg/day

Dosage altered for renal impairment

**Absorption and Fate:** Peak level: IM, 15 to 60 minutes; IV, 15 minutes after end of infusion. Half-life: 80 minutes but it is inversely proportional to age. 33 to 50% bound to proteins and widely distributed to body tissues and fluids. Drug absorption into cerebral spinal fluid at higher levels when meninges are inflamed. Not metabolized and excreted unchanged in urine.

**Contraindications and Precautions:** Pregnancy category B. Excreted in breast milk; use caution during lactation. Do not use if infant under 3 months old. Contraindicated if hypersensitive to drug or other cephalosporins. Use caution in sensitivity to penicillins, allergy to other drugs, renal disease, or history of GI disease

**Side Effects:**
*GI:* nausea, vomiting, diarrhea, **pseudomembranous colitis** (rare). *Hepatic:* transient rise in SGOT, SGPT, LDH, alkaline phosphatase levels, bilirubin. *GU:* elevated serum creatinine, BUN; decrease in creatinine clearance (relationship unknown); vaginitis, pruritus. *Hemic:* decreased hemoglobin and hematocrit, transient eosinophilia, transient neutropenia and leukopenia. *Other:* Hypersensitivity: maculopapular and erythematous rashes, urticaria, **drug fever, dyspnea**; Local: IM: pain mild to moderate usually lasting 5 minutes, induration, sterile abscesses, temperature elevations, **tissue sloughing**; IV: **thrombophlebitis, phlebitis**.

**Nursing Implications:**
*Assess:* For previous allergy to cefuroxime, cephalosporins, and penicillins. Obtain cultures and sensitivity before treatment, but can start treatment before results. Obtain baseline data on renal function.
*Administer:* Reconstituted solution is light yellow to amber color due to diluent and concentration. Powder and solution may darken with storage; does not appear to affect potency. IM: Reconstitute powder with sterile water; it results in a thick suspension. Injection painful for about 5 minutes afterward. *IV:* Reconstitute according to package inserts with sterile water, 0.9% sodium chloride, or 5% dextrose. Can be given slow IV push 1 g over 3 to 5 minutes. Intermittent infusion (perferred), minimum dilution is 1.5 g/5O ml infused over 30 to 60 minutes. Compatible with $D_5W$, $D_5W/NS$, $D_5W/0.5\%NS$, $D_5W/0.2\%NS$, $D_{10}/W$, NS, lactated Ringer's and Ringer's. Do not premix with other medications and infuse separately.
*Monitor:* Observe IM site for induration and sterile abscesses. IV site for vein irritation, extravasation, and change site every 72 hours. Cefuroxime contains sodium may affect child if on sodium restrictions. Therapy course usually continued for 48 to 72 hours after symptoms subside. (See Defuroxime axetil, Monitor under *Nursing Implications*.)

**Drug Interactions:** Cefuroxime contains sodium bicarbonate making incompatible in solutions containing magnesium or calcium ions. In combination with aminoglycosides, colistins, potassium-depleting diuretics, e.g., furosemides, probenecid, polymyxin B, sulfinpyrazone, vancomycin; nephrotoxicity may result. Aminoglycosides, chloramphenicol, and penicillins in combination with cefuroxime may cause a synergistic effect with certain organisms.

**Laboratory Test Interferences:** See Cefuroxime axetil.

**Storage Requirements:** Store powder at 15 to 30°C (59 to 86°F), protect from light. Reconstituted solution stable room temperature for 24 hours and 48 hours if refrigerated. Store frozen preparation below −20°C.

---

# □ CEPHALEXIN HYDROCHLORIDE

(sef-a-lex′in)

(Cefanex, Ceporex, Keflet, Keflex, Novolexin)

**Classification:** cephalosporin, first generation

## Available Preparations:
- 100 mg/ml; 125, 250 mg/5 ml
- 250 mg, 500 mg, 1-g tablets
- 250, 500-mg capsules

**Action and Use:** Semisynthetic that inhibits mucopeptide synthesis in bacterial cell wall; generally considered a broad-spectrum antibiotic active against most gram-positive bacteria (*Staphylococcus* and *Streptococcus*) and limited strains of gram-negative bacteria (e.g., *Escherichia coli, Haemophilus influenzae, Proteus, Klebsiella, Enterobacter*). Used to treat infections of respiratory and GU tract, skin, bone, and middle ear.

## Routes and Dosage:
*PO:* 25 to 50 mg/kg/day in 3 to 4 divided doses or 0.75–1.5 g/m²/day in 4 divided doses. (Maximum dosage 3 g/day)
Otitis Media: 75–100 mg/kg/day in 4 divided doses.
Reduced dosage in renal impairment

**Absorption and Fate:** Rapidly and completely absorbed from GI tract but neonates absorption may be delayed up to 50% of that of older children and adults. Peak levels: infants under 6 months, 3 hours; infants 9 to 12 months, 2 hours; older children, 1 hour. Half-life: neonates, 5 hours; infants 3 to 12 months, 2.5 hours; older children, 30 to 90 minutes. Therapeutic level: 2 to 8 μg/ml. Excreted unchanged in urine.

**Contraindications and Precautions:** Pregnancy category B. Excreted in breast milk; use with caution during lactation. Contraindicated in hypersensitivity to this drug or cephalosporins. Use with caution if allergic to penicillins, in allergy to other drugs, impaired renal function and GI disease especially colitis.

## Side Effects:
*CNS:* vertigo, fatigue, headache. *GI:* diarrhea, abdominal pain, **pseudomembranous colitis**, nausea, vomiting. *Hepatic:* slight elevations SGOT, and SGPT. *GU:* pruritus, genital moniliasis, vaginitis, vaginal discharge. *Skin:* hypersensitivity: rash, urticaria, angioedema. *Hemic:* eosinophilia, neutropenia. *Other:* Hypersensitivity: **Anaphylaxis**.

## Nursing Implications:
*Assess:* Assess if previous allergy to cephalexin, penicillins, or cephalosporins. Obtain cultures and sensitivity before treatment, but can start treatment before results. Baseline data for long-term therapy: BUN, creatinine, CBC, Hct, AST, ALT, and alkaline phosphatase.

*Administer: PO:* Suspension: refrigerate and shake well. Capsules may be taken apart or tablet crushed, given with a small amount of food or fluid. May be given with food or without food, if nausea occurs give with food or milk.

*Monitor:* Observe for superinfections: black tongue, sore month, itching, loose stools, fever. Yogurt (4 oz) daily may maintain normal intestinal flora. Take for 10 days especially if given for A β-hemolytic streptococcal infection to reduce incidence of rheumatic fever and glomerulonephritis.

*Patient Teaching:* Take as scheduled and prescribed for full course of therapy. Observe for side effects. Store suspension in refrigerator. Reconstituted suspension should be discarded after 14 days if refrigerated.

**Drug Interactions:** Probenecid in combination with cephalexin inhibits renal excretion of cephalosporin thus prolonging serum levels.

**Laboratory Test Interference:** Gives false-positive direct Coombs' (may interfere with cross-matching and other hematologic tests),and urine glucose by copper sulfate reduction (Clinitest, Benedict's reagent)

**Storage Requirements:** Store tablets and capsules at 15 to 30°C (59 to 86°F). Reconstituted suspension stable for 14 days refrigerated, 7 days at room temperature. Label suspension at time of reconstitution with date and time.

---

# □ CHLORAL HYDRATE                    (klor'al hye'drate)

(Aquachloral, Noctec)

## Classification: sedative, hypnotic

## Available Preparations:
- 250, 500-mg capsules
- 250, 500 mg/5 ml syrup

- crystals
- 325, 500, 650-mg suppositories

## Action and Use:
Central nervous system depressant creates deep sleep by a mechanism not fully described. Used to treat insomnia. Major uses in children include preoperatively to reduce anxiety and produce sedation, postoperatively in conjunction with analgesics, and to produce sedation for tests such as EEG, CT scan, MRI, and for some dental work.

## Routes and Dosages:
*PO, PR:*
- Hypnotic: 50 mg/kg *or* 1.5 g/m$^2$; not to exceed 1 g/dose
- Sedative: 8.3 mg/kg *or* 250 mg/m$^2$ TID; not to exceed 500 mg TID
- EEG Premedication Sedation: 20 to 25 mg/kg

## Absorption and Fate:
Absorbed rapidly from both oral and rectal routes. Distributed widely in body tissues but only small amounts present in breast milk. Metabolized by the liver to trichloroethanol, which is an active metabolite, causing drug effects. Slowly excreted primarily in the urine. Onset of action in 30 minutes; peak level in 20 to 60 minutes; sleep occurs in 30 to 60 minutes and lasts 4 to 8 hours. Half-life is 8 to 11 hours. Therapeutic level is 7 to 10 μg/ml.

## Contraindications and Precautions:
Pregnancy category C. Crosses placenta; effects on fetus unknown. May lead to withdrawal in infant if pregnant mother on chronic use. Contraindicated in those with prior hypersensitivity to the drug, persons with hepatic or renal dysfunction, and those with inflammation or ulcers of GI tract. Cautious use in those with cardiac disease, porphyria, depression, drug abuse, and in lactating women. Rectal form may irritate mucosa, especially of those with colitis.

## Side Effects:
*CNS:* continued sedation, disorientation, paranoia, paradoxical excitement, dizziness, headache, gait disturbance. *CV:* cardiac arrhythmia with overdose, bradycardia. *GI:* nausea, vomiting, diarrhea, stomach pain, flatulence; gastritis and GI hemorrhage with overdose. *Respiratory:* respiratory depression with overdose. *Hepatic:* jaundice with overdose. *GU:* porphyria, rare ketonuria; albuminuria with overdose. *Skin:* rash, urticaria, purpura, eczema (all uncommon). *Hemic:* leukopenia, eosinophilia. *Other:* chronic overdose causes drowsiness, lethargy, speech slurring, incoordination, nystagmus; acute overdose causes hypotension, muscle weakness, arrhythmia, vomiting, renal and hepatic dysfunction, coma.

## Nursing Implications:
*Assess:* Establish baseline vital signs. Take history of other drugs. Obtain history of gastric or anal problems.
*Administer:* Schedule IV drug in Federal Controlled Substances Act. Avoid contact with skin. Administer PO form with a meal or snack, to decrease

gastric distress. Check anal area for tissue irritation before PR administration. Put side rails of bed up after administration and take any dangerous materials (machines, cigarettes) away from patient.

*Monitor:* Observe patient for onset of sleep. Watch for drug side effects. If patient continues on drug be observant for signs of chronic overdose or lessening effects. Habituation requiring increasingly larger doses can occur. Withdrawal from the drug for the person with chronic use often requires hospitalization.

*Patient Teaching:* Drug can alter mental alertness, therefore avoid driving and adjust other activities accordingly. Take drug with food to decrease gastric irritation. Avoid alcohol, street drugs, or other medications unless ordered by physician. Continued use can be habit-forming; see health-care provider regularly.

**Drug Interactions:** Other CNS depressants, such as alcohol, barbiturates, tranquilizers, cause additive CNS depression. When given with IV furosemide, diaphoresis, flushing, and alteration in blood pressure, particularly hypertension can occur. When given with oral anticoagulant, namely warfarin, hypoprothrombinemia can occur.

**Laboratory Test Interferences:** False-positive urine glucose by some tests (Clinistix; Tes-Tape not affected). Alters fluorometric test results for urine catecholamines (do not give chloral hydrate for 48 hours before the test) and urine 17-hydroxycorticosteroids. Causes false-positive phentolamine test.

**Storage Requirements:** Store at 15 to 30°C (59 to 86°F) in tightly covered, light-resistant containers.

---

☐ **CHLORAMPHENICOL,**                    (klor-am-fen'i-kole)
**CHLORAMPHENICOL**
**PALITATE,**
**CHLORAMPHENICOL**
**SODIUM SUCCINATE**

(Ak-Chlor, Chlorofair, Chloromycetin, Chloroptic, Chloroptic, S.O.P, Fenicol, Isopto Fenicol, Mychel, Novochlorocap, Ophthochlor, Pentamycetin)

**Classification:** antiinfective, antibiotic

**Available Preparations:**
- 150 mg/5ml oral suspension
- 250-mg capsules
- 1 g for parenteral administration
- 0.25%, 0.5% ophthalmic solution and 0.1% ophthalmic ointment
- 0.5% otic solution

■ 1% topical cream

**Action and Use:** Inhibits ribosomal protein synthesis by binding to 50S ribosomal subunit inhibiting peptide bond formation. Considered a broad-spectrum antibiotic. Has no activity against fungus, yeast, viruses, protozoa, or *Pseudomonas*. Only used in treatment of serious infections, e.g., *Rickettsia*, *Haemophilus influenzae*, *Chlamydia*, *Salmonella typhi*, when less toxic drugs are ineffective.

## Routes and Dosage:
*PO, IV:*
Loading Dose: 20 mg/kg/dose times one
Maintenance:
  ■ prematures: 10–25 mg/kg/day in equally divided doses every 12 to 24 hours.
  ■ term neonates <2 weeks: 25 mg/kg/day in equally divided doses every 8 to 12 hours
  ■ term neonates >2 weeks: 25–50 mg/kg/day in equally divided doses every 6 to 12 hours
  ■ children, adults: 50 to 75 mg/kg/day equally divided doses every 6 hours. (Up to 100 mg/kg/day may be used with caution due to increase chance for toxicity.)
(Maximum dosage is 2 g/day)
Ophthalmic:
  ■ Drops: Instill 1 to 2 drops to conjunctiva every 3 to 6 hours
  ■ Ointment: Instill 1-cm strip into conjunctiva sac every 4 to 6 hours
  ■ Otic: Instill 2 to 3 drops into external ear canal 3 times per day
  ■ Topical: Apply sparingly to clean wound 3 to 4 times per day

**Absorption and Fate:** Absorption: GI tract absorption rapid, but slowly and erratically absorbed in neonates; may be absorbed into aqueous humor; unknown if absorbed significantly from mucous membranes, intact or broken skin. Peak levels: 1 to 3 hours PO; IV highly variable. Distributed to body tissues, 60% bound to plasma proteins. Half-life: neonates 1 to 2 days old, 24 hours; infants 10 to 16 days, 10 hours; adults, 1.5 to 4.1 hours. Liver inactivates this drug by glucuronyl transferase. 68 to 99% drug excreted into urine over 3 days. Therapeutic plasma level 5 to 20 µg/ml.

**Contraindications and Precautions:** Pregnancy category C. Excreted into breast milk; use extreme caution during lactation. Use caution with prematures, neonates, and infants. Contraindicated if allergic to this drug, final stages labor and delivery, treatment or prophylaxis of minor infections or typhoid carrier state. Use caution with impaired liver or renal function.

## Side Effects:
*CNS:* headache, mental depression confusion, delirium, **optic neuritis and peripheral neuritis** (usually with long-term high-dose therapy). *GI:* nausea, vomiting, diarrhea, unpleasant taste, stomatitis, enterocolitis. ***Hepatic:*** jaun-

dice (rare). **Hemic:** **bone marrow depression** (2 types) (1) nondose-related, occurring after first dose to weeks or months after drug stopped: **irreversible bone marrow depression, aplastic anemia, pancytopenia, 50% or greater mortality rate**, (2) dose-related, usually reversible if drug stopped: anemia, vacuolation of erythroid cells, reticulocytopenia, **thrombocytopenia**, leukopenia. **Other:** Hypersensitivity: fever, macular and vesicular rashes, urticaria, angioedema, hemorrhage skin, mucosal, serosal surfaces of intestine, bladder, mouth, **anaphylaxis**. **Gray Syndrome:** premature and neonates (usually, first 48 hours of life) but can occur to 2 years: **circulatory collapse**, refusal to suck, abdominal distention with or without emesis, **progressive pallid cyanosis, vasomotor collapse** (possible), **irregular respiration, death in few hours of symptoms**.

## Nursing Implications:

**Assess:** Assess previous allergy to this drug, any renal or hepatic impairment. Obtain cultures and sensitivity before treatment, but can start treatment before results, especially if suspect organisms requiring treatment are present. Obtain baseline hematological (CBC, platelets, reticulocyte counts) and renal function data. Observe and record appearance of wound or eye if used topically.

**Administer: PO:** Give 1 hour before or 2 hours after meals. Suspension; shake well, take suspension through nipple. Capsules may be taken apart and mixed with food or fluid. **IV:** Reconstitute with sterile water or 5% dextrose. Give IV push in concentrations no greater than 100 mg/ml over 1 minute. Intermittent infusion infused over 30 to 60 minutes; minimum dilution of 1 g/50ml. Compatible with $D_5W$, $D_{10}W$, $D_5W/0.5\%$ NS, $D_5W/0.2\%$ NS, $D_5W/NS$, NS, LR, ionosol and dextran solutions. Do not premix with phenothiazines, vancomycin, or tetracyclines. Do not use solutions if cloudy. **Ophthalmic:** See Part I for instillation of drops or ointments. Clean exudate from eye before instillation. Following administration of drops apply finger to lacrimal sac using light pressure for 1 to 2 minutes to minimize systemic absorption. Use only for treatment of infections of susceptible organisms. **Otic:** See Part I for instillation. Use only for treatment of infections of susceptible organisms. **Topical:** Clean wound according to physician's directions. Apply sparingly.

**Monitor:** **Lethal drug especially for children under 2 years**. Monitor prematures, newborns, infants, and children under 2 years for Gray syndrome. If newborn's mother received this drug during labor or delivery closely monitor infant for drug's side effects. Assess CBC, platelets, and reticulocyte counts every 48 hours to detect bone marrow depression and observe for any symptoms of bleeding. If either occurs, discontinue drug. Serum drug concentrations should be 5 to 20 µg/ml; higher levels could indicate toxicity. If symptoms of optic or peripheral neuritis occur, discontinue drug immediately. Assess renal function by I & O, weights, BUN, and serum creatinine. If symptoms of nephrotoxicity occur notify physician. Watch for symptoms of superinfections. Maintain fluid I & O for age group. If rash, itching, or swelling occurs with ophthalmic, otic, or topical preparations, discontinue medication. Topical applications can cause systemic symptoms.

**Patient Teaching:** Teach proper instillation and application of topical, otic, or ophthalmic preparations. Strict adherence to oral dosing schedule; need close medical supervision while on this drug. Discontinue and inform physician of any side effects.

**Drug Interactions:** Avoid giving with other drugs that may also cause bone marrow depression. This drug may inhibit hepatic microsomal enzyme activity of chlorpropamide, dicumarol, phenytoin, tolbutamide, and rifampin, thus prolonging their half-lives. Chloramphenicol can interfere with vitamin K production of intestinal bacteria. Concurrent use with phenobarbital may lower plasma levels of antibiotic. Utilization of this drug with iron preparations, folic acid, or vitamin $B_{12}$ causes delay in these drugs' actions. In vitro the use of penicillins and aminoglycosides with this drug antagonizes bactericidal actions, however, they have been used in practice; therefore use with caution.

**Storage Requirements:** Store sterile powder, capsules, suspension, topical, otic at 15 to 30°C in tight containers; protect from freezing. Reconstituted solutions of 100 mg/ml stable for 30 days at room temperature. Consult package insert for storage of ophthalmic preparations.

---

## □ CHLOROTHIAZIDE                                    (klor-oh-thye'a-zide)

(Diuril)

**Combination Products:** Aldochlor, Chloro-Res, Chloroserp, Chloroserpine, Diupres

**Classification:** thiazide diuretic, antihypertensive

**Available Preparations:**
- 250, 500-mg tablets
- 250 mg/5 ml oral suspension
- 500-mg vial for parenteral use

Also available in combination tablets with reserpine, methyldopa.

**Action and Use:** This short-acting thiazide diuretic interferes with sodium reabsorption and promotes potassium secretion in the distal convoluted tubules, thus reducing plasma and extracellular fluid volume. Also decreases excretion of calcium. Used to treat hypertension and in conjunction with digitalis, to treat congestive heart failure. Use not approved by the FDA: prevention of calcium renal stones.

**Routes and Dosages:**
*PO:*
- under 6 months: 10 to 33 mg/kg/day in 1 to 2 doses
- over 6 months: 10 to 22 mg/kg/day or 600 mg/m²/day in 1 to 2 doses

Daily dose range for children under 2 years is 125 to 375 mg/day and for children 2 to 12 years is 375 mg to 1g/day.
*IV:* Route not recommended for children

**Absorption and Fate:** Incompletely absorbed from PO route with considerable variability. Food increases drug absorption. Crosses the placenta and present in breast milk. Variably (20 to 80%) bound to plasma proteins. Excreted primarily in urine in unchanged form. Onset of action is within 2 hours, peak effect in 2 hours, and duration of action is up to 24 hours, more commonly 6 to 12 hours. Therapeutic effect: best after 3 to 4 days of therapy. Half-life is 13 hours.

**Contraindications and Precautions:** Pregnancy category B. No known teratogenesis in animals. Present in breast milk, not advised during lactation. Contraindicated in those with allergy to thiazides or sulfonamide derivatives, in anuric patients. Cautious use in infants with jaundice, electrolyte imbalance, renal dysfunction, hepatic dysfunction, diabetes, hyperuricemia, hypercalcemia, lupus, pancreatitis.

**Side Effects:**
*CNS:* fatigue, headache, weakness, mood change. *CV:* orthostatic hypotension, irregular pulse. *GI:* nausea, vomiting, anorexia, abdominal cramping, dry mouth, thirst. *Hepatic:* dysfunction, yellowish eye sclera and skin. *Metabolic:* hypokalemia and hyponatremia manifested by fatigue, lethargy, muscle weakness, anorexia, constipation; hypochloremic alkalosis, hyperuricemia, hypercalcemia, hypophosphatemia, hyperglycemia, glycosuria in diabetics. *Hemic:* thrombocytopenia leading to bruising, eosinophilia leading to fever and sore throat. *Other:* hypersensitivity manifested by urticaria, purpura, photosensitivity, rash, fever, anaphylaxis.

**Nursing Implications:**
*Assess:* Establish baseline CBC, serum electrolytes, blood glucose, uric acid, weight, and vital signs, particularly blood pressure. Injection powder contains thimerosal, a mercury derivative used as preservative; be alert to patient history of mercury hypersensitivity.
*Administer: PO:* Schedule early in day (before 3 P.M.) and after eating to avoid nocturia and stomach upset. *IV:* route not generally recommended for pediatrics. When used, at least 18 ml normal saline or sterile water are added to vial for reconstitution. Solution will contain 25 mg/ml and is stable for 24 hours at room temperature. Further diluted in 5% dextrose or saline for administration. Incompatible with many drugs; do not administer with blood or blood products. Avoid extravasation.
*Monitor:* Monitor CBC, serum potassium and sodium, other serum electrolytes, daily weight, vital signs, I & O, and check hydration status. Evaluate BUN and uric acid periodically. Monitor blood glucose and status of the diabetic patient carefully as hyperglycemia may occur and necessitate insulin adjustment. Watch for signs of hypokalemia such as confusion, weakness, muscle cramps, dry mouth, and anorexia.

***Patient Teaching:*** Take at same time each day; early in day to avoid nocturia; may take with food. Eat potassium rich foods such as orange juice, tomatoes, apricots, figs, prunes, avocados, raisins, banana, meat, and potatoes. Diet with sodium restriction may be ordered. Teach to get up slowly to avoid orthostatic hypotension. Avoid OTC medications unless recommended by physician; many contain sodium. Weigh and report changes to physician. Continue to take as directed; do not discontinue unless instructed. Avoid exposure to sun. Watch for and report nausea, vomiting, diarrhea. Careful blood glucose monitoring for diabetic patients.

**Drug Interactions:** Hypokalemia such as that resulting from this drug increases susceptibility to digitalis toxicity and increases blocking effect of neuromuscular blocking agents. Additive effect of hypokalemia with other drugs that lower potassium such as corticosteroids and amphotericin B. Reduced lithium clearance. Caution when given to patient on insulin due to hyperglycemia. Increased antihypertensive effect with other antihypertensives. Probenecid decreases uric acid retention. Alkalinization of urine caused by the drug may lead to decreased excretion of some amine drugs such as quinidine and amphetamine. Other drugs that cause orthostatic hypotension, such as alcohol and barbiturates, may lead to additive effect. Cholestyramine and colestipol may bind thiazides and decrease their absorption, therefore, should be given at least 1 hour later. Increased diuresis with other diuretics. Hypercalcemia when given with calcium-containing medications. Increased potential for renal dysfunction if given with nonsteroidal antiinflammatories.

**Laboratory Test Interferences:** Increased serum amylase. False-negative tyramine and phentolamine tests and histamine test for pheochromocytoma. Decreased urinary corticosteroid. Invalidates bentiromide test. Increases serum and urine glucose in diabetics. Increased serum cholesterol, triglyceride, low density lipoprotein, bilirubin, uric acid, magnesium, and potassium. May decrease serum PBI, sodium. Decreases urinary calcium. Decrease 3 days before parathyroid function test due to effect on calcium excretion.

**Storage Requirements:** Store tightly closed at 15 to 30°C (59 to 86°F). Avoid freezing oral suspension.

---

## □ CHLORPHENIRAMINE MALEATE

(klor-fen-eer'a-meen)

(Aller-Chlor, AL-5, Chlo-Amine, Chlor-Pro, Chlormene, Chlorotab, Chlor-Trimeton, Histaspan, Novopheniram, Phenetron, Pyranistan, Teldrin)

**Combination Products:** Chlorpheniramine maleate with many other drugs such as: pseudoephedrine HCl, pseudoephedrine sulfate, acetaminophen, phenylpropanolamine HCl, and aspirin.

**Classification:** antihistamine

## Available Preparations:
- 2 mg/5 ml oral solution
- 4-mg tablet
- 2-mg chewable tablets
- 8, 12-mg extended-release tablets
- 6, 8, 12-mg extended-release capsules
- 10, 100 mg/ml for parenteral administration

**Action and Use:** Propylamine derivative that competes with histamine for $H_1$-receptor sites of effector cells. By blocking the histamine it decreases the allergic reactions. Used to relieve rhinitis and allergy symptoms. Parenteral form given to prevent allergic reactions to blood, plasma, and in anaphylactic reactions.

## Routes and Dosages:
*PO:*
- 0.35 mg/kg/day equally divided doses every 6–12 hours
- 2 to 6 years: 1 mg every 4 to 6 hours
- 6 to 12 years: 2 mg every 4 to 6 hours or one 8 or 12 mg extended-release tablets every 12 hours. (Maximum dosage 12 mg/day)
- over 12 years: 4 mg every 4 to 6 hours or one 8 or 12 mg extended-release tablet every 12 hours. (Maximum dosage 24 mg/day)

*SC, IM, IV:*
- under 12 years: 0.0875 mg/kg or 2.5 mg/m² 4 times/day
- over 12 years: 5 to 20 mg as single dose. (Maximum dosage 40 mg/day)

**Absorption and Fate:** Absorbed well from GI tract. Peak level: 2 to 6 hours. Elimination half-life: 5.2 to 23.1 hours. Excreted primarily in urine.

**Contraindications and Precautions:** Pregnancy category B. Use during lactation not recommended. Do not use in neonates or prematures, extended-release tablets or injection in children under 12 years; in those under 6 years drug should be given only under physician's direction. Contraindicated if hypersensitivity to drug, acute asthma attack. Use caution with cardiovascular or renal diseases; asthma, hypertension, increased intraocular pressure, bladder neck obstruction, urinary retention, hyperthyroidism, stenosed peptic ulcers.

## Side Effects:
*CNS:* drowsiness, paradoxical excitement, dizziness, headaches, nervousness, insomnia, tremors, **seizures**. *CV:* palpitations, **hypotension**. *GI:* anorexia, nausea, vomiting, diarrhea, dry mouth and throat. *Hepatic:* mild increase, SGOT, SGPT. *Resp:* increased thick secretions, **wheezing, chest tightness**. *GU:* urinary retention or frequency. *Skin:* rash, urticaria. *Other:* Local: IV: stinging at injection site, sweating, hypotension.

## Nursing Implications:

*Assess:* Obtain CBC before long-term therapy.

*Administer: PO:* Solution contains 7% alcohol. Can crush tablet, mix with small amounts of food or fluid. Extended-release tablets or capsules are not to be crushed or chewed but swallowed whole. Chew chewable tablets. *SC, IM:* Give as undiluted injection. *IV:* 100 mg/ml is not recommended for IV usage. May be given undiluted or dilute to desired amount and infuse over at least 3 to 5 minutes. Compatible with most IV fluids but check with pharmacist before infusion. Incompatible with calcium chloride, pentobarbital, iodipamide meglumine, levarterenol, and kanamycin. Do not add directly to blood units. Because local reaction to IV may occur (hypotension, sweating, syncope), observe child carefully and stop infusion if these reactions occur.

*Monitor:* Assess for side effects. Periodic CBC if on long-term therapy.

*Patient Teaching:* Take only as directed. Give only under physician's supervision in those under 6 years. Observe for side effects and maintain hydration. Assess relief of symptoms. If CNS symptoms occur, may require adjustment of behavior, e.g., skate boarding, bike riding, and other activities requiring mental alertness. Do not use alcohol or take other OTC drugs that may increase CNS symptoms while on this drug. Chewing sugarless gum or sucking sugarless candy may relieve dry mouth.

**Drug Interferences:** This drug may increase CNS depression of alcohol, other CNS drugs, and barbiturates. Use of this drug and MAO inhibitors may cause increased anticholinergic effects. May increase effects of phenytoin.

**Laboratory Test Interferences:** May suppress reactions to skin testing; discontinue drug 4 days before testing.

**Storage Requirements:** Store at 15 to 30°C (59 to 86°F), in tight containers. Solution and parenteral form: protect from light and avoid freezing.

---

## □ CHOLESTYRAMINE                    (koe-less-tear'a-meen)

(Questran)

**Classification:** antilipemic, antipruritic, antidiarrheal

**Available Preparations:** powder for oral suspension; 9 g powder = 4 g cholestyramine (one scoop)

**Action and Use:** This bile acid sequestrant binds with bile acids in the GI tract so the body uses cholesterol to manufacture more bile acids. Serum cholesterol and low density lipoprotein fall in persons with hyperlipoproteinemia. Serum triglycerides may also decrease. Causes decrease in pruritus probably by decreased bile acids available for deposit in the skin. Also releases chloride ions into the intestine. Used in treatment of type IIa hyperlipidemia to decrease cardiovascular risk and to relieve pruritus in those with biliary obstruction. It is used without FDA approval in treatment of digitalis overdose, to relieve diarrhea caused by increased bile acids, and in hyperoxaluria.

## Routes and Dosages:
*PO:*
- under 6 years: dosage not established
- over 6 years: 80 mg/kg or 2.35 g/m$^2$ TID; Alternatively 2 to 4 g BID before meals may be used initially and increased until serum cholesterol is lowered below 250 mg/dl; general dosage range is 8 to 16 g/day

Dosages established by clinicians rather than the manufacturer.

## Absorption and Fate:
Not absorbed from GI tract. Onset of action on cholesterol occurs in 24 to 48 hours but may continue to decrease cholesterol up to 1 year. Once withdrawn, cholesterol returns to usual levels in 2 to 4 weeks. Onset of action for pruritus occurs in 1 to 3 weeks after therapy begins and pruritus returns 1 to 2 weeks after therapy ends. Diarrhea relief occurs in 24 hours.

## Contraindications and Precautions:
Pregnancy category C. Because the drug is not absorbed, it is unlikely to cause fetal harm; however, studies with pregnant women have not been done and as the drug decreases absorption of fat soluble vitamins it is not recommended during pregnancy or lactation. Studies to demonstrate long-term effects on children have not been performed. Contraindicated in complete biliary obstruction, and in those with hypersensitivity to the drug. Questran contains tartrazine (yellow dye #5), therefore, should not be used in those with allergy to the dye. Cautious use in GI dysfunction, bleeding problems, constipation, malabsorption, renal dysfunction, coronary artery disease, and gallstones.

## Side Effects:
*GI:* constipation, GI bleeding, abdominal pain, nausea, vomiting, indigestion, bloating, belching, diarrhea. *Hemic:* bleeding tendency due to vitamin K deficiency. *Metabolic:* hyperchloremic acidosis especially in children.

## Nursing Implications:
*Assess:* Take weight. Serum cholesterol and triglyceride levels are measured. Inquire about history of tartrazine (yellow dye #5) allergy.
*Administer:* Place powder in 60 to 180 ml of noncarbonated liquid such as juice, milk, water, soup, or along with milk in cereal. Allow to sit for 1 to 2 minutes and then mix; a suspension with undissolved drug will be produced. Do not take dry to avoid constipation. Take at meal time.
*Monitor:* Serum cholesterol and triglyceride levels are taken at least every 3 to 6 months; more often during early therapy. Take child's height and weight and record on growth grid. Monitor for signs of vitamin deficiency. Serum concentrations of fat soluble vitamins and prothrombin time and periodically

measured. Record bowel movements and institute measures to prevent constipation as necessary.

**Patient Teaching:** Teach correct method for mixing dose in liquid. Continue to take unless instructed otherwise by prescriber. Keep scheduled health care visits so monitoring of cholesterol and triglyceride levels can be done. Dietary teaching to encourage low cholesterol diet should be part of the therapy. Dietary vitamin supplements may be ordered. Take other oral drugs at least 1 hour before or 4 hours after cholestyramine.

**Drug Interactions:** Cholestyramine binds to many drugs, slowing or interfering with their absorption. It is particularly likely to bind with acidic drugs. Examples of drugs known to be bound are digitalis preparations, thyroid, warfarin, thiazide diuretics, propranolol, penicillin G, tetracycline, vancomycin. Other drugs should be taken a minimum of 1 hour before or 4 hours after cholestyramine. The drug interferes with fat-soluble vitamin and folic acid absorption and with vitamin K synthesis. Supplements may need to be taken.

**Laboratory Test Interferences:** Increases alkaline phosphatase, SGOT, chloride, phosphorus. Decreases calcium, potassium, sodium. Desired effect is decreased serum cholesterol and triglycerides.

**Storage Requirements:** Store tightly closed at 15 to 30°C (59 to 86°F).

---

## □ CIMETIDINE                                    (sye-met′i-deen)

(Apo-Cimetidine, Novocimetine, Peptol, Tagamet)

**Classification:** antihistamine, $h_2$-receptor antagonist

### Available Preparations:
- 300 mg/5ml oral syrup
- 200, 300, 400, 800-mg tablet
- 150 mg/ml for parenteral administration

**Action and Use:** $H_2$-histamine receptor antagonist that suppresses histamine and pentagastrin-stimulated acid secretion in the stomach. Used prophylactically for treatment of active GI hemorrhage or peptic ulcer disease, hypersecretory syndrome, gastroesophageal reflux; or as adjunct therapy in the management of severe pancreatic insufficiency in patients who fail to respond to oral pancreatic enzyme supplements.

### Routes and Dosage:
**PO:** 20 to 40 mg/kg/day in divided doses 4 times per day, after meals and at bedtime
**IM, IV:** 20 to 40 mg/kg/day in equally divided doses every 6 hours
Maximum dosage, 2400 mg/day

**Absorption and Fate:** Well adsorbed from GI tract. Peak level: PO, 60 to 90 minutes; IV, following infusion. 15 to 20% bound to plasma proteins. Half-life: 2 to 2.5 hours. Metabolized in liver, primarily excreted in urine, 10% in feces. Therapeutic level: 0.5 $\mu g/ml$ to produce 50% inhibition gastric acid secretion.

**Contraindications and Precautions:** Pregnancy category B. Excreted in breast milk and not recommended during lactation. Safe use in those under 16 years not established due to lack of controlled studies, thus risk versus benefit must be evaluated. Contraindicated if hypersensitivity to this drug. Use caution with hepatic or renal function impairment.

**Side Effects:**
**CNS:** dizziness, headache, agitation, restlessness, mental confusion, depression, **delirium, hallucinations**. **CV:** bradycardia, hypotension. **GI:** mild and transient diarrhea. **Hepatic:** increase in SGOT, SGPT, alkaline phosphatase. **GU:** transient elevation serum creatinine, BUN, **interstitial nephritis** (rare). **Skin:** maculopapular rash, acnelike, urticaria. **Hemic:** neutropenia, agranulocytosis, thrombocytopenia, **aplastic anemia**. **Endocrine:** mild gynecomastia after being on drug over 1 month. **Other:** muscular pain; Local: IM: transient pain at site.

**Nursing Implications:**
**Assess:** In cystic fibrosis management, assess stool quantity and quality, and obtain weight. If on warfarin therapy, obtain prothrombin time.
**Administer: PO:** Unaffected by food, usually given before meals; do not give within 1 hour of antacids. Tablet may be crushed, mixed with small amounts of food or fluid. Physician should specify dosing schedule; for peptic ulcer a larger bedtime dose may be required to suppress gastric secretion during sleep. **IM:** Do not use if discolored or has precipitate. Injection painful. **IV:** Manufacturers prefilled syringe is not given as direct IV bolus, must be diluted. Dilute with 20 ml of 5% dextrose, 0.9% sodium chloride, or other compatible IV solutions; infuse slowly over at least 2 minutes. If given too rapidly, sudden hypotension, arrhythmias, **cardiac arrest** may result. Preferred route, intermittent infusion with dilution of 300 mg/50 ml infused over 15 to 20 minutes. Compatible with $D_5W$, $D_5W/0.2\%NS$, $D_5W/0.5\%NS$, $D_5W/NS$, $D_{10}W$, NS, LR, ionosol products, normosol, parenteral nutrition solutions. Incompatible with aminophylline, barbiturates, cephalosporins, amphotericin B. Do not add any drugs to manufacturer-prefilled plastic syringes of cimetidine.
**Monitor:** Assess for side effects; notify physician if they occur. Monitor blood counts, renal and hepatic function during therapy. Assess medication effectiveness by assessing symptoms of entity being treated. Oral therapy for peptic ulcer continues for 4 to 6 weeks. Duodenal ulcers usually recur after medication stopped and it appears that gradual withdrawal of drug may reduce some recurrences.
**Patient Teaching:** Drug dosage must be followed and given at time ordered. Sudden stoppage of drug may cause ulcer perforation. Notify physician if side effects occur; importance of close medical follow-up while on this medication.

Gynecomastia can occur, usually reversible when cimetidine discontinued. Parent and child need to understand diet, drug therapy, and disease entity for effective treatment of ulcers. Do not take any OTC drugs without consulting physician or pharmacist.

**Drug Interactions:** Antacids decrease action of this drug, give 1 hour before or 1 hour after cimetidine. Cimetidine may accentuate hypoprothrombinemia when child is on warfarin therapy. Reduces the hepatic microsomal metabolism of many drugs such as phenytoin, lidocaine, metronidazole, theophylline, bone marrow depressants, and many others check with pharmacist before adding any drugs to child's therapy. Smoking decreases this drug's effectiveness.

**Laboratory Test Interference:** False-positive gastric acid test for blood (hemoccult) if obtained within 15 minutes of drug dosage. May inhibit cutaneous histamine response of skin allergens causing false-positive results.

**Storage Requirements:** Store at 15 to 30°C (59 to 86°F) in light-resistant containers. Diluted parenteral form stable 48 hours at room temperature.

---

☐ **CISPLATIN**                                          (cis′pla-tin)

(Platinol)

**Classification:** antineoplastic

**Available Preparations:** 10, 50-mg vials for parenteral use

**Action and Use:** This platinum-containing drug binds to DNA and inhibits its synthesis; it is cell phase nonspecific. May also act by enhancing tumor immunogenicity. Used for solid tumors such as those of head, neck, and cervix. Is used experimentally for osteogenic sarcoma, neuroblastoma, brain tumors, lymphomas, although it is not approved by the FDA for these purposes.

**Routes and Dosages:** IV. Experimental intraarterial and intraperitoneal use.
*IV:*

- Osteogenic Sarcoma and Neuroblastoma: 90 mg/m² once every 3 weeks *or* 30 mg/m² weekly
- Brain Tumors: 60 mg/m² daily for 2 days every 3 to 4 weeks *or* 90 mg/m² q42 days.

These pediatric doses have been established by clinicians rather than the manufacturer.

**Absorption and Fate:** Rapidly absorbed after IV administration and widely distributed to body tissues, especially liver, kidneys, and prostate. Does not penetrate CNS in therapeutic levels. Excreted mainly in urine as intact drug. Peak level of 2.3 μg/ml after 50 mg/m$^2$ dose and 3.3 μg/ml after 100 mg/m$^2$ dose reached after 30 minutes. Lower peak levels observed after 1 hour infusion rather than bolus dose. Half-life is biphasic with 25 minutes initially and 60 to 70 hours in terminal phase.

## Contraindications and Precautions:
Pregnancy category D. Not recommended for use in lactation. Safety in children is not yet established. Contraindicated in those with prior history of hypersensitivity to the drug or platinum or those with preexisting renal impairment or with chicken pox or herpes zoster infection. Decreased leukocyte and platelet counts and auditory side effects may necessitate reduction or stopping drug. Use with caution in those with previous chemotherapy or radiation therapy; those with infections.

## Side Effects:
**CNS:** peripheral neuropathy, reduced deep tendon reflexes, weakness, headache. **CV:** bradycardia, EKG changes, left bundle branch block, congestive heart failure, thrombus, coronary artery disease, CVA. **GI:** nausea, vomiting, and anorexia occurs in nearly everyone 1 to 4 hours after dose; vomiting persists 24 hours, nausea and anorexia last 1 week; antiemetics minimally effective; diarrhea. **Hepatic:** transient, mild SGOT and SGPT elevations. **GU:** renal toxicity manifested by elevated creatinine, BUN, uric acid; related to high cumulative levels of drug; often occurs 2 weeks after drug therapy begins; hyperuricemia. **Skin:** rash, mild alopecia, phlebitis at IV site. **Hemic:** myelosuppression with leukopenia, thrombocytopenia, and anemia. WBC and platelet levels are lowest at 18 to 23 days and normal at 39 days. **Metabolic:** hypomagnesemia, hypocalcemia, hypokalemia. **Sensory:** ototoxicity, tinnitus, hearing loss, deafness with these effects most common in children. These effects may not be reversible when drug is stopped. **Other:** anaphylaxis manifested by dyspnea, facial edema and flushing, hypotension, tachycardia.

## Nursing Implications:
**Assess:** Obtain history of prior courses of this or other antineoplastic drug or radiation therapy. Establish baseline renal studies such as BUN, creatinine clearance, uric acid. Perform audiometry. CBC and serum electrolytes are measured.

**Administer:** This drug has potentially severe toxic effects and should be given only under the supervision of a physician with training and experience in cancer chemotherapy. The drug's potential for toxic effects on health-care personnel as well as patients necessitates careful handling during preparation and administration. Generally during preparation of antineoplastics, latex gloves, a mask, and a solid front gown are worn and a laminar flow hood is used. Gloves and gown may also be recommended for administration. Contaminated equipment such as needles, syringes, vials and unused medication is disposed of properly. Clean up of spills is carefully performed and accidental contact by patient or personnel receives prompt flushing and cleaning. **IV:** Begin hydration

8 to 12 hours before therapy with IV fluids, possibly mannitol and a diuretic, and insert a Foley catheter. Creatinine clearance of 10 to 50 ml/minute may necessitate lowering dose by 25%; if under 10 ml/minute a dose may be lowered by 50%. Do not use administration equipment with aluminum parts. Reconstitute powder with saline, 5% dextrose, or bacteriostatic water; sodium bicarbonate and other alkaline solutions should not be used. Reconstituted solutions are stable for 20 hours at 27°C (80°F); do not refrigerate. The dose is then further diluted in 2 L of saline or 5% dextrose with 18.75 g mannitol/L and given IV in 6 to 8 hours. Continuous 1- or 5-day infusions are also used. Administration more rapid than recommended leads to an increased risk of nephrotoxicity and ototoxicity.

*Monitor:* Observe during and for 30 minutes after infusion for signs of anaphylaxis. Keep emergency drugs and equipment readily available. Intake and output and urine specific gravity are monitored during and for 24 hours after drug administration. Creatinine, creatinine clearance, and BUN are checked before each dose and additional doses are withheld if serum creatinine is over 1.5 mg/dl, if creatinine clearance is less than 50 ml/minute, or if BUN is more than 25 mg/dl. SGPT, SGOT, bilirubin, uric acid may also be monitored. Watch IV site as IV hydration is usually continued for 24 hours after dose. Serum electrolytes such as potassium, magnesium, calcium, phosphate, and sodium are monitored. Perform neurological testing daily and report changes. Audiometry is performed before each subsequent dose and dose is not given until hearing is normal. Be alert for other signs of ototoxicity such as tinnitus. CBC is regularly monitored. The patient is observed for nausea and vomiting and antiemetics are administered as needed. Monitor respiratory status. Weigh daily.

*Patient Teaching:* Report signs of hearing loss or unusual symptoms related to ears. Continue increased hydration for several days after dose. Avoid persons with infections such as colds, influenza, chicken pox. Report signs of infection, such as fever, sore throat, cough, malaise. Report bleeding and bruising. Perform good oral hygiene. Report wheezing or fast heart beat. Increase fluid intake. Encourage adequate nutritional intake with small, frequent, nutritious meals.

**Drug Interactions:** Risk of nephrotoxicity is increased with aminoglycoside antibiotics concurrently administered or given up to 2 weeks after cisplatin. Possible synergistic antineoplastic activity with other antineoplastics, such as etoposide, bleomycin, doxobubicin, fluorouracil, methotrexate, vinblastine, vincristine, may occur. May alter renal elimination of drugs such as bleomycin and methotrexate. Potential increased risk of ototoxicity when given with other ototoxic drugs. Suppresses immune response to immunizations. Live virus vaccines must not be given, nor oral polio vaccine to those in close contact with the patient on this drug due to the chance of infection with a virus; these vaccines are delayed at least 3 months after chemotherapy when the patient is in remission.

**Laboratory Test Interferences:** Transient elevated SGOT, SGPT, bilirubin, alkaline phosphatase

**Storage Requirements:** Store powder at 15 to 30°C (59 to 86°F) and protected from light. Once reconstituted store solution at 27°C; it is stable for 20 hours. Do not refrigerate reconstituted solutions as this will form a precipitate.

---

□ **CLINDAMYCIN**                                                   (klin-da-mye′sin)
**HYDROCHLORIDE,**
**CLINDAMYCIN**
**PALMITATE**
**HYDROCHLORIDE,**
**CLINDAMYCIN**
**PHOSPHATE**

(Cleocin Hydrochloride, Cleocin Pediatric, Cleocin Phosphate, Cleocin T, Dalacin)

**Classification:** antibiotic, antiinfective

## Available Preparations:
- 75 mg/5 ml oral solution
- 75, 150-mg capsules
- 150 mg/ml for parenteral administration
- 1% topical gel, topical solution, topical lotion

**Action and Use:** Semisynthetic derivative of lincomycin that inhibits protein synthesis by binding to 50S ribosomal subunit inhibiting peptide formation. Active against many gm + organisms (staphylococci, pneumococci, and streptococci), anaerobes (such as *Bacteroides*), but is relatively inactive against gm − bacteria. More active against susceptible organisms than lincomycin. Topical form used for acne vulgaris.

## Routes and Dosage:
*PO:*
- weighing under 10 kg: 37.5 mg 3 times a day
- over 10 kg: 8 to 25 mg/kg/day in equally divided doses every 6 to 8 hours

*IM, IV:*
- prematures, small neonates: 15 mg/kg daily
- under 1 month: 15 to 20 mg/kg/day equally divided doses every 6 to 8 hours
- over 1 month: 15 to 40 mg/kg/day or 350–450 mg/m$^2$/day equally divided doses every 6 to 8 hours

*Topical:* Apply as thin film to cleansed affected area twice daily

**Absorption and Fate:** 90% of PO dose rapidly absorbed from GI tract. About 10% of topical form absorbed into stratum corneum. Peak levels: PO, 1 hour; IM, 2 hours; IV, at end of infusion. Distributed to body tissues and fluid with minimal amounts in CSF even if meninges inflamed. Half-life: 2 to 3 hours children; 8.7 hours prematures; 3.6 hours neonates; and 3 hours infants 1 month to 1 year. Excreted in urine, bile, and feces.

**Contraindications and Precautions:** Pregnancy category B and use during lactation not recommended. Use with caution in prematures, neonates and infants. Contraindicated in hypersensitivity to this drug, lincomycin, or dye tartrazine (yellow dye #5) found in clindamycin hydrochloride capsules. Use with caution in history of GI disease especially colitis, renal, or hepatic impairment and atopic children.

## Side Effects:
*GI:* nausea, vomiting, abdominal pain, diarrhea, flatulence, esophagitis **pseudomembranous colitis**. *Hepatic:* transient increase SGOT, serum bilirubin, alkaline phosphatase. *GU:* azotemia, oliguria, proteinuria (rare and relationship to drug not established). *Skin:* topical: dryness, erythema, burning, peeling, pruritus. *Hemic:* transient leukopenia, neutropenia, thrombocytopenia, eosinophilia, agranulocytosis. *Musculoskeletal:* polyarthritis (rare). *Other:* Hypersensitivity: maculopapular rash, urticaria, pruritus erythema multiforme resembling Stevens-Johnson syndrome (rare); Local: IM: pain, induration sterile abscess; IV pain, swelling, erythema, thrombophlebitis, **hypotension and cardiac arrest if infused too rapidly**.

## Nursing Implications:
*Assess:* Assess previous allergy to this drug or lincomycin. Obtain cultures and sensitivity before treatment, but can start treatment before results. Obtain baseline hematological, renal, and hepatic data before long-term therapy or in prematures and neonates. With topical use, observe and record appearance of skin.

*Administer: PO:* Give without regard to food; however, if given with meals the peak serum levels may be delayed. Solution; shake well. Do not refrigerate, thickens solution causing difficulty in measuring. Capsules may be taken apart and mixed with a small amount of food or fluid. Give oral forms with as much fluid as child will take to decrease possibility of esophageal irritation. *IM:* Injection is painful. Do not give over 600 mg per injection site. *IV:* Do not give IV push. May dilute medication further with compatible IV solution. Intermittent infusion concentration not to exceed 6 mg/ml infused at rate not to exceed 30 mg/minute. Too rapid infusion can cause hypotension and cardiac arrest. Compatible with $D_5W$, $D_{10}W$, $D_5W/0.5\%$ NS, $D_5W/0.2\%$NS, $D_5W/NS$, NS, LR, amino acids 4.25%/D 25%, Isolyte M/$D_5W$. Do not premix with aminophylline, ampicillin, barbiturates, calcium, magnesium, and phenytoin. *Topical:* Clean face according to physician's directions. Apply sparingly, avoid eye area, contains alcohol that may irritate eyes and mucous membranes.

*Monitor:* Observe IM site for induration and abscess; IV site for extravasation and thrombophlebitis. Monitor prematures, newborns, and infants for organ function. During long-term therapy assess CBC, liver and renal function. If symptoms of severe diarrhea, abdominal cramps, and passage of blood or mucus occur, notify physician, and discontinue drug until assessment of pseudomembranous colitis is obtained. Symptoms of colitis develop 2 to 9 days after therapy is initiated or can start several weeks after drug is stopped. Watch for symptoms of superinfections primarily yeasts. Maintain fluid intake and output for age group. If rash, itching, or swelling occurs with topical preparations, discontinue medication. Topical applications can cause systemic symptoms.

*Patient Teaching:* Teach proper application of topical preparations. Strict adherence to oral dosing schedule; need for close medical supervision while on this drug. Inform physician of any side effects, especially diarrhea.

**Drug Interactions:** Clindamycin may enhance neuromuscular blocking properties of nondepolarizing muscle relaxants such as ether, tubocurarine, pancuronium, atracurium. In vitro antagonism between this drug and aminoglycosides has occurred, however, clinically this has not been demonstrated.

**Laboratory Test Interference:** Creatine phosphokinase increased following IM administration.

**Storage Requirements:** Store capsules, solution, topical at 15 to 30°C (59–86°F). Consult package insert for storage of parenteral preparations.

---

# ☐ CLONAZEPAM                                    (kloe-na'zi-pam)

(Klonopin)

**Classification:** anticonvulsant, benzodiazepine

**Available Preparations:** 0.5, 1, 2-mg tablets

**Action and Use:** Related to other benzodiazepine derivatives such as diazepam and flurazepam. Acts at limbic and subcortical levels to suppress certain types of seizures. Used in absence (petit mal), akinetic, and myoclonic seizures. Used without FDA approval in tonic–clonic (grand mal), psychomotor, and infantile spasm seizures. IV form is not available in U.S. but has been used for status epilepticus.

**Routes and Dosages:**
*PO:*
- under 10 years or 30 kg: 0.01 to 0.03 mg/kg/day initially in 2 to 3 doses; initial dosage not to exceed 0.05 mg/kg/day in 2 to 3 doses;

dosage increased no more than 0.5 mg q3d; maintenance dose not to exceed 0.2 mg/kg/day
- adult dose (and older children): 1.5 mg/day initially; dosage increased 0.5 to 1.0 mg q3d; maintenance dose not to exceed 20 mg/day.

## Absorption and Fate:
Well absorbed from GI tract. Distribution in body unknown. Metabolized in the liver and excreted in urine. Peak level reached in 1 to 2 hours or longer; duration of action 6 to 8 hours in children. Half-life is 19 to 40 hours. Therapeutic level is 20 to 80 ng/ml.

## Contraindications and Precautions:
Pregnancy category C. Not used in pregnancy unless clearly needed for mother's seizure control. Not recommended for use in lactation. Used in pediatric patients only if clearly needed as effects on development have not been tested. Contraindicated in those with hepatic dysfunction, sensitivity to benzodiazepines, and those with acute angle-closure glaucoma. Cautious use in those with respiratory disease, renal dysfunction, or those in whom increased secretions could be harmful.

## Side Effects:
*CNS:* sedation, drowsiness, ataxia, behavior changes especially in those with brain damage or mental retardation or mental illness, aggression, irritability, hyperactivity, confusion, depression, headache, dizziness, tremor, vertigo, insomnia. *CV:* palpitation. *GI:* constipation, gastritis, anorexia, nausea, dry mouth, thirst, sore gums. *Respiratory:* increased airway secretions, dyspnea, difficulty swallowing. *Hepatic:* hepatomegaly, liver enzyme changes. *GU:* dysuria, enuresis, retention, nocturia. *Skin:* hirsutism or hair loss, rash. *Hemic:* anemia, leukopenia, thrombocytopenia, eosinophilia. *Other:* fever, dehydration, lymphadenopathy.

## Nursing Implications:
*Assess:* Establish height and weight before therapy. Perform baseline liver function studies and CBC.
*Administer:* Schedule IV drug under Federal Controlled Substances Act. Give orally in 1 to 2 doses as ordered.
*Monitor:* Record seizure activity. Tolerance may develop in 3 months or longer, therefore, increasing seizure activity may require medication adjustment. Measure height and weight regularly. Periodic measures of liver function and CBC are needed. Record I & O during establishment of dosage. Monitor behavior changes.
*Patient Teaching:* Take drug as directed. Do not discontinue suddenly as increased seizure activity can occur. Do not operate machinery or drive car. Report continuing disturbing symptoms of drowsiness and ataxia as they usually decrease as therapy continues. Avoid alcohol, CNS depressants, or other drugs unless ordered by prescriber. Wear bracelet stating person has seizures and is on anticonvulsant medication.

## Drug Interactions:
Additive CNS depression with other CNS depressants. Increases serum phenytoin level when given together. Increased blood levels

may occur in patients also on cimetidine or disulfiram. Decreased serum levels of both drugs when given with carbamazepine.

**Laboratory Test Interferences:** Elevation of serum transaminase and alkaline phosphatase.

**Storage Requirements:** Store in tightly covered, light-resistant containers at 15 to 30°C (59 to 86°F).

---

## □ CLOTRIMAZOLE                                      (kloe-trim′a-zole)

(Canesten, Gyne-Lotrimin, Lotrimin, Mycelex, Mycelex-G)

**Combination Products:** Clotrimazole with betamethasone dipropionate

**Classification:** antiinfective, antifungal

### Available Preparations:
- 10 mg oral lozenges
- 1% solution, lotion, cream for topical application
- 100, 500-mg vaginal tablets
- 1% vaginal cream

**Action and Use:** Binds with phospholipids in fungal cell wall membrane increasing its permeability, causing loss of potassium and other cellular components. Fungicidal action used to treat tinea, pedis, cruris, tinea corporis, as well as vulvovaginal and oropharyngeal candidiasis.

### Routes and Dosage:
*PO:* Lozenge: dissolve 10 mg completely in mouth 5 times per day for 14 days
*Topical:* Apply solution, lotion, cream 2 times per day morning and evening
*Vaginal:*
- Cream: 1% insert 1 applicatorful 1 time per day at bedtime for 7 to 14 days;
- Tablet: Insert 500-mg tablet 1 time only at bedtime; insert 200-mg tablet once per day at bedtime for 3 days; or insert 100-mg tablet once per day at bedtime for 7 days

**Absorption and Fate:** Minimal adsorption from all preparations. PO form appears to be bound to oral mucosa where it is slowly released and inhibits most *Candida* strains for 3 hours. Vaginal peak serum concentrations 24 hours after 100-mg tablet.

**Contraindications and Precautions:** Pregnancy category B. Use with caution during lactation. Safe use in children under 3 years not established.

Contraindicated if hypersensitivity to drug, ophthalmic usage. Use with caution with hepatic impairment.

## Side Effects:
*GI:* lozenges: nausea, vomiting. *Hepatic:* Elevated SGOT. *GU:* vaginal: mild burning, skin rash, itching, lower abdominal cramps, vulval irritation. *Skin:* burning, stinging, erythema, blistering, itching, edema, peeling, urticaria, skin fissures.

## Nursing Implications:
*Assess:* Establish diagnosis through cultures before therapy.
*Administer: PO:* Lozenge should be held in mouth until it dissolves (15 to 30 minutes) and do not chew or swallow whole. Child must understand this or drug will not be effective. *Topical:* Shake lotion before use. Clean skin according to physicians direction. Apply sparingly, using gloves, to thoroughly dried skin; avoid contact with eyes. Do not use occlusive dressings. *Vaginal:* For instillation of vaginal medication, see Part I. Drug should be given when child is put to bed.
*Monitor:* Assess affected skin response to medication; usually improvement is apparent in 7 days. If signs of irritation develop or condition worsens after 2 weeks, contact physician. Hepatic function should be evaluated if on long-term therapy.
*Patient Teaching:* Teach parent or child how to give, apply, or instill. Observe for side effects and effectiveness of drug and contact physician as necessary. If no improvement in 4 weeks, contact physician. Child's clothes, linens, towels should be kept separate and laundered in hot water.

**Storage Requirements:** Store at 15 to 30°C (59 to 86°F).

---

## □ CLOXACILLIN SODIUM                (klox-a-sill'in)

(Apo-Cloxi, Bactopen, Cloxapen, Cloxilean, Novocloxin, Orbenin, Tegopen)

**Classification:** penicillins, penicillinase-resistant

## Available Preparations:
- 125 mg/5ml oral solution
- 250, 500-mg capsules

**Action and Use:** Similar to penicillin in action but resistant to inactivation by penicillinase; also active against *Streptococcus pyogenes* and *Pneumococcus*. Drug of choice for oral use in treating penicillinase-producing *Staphylococcus aureus* and *S. epidermidis* infection.

## Routes and Dosage:
*PO:*
- over 1 month, < 20 kg: 50 to 100 mg/kg/day in equally divided doses every 6 hours
- over 20 kg: 250 mg every 6 hours

(Maximum dosage 4 g/day)

**Absorption and Fate:** Rapidly, incompletely absorbed from GI tract. Distributed in liver, kidneys, synovial and pleural fluid, bone, bile. Peak level: 1 to 2 hours. Half-life: neonates, 0.8 to 1.5 hours; children, 0.4 to 0.8 hours. 90 to 96% bound to plasm proteins. Drug and metabolites excreted urine (30 to 45%), feces (9 to 22%).

**Contraindications and Precautions:** Pregnancy category B. Use caution during lactation. Manufacturer states that safe use in neonates not established. Contraindicated if hypersensitivity to drug, penicillins, cephalosporins, or cephamycins. Use caution with allergies, asthma, family history of allergies, impaired renal or hepatic function.

## Side Effects:
*GI:* nausea, vomiting, epigastric pain, loose stools, diarrhea, flatulence. *Hepatic:* transient rise SGOT, SGPT, and alkaline phosphatase, intrahepatic cholestasis. *GU:* transient hematuria, **interstitial nephritis**. *Skin:* morbilliform, maculopapular, urticarial, or erythematous, rashes, pruritus (hypersensitivity). *Hemic:* **eosinophilia, anemia, neutropenia, thrombocytopenia, leukopenia, agranulocytosis**. *Other:* Hypersensitivity: drug fever, **anaphylaxis** (rare).

## Nursing Implications:
*Assess:* Assess previous allergy to drug, penicillins, cephalosporins, other drugs, asthma, or family history of allergies. Obtain cultures and sensitivity before treatment, but can start treatment before results.

*Administer: PO:* Food interferes with drug absorption, give 1 hour before or 2 hours after meals. Refrigerate solution. Capsules may be taken mixed with small amount of food or fluid.

*Monitor:* Monitor child for hypersensitivity (especially in first 20 minutes of first dosage), rash (onset and characteristics), and side effects. Watch for symptoms of superinfections or diarrhea (may indicate pseudomembranous colitis, which can occur while on drug or 4 days to 6 weeks after drug discontinued). Assess renal, hepatic, and hematological functions in prolonged or high-dose therapy. Maintain fluid intake for age group. Therapy course continued for 48 to 72 hours after negative bacterial cultures or symptoms subside. If given for **A β-hemolytic streptococcal infection**, 10-day course need to prevent risk of acute rheumatic fever or glomerulonephritis.

*Patient Teaching:* Take as prescribed for full course of therapy. Observe for side effects especially diarrhea or rash, and report to physician. Do not take OTC drugs without consulting physician. Store solution in refrigerator out of reach of children. Reconstituted solution should be discarded after 14 days if refrigerated.

**Drug Interactions:** Erythromycin, tetracycline, chloromycetin, and antacids decrease the effects of cloxacillin.

**Storage Requirements:** Store capsules at 15 to 30°C (59 to 86°F). Reconstituted suspensions stable for 14 days if refrigerated. Label with time and date at time of reconstitution.

---

## □ CODEINE                                         (koe'deen)

**Combination Products:** Codeine combined with other drugs such as; Actifed, Ascriptin, Empirin, Guiatussin, Phenergan and Tylenol

**Classification:** narcotic analgesic, opiate agonist, antitussive

### Available Preparations:
- 15 mg/5 ml oral solution
- crystals
- powder
- 15, 30, 60-mg tablets
- 15, 30, 60 mg/ml vials for parenteral use

Available in many combination forms with aspirin, butabarbital, caffeine, acetaminophen, phenylephrine, chlorpheniramine, pseudoephedrine, potassium iodide, bromodiphenhydramine, brompheniramine, phenylpropanolamine, carbetapentane, guaifenesin, ephedrine, iodinated glycerol, promethazine, triprolidine, papaverine, terpin hydrate.

**Action and Use:** A phenanthrene derivative of opium. Acts on the CNS by using neurotransmitters to create analgesia; suppresses cough by action on the medulla cough center, depresses respiration by acting on respiratory center in brainstem, delays gastric secretion and digestion, causes smooth muscle spasm such as of the urinary tract, stimulates vasopressin release. Used for treatment of mild to moderate pain and to suppress cough.

**Routes and Dosages:** PO (codeine sulfate), IM, SC (codeine phosphate)
***PO, IM, SC:*** Pain: 3 mg/kg or 100 mg/m$^2$/day in 6 divided doses; or 0.5 mg/kg or 15 mg/m$^2$ q4–6h.
***PO:*** Antitussive:
- 2 to 6 years: 1 mg/kg/day in 4 doses not more than q4–6h
- 6 to 11 years: 5 to 10 mg q4–6h; not to exceed 60 mg/day
- 12 years and over: 10 to 20 mg q4–6h; not to exceed 120 mg/day

Alternatively:
- 2 years (12 kg): 3 mg q4–6h; not to exceed 12 mg/day
- 3 years (14 kg): 3.5 mg q4–6h; not to exceed 14 mg/day
- 4 years (16 kg): 4 mg q4–6h; not to exceed 16 mg/day
- 5 years (18 kg): 4.5 mg q4–6h; not to exceed 18 mg/day

Extended-release Oral Suspension:
- 6 to 11 years: 10 mg q12h; not to exceed 20 mg/day
- over 12 years: 20 to 30 mg q12h; not to exceed 60 mg/day

**Absorption and Fate:** Well absorbed after PO and injection. Metabolized in the liver and excreted principally in urine. Onset of action: 15 to 30 minutes; peak level: 60 to 90 minutes; duration of action: 4 to 6 hours.

**Contraindications and Precautions:** Pregnancy category C. Not used as an antitussive in children under 2 years, extended-release oral suspension not used in children under 6 years. Contraindicated in those with hypersensitivity to the drug, preparations with bisulfite are contraindicated in those with sulfite hypersensitivity, avoid in patients with respiratory depression, comatose, elevated CSF pressure. Cautious use in asthma, hepatic or renal dysfunction, colitis, hypothyroidism, neonates.

**Side Effects:**
**CNS:** sedation, dizziness, depression, coma, euphoria, restlessness, insomnia. **CV: circulatory depression** is potentially life threatening; orthostatic hypotension, palpitation, bradycardia, tachycardia. **GI:** nausea, vomiting, constipation. **Respiratory:** respiratory depression is a serious side effect. **Hepatic:** biliary spasm, increased serum amylase and lipase. **GU:** urinary retention, oliguria, stimulates release of vasopressin; impotence. **Skin:** rash, erythema, urticaria, pruritus, facial flushing indicate hypersensitivity reaction

**Nursing Implications:**
**Assess:** Assess type and degree of pain; use other pain control methods in addition to analgesic. Take baseline vital signs.
**Administer:** Codeine is a Schedule II drug under the Federal Controlled Substances Act; combination capsules are Schedule III; liquids are Schedule V. Check time of last dose carefully before giving. **PO:** Give PO form with milk or food to decrease GI discomfort. **IM, SC:** Rotate injection sites. Incompatible with aminophylline, heparin, methicillin, nitrofurantoin, phenobarbital, sodium bicarbonate, and some other drugs. Consult references or pharmacologist before placing in other solutions.
**Monitor:** Monitor vital signs every 15 to 30 minutes after administration. If hypotension occurs, or patients feel nausea or dizziness, have them lie down. After parenteral forms, patient is generally left in bed with side rails up. Evaluate pain in 30 minutes and record results. If giving antitussive dose, record type and amount of cough.
**Patient Teaching:** Take drug only as directed and only for patient prescribed. Drug can alter mental alertness; therefore, avoid driving and adjust other activities accordingly. Parents should be advised of age limitations of antitussive

medication so they do not administer codeine under 2 years at home and do not give extended-release syrup under 6 years. If excessive drowsiness or other symptoms occur, the drug should be withheld and health care sought. Often one dose of antitussive a short time before bedtime will enable the child with a cough to sleep well and the drug is not needed all day. Prolonged use can be habit forming and the drug should not generally be used for more than 1 week for a child at home.

**Drug Interactions:** Additive CNS effects with alcohol and other CNS depressants. Phenothiazines may antagonize action. Increased effects if given with dextroamphetamine, may increase effects of neuromuscular-blocking agents. Codeine may decrease effects of diuretics in congestive heart failure.

**Diagnostic Test Interferences:** Increases serum amylase and lipase; delay drawing blood for these tests for 24 hours after the drug. Decreased serum and urine 17-ketosteroids, 17-hydroxysteroids.

**Storage Requirements:** Store in tightly covered, light-resistant containers at 15 to 30°C (59 to 86°F). Avoid freezing injection solution.

---

□ **COLISTIMETHATE SODIUM, COLISTIN SULFATE**     (koe-lis-ti-meth'ate and koe-lis'tin)

(Coly-Mycin M, Coly-Mycin S, Polymyxin E)

**Combination Products:** 3 mg Colistin Sulfate, 3.3 mg Neomycin Sulfate, and 10 mg Hydorcortisone, otic (Coly-Mycin S)

**Classification:** antibacterial, polymyxin

**Available Preparations:**
- 25 mg (colistin) /5 ml oral suspension
- 150 mg (colistin) for parenteral administration
- 3 mg (colistin) otic

**Action and Use:** Obtained from cultures of *Bacillus polymyxa* var. *colistinus*, whose action is similar to polymyxin B. Damages the cytoplasmic membrane of bacteria by cationic detergent action causing leakage of the essential intracellular metabolites. Treats susceptible strains of gm− bacteria such as *Pseudomonas, Klebsiella, Enterobacter,* and *E. coli.* Used to treat diarrhea, gastroenteritis, urinary infections, and (otic) external ear infections.

**Routes and Dosage:**
*PO:* 5 to 15 mg/kg/day in equally divided doses every 8 hours

*IM, IV:* 2.5 to 5 mg/kg/day in equally divided doses every 8 hours (Maximum parenteral dose is 5 mg/kg)
Dosage and frequency decreased in patients with renal impairment.

**Absorption and Fate:** Colistin sulfate minimally absorbed from GI tract except in infants. Colistimethate sodium given parenterally. Peak level: IM, 2 hours; IV, within 10 minutes of infusion. 50% bound to plasma proteins; half-life: 1.5 to 8 hours. Drug and metabolites excreted in urine.

**Contraindications and Precautions:** Safe use during pregnancy not established; distributed into breast milk. Use caution in neonates, infants, or impaired renal function. Contraindicated in hypersensitivity to drug or renal failure.

**Side Effects:** More likely seen with high dosages or impaired renal function. *CNS:* circumoral or peripheral paresthesia, numbness, tingling, slurring of speech, dizziness, vertigo, ataxia, blurred vision, coma, psychosis, **seizures, neuromuscular blockade**. *GI:* GI disturbances. *Resp:* **respiratory arrest following IM injection**. *Hepatic:* **hepatotoxicity** (rare). *GU:* **nephrotoxicity:** decreased urine output, increase BUN or serum creatinine, proteinuria, hematuria, casts, **acute tubular necrosis**. *Skin:* pruritus, urticaria, rash. *Hemic:* leukopenia, granulocytopenia. *Other:* drug fever; Local: pain at injection site.

**Nursing Implications:**
*Assess:* Assess previous allergy to this drug. Obtain cultures and sensitivity before treatment, but can start treatment before results. Obtain baseline renal function data.
*Administer: PO:* Suspension; refrigerate and shake well. *IM, IV:* Reconstitute with 2 ml of sterile water for injection. After diluent added swirl gently to avoid frothing. *IM:* Injection painful. Have emergency equipment if necessary for respiratory arrest. *IV:* Can give ½ of dose or 75 mg IV push over 3 to 5 minutes. Intermittent infusion infused at rate not exceeding 5 to 6 mg/hour. Compatible with D₅W, LR, 10% invert sugar solution. Do not premix with other drugs or solutions.
*Monitor:* **Respiratory arrest can follow IM injection**. Observe IV site for extravasation. Monitor for nephrotoxicity and neurotoxicity (symptoms usually occur in first 4 days of therapy). Assess renal function by I & O, BUN, and serum creatinine. Neurotoxicity can be difficult to detect in infants and young children because of their inability to verbalize. Watch for symptoms of superinfections. Maintain fluid intake for age group.
*Patient Teaching:* Take as scheduled and prescribed for full course of therapy. Observe for side effects especially nephrotoxicity and neurological symptoms and report to physician. If given for diarrhea inform about enteric precautions. Maintain adequate hydration for age group. Store suspension in refrigerator. Reconstituted suspension should be discarded after 14 days if refrigerated. Do not take OTC without consulting with physician.

**Drug Interactions:** Avoid giving with other neurotoxic drugs aminoglycosides; amphotericin B, capreomycin, methoxyflurane, polymyxin B sulfate, vancomycin. Curariform muscle relaxants (ether, tubocurarine, succinylcholine, gallamine, decamethoniuma, and sodium citrate) may enhance neuromuscular reactions of colistimethate sodium. Cephalothin and this drug may cause increased nephrotoxic effect.

**Storage Requirements:** Store at 15 to 30°C. Parenteral form stable either refrigerated or at room temperature for 7 days; however, if further diluted for IV use, stable for 24 hours. Oral suspension stable for 14 days if refrigerated. Protect all solutions from light.

---

## □ CORTISONE ACETATE                                    (kor'ti-sone)

(Cortelan, Cortistab, Cortistan, Cortone Acetate)

**Classification:** corticosteroid, glucocorticoid, mineralocorticoid

### Available Preparations:
- 5, 10, 25-mg tablets
- 25, 50 mg/ml for parenteral administration

**Action and Use:** Synthetic and naturally occurring glucocorticoids that can cause profound and varied metabolic effects, modifies the body's immune response to diverse stimuli and causes potent antiinflammatory effects. Treats diseases such as collagen, dermatologic, allergy, acute leukemia, and others. It is used with mineralocorticoids in treatment of adrenocortical deficiencies.

### Routes and Dosage:
*PO:* 0.7 to 10 mg/kg/day or 20 to 300 mg/m²/day in 4 divided doses
*IM:* 12.5 mg/m² once daily (highly individualized doses)
Note: Dosage determined by severity of condition and child's response. High dosage daily therapy may inhibit child's growth. Combining with other oral intermediate-acting glucocorticoid (prednisone, prednisolone, methylprednisolone, triamcinolone) on alternate day therapy may decrease growth suppression effects.

**Absorption and Fate:** Absorption: PO, rapid, almost complete; IM, slow but complete. Peak level: PO, 2 hours; IM, 20 to 48 hours. Duration: both forms, 1.25 to 1.5 days. Metabolized by liver and excreted primarily in urine.

**Contraindications and Precautions:** Pregnancy category C and safety during lactation not established. Use caution in children and adolescents; possible growth suppression. Contraindicated if hypersensitivity to drug or its components, sensitivity to corticosteroids, varicella, systemic fungal infections, acquired immune deficiency syndrome (AIDS); fetal respiratory distress syndrome, do not use if delivery is imminent; immunizations with live virus vaccines and oral polio virus vaccine or contact with those who have had the vaccine. Use with caution in renal disease, hypertension, congestive heart failure, cardiac disease, diabetes, ulcerative colitis, gastrointestinal ulceration, hyperthyroidism, impaired hepatic function, systemic lupus erythematosus, osteoporosis, vaccinia, exanthema, Cushing's syndrome, seizures, myasthenia gravis, tuberculosis, ocular herpes simplex, hypoalbuminemia, emotional or psychotic tendencies.

**Side Effects:** Usually dependent on dosage and duration of treatment. **CNS:** headaches, vertigo, euphoria, insomnia, **increased intracranial pressure** (papilledema), **psychotic behavior, seizures.** **CV:** edema, **hypertension, congestive heart failure.** **GI:** nausea, vomiting, change in appetite, gastrointestinal irritation, abdominal distention, pancreatitis, ulcerative esophagitis, peptic ulcer. **Skin:** impaired wound healing, thin fragile skin, petechiae, ecchymosis, acne, facial erythema, increased sweating, may mask infections. **Hemic: thrombocytopenia.** **Endocrine: HPA-axis suppression,** menstrual irregularities, Cushing's states, **secondary adrenocortical, pituitary unresponsiveness.** **Musculoskeletal: suppression of bone growth, osteoporosis,** muscle weakness, **aseptic necrosis of femoral and humeral heads.** **Sensory:** Ophthalmic: **posterior subcapsular cataracts, increased intraocular pressure.** **Other: negative nitrogen balance, hypokalemia, hyperglycemia,** sodium retention, potassium loss, susceptibility to infections; Withdrawal symptoms: rebound inflammation, fatigue, weakness, arthralgia, fever, dizziness, lethargy, depression, fainting, orthostatic hypotension, dyspnea, anorexia, hypoglycemia, nausea and vomiting, shortness of breath, unusual weight loss, **death**.

**Nursing Implications:**
**Assess:** Obtain baseline weight, height; before long-term therapy: ECG, chest and spinal x-rays, glucose tolerance test, evaluation of HPA-axis function and BP.
**Administer:** Best to calculate drug dosage on mg/m²; reduces overdosage possibilities in very short or heavy children. **PO:** Take with food or milk to reduce GI irritation. Best to give daily dosage before 9 AM; it suppress adrenal cortex activity less, this may reduce risk of HPA-axis suppression. Alternate-day therapy recommended to reduce growth retarding effects. Tablet can be crushed, mixed with small amount of food or fluid. **IM:** Oral therapy is preferred. Shake well before withdrawal. Do not mix with other drugs because rate of absorption or state of suspension of drug may be altered. Preparation is not for IV usage.
**Monitor:** Carefully assess child's response to drug; necessary for dosage adjustments. Observe for side effects, especially hypocalcemia, signs of adrenal insufficiency, symptoms of infections, or worsening of condition. Children

more prone to muscular skeletal side effects; repeat any pain or gait changes to physican immediately. Monitor BP and daily weights, report any sudden weight gain to the physician. With long-term usage monitor serum electrolytes and height. Encourage well-balanced diet low in sodium, rich in calcium and potassium, and encourage good hygiene and dental care (possible oral fungal infections). Tonometry (eye) examinations every 6 weeks. Discontinuing drug: dosage should be reduced gradually, especially after long-term usage, so it does not cause acute life-threatening adrenal insufficiency. After discontinuation of short-term therapy (up to 5 days) with high dosage, adrenal recovery may occur within 1 week. After prolonged high-dose therapy, complete recovery of adrenal function may require up to 1 year. Adrenal suppressed patients need to be supplemented with higher doses of drug at times of severe stress.

**Patient Teaching:** Do not alter dosage or stop drug abruptly, it could cause very serious side effects, even death. Gradual tapering of dosage is necessary. Increasing amount of medication will not hasten healing process. Discuss dosing schedule for oral form. Monitor signs and symptoms of medication, symptoms of adrenal insufficiency, or worsening of condition and report to physician. Obtain daily weights; report any sudden weight gains to physician. Importance of close medical supervision and follow-up. Regular ophthalmic examinations if on long-term therapy. Caution about receiving skin tests, vaccinations or other immunizations, or coming in contact with persons receiving oral polio virus vaccine. Inform any health-care provider, including dentists, surgeons, or emergency care personnel that child is on this medication. Child should carry a medical identification card. Observe for symptoms of infections. Do not use OTC medications without contacting health care provider.

**Drug Interactions:** This drug, in combination with high dosage of acetaminophen, may increase risk of hepatotoxicity. With analgesics and antiinflammatory drugs, it may increase the risk of gastric ulceration. Amphotericin B and potassium-depleting diuretics increase risk of hypokalemia. Use with anabolic steroids may increase the risk of edema and acne. Drug in combination with anticoagulants may decrease anticoagulant effect. This drug used with anticonvulsants (phenytoin) may lower seizure threshold. This drug's glucocorticoid metabolism may be increased when used with barbiturates, phenytoin, or rifampin. Use with vaccines, live virus, or other immunizations may potentiate replication of the vaccine virus, increasing chance for developing the viral disease.

**Laboratory Test Interferences:** May decrease serum calcium, potassium, $T_4$, and reduce $^{131}I$ uptake, urine 17 hydroxysteroid and 17 ketosteroids. Tends to suppress skin tests; may give a false-negative result with nitroblue–tetrazolium for bacterial infection.

**Storage Requirements:** Store at 15 to 30°C (59 to 86°F). IM preparation sensitive to heat; do not autoclave.

# ☐ CO-TRIMOXAZOLE                    (koe-try-mox'a-zole)

(Apo-Sulfatrim, Bactrim, Bactrim DS, Bactrim I.V. Infusion, Bethaprim, Cotrim, Cotrim DS, Septra, Septra DS, Septra I.V. Infusion, Sulfatrim)

**Classification:** antibiotic, sulfonamide

**Available Preparations:**
- 200 mg (SMZ) and 40 mg (TMP) / 5ml suspension
- 400 mg (SMZ) and 80 mg (TMP); 800 mg (SMZ) and 160 mg (TMP) tablets
- 80 mg/ml (SMZ) and 16 mg/ml (TMP) for parenteral administration

**Action and Use:** Combination of trimethoprim (TMP) and sulfamethoxazole (SMZ), which acts synergistically in inhibiting folic acid metabolism in bacteria. Its spectrum of activity covers a wide variety of bacteria except *Pseudomonas*, enterococci, mycobacteria, *Clostridia*. Treats *Pneumocystis carinii* pneumonia.

**Routes and Dosage:** (Dosage based on trimethoprim)
*PO, IV:*
Minor Infections:
- less than 40 kg: 8 to 10 mg/kg/day in equally divided doses every 12 hours
- over 40 kg: 320 mg/day equally divided every 12 hours

Severe Infections: 20 mg/kg/day equally divided doses every 6 to 8 hours

**Absorption and Fate:** Rapidly, well absorbed from GI tract. Peak level: 1 to 4 hours. Well distributed into body tissues and fluids. Half-life: (TMP) 11 hours; (SMZ) 14.5 hours. Therapeutic level is ratio of 1:20 or 0.1 to 1 µg/ml (TMP) and 1 to 50 µg/ml (SMZ). Metabolized in liver; excreted in urine with small amount in bile.

**Contraindications and Precautions:** Pregnancy category C, near term D. Contraindicated during lactation, first 2 months life (may cause kernicterus in infants), hypersensitivity to either drug, sulfonamides, megaloblastic anemia, or creatinine clearances under 15 ml/minute. Use with caution in impaired renal or hepatic function, bronchial asthma, allergies, folate or G-6-PD, blood dyscrasias, acquired immunodeficiency syndrome (AIDS), or X chromosome mental retardation.

**Side Effects:**
*CNS:* headache, lethargy, nervousness, ataxia, mental depression, **seizures**, hallucinations. *GI:* nausea, vomiting, diarrhea, GI pain, stomatitis, **pseudomembranous enterocolitis**, pancreatitis. *Hepatic:* **hepatitis.** *GU:* increased BUN and serum creatinine, crystalluria, and rarely **interstitial nephritis, toxic nephrosis with oliguria, anuria.** *Skin:* erythematous, maculopapular, morbil-

liform rashes, urticaria. *Hemic:* **agranulocytosis, aplastic anemia, leukopenia, neutropenia, thrombocytopenia, hemolytic anemia**. *Other:* Hypersensitivity: **epidermal necrolysis, Stevens-Johnson syndrome, exfoliative dermatitis, allergic myocarditis**, arthralgia, pruritus, photosensitivity, **anaphylaxis**; Local: pain, irritation and inflammation, thrombophlebitis (rare).

## Nursing Implications:

*Assess:* Assess if previous allergy to drug combination or sulfonamides. Obtain cultures and sensitivity before treatment, but can start treatment before results. Obtain baseline CBC, UA, renal function tests, especially if on long-term therapy.

*Administer: PO:* Shake suspension well. Tablet may be crushed, mixed with a small amount of food or fluid. Give on empty stomach. *IV:* Do not use if solution cloudy or has crystals. Do not give IV push or rapid infusion. Usually diluted with 75 or 125 ml of 5% dextrose. Intermittent infusion (minimum dilution of 1 ml in 15 ml) infused over 60 to 90 minutes. Must be used within 2 hours of dilution. Compatible with $D_5W$, $D_5W$/0.5% NS, NS, 0.5% NS, LR. Do not premix with other medications or solutions.

*Monitor:* Observe IV site for vein irritation and extravasation and change site every 72 hours. Observe for sore throat, fever, skin rash, and sore mouth; signs of blood dyscrasias. Observe for side effects. Side effects of rash, fever, and hematological changes seen most frequently with caucasian AIDS patients, occurring second week of therapy; symptoms usually reversible. Assess CBC and renal function during therapy. Report hematological symptoms immediately; stop medication. Maintain daily hydration level for child's age.

*Patient Teaching:* Take as prescribed for full course of therapy. Observe for side effects and maintain hydration levels. Protect child from sun.

## Drug Interactions:
Probenecid increases chance for sulfinpyrazone toxicity. Used in combination with warfarin may prolong prothrombin time. Can displace methotrexate from binding sites when used together. Interferes with bactericidal effects of penicillins. This drug may inhibit the hepatic metabolism of phenytoin.

## Storage Requirements:
Store at 15 to 30°C (59 to 86°F), light-resistant containers. Injectable form storage affected by further dilution, check with package inserts for storage time.

---

## ☐ CROMOLYN SODIUM                                        (kroe'moe-lin)

(Disodium Cromoglycate, Fivent, Intal, Nasalcrom, Opticrom, Rynacrom)

**Classification:** antiasthmatic, mast cell stabilizer

## Available Preparations:
- 4% solution for ophthalmic administration
- 800 μg/metered aerosol spray for oral inhalation
- 20 mg/2 ml solution for nebulization
- 20 mg powder (contained in capsules) for inhalation
- 5.2 mg/metered spray (40 mg/ml) for nasal inhalation

**Action and Use:** Inhibits release of chemical mediators (such as histamine or slow-reacting substance) from mast cells as result of IgE-mediated antigen-antibody reaction. This drug has no direct bronchodilating effect, but is useful in the prevention of an asthma attack. Ophthalmic form treats allergic conjunctivitis and keratoconjunctivitis, vernal keratoconjunctivitis, and keratitis. Allergic rhinitis is treated with nasal form.

## Routes and Dosage:
*Ophthalmic:* over 4 years: instill 1 to 2 drops of 4% solution into conjunctival sac 4 to 6 times per day at regular intervals
*Nasal:* Allergic Rhinitis: over 6 years: 5.2 mg delivered per metered spray; give 1 spray, 3 to 4 times at regular intervals
*Inhalation:*
- Bronchial Asthma: over 2 years: oral inhalation solution, 20 mg inhaled 4 times per day at regular intervals
- Aerosol: over 5 years: two inhalations 4 times a day at regular intervals
- Capsule in Oral Inhaler: over 5 years: 20 mg inhaled 4 times daily at regular intervals

**Absorption and Fate:** Minimal amount absorbed systemically from GI tract, eye or nasal routes (about 8 to 10% absorbed from lungs). Half-life: 80 minutes. Excreted equally in urine and biliary tract.

**Contraindications and Precautions:** Pregnancy category B. Use with caution during lactation. Preparations of cromolyn are contraindicated in oral inhalation solution under 2 years, ophthalmic solution under 4 years, powder or aerosol under 5 years, and nasal solution under 6 years. Contraindicated in hypersensitivity to drug or its ingredients (lactose), relief of acute bronchospasm, status asthmaticus. Use with caution in coronary artery disease, history of cardiac arrhythmias, hepatic or renal function impairment.

## Side Effects:
*CNS:* headache, dizziness, **peripheral neuritis**. *GI:* nausea. *Resp:* throat and tracheal irritation, cough, bronchospasm (powder), bad taste, hoarseness, wheezing (aerosol), esophagitis, hemoptysis, epistaxis. *GU:* dysuria, urinary frequency. *Skin:* rash, urticaria, angioedema, **exfoliative dermatitis** (rare). *Musculoskeletal:* joint pain, swelling. *Sensory:* Ophthalmic: burning or stinging, dryness, eye irritation styes, edema of tissue surrounding eyes, lacrimation. *Other:* swelling parotid gland, myalgia, **nephrosis, pericarditis, anemia, anaphyaxis**.

## Nursing Implications:

*Assess:* Ability of child to follow directions for using hand-held inhalers. A neubulizer can be used for child who is unable to use inhaler. Assess for lactose intolerance (capsule) before its usage. Pulmonary function test to assess significant bronchodilator-reversible component to airway obstruction is recommended before therapy.

*Administer: Ophthalmic:* For instillation, see Part I. Do not touch dropper tip to eye or adjacent structures. Manufacturer recommends that this preparation not be used with soft contact lenses due to preservative benzalkonium chloride; however, some medical experts believe this is not necessary. Check with child's ophthalmologist. *Nasal:* Administer with special nasal inhaler. Before use, clear nasal passages of mucus. Follow package insert for priming and assembly of inhaler. Have child inhale through nose during administration. Manufacturer recommends not cleaning device after each use. Instead, replace device every 6 months. *Inhalation:* If an inhaler for bronchodilation is also prescribed, use 5 minutes before cromolyn. If used for exercise-induced bronchospasm, cromolyn should be administered 30 minutes before exercise. Drug (solution) can be administered through power-operated nebulizer; dosage and duration of treatment should be ordered by physician. To use aerosol inhaler, invert and shake well. Assemble and load capsule into oral inhaler according to package insert. Both inhalers are used as described in Part I. Remove inhaler, hold breath for a few seconds, then exhale slowly. Capsule inhaler is used until all of powder is gone from inhaler. Do not exhale into inhaler because moisture from breath can interfere with operation of inhaler. Capsule inhaler is cleaned by dismantling and cleaning it in warm water once a week. Aerosol mouth piece is removed from canister and cleaned with warm water after use.

*Monitor:* Monitor for side effects. Eosinophil count is an indicator of developing hypersensitivity to drug. Lactose intolerance side effects include nausea, bloating, abdominal cramps, and flatulence. These symptoms may follow inhalation of capsules and may occur within 2 hours of inhalation. Therapeutic effects of drug may occur in several days; however, results are usually seen within 1 to 2 weeks. If child is on concurrent corticosteroid therapy, do not withdraw either drug rapidly because it may cause exacerbation of asthmatic symptoms; withdrawal of either drug should be gradual and under physician's supervision. Not all children respond to this drug. If no effect is seen after 1 month trial, it should be discontinued.

*Patient Teaching:* Proper use and care of inhaler should be taught. It is beneficial to have child demonstrate inhaler use. Use inhaler only as prescribed and do not use during acute asthmatic attack. Symptoms of throat irritation may be relieved by rinsing mouth or sucking on sugarless hard candy after use. Caution parents that capsule should not be swallowed.

**Storage Requirements:** Store at 2 to 30°C (36 to 86°F) and protect from flame or heat above 102°F. Do not puncture or discard inhaler into fire or incinerator.

# ☐ CROTAMITON                                    (kroe-tam'i-tonn)

(Eurax)

## Classification: scabicide

## Available Preparations:
- 10% topical lotion
- 10% topical cream

## Action and Use: A synthetic chloroformate whose action is unknown; used to eradicate parasitic mite *Sarcoptes scabiei*.

## Routes and Dosage:
*Topical:* Apply a thin layer of 10% preparation to all body parts from chin downward to feet. Reapply in 24 hours (see *Administer* on how to apply)

## Contraindications and Precautions: Pregnancy category C. Safe use in children not established. Contraindicated if hypersensitivity to drug or its components, acutely inflamed, raw, or weeping skin surfaces.

## Side Effects:
*Skin:* local irritation, rash

## Nursing Implications:
*Assess:* Carefully inspect and note extent and amount of infestation. Diagnosis confirmed by examining of material from burrow track area.

*Administer: Topical:* Shake lotion before usage. Bathe child with soap and water gently removing scales and crusts; towel dry. Apply very thin layer of medication from chin downward making sure that all skin surfaces covered e.g., folds of skin, hands, fingers, feet including toes and soles of feet. Do not apply to face, eyes, mucous membranes, or urethral meatus. Do not bathe child. A second coat should be applied in 24 hours and left on for 48 hours, child should not bathe during treatment. After this 48-hour period, give cleansing bath. Fresh bedding should be placed on bed; then all bedding, towels and other personal items used should be washed in hot water and dried on hot dryer setting. Items that cannot be washed should be dry cleaned (stuffed animals, etc.) or placed in dryer for 20 minutes on hot setting. If child sleeps with another child, he too should be treated. Some clinicians believe the entire household should be treated.

*Monitor:* If child is hospitalized during this infestation take proper isolation precautions used by agency. Assess skin for healing and notify physician if condition does not improve or worsens. Notify preschools, nursery schools, day-care centers, or schools of infestation.

*Patient Teaching:* Parent and child should understand that this is a contagious condition and why it has to be treated. Explain how to apply and prevent reinfestations or spreading of scabies. Thick applications will not hasten healing and may cause irritation. The child should be kept home from school, day-care centers, preschool until treatment rendered and these agencies should be informed of infestation. If child is sexually active, sexual partner also needs treatment.

**Storage Requirements:** Store at 15 to 30°C (59 to 86°F) in light-resistant containers.

---

## □ CYCLOPHOSPHAMIDE                  (sye-kloe-foss'fa-mide)

(Cytoxan, Neosar)

**Classification:** antineoplastic, alkylating agent

**Available Preparations:**
- 25, 50-mg tablets
- 100, 200, 500-mg, 1, 2-g vials for injection
- Injection vials also available in combination with mannitol

**Action and Use:** This alkylating agent interferes with nucleic acid function by inhibiting DNA synthesis and RNA function, thereby preventing cell division after it is turned to active metabolites (phosphoramide mustard) by the liver. It is used in a variety of malignancies such as acute lymphoblastic leukemia, Hodgkin's and non-Hodgkin's lymphoma, Burkitt's lymphoma, neuroblastoma, retinoblastoma, and Ewing's sarcoma. It is also a potent immunosuppressant and has been used (although not approved by the FDA for these purposes) in treatment of recurrent glomerulonephritis and nephrotic syndrome and to prevent rejection after organ transplant.

**Routes and Dosages:** PO, IV; occasionally IM, intracavitary, direct perfusion
**PO, IV:** Induction Dose: 2 to 8 mg/kg or 60 to 250 mg/m²/day in divided doses for 6 or more days
**PO:** Maintenance Dose: 1 to 5 mg/kg or 50 to 150 mg/m² twice weekly
Clinicians give one large dose at one time or over 2 to 4 days (i.e., 500 to 1200 mg/m² or 30 to 40 mg/kg every 2 to 4 weeks) or a smaller dose over a longer period of time.
Dosages vary according to the disease and other drugs being used simultaneously. Some examples of doses used by clinicians are:
- Rhabdomyosarcoma: 10 to 40 mg/kg/day for 3 days
- Hepatoblastoma: 500 mg/m² every 21 days
- Neuroblastoma: 750 mg/m² every 28 days
- Non-Hodgkin's Lymphoma: 1000 mg/m² every 6 weeks
- Acute Lymphocytic Lymphoma: 1000 mg/m² every 14 days
- Ewing's Sarcoma: 1200 mg/m² for 3 days every 6 weeks

**Absorption and Fate:** Oral form well absorbed from GI tract. Distributed to all body tissues. Crosses placenta and present in breast milk. Metabolized by the liver and excreted mainly in the urine. Peak level: 1 hour after PO, immediate after IV. Half-life: 2.4 to 6.5 hours (average 4.1 hours); present in blood 72 hours after administration.

**Contraindications and Precautions:** Pregnancy category C. Use during pregnancy especially the first trimester is avoided unless clearly necessary. Patients should avoid pregnancy for at least 4 months after discontinuation of the drug. Breast-feeding should be avoided while on the drug. The drug is generally discontinued if the patient develops a life-threatening infection such as chicken pox or herpes zoster, and resumed after successful treatment of the infection. Use with caution in those with previous antineoplastic therapy, impaired renal or hepatic function, infections. Hemorrhagic cystitis is dose limiting.

**Side Effects:**
***CNS:*** headache, dizziness; faintness and flushing after IV especially if administered too quickly. ***CV:*** heart toxicity with large doses and if given concomitantly with doxorubicin or daunomycin or with irradiation involving cardiac vessels. ***GI:*** nausea, vomiting, anorexia especially at high doses; about 6 hours after drug administration, may last 4 hours. Diarrhea, mucosal irritation such as stomatitis, ulceration, colitis are less common. ***Respiratory:*** interstitial pulmonary fibrosis (rare but potentially fatal). ***Hepatic:*** hepatic toxicity (rare). ***GU:*** hemorrhagic cystitis especially in children (dose-limiting effect); hyperuricemia; nephrotoxicity (rare); altered ADH secretion can lead to retained water, weight gain, edema, hyponatremia. Gonadal suppression and sterility of both sexes can occur. ***Skin:*** alopecia (common, occurs in about 33% about 3 weeks after treatment begins), abnormal fingernail growth, dermatitis, hyperpigmentation, suppression of TB test results. ***Hemic:*** leukopenia, thrombocytopenia (common and major dose-limiting effects), nadir is 7 to 12 days for leukopenia, 10 to 15 days for thrombocytopenia; hypoprothrombinemia and anemia (rare). ***Other:*** hyperkalemia; secondary malignancies such as bladder and lymph carcinomas may occur, even several years after therapy.

**Nursing Implications:**
***Assess:*** Establish baseline weight, vital signs, CBC with differential, urinalysis.
***Administer:*** This drug has potentially severe toxic effects and should be given only under the supervision of a physician with training and experience in cancer chemotherapy. The drug's potential for toxic effects on health-care personnel as well as patients necessitates careful handling during preparation and administration. Generally during preparation of antineoplastics, latex gloves, a mask, and a solid front gown are worn, and a laminar flow hood is used. Gloves and gown may also be recommended for administration. Contaminated equipment, such as needles, syringes, vials, ampules, and unused medication,

should be disposed of properly. Clean-up of spills is carefully performed and accidental contact by patient or personnel receives prompt flushing and cleaning. *PO:* Give between meals if nausea and vomiting are not a problem; otherwise give during or immediately after a meal. Give no later than 4 PM to reduce amount in bladder at night. Increase fluid intake about three times normal. *IV:* Add sterile or bacteriostatic water for injection (5 ml for 100 mg, 10 ml for 200 mg, 25 ml for 500 mg, 50 ml for 1g, or 100 ml to 2 g for a solution of 20 mg/ml). Solution takes time to dissolve; shake well. May be added to normal saline, 5% dextrose, lactated Ringer's solution for administration. Given in 15 to 30 minutes. Reconstituted solutions are stable 24 hours at room temperature or 6 days if refrigerated.

*Monitor:* Monitor I & O. Observe for hematuria and dysuria. Monitor CBC, uric acid, serum electrolytes, urinary specific gravity, SGOT, SGPT, bilirubin, creatinine, LDH. These laboratory tests are done periodically or several hours after an IV dose. Protect patient from sources of infection. Leukopenia may necessitate reverse isolation. Weigh at least twice weekly. Take vital signs regularly. Look for signs of infection such as fever, purulent wounds, varicella or herpes infection. Check diet by nutritional analysis.

*Patient Teaching:* Talk about possibility of nausea and vomiting, and emphasize effectiveness of antiemetic therapy. Encourage increase in fluid intake and frequent voiding. Patient should inform physician if there is no voiding within 2 hours after oral cyclophosphamide is taken. Inform patient to report signs of possible infection or bleeding such as fever, chills, cough, skin irritation, bloody urine, tarry stools. Avoid persons with illness such as colds, chicken pox, influenza. Prepare patient for possibility of alopecia and make plans for wig or hat use if appropriate. Plan for nutritious, appetizing meals. Explain importance of monitoring during therapy as well as long-term follow-up for signs of secondary cancer, especially bladder.

## Drug Interactions:
Several drugs enhance the effects of cyclophosphamide, increasing chance of bone marrow toxicity; these include allopurinol, barbiturates, chloramphenicol, corticosteroids. Potential for cardiac complications increases when given with other cardiotoxic drugs such as doxorubicin and daunorubicin. Succinylcholine effects may be prolonged in patients on cyclophosphamide. Immune response may be insufficient if given immunizations while on this drug. Live virus vaccines must not be given, or oral polio vaccine to those in close contact with the patient on cyclophosphamide due to the chance of infection with a virus; these vaccines delayed until at least 3 months after chemotherapy when patient is in remission.

## Laboratory Test Interferences:
Suppresses positive TB test; increases uric acid levels in blood and urine. Occasionally produces positive direct antiglobulin (Coombs') test.

## Storage Requirements:
Store at 15 to 30°C (59 to 86°F). Keep containers tightly closed.

---

# □ CYPROHEPTADINE

(si-proe-hep'ta-deen)

(Periactin)

**Classification:** antihistamine, appetite stimulant

## Available Preparations:
- 4-mg tablets
- 2 mg/5 ml oral solution

**Action and Use:** Competes with histamine for $H_1$ receptor sites. Also competes with serotonin for receptor sites in smooth muscle. Also acts as an anticholinergic, sedative, and calcium-channel blocker. Used for its antihistamine effect in treatment of cold urticaria and for a variety of unapproved uses such as in treatment of anorexia nervosa, somatotropin deficiency, and Cushing's syndrome.

## Routes and Dosages:
*PO:* Allergy:
- 2 to 6 years: 2 mg BID or TID; not to exceed 12 mg/day
- 7 to 14 years: 4 mg BID or TID; not to exceed 16 mg/day
- Alternative childhood dose: 0.25 mg/kg/day or 8 mg/m²/day in divided doses

Anorexia Nervosa: 13 years and over: 2 mg QID; increased over 3 weeks to 8 mg QID

**Absorption and Fate:** Well absorbed from GI tract. Distribution unknown. Metabolized by liver and metabolites excreted in urine. Peak levels reached in 6 to 9 hours.

**Contraindications and Precautions:** Pregnancy category B. Not recommended during lactation as it can inhibit lactation and effects on the infant can include paradoxical excitement. Contraindicated in newborns and safety in children under 2 years is not established. Contraindicated with antihistamine allergy history.

## Side Effects:
*CNS:* drowsiness, dizziness, incoordination, paradoxical excitement in children with insomnia, tremors, palpitation, seizures. *GI:* nausea, vomiting, diarrhea, constipation, anorexia, epigastric discomfort. *Respiratory:* dyspnea, nasal stuffiness. *Skin:* rash, pruritis, eczema, inflammation

## Nursing Implications:
*Assess:* Baseline height and weight.
*Administer:* May give with food to decrease GI upset. May crush tablet and give in small amount of food or fluid.

*Monitor:* When given for anorexia nervosa, record food and fluid intake and urinary output. Daily weight.

*Patient Teaching:* Take as directed and report changes in appetite or weight. Drug can alter mental alertness therefore avoid driving and adjust activities accordingly.

**Drug Interactions:** Increased CNS depression with other CNS depressants. Increased antimuscarinic effects with other antimuscarinics. Increased anticholinergic effects with MAO inhibitors.

**Laboratory Test Interferences:** Increased serum amylase and prolactin. May inhibit response to skin tests; discontinue drug at least 72 hours before skin test.

**Storage Requirements:** Store in tightly closed container between 15 and 30°C (59 and 86°F). Protect syrup from freezing.

---

## □ CYTARABINE                                     (sye-tare′a-been)

(ARA-C, Cytosar-U, Cytosine arabinoside)

**Classification:** antineoplastic, antimetabolite

**Available Preparations:** 100, 500-mg vials for parenteral use

**Action and Use:** Inhibits DNA synthesis and may be incorporated into DNA and RNA molecules. Cell cycle specific for S phase of cell division. Also has a powerful immunosuppressant effect. Used in treatment of leukemia such as acute myelocytic and acute lymphocytic leukemia, and meningeal leukemia and other meningeal neoplasms; used in lymphoma.

**Routes and Dosages:** IM, IV, IT; SC and IM experimentally
Dosage is highly individualized depending on type and timing of treatment. Examples of treatment follow.
*IV:* 100 to 200 mg/m² by continuous IV infusion for 5 days at 2-week intervals; or 25 mg/m²/day for 5 days; or 75 mg/m²/day for 8 days
  ■ Combination Therapy: 2 to 6 mg/kg/day or 100 to 200 mg/m²/day by continuous IV infusion of 5 to 10 days or divided into 2 to 3 injections daily
  ■ High Dose Treatment for AML: Capezzi treatment: 3000 mg/m² over 4 hours, given every 12 hours for 4 doses
  ■ Maintenance Therapy: 70 to 200 mg/m²/day or same amount in 2 to 5-day infusion each month
*IM, SC:* Maintenance Therapy: 1 to 1.5 mg/kg q1–4wk

*IT:* 5 to 75 mg/m$^2$ or 30 to 100 mg q2–7d. Commonly used IT doses for young children are:
- under 1 year: 20 mg
- 1 to 2 years: 30 mg
- 2 to 3 years: 50 mg
- 3 years and over: 50 mg

## Absorption and Fate:
Absorbs poorly from GI tract; not effective as oral drug. Widely distributed in body tissues. Metabolized in liver, kidneys, and other sites. Excreted in urine. Peak level after SC and IM is 20 to 60 minutes; peak levels are lower after these routes than IV. Half-life is biphasic with initial in 10 minutes, terminal in 1 to 3 hours. Half-life in CSF is 2 hours.

## Contraindications and Precautions:
Pregnancy category C. Should not be used in pregnancy especially first trimester unless clearly needed. Possibility of fetal anomaly must be discussed. Should not be used during lactation. Safety in infants and children is not established although it is used in these age groups when needed. Contraindicated during chicken pox or herpes zoster infection. The preparation with benzyl alcohol preservative should not be used in neonates or for high dose or intrathecal administration. Cautious use in those with hepatic or renal disease or with myelosuppression.

## Side Effects:
*CNS:* headache, paresthesia, paralysis, seizures; most common with high dose or IT use. *GI:* nausea, vomiting (especially after rapid IV infusion), diarrhea, anorexia, stomatitis, GI hemorrhage. *Hepatic:* jaundice, elevated bilirubin, transaminase, alkaline phosphatase; all more common with high dose. *GU:* hyperuricemia due to cell breakdown; effect treated by allopurinol and increased fluid intake. *Skin:* rash, alopecia, freckling, irritation at injection site. *Hemic:* leukopenia from granulocyte suppression, anemia, thrombocytopenia. Leukopenia occurs in two phases: one, 24 hours after therapy begins; the second, at 15 to 24 days. Thrombocytopenia begins 5 days after therapy and continues until about day 15 after which platelet levels rise. *Other:* fever, myalgia, bone and joint pain, chest pain; this combination of symptoms occurs 6 to 12 hours after drug administration and may be treated with corticosteroids. **High dose** may cause somnolence, coma, hemorrhagic conjunctivitis, GI and pulmonary toxicity, peripheral neuropathies, and more commonly leads to the CNS and hepatic symptoms listed above. **High-dose toxicities** may be fatal.

## Nursing Implications:
*Assess:* Establish baseline vital signs, CBC, platelet count, UA, weight.
*Administer:* This drug has potentially severe toxic effects and should be given only under the supervision of a physician with training and experience in cancer chemotherapy. The drug's potential for toxic effects on health-care personnel as well as patients necessitates careful handling during preparation and administration. Generally, during preparation of antineoplastics, latex gloves, a mask, and a solid front gown are worn, and a laminar flow hood is used. Gloves and gown may also be recommended for administration. Contaminated

equipment, such as needles, syringes, vials, and unused medication, is disposed of properly. Clean-up of spills is carefully performed and accidental contact by patient or personnel receives prompt flushing and cleaning. Increase fluid intake to assist with cell and drug elimination. *IV:* Reconstitute with bacteriostatic water with 5 ml for 100-mg vial or 10 ml for 500-mg vial for a preparation of 20 mg/ml or 50 mg/ml, respectively. Reconstituted solution stable for 2 days at room temperature unless a preservative free solution is used; then it is best to discard excess drug. May be diluted in water for injection, 5% dextrose, or saline if given as IV infusion. Incompatible in IV solutions with several other drugs such as fluorouracil. Benzyl alcohol preservative preparations are not to be used for neonates or high-dose therapy. *IT:* Reconstitute with preservative free saline, Elliot's B solution, or with patient's own spinal fluid. Preparations with benzyl alcohol must not be used for IT administration. Given in 5 to 15 ml of solution after removing an equal amount of CSF.

*Monitor:* Leukocyte, granulocyte, and platelet counts should be done daily during remission therapy and regularly during maintenance therapy. Notify physician of polymorphonuclear granulocyte or leukocyte counts below 1000/mm³ or platelet counts below 50,000/mm³ as this may be cause for discontinuation or modification of therapy. Therapy may begin again after counts have reached the levels above. Bone marrow tests are done every 1 to 2 weeks. Monitor for signs of drug toxicity and infections. Monitor for nausea and use ordered antiemetics as needed. Observe for fluid and elctrolyte disturbances; monitor I & O, daily weight, electrolytes. Monitor liver and kidney function tests such as bilirubin, BUN, SGPT, SGOT, creatinine, LDH, uric acid. **High dose:** Watch for peripheral neuropathy (weakness, gait changes, handwriting problems, numbness, myalgia) and report to the physician immediately as these effects may be irreversible. Antiemetic and diet alteration (such as small frequent meals) can improve nutritional status; administer antiemetic routinely. Observe for fluid and electrolyte imbalances. Monitor I & O; take weight once or twice daily especially if vomiting is severe; monitor electrolyte levels. Observe for changes in level of consciousness. Take vital signs regularly; temperature elevation may occur. Observe for hemorrhagic conjunctivitis; administer eye ointments or drops as ordered. Observe for hyperuricemia; allopurinol may be ordered.

*Patient Teaching:* The patient should be alert for and report signs of infection or bleeding such as fever, sore throat, cough, bruising, and tarry stools. Report skin problems and bone or joint pain. Encourage increased fluid intake and nutritious food. Hair loss may occur. Flulike symptoms may occur 6 weeks or more after drug therapy begins. Have patient report changes in urine output. Close monitoring is essential so patient must return for follow-up visits.

**Drug Interactions:** Suppresses immune response to immunization. Live virus vaccines must not be given, nor oral polio vaccine to close contacts, when the patient is on this drug due to the chance of infection with a virus; these vaccines are delayed until at least 3 months after chemotherapy when the patient is in remission.

**Laboratory Test Interferences:** Increases bilirubin, transaminase, alkaline phosphatase results.

**Storage Requirements:** Store powder at 15 to 30°C (59 to 86°F). Solutions may be stable at room temperature for 2 days after reconstitution; if solution develops a slight haze, it should not be used.

---

## □ DACARBAZINE                                     (da-kar'ba-zeen)

(DTIC-Dome, DTIC)

**Classification:** antineoplastic, alkylating agent

**Available Preparations:** 100, 200-mg vials for parenteral use

**Action and Use:** Exact mechanism of action is unknown but appears to inhibit DNA, RNA, and protein synthesis. Cell cycle nonspecific. Used in treatment of Hodgkin's disease. Used experimentally in rhabdomyosarcoma and neuroblastoma and some brain tumors, such as astrocytomas, although not approved by the FDA for these tumors.

### Routes and Dosages:
Pediatric dosages not established. Examples of doses used by clinicians are:
*IV:*
- 3.5 mg/kg or 250 mg/m²/day for 1 to 10 days; repeat every 28 days
- 150 mg/m² q28d
- 500 mg/m² q3–4wk
- Hodgkin's Disease: adult dose: 150 mg/m²/day for 5 days, repeated every 4 weeks *or* 375 mg/m² on day 1, repeated day 15; *or* 2 to 4.5 mg/kg/day for 10 days repeat q28d; *or* up to 250 mg/m²/day for 5 days, repeat q21d; given with other agents

**Absorption and Fate:** Absorbed rapidly after IV administration. Distributed in body with possible storage in liver; slightly bound (5%) to plasma proteins; present in low levels in CNS. Metabolized and excreted in urine by tubular secretion. Peak level of 8 μg/ml reached immediately after IV administration. Biphasic half-life with 19 minutes initially and 5 hours terminally. Prolonged in renal or hepatic dysfunction to 55 minutes and 7.2 hours.

**Contraindications and Precautions:** Pregnancy category C. Used only if clearly needed in pregnancy as it has been teratogenic in laboratory animals. Not recommended during lactation as its distribution in breast milk is unknown. Contraindicated in those with a known hypersensitivity to the drug and those with chicken pox or herpes zoster infection. Drug is modified if WBC count falls below 3000/mm³ or platelet count falls below 100,000/mm³ or in infections.

## Side Effects:
*CNS:* confusion, headache, seizures. *GI:* nausea, vomiting, anorexia (common in 90% of patients; symptoms improve after first 2 days); diarrhea, stomatitis. *Hepatic:* elevated SGOT, SGPT, BUN, hepatic vein thrombosis. *Skin:* alopecia, facial flushing, pain and necrosis with extravasation. *Hemic:* leukopenia, thrombocytopenia 2 to 4 weeks after last dose. *Other:* flulike syndrome about 7 days after dose

## Nursing Implications:
*Assess:* Take baseline CBC and liver studies. Question prior hypersensitivity to drug.

*Administer:* This drug has potentially severe toxic effects and should be given only under the supervision of a physician with training and experience in cancer chemotherapy. The drug's potential for toxic effects on health-care personnel as well as patients necessitates careful handling during preparation and administration. Generally, during preparation of antineoplastics latex gloves, a mask, and a solid front gown are worn, and a laminar flow hood is used. Gloves and gown may also be recommended for administration. Contaminated equipment, such as needles, syringes, vials, and unused medication, is disposed of properly. Clean-up of spills is carefully performed and accidental contact by patient or personnel receives prompt flushing and cleaning. *IV:* Solution reconstituted with 9.9 ml (for 100-mg vial) or 19.7 ml (for 200-mg vial) sterile water and injected IV over 1 to 2 minutes or added to 250 ml of saline or 5% dextrose and infused over 15 to 30 minutes. Solutions reconstituted with sterile water are stable for 72 hours if refrigerated or 8 hours at room temperature. Solutions in 5% dextrose or saline are stable 24 hours if refrigerated or 8 hours at room temperature. Decomposition is indicated by color change from clear or pale yellow to pink. Avoid extravasation as tissue damage and severe pain can occur. Local pain and irritation at injection site may occur even without extravasation and may be treated with application of heat. Increased or decreased hydration is used to decrease nausea depending on clinician. (Some restrict fluid 4 to 6 hours before a dose, whereas others increase hydration until 1 hour before a dose.)

*Monitor:* CBC is monitored regularly and drug dosage may be altered if WBC count is under 3000/mm³ or platelet count is below 100,000/mm³. Monitor I & O. Observe injection site carefully to avoid extravasation. Renal and hepatic function may be monitored with BUN, SGPT, SGOT, LDH, bilirubin, creatinine, uric acid, UA.

*Patient Teaching:* Take ordered antiemetic for nausea. If nausea and vomiting continue, report this. Encourage nutritious intake and adequate fluids. Avoid persons with infections such as colds, influenza, chicken pox. Report signs of infection such as fever, malaise, sore throat, cough and signs of bleeding and bruising. Avoid sun exposure.

## Drug Interactions:
Suppresses immune response to immunization. Live virus vaccines must not be given, nor oral polio vaccine to those in close contact with the patient on this drug due to the chance of infection with a virus; these vaccines are delayed until at least 3 months after chemotherapy when the patient is in remission.

**Laboratory Test Interferences:** Elevated SGOT, SGPT, BUN

**Storage Requirements:** Store at 2 to 8°C (35 to 46°F) and protect from light. Do not use pink solutions.

---

# □ DACTINOMYCIN    (dak-tin-oh-mye'sin)

(Actinomycin D)

**Combination Products:** Cosmegen

**Classification:** antineoplastic, antibiotic

## Available Preparations:
- 500-μg vial for parenteral use
- Available with 20 mg mannitol

**Action and Use:** Binds to DNA and inhibits RNA synthesis and is cell-phase nonspecific. It has immunosuppressive and hypocalcemic actions. Effective against gram-positive organisms but is not used as an antibiotic due to its toxicity. Used to treat Wilms' tumor, rhabdomyosarcoma, and Ewing's sarcoma. It has been used to prevent rejection in those with organ transplant, although this use is not approved by the FDA.

## Routes and Dosages:
*IV:* 10 to 15 μg/kg/day for 5 days; or 450 μg/m²/day for 5 days; or 500 μg/m²/day for 4 days; or 2.5 mg/m² as a cumulative dose divided into several doses and given over 1 week. Additional courses may be used each 2 to 4 weeks, if drug toxicity is not evident. A single dose must not exceed 500 μg. Dosages may need to be lowered in the obese patient or one who has received prior chemotherapy or radiation therapy.
*Regional perfusion (uncommon):* 50 μg/kg for pelvis and lower extremity; 35 μg/kg for upper extremity.

**Absorption and Fate:** Absorbed poorly from GI tract; no oral form available. Rapidly distributed to body tissues after IV administration. Present in bone marrow and blood cells, not present in therapeutic amounts in CNS. Excreted mainly as unchanged drug in feces and urine. Peak level is immediate. Half-life is 36 hours.

**Contraindications and Precautions:** Pregnancy category C. Use in pregnancy only if clearly needed as the drug is teratogenic in animals. Do not use during lactation. Used only in children over 6 months; children from 6 to 12 months should have reduced dosages and frequent checks of hemic status. Contraindicated in chicken pox or herpes zoster infections. Cautious use in obese and edematous patients, those with hepatic or renal dysfunction, those with previous chemotherapy or radiation therapy, with infections, or who are immunosuppressed.

## Side Effects:
**CNS:** fatigue, malaise. **GI:** nausea, vomiting for 24 hours after administration; oral and GI ulcers as well as diarrhea are signs of toxicity and may necessitate dosage adjustment. **Hepatic:** elevated SGOT, ascites, hepatomegaly (rare). **GU:** hyperuricemia. **Skin:** alopecia 7 to 10 days after administration, can involve eyebrows; hyperpigmentation, rash; pain and erythema at injection site; tissue necrosis with extravasation. **Hemic:** myelosuppression 1 to 7 days after therapy with blood values returning to normal by about 21 days; leukopenia, thrombocytopenia, anemia. **Other:** fever, rare anaphylaxis. When given up to several months after radiation therapy, radiation recall may occur (erythema, desquamation, hyperpigmentation). Regional perfusion can lead to edema and damage to tissues in area of perfusion; systemic effects can occur if absorbed.

## Nursing Implications:
**Assess:** Establish history of previous chemotherapy and radiation therapy. Baseline CBC.

**Administer:** This drug has potentially severe side effects and should be given only under the supervision of a physician with training and experience in cancer chemotherapy. The drug's potential for toxic effects on health-care personnel as well as patients necessitates careful handling during preparation and administration. Generally, during preparation of antineoplastics, latex gloves, a mask, and a solid front gown are worn, and a laminar flow hood is used. Gloves and gown are recommended for administration. Contaminated equipment, such as needles, syringes, vials, and unused medication, is disposed of properly. Clean-up of spills is carefully performed and accidental contact by patient or personnel receives prompt flushing and cleaning. **IV:** Give IV as drug is irritating to tissues. Reconstitute with sterile water without preservatives as bacteriostatic water and normal saline solutions may cause precipitation. May be added to 5% dextrose or normal saline IV solution for administration. Give directly into sidearm of running IV over several minutes and use 5 to 10 ml of IV fluid to flush tubing after use. If administered directly into the vein, apply a new needle after drawing up solution before administration. Administer immediately after reconstitution and discard unused solution as the drug contains no preservative. Do not use cellulose ester membrane IV filters as they may remove some of the drug. If extravasation occurs, treatment may involve infiltration of site with 50 to 100 mg hydrocortisone, thiosulfate, or 1 ml of 5% ascorbic acid injection and application of cool compresses to site.

**Monitor:** Monitor infusion carefully to avoid extravasation. Watch for nausea and vomiting and administer antiemetics as needed. Administer IV fluids as ordered to avoid fluid and electrolyte imbalances. Monitor vital signs and watch for signs of infection. Platelet and WBC counts are done during and for 2 to 3 weeks after therapy; marked drops require delay of therapy. Renal and hepatic function are monitored regularly with tests such as BUN, SGPT, SGOT, bilirubin, creatinine, LDH, and uric acid. Inspect oral mucosa and watch for signs of bleeding in stool. Look for ecchymosis.

*Patient Teaching:* Prepare for the potential of alopecia, which may include eyebrows. Teach methods to ensure nutritious food intake. Instruct to watch for and report signs of bleeding and of infection such as fever, sore throat, bruising, black tarry stools. Avoid contact with persons with infections such as colds, chicken pox, influenza.

**Drug Interactions:** Increased bone marrow suppression when used with or after other chemotherapy. If given within 2 months after radiation therapy erythema, stomatitis, elevated SGOT, ascites, myelosuppression may occur. May interfere with vitamin K effects. Can suppress immune response to immunizations. Live virus vaccines must not be given, nor oral polio vaccine to those in close contact with the patient on this drug due to the chance of infection with the virus; these vaccines are delayed at least 3 months after chemotherapy when the patient is in remission.

**Storage Requirements:** Store at 15 to 30°C (59 to 86°F) and protect from light. Use reconstituted solution immediately and discard unused portion.

---

## ☐ DAUNORUBICIN                                    (daw-noe-roo'bi-sin)

(daunomycin)

**Combination Products:** Cerubidine

**Classification:** antineoplastic, antibiotic, anthracycline

### Available Preparations:
- 20-mg vials for parenteral use
- Available with 100 mg mannitol

**Action and Use:** This antibiotic interferes with DNA and RNA synthesis by forming a complex with DNA. Most active during S phase of cell division. Not used for its antibacterial effects due to its toxicity. Used for remission induction in acute lymphocytic leukemia and acute myelocytic leukemia. May be used in neuroblastoma or some other tumors, such as lymphoma, Ewing's sarcoma, and rhabdomyosarcoma, although those uses are not approved by the FDA.

### Routes and Dosages:
*IV:* 25 to 45 mg/m$^2$ once weekly; or 1 mg/kg/day for 5 days. For those under 2 years or under 0.5 m$^2$, calculate dosage on mg/kg rather than square meter. Total anthracycline cumulative lifetime dose should not exceed 500 mg/m$^2$. Total cumulative dose may be kept at 300 mg/m$^2$ in children over 2 years; 10 mg/kg for those under 2 years to decrease chance of cardiotoxicity.

**Absorption and Fate:** Rapidly absorbed and widely distributed in body tissues such as spleen, liver, kidney, lung. Metabolized by the liver and excreted in urine and bile. Peak level is immediate. Half-life is 45 minutes initially, 18.5 hours in terminal phase.

## Contraindications and Precautions:
Pregnancy category D. Contraindicated in pregnancy, during chicken pox or herpes zoster infection. Use with caution in hepatic or renal dysfunction, heart disease, or bone marrow depression. Treatment stopped if signs of congestive heart failure occur.

## Side Effects:
*CV:* acute, transient EKG changes that are not serious; **congestive heart failure** that can be fatal. Heart failure is related to total cumulative dosage and is a low risk if total dosages do not exceed 300 mg/m$^2$ in children over 2 years or 10 mg/kg under 2 years or whose body surface area is under 0.5 m$^2$. Heart failure is more common in those under 2 years or over 70 years. *GI:* nausea, vomiting after drug administration lasting up to 48 hours; stomatitis, esophagitis, diarrhea, abdominal pain are rare. *GU:* hyperuricemia, causes urine to be red in color. *Skin:* alopecia, rash, itching, hyperpigmentation especially if patient had prior radiation; severe necrosis with extravasation. *Hemic:* leukopenia, thrombocytopenia, anemia; WBC and platelet counts are lowest 10 days to 2 weeks after therapy and are normal by third week

## Nursing Implications:
*Assess:* Assess history of previous therapy with cyclophosphamide or doxorubicin. Evaluate hepatic and renal function. Evaluate cardiac function with EKG and ECHO.

*Administer:* This drug has potentially severe side effects and should be given only under the supervision of a physician with training and experience in cancer chemotherapy. The drug's potential for toxic effects on health-care personnel as well as patients necessitates careful handling during preparation and administration. Generally, during preparation of antineoplastics, latex gloves, a mask, and a solid front gown are worn, and a laminar flow hood is used. Gloves and gown may also be recommended for administration. Contaminated equipment, such as needles, syringes, vials, and unused medication, is disposed of properly. Clean-up of spills is carefully performed and accidental contact by patient or personnel receives prompt flushing and cleaning. *IV:* Reconstitute with 4 ml sterile water for injection, shake gently to dissolve, and infuse in 5% dextrose or saline solution over several minutes into sidearm of IV or add to 100 ml and infuse over 30 to 45 minutes. Do not add to other drugs as it is incompatible with many drugs such as heparin, fluorouracil, cexamethasone, hydrocortisone, aminophylline, caphalothin. Flush IV lines with saline solution after infusing. Do not use veins that are small, swollen, or over joints. Avoid extravasation. Reconstituted solutions should be protected from sunlight and are stable for 24 hours at room temperature or 48 hours if refrigerated.

*Monitor:* Monitor IV site carefully to avoid extravasation. Discontinue IV if patient complains of burning or pain and infuse at another site. Monitor platelet, WBC, and RBC counts during and up to 3 weeks after therapy. Check vital signs frequently and watch for signs of infection. Monitor patient for signs of congestive heart failure and report promptly as drug must be stopped (EKG changes, weight gain, fatigue, breathing difficulty); regular EKG and serial ECHOs are done. Monitor hepatic and renal function with tests such as BUN, bilirubin, SGPT, SGOT, creatinine, LDH, and uric acid.

*Patient Teaching:* Avoid contact with persons with infections such as colds, chicken pox, influenza. Report signs of infection such as fever, sore throat, malaise. Report bruising and other signs of bleeding. Urine may turn red in color for 1 to 2 days after each dose. If pain or other urinary symptoms occur, report them. Increase fluid intake. Because congestive failure may occur even months after therapy, the patient should return for follow-up visits and should report increasing weight, difficulty breathing, and edema.

**Drug Interactions:** Previous treatment with cyclophosphamide or doxorubicin increases possibility of cardiac toxicity. Increased chance of hepatotoxicity with other hepatotoxic drugs. Increased cardiac toxicity with radiation to mediastinum. Suppresses immune response to immunization. Live virus vaccines must not be given, nor oral polio vaccine to those in close contact with the patient on this drug due to the chance of infection with the virus; these vaccines are delayed at least 3 months after chemotherapy when the patient is in remission.

**Laboratory Test Interferences:** Increases uric acid levels, bilirubin, SGOT, alkaline phosphatase

**Storage Requirements:** Store vial at 15 to 25°C (59 to 77°F). Protect reconstituted solution from sunlight. Reconstituted solution is stable for 24 hours at room temperature or 48 hours if refrigerated.

---

# ☐ DESMOPRESSIN ACETATE

(des-moe-press'in)

(DDAVP)

## Classification: antidiuretic

## Available Preparations:
- 0.1 mg/ml nasal solution
- 0.004 mg/ml for parenteral administration

**Action and Use:** Synthetic vasopressin compound that has increased antidiuretic and decreased vasopressor activity. Used to treat diabetes insipidus by increasing the reabsorption of water in the kidney collecting tubules. Injectable form used to treat bleeding patients with mild hemophilia or moderate von Willebrand's disease, type I whose plasma factor VIII activity is greater than 5%.

## Routes and Dosage:
*SC, IV:* over 3 months: > 10 kg: 0.3 μg (0.0003 mg)/kg 30 minutes before procedure
*Nasal:* 3 months to 12 years:
- Initial: 5 μg (0.005 mg) at bedtime; can increase dosage nightly in increments of 2.5 μg (0.0025 mg) until a satisfactory sleep response obtained. If urine volume remains large, 5 μg (0.005 mg) morning dose may be added and adjusted to obtain desired response.
- Maintenance: 2 to 4 μg (0.002 to 0.004 mg)/kg/day or 5 to 30 μg (0.005 to 0.03 mg) per day, as a single dose or in two divided daily doses.

Note: Young children have increased sensitivity to antidiuretic effects and risk of water intoxication and hyponatremia.

## Absorption and Fate:
10 to 20% absorbed slowly from nasal mucosa. Peak level: intranasal, 1 to 5 hours (antidiuretic); IV, within 90 minutes to 3 hours (antihemorrhagic). Duration of action: variable, about 10 to 20 hours.

## Contraindications and Precautions:
Pregnancy category B and safety during lactation not established. Contraindicated in infants under 3 months, IV form for diabetes insipidus those under 12 years, and under 3 months for hemophilia A. Use with caution in coronary artery insufficiency, hypertensive cardiovascular disease.

## Side Effects:
Infrequent and dose related.
*CNS:* transient headache. *CV:* slight increase in blood pressure. *GI:* nausea, mild abdominal cramps. *GU:* vulval pain. *Other:* nasal irritation, nasal congestion, rhinitis, flushing.

## Nursing Implications:
*Assess:* Assess pattern and amount of polyuria and nocturia. Obtain accurate body weight.
*Administer: Nasal:* Discard any solution that is outdated, discolored, or contains particulate matter. Place measured quantity of solution in one end of flexible plastic tubing supplied by manufacturer. Administered by inserting open end into child's nostril and placing other end into mouth. Blow the contents onto the nasal mucosa. An air-filled syringe can be placed onto oral end of tube for delivering drug into an infant or young child's nasal mucosa. Child should be in an upright sitting position so medication is delivered to nasal mucosa not down the throat. *SC, IV:* Rarely used for diabetes insipidus. IV: in those weighing over 10 kg, dilute in 10 ml of 0.9% sodium chloride injection and infuse slowly over 15 to 30 minutes. For those over 10 kg, dilute in 50 ml of 0.9% sodium chloride for injection and infuse slowly over 15 to 30 minutes. Dosage may be repeated, remembering that tachyphylaxis (decreasing responsiveness) can occur with more frequent administration than every 24 to 48 hours.

*Monitor:* Monitor BP and P during infusion. May cause erythema, burning and swelling at injection site. Assess drugs effectiveness by I & O, weights, urinary osmolality that determines urine concentration (check normal range for age group), and freedom of nocturia. Weigh child using same scale at same time of day. Monitor for symptoms of hyponatremia and water intoxication, e.g., subtle changes in mental status, confusion, lethargy, and neuromuscular excitability. Report any nasal irritation or URI development to physician. Medication usually requires dosage adjustment. Monitor response to medication; hemophilia A: monitor factor VIII concentration; and in von Willebrand's disease, monitor bleeding times, factor VIII, ristocetin factor, and Willebrand's factor.

*Patient Teaching:* Teach parents proper instillation; medication is ineffective if not given correctly. Signs and symptoms of overdosage, hyponatremia, and water intoxication. Monitor I & O and the importance of accurate weights. Do not give more frequently or alter dosage without consulting physician.

**Drug Interactions:** Use with caution in combination with other pressor agents. May increase antidiuretic effect with carbamazepine, chlorpropamide, clofibrate, fludrocortisone, urea. May decrease antidiuretic effect with alcohol, demeclocycline, epinephrine, heparin, lithium carbonate.

**Storage Requirements:** Store at 4°C (39.2°F), protect from freezing. Solution has a 1-year expiration from date of manufacture.

---

# □ DEXAMETHASONE

(Aeroseb-Dex, Decaderm, Decadron, Decadron Phosphate Respihaler, Decaspray, Deronil, Dexameth, Dexasone, Dexone, Hexadrol, Maxidex, SK-Dexamethasone, Turbinaire)

# □ DEXAMETHASONE ACETATE

(Dalalone-DP, Dalalone-LA, Decadron-LA, Decaject-LA, Dexacen-LA, Dexasone-LA, Dexon-LA, Dexone-LA, Solurex-LA)

# □ DEXAMETHASONE SODIUM-PHOSPHATE

(AK-Dex, Dalalone, Decadrol, Decadron Phosphate, Decadron Phosphate Respihaler, Decaject, Decameth, Dexacen-4, Dexair, Dexason, Dexon, Dexone, Hexadrol Phosphate, I-Methasone, Maxidex, Ocu-Dex, Oradexon, Savacort-D, Solures, Turbinaire, Wexaphos "4")

**Combination Products:** Dexamethasone with neomycin sulfate, polymyxin B sulfate (Ak-trol, Dexacidin, Des-Ide, Ocu-Trol); dexamethasone with tobramycin (TrobraDex); dexamethasone sodium phosphate with lidocaine HCl (Decadrone Phosphate with Xylocaine); dexamethasone sodium phosphate with neomycin sulfate (Neodecadron)

**Classification:** corticosteroid, glucocorticoid

## Available Preparations:
- 0.5 mg/5 ml oral elixir and solution
- 0.25, 0.5, 0.75, 1, 1.5, 2, 4, 6-mg tablets
- 8, 10, 16, 20, 24 mg/ml for parenteral administration
- 0.1% ophthalmic solution
- 0.05% ophthalmic ointment
- 100 g/m spray for oral inhalation
- 0.1% topical cream and gel
- 0.01%, 0.04% topical aerosol

**Action and Use:** Natural or synthetic, short-acting glucocorticoids that have strong antiinflammatory, immunosuppressant, and metabolic actions. Used to treat diseases such as collagen, dermatologic, allergy, acute leukemia, and fetal respiratory distress syndrome. Used with mineralocorticoids as replacement therapy in adrenocortical deficiencies. Used as a diagnostic aid in Cushing's syndrome and antiemetic in cancer chemotherapy. Topical form is low potency and fluorinated. Inhaler used to control symptoms of bronchial asthma, seasonal or perennial rhinitis (cases poorly responsive to conventional treatments).

## Routes and Dosage:
*PO:* 0.024 to 0.34 mg/kg/day or 0.66 to 10 mg/m²/day in equally divided doses 4 times a day
*IM, IV:*
- Dexamethasone Sodium Phosphate: 6 to 40 μg/kg or 0.235 to 1.25 mg/m²/day in 1 or 2 doses
- Increased Intracranial Pressure: Loading dose: 0.5 to 1.5 mg/kg, then 0.2 to 0.5 mg/kg/day every 6 hours for 5 doses then dosage tapered over 5 days
- Airway Edema: 0.25 to 0.5 mg/kg/day every 6 hours as needed for croup or 24 hours before planned extubation, then times 4 to 6 doses
- Antiemetic: Loading dose: 4 to 8 mg/m² then 2 to 4 mg/m² every 6 hours
*Ophthalmic:*
- Drops: instill 1 drop 3 to 4 times a day; up to 6 times per day
- Ointment: instill 1 cm 3 to 4 times per day
*Otic:* install 3 to 4 drops (ophthalmic solution) 2 to 3 times per day
*Inhalation:* 2 inhalations 3 to 4 times a day. (Maximum 8 inhalations daily)
*Topical:* apply as thin film, rubbing in 1 to 4 times per day; Aerosol: apply 1 to 2 times per day
Note: Dosage determined by severity of condition and child's response.

**Absorption and Fate:** Absorption: oral, rapid, complete; IM sodium phosphate, rapid; IM acetate, slow but complete; topical, increased in inflamed or diseased skin or use of occlusive dressings; inhalation, increased if inadvertently swallowed. Peak level: oral, 1 to 2 hours; IM sodium phosphate or succinate, 1 hour. Half-life 3 to 4.5 hours. Duration: oral, 2.75 days; IM acetate, 6 to 8 days. Metabolized by liver and excreted primarily by kidney.

**Contraindications and Precautions:** Pregnancy category C and safety during lactation not established. IM (acetate) not recommended for those under 12 years. Use caution in children; possible growth suppression, not recommended for long-term usage. Contraindicated if hypersensitivity to drug or its components, sensitivity to corticosteroids, varicella, systemic fungal infections, latent amebiasis, acquired immune deficiency syndrome (AIDS), fetal respiratory distress syndrome (do not use if delivery is imminent), immunizations with live virus vaccines and oral polio virus vaccine or contact with those who have had the vaccine. Use with caution in renal disease, hypertension, congestive heart failure, diabetes, ulcerative colitis, gastrointestinal ulceration, hyperthyroidism, systemic lupus erythematosus, impaired hepatic function, osteoporosis, vaccinia, exanthema, Cushing's syndrome, seizures, myasthenia gravis, tuberculosis, ocular herpes simplex, hypoalbuminemia, emotional or psychotic tendencies.

**Side Effects:** Usually dependent on dosage and duration of treatment.
*CNS:* headache, vertigo, euphoria, insomnia, **increased intracranial pressure** (papilledema), **psychotic behavior, seizures**. *CV:* edma, **hypertension, congestive heart failure**. *GI:* nausea, vomiting, change in appetite, gastrointestinal irritation, abdominal distention, pancreatitis, ulcerative esophagitis, peptic ulcer. *Skin:* impaired wound healing, thin fragile skin, petechia, ecchymosis, acne, facial erythema, increased sweating, may mask infections; Topical: burning, itching, irritation, dryness, folliculitis, hypertrichosis, hypopigmentation, allergic contact dermatitis, maceration of the skin, secondary infection, **skin atrophy, striae, miliaria**. *Hemic:* **thrombocytopenia**. *Endocrine:* **HPA-axis suppression**, menstrual irregularities, Cushing's states, **secondary adrenocortical, pituitary unresponsiveness**. *Musculoskeletal:* **suppression bone growth, osteoporosis**, muscle weakness, **aseptic necrosis of femoral and humeral heads**. *Sensory:* Ophthalmic: **posterior subcapsular cataracts, increased intraocular pressure**. *Other:* sodium retention, potassium loss, **negative nitrogen balance, hypokalemia, hyperglycemia**, susceptibility to infections; Withdrawal symptoms: rebound inflammation, fatigue, weakness, fever, arthralgia, dizziness, lethargy, depression, fainting, orthostatic hypotension, dyspnea, anorexia, hypoglycemia, nausea and vomiting, shortness of breath, unusual weight loss.

**Nursing Implications:**
*Assess:* Obtain baseline weight, height; before long-term therapy ECG, chest and spinal x-rays, glucose tolerance test, evaluation of HPA-axis function and BP before therapy. *Ophthalmic:* do not use if eye is infected. *Inhalation:* do not use during an acute asthma attack, patient should be stabilized on systemic steroids. If child has an asthma attack, contact physician immediately so that systemic corticosteroid may be started. *Topical:* observe, record appearance of involved area for baseline information.

***Administer:*** Best to calculate drug dosage on mg/m$^2$; reduces overdosage possibilities in very short or heavy children. ***PO:*** Take with food or milk to reduce GI irritation. Best to give daily dosage before 9 AM; it suppress adrenal cortex activity less, which may reduce risk of HPA axis suppression. Elixir contains 5% alcohol. Tablet can be crushed, mixed with small amount of food or fluid. ***IM:*** Shake well (acetate only) before withdrawal. Do not use deltoid muscle. Drug may produce muscle atrophy. ***IV:*** Dexamethasone sodium phosphate is form of drug used IV. Sodium phosphate is commercially diluted. Can give IV push slowly over 3 to 5 minutes. Intermittent infusion dilute with equal volume of IV solution and infuse over 10 to 20 minutes. Compatible solutions D$_5$W or NS. Compatible with aminophylline, and lidocaine; incompatible with amikacin, daunorubicin, doxorubicin, metaraminol, prochlorperazine, vancomycin. Consult pharmacist for others. ***Ophthalmic:*** See Part I for instillation. Shake solution before usage. Remove contact lenses before usage and consult physician when child may begin wearing them again. ***Otic:*** See Part I for instillation. Ophthalmic solution used. ***Inhalation:*** See Part I for instillation. Shake before usage. ***Topical:*** Cleanse with water before application or as physician prescribes. Apply thin coat as described in Part I. Do not cover with occlusive dressing unless directed by physician. If used, occlusive dressings should not remain in place for more than 16 hours; they increase incidence of side effects. Disposable diapers or plastic pants act as an occlusive dressing if covering medicated groin area. Aerosol: spray for no more than 2 seconds from distance of no less than 6 inches. When using on scalp, apply to dry scalp and prevent from getting medication into eyes.

***Monitor:*** Monitor BP during infusion. Careful assessment of child's response to drug, necessary for dosage adjustments. Observe for side effects, especially hypocalcemia, signs of electrolyte imbalance, signs of adrenal insufficiency, symptoms of infections, or worsening of condition. Monitor BP and daily weights, report any sudden weight gain to the physician. With long-term usage, monitor serum electrolytes and height. Encourage well balanced diet low in sodium, rich in potassium, calcium, vitamin K and D. Observe for ulcer development; if on long-term therapy, prophylactic antacids may be used. Encourage good hygiene and dental care (possible oral fungal infections). Tonometry (eye) examinations every 6 weeks. Diabetics may need increase in insulin due to steroid-induced hyperglycemia. Discontinuing of drug dosage: should be reduced gradually, especially after long-term usage, so it does not cause acute life-threatening adrenal insufficiency. After discontinuation of short-term therapy (up to 5 days) with high dosage, adrenal recovery may occur within 1 week. After prolonged high-dose therapy, complete recovery of adrenal function may require up to 1 year. If infection occurs (topical, ophthalmic, otic), discontinue drug and inform physician. Itching can lead to scratching and introduction of infections, so younger children may need restraining especially during naps or at night. Keep nails short and clean. Contact physician if itching persists. Rinse mouth after each inhalation.

***Patient Teaching:*** Do not alter dosage or stop drug abruptly; it could cause very serious side effects, even death. Gradual tapering of dosage is necessary. Increasing amount of medication will not hasten healing process. Demonstrate how to apply topical medication, use inhaler, instill ophthalmic or otic forms, or dosing schedule for oral form. Monitor signs and symptoms of medication, symptoms of adrenal insufficiency, or worsening of condition and report to physician. Obtain daily weights; report any sudden weight gain to physician. Importance of close medical supervision and follow-up. Regular ophthalmic examinations if on long-term therapy. Caution about receiving skin tests, vaccinations or other immunizations, or coming in contact with persons receiving oral polio virus vaccine. Inform any health-care provider, including dentists, surgeons, or emergency care personal that child is on this medication. Child should carry a medical identification card. Observe for symptoms of infections. Do not use OTC medications without contacting health-care provider. Topical: Do not use medication on other areas than those prescribed by physician. Do not use inhaler during acute asthma attack.

**Drug Interactions:** This drug in combination with high dosage of acetaminophen may increase risk of hepatotoxicity. With analgesics and antiinflammatory drugs, it may increase the risk of gastric ulceration. Amphotericin B and potassium-depleting diuretics increase risk of hypokalemia. Aminoglutethimide may accelerate metabolization of dexamethasone so that its half-life is reduced by twofold. Use with anabolic steroids may increase the risk of edema and acne. Drug in combination with anticoagulants may decrease anticoagulant effect. This drug used with anticonvulsants (phenytoin) may lower seizure threshold. Use with vaccines, live virus, or other immunizations may potentiate replication of the vaccine virus, increasing chance for developing the viral disease.

**Laboratory Test Interferences:** May increase serum cholesterol, sodium and blood glucose. May decrease serum calcium, potassium, $T_4$, $^{131}I$ uptake, urine 17-hydroxysteroid and 17-ketosteroids. Tends to suppress skin tests; may give a false-negative result with nitroblue-tetrazolium for bacterial infection. Adrenal function assessed by ACTH stimulation or plasma cortisol may be decreased.

**Storage Requirements:** Store at 15 to 30°C (59 to 86°F). Protect from light and freezing. Do not puncture or dispose of aerosol preparations into fire or incinerator. Consult package inserts for storage of parenteral forms.

---

## □ DEXTROAMPHETAMINE                    (dex-troe-am-fet′a-meen)

(Biphetamine, Dexedrine, Ferdex, Oxydess)

**Classification:** cerebral stimulant, amphetamine

**Available Preparations:**
- 5 mg/5 ml elixir
- 5, 10, 15-mg tablets
- 5, 10, 15-mg extended-release capsules

- 6.25-mg capsules with 6.25 mg amphetamine and 10 mg capsules with 10 mg amphetamine

**Action and Use:** This drug acts similarly to ephedrine, causing CNS stimulation, respiratory stimulation, and sympathomimetic effects. Its action in attention-deficit disorder is unclear but it modulates cortical functions through enhancement of catecholamine effects in the reticular activating system, thereby resulting in improvement of attention span and task performance. This may also prevent the flooding of sensory impulses into the cortex and allow them to enter in a more integrated manner. Used in children to treat attention deficit disorder and for children over 12 years for short-term obesity control.

**Routes and Dosages:**
*PO:* Attention-Deficit Disorder:
- 3 to 5 years: 2.5 mg initially; increased by 2.5-mg increments weekly PRN
- over 6 years: 5 mg initially; increased by 5-mg increments weekly PRN; not to exceed 40 mg/day

Exogenous Obesity: over 12 years: 5 to 30 mg/day
Tablets are given with dose divided to be administered 30 to 60 minutes before meals; extended-release capsules are given once daily in AM; capsule combinations with amphetamine is given one daily 10 to 14 hours before bedtime.

**Absorption and Fate:** Well absorbed from GI tract. Distributed in most body tissues with high amounts crossing the blood-brain barrier. Metabolism unknown; excreted in urine. Peak action unknown; duration: 4 to 24 hours. Half-life: about 6.5 hours.

**Contraindications and Precautions:** Pregnancy category C. Contraindicated in pregnancy, especially in first trimester. Not to be used for treatment of obesity in children under 12 years or for attention-deficit disorder in children under 3 years. Contraindicated in hyperthyroidism, hypertension, agitation, cardiovascular disease, glaucoma, history of hypersensitivity to sympathomimetic amines, within 14 days of administration of monoamine oxidase inhibitors, psychosis. The extended-release capsules and 5-mg tablets contain yellow dye #5 (tartrazine), which produces allergic reactions in some persons. These preparations should not be given to those persons.

**Side Effects:**
*CNS:* nervousness, insomnia, hyperactivity, headache, irritability, euphoria, depression, psychosis. *CV:* tachycardia, palpitation, hypertension, hypotension, arrhythmia. *GI:* anorexia, nausea, vomiting, metallic taste, abdominal cramps, dry mouth. *Musculoskeletal:* twisting, purposeless movement, tremors. *Sensory:* mydriasis.

**Nursing Implications:**
*Assess:* Establish baseline vital signs. Obtain history of hypersensitivity to other drugs such as aspirin and to yellow dye #5 (tartrazine).

*Administer:* Schedule II drug under Federal Controlled Substances Act. Extended-release tablet should not be chewed or crushed. When used for obesity, doses are divided and given 30 to 60 minutes before meals. When used for attention deficit disorders, the first dose is given on wakening and the remaining 1 to 2 doses are given at 4 to 6-hour intervals, with the last dose no later than 6 hours before bedtime.

*Monitor:* Take vital signs, particularly pulse and blood pressure regularly. Monitor food intake, height, and weight. For the child with attention deficit disorder, obtain parent and teacher reports about behavioral performance of child. The child is usually given drug-free holidays occasionally to be certain that the drug is still necessary.

*Patient Teaching:* Take drug as directed and keep locked securely. When given for obesity, therapy is short-term and needs to be accompanied by dietary teaching and management. If drowsiness or other side effects occur, report them so that drug or dosage can be adjusted. Report improvement or worsening of behavioral symptoms at home and school.

**Drug Interactions:** Potentiation of effects with MAO inhibitors, possibly leading to hypertensive crisis. Barbiturates may interfere with action.

**Laboratory Test Interferences:** Increases serum corticosteroids and urinary epinephrine.

**Storage Requirements:** Store in tightly covered light-resistant containers at 15 to 30°C (59 to 86°F). Protect elixir from freezing.

---

## □ DIAZEPAM  (dye-aze′ah-pam)

(Intensol, Q-pam, Valium, Valrelease)

**Classification:** anxiolytic, sedative, anticonvulsant, benzodiazepine

## Available Preparations:
- 2, 5, 10-mg tablets
- 15-mg extended-release capsules
- 5 mg/5 ml solution
- 5 mg/ml concentrate
- 5 mg/ml ampules and vials for parenteral use

**Action and Use:** This benzodiazepine has sedative effects on the CNS and prevents the propagation and generalization of seizure activity originating from the seizure foci. Its muscle relaxant activity is believed to be mediated by both distal and central effects at the neuromuscular junctions. Used as an antianxiety agent, often preoperatively, as a muscle relaxant such as in tetanus, and to treat status epilepticus. Experimental use in neonates in withdrawal from opiates.

## Routes and Dosages:

*PO:* over 6 months: 1 to 2.5 mg TID or QID *or* 0.04 to 0.2 mg/kg TID or QID *or* 1.17 to 6 mg/m$^2$ TID or QID. Smallest dose necessary to produce therapeutic results is used.

Epilepsy: 6 to 15 mg/day in divided doses; not to exceed 30 mg/day.

Note: If a child's dose is 5 mg TID, the 15-mg extended-release capsule may then be used.

*IV:*

Status Epilepticus:
- 30 days to 5 years: 0.2 to 0.5 mg q2–5min; not to exceed total of 5 mg; repeat in 2 to 4 hours PRN
- over 5 years: 1 mg q2–5min; not to exceed total of 10 mg; repeat in 2 to 4 hours PRN

Tetanus:
- 30 days to 5 years: 1 to 2 mg q3–4h PRN
- over 5 years: 5 to 10 mg q3–4h PRN

Acute Anxiety Reaction: 0.04 to 0.2 mg/kg, repeat in 3 to 4 hours; not to exceed 0.6 mg/kg total in 8 hours

Note: If IV route is unavailable, IM may be substituted.

*IM* (rarely):

Preoperative: over 2 years: 0.4 mg/kg 1 to 2 hours before surgery

Neonate Opiate Withdrawal: 0.5 to 2.0 mg q8h; slow dosage reduction

**Absorption and Fate:** Oral absorption is rapid. IM absorption unpredictable, slow; best absorbed from deltoid. Highly protein bound. Metabolized in liver, excreted mainly in urine. Peak level after PO is 1 to 2 hours; after IM is 15 to 30 minutes; after IV is 1 to 5 minutes. Half-life is biphasic with terminal half-life at 20 to 70 hours; half-life prolonged in infants. Therapeutic level is 0.5 μg/ml for seizure control.

**Contraindications and Precautions:** Pregnancy category D. Contraindicated in pregnancy especially in first trimester as congenital malformation can occur. Not recommended for use in the laboring patient due to lasting effects in the neonate. Not recommended during lactation. Safety of the oral drug in children under 6 months or parenteral form in infants under 30 days has not been established although it is sometimes used clinically in the younger age groups. Contraindicated in those with acute closed-angle glaucoma, shock, coma. Cautious use in those with hepatic or renal dysfunction, epilepsy, depression, drug or alcohol abuse, hyperkinesis, hypoalbuminemia, porphyria.

## Side Effects:

*CNS:* drowsiness, paradoxical excitement, dizziness, ataxia, confusion, weakness, tremor, vertigo, syncope; young children and particularly newborns are more likely to show CNS side effects; excitement more common in hyperactive children. *CV:* hypotension, bradycardia, **cardiac arrest** with rapid IV administration. *GI:* nausea, vomiting, constipation, diarrhea, appetite and weight changes, increased salivation, metallic taste, decreased gag reflex. *Respiratory:* apnea with rapid IV administration. *GU:* retention, incontinence. *Skin:* rash, urticaria, pruritus, photosensitivity. *Musculoskeletal:*

bone pain, muscle cramps, paresthesia. *Sensory:* blurred vision, nystagmus, diplopia.

## Nursing Implications:

*Assess:* Take baseline vital signs.

*Administer:* Schedule IV drug under Federal Controlled Substances Act. *PO:* Tablet may be crushed and mixed with small amount of food or drink. *IV:* Have resuscitative drugs and equipment readily available; be prepared for insertion of airway if needed. Do not mix with other drugs or solutions as incompatibility is likely. It also interacts with plastic IV tubing, therefore, is given directly into vein or as close as possible to IV site. Small veins and extravasation should be avoided. Give slowly at 0.25 mg/kg over 3 minutes or slower. *IM:* Not preferred route as action is less predictable. If used give deep IM, aspirating carefully before injection.

*Monitor:* Take vital signs frequently. Respirations must be constantly monitored during IV administration. Children are most prone to respiratory depressant effects of this medication, therefore, small doses are used initially. Monitor I & O. If on long-term therapy, CBC, liver function tests, nutrition, and weight are monitored periodically. If drug is taken for seizure control, monitor presence of seizures; particular care needed when dosage is changed.

*Patient Teaching:* Avoid OTC drugs, alcohol, or illicit drugs. Do not change or discontinue medicine without consulting physician. Report drowsiness, dizziness, excitement or other unusual effects. Return to physician for scheduled visits. Wear identification if taking the drug for seizures.

**Drug Interactions:** Increased CNS depressant effects with other CNS depressants. Lowered seizure threshold with tricyclic antidepressants. Decreased levels of both drugs when taken with carbamazepine. Decreased clearance and increased drug level if taken with cimetidine and disulfiram. Increased hypotensive effect with other medications having this effect. Antacids can decrease rate of GI absorption of drug. Smoking may increase the drug's sedative effects. Diazepam may reduce digoxin excretion. Excretion enhanced by rifampin. Serum phenytoin levels may increase when given with this drug. Effects of this drug increase with MAO inhibitors.

**Laboratory Test Interferences:** Increased CK, CPK. Elevated SGOT, SGPT, LDH, alkaline phosphatase, bilirubin. Changes in blood studies and renal function may occur.

**Storage Requirements:** Store in tightly covered, light-resistant containers at 15 to 30°C (59 to 86°F). Avoid freezing.

---

## □ DICLOXACILLIN SODIUM

(dye-klox-a-sill′in)

(Dycill, Dynapen, Pathocil)

**Classification:** antibiotic, penicillinase-resistant

## Available Preparations:
- 62.5 mg/5ml oral suspension
- 125, 250, 500-mg capsules

**Action and Use:** Similar to penicillin in action but resistant to inactivation by penicillinase; also active against *Streptococcus pyogenes* and *Pneumococcus*. Drug of choice for oral use in treating penicillinase-producing *Staphylococcus aureus* and *S. epidermidis* infections. Capsules contain about 0.6 mEq sodium and suspension 2.9 mEq sodium per 5 ml.

## Routes and Dosage:
*PO:*
- over 1 month, < 40 kg: 12.5 to 25 mg/kg/day in equally divided doses every 6 hours
- over 40 kg: 125 to 250 mg every 6 hours

**Absorption and Fate:** Rapidly, incompletely absorbed from GI tract. Distributed: synovial and pleural fluids, bone, bile. Peak level: 1 hour. Half-life: 0.5 to 1.9 hour. Therapeutic level for staphylococci is 0.1 to 0.3 μg/ml. 95 to 99% bound to serum proteins. Drug and metabolites excreted in urine.

**Contraindications and Precautions:** Pregnancy category B. Use caution during lactation. Manufacturer states safe use in neonates is not established. Contraindicated if hypersensitivity to drug, penicillins, cephalosporins, or cephamycins. Use caution with allergies, asthma, family history of allergies, acute GI upsets, cardiospasm, or intestinal hypermotility.

## Side Effects:
*GI:* nausea, vomiting, epigastric pain, loose stools, diarrhea, flatulence, hemorrhagic colitis, **pseudomembranous colitis** (rare). *Hepatic:* transient rise in SGOT, SGPT. *Skin:* morbilliform, maculopapular, urticarial, or erythematous, rashes, pruritus (hypersensitivity). *Hemic:* **eosinophilia, anemia, neutropenia, thrombocytopenia, leukopenia**. *Other:* Hypersensitivity: drug fever, **anaphylaxis** (rare).

## Nursing Implications:
*Assess:* Assess previous allergy to drug, penicillins, cephalosporins, other drugs, asthma, or family history of allergies. Obtain cultures and sensitivity before treatment, but can start treatment before results.
*Administer: PO:* Food interferes with drug absorption, give 1 hour before or 2 hours after meals. Refrigerate solution and shake well. Capsules may be taken apart; mixed with small amount of food or fluid.
*Monitor:* Monitor child for hypersensitivity (especially in first 20 minutes of first dosage), rash (onset and characteristics), and side effects. Watch for symptoms of superinfections or diarrhea (may indicate pseudomembranous colitis, which can occur while on drug or 4 days to 6 weeks after drug is

discontinued). Assess renal, hepatic, and hematological functions with prolonged or high-dose therapy. Maintain fluid intake for age group. Therapy course continued for 48 to 72 hours after negative bacterial cultures or symptoms subside. If given for β-**hemolytic streptococcal infection**, 10-day course needed to prevent risk of acute rheumatic fever or glomerulonephritis.

*Patient Teaching:* Take as prescribed for full course of therapy. Observe for side effects especially diarrhea or rash and report to physician. Do not take OTC drugs without consulting physician. Store solution in refrigerator out of reach of children. Reconstituted solution should be discarded after 14 days if refrigerated.

**Drug Interactions:** Erythromycin, tetracycline, chloromycetin may decrease the antibacterial effects of dicloxacillin.

**Storage Requirements:** Store capsules at 15 to 30°C (59 to 86°F). Reconstituted suspensions, if refrigerated stable for 14 days. Label with time and date at time of reconstitution.

---

## □ DICYCLOMINE HYDROCHLORIDE                    (dye-sye'kloe-meen)

(Antispas, Bentyl, Bentylol, Cyclocen, Dibent, Dicen, Di-spaz Formulex, Neoquess, Nospaz, Or-Tyl, Rocyclo, Rotyl HCL, Stannitol, Viscerol)

**Combination Products:** Dicyclomine hydrochloride with phenobarbital

**Classification:** anticholinergic, gastrointestinal antispasmodic

### Available Preparations:
- 10 mg/5ml oral syrup
- 20-mg tablets
- 10-mg capsules
- 10 mg/ml for parenteral administration

**Action and Use:** Amino alcohol ester that has anticholinergic properties; actions are primarily on the smooth muscle of the GI and biliary tracts. Used in treatment of infantile colic or irritable colon.

### Routes and Dosage:
*PO:*
- under 6 months: not recommended
- 6 month to 2 years: 5 to 10 mg 3 to 4 times per day
- over 2 years: 10 mg 3 to 4 times per day

*IM:* Dosage has not been established

**Absorption and Fate:** Half-life: 1.8 hours, initial; 9 to 10 hours, secondary. Appears to be excreted by urine and feces.

**Contraindications and Precautions:** Pregnancy category B and safety during lactation not established. Contraindicated in infants under 6 months, hypersensitivity to drug, obstruction of bladder or GI tract, paralytic ileus, intestinal atony, unstable cardiac conditions in acute hemorrhage, toxic megacolon, and narrow-angle glaucoma. Use caution with autonomic neuropathy, hepatic or renal impairment, ulcerative colitis, hyperthyroidism, coronary heart disease, congestive heart failure, hypertension, cardiac arrhythmias, hiatal hernia, biliary tract disease, spastic paralysis, or brain damage.

**Side Effects:**
*CNS:* dizziness, light-headedness, drowsiness, weakness, headache, insomnia, confusion, hyperexcitability. *CV:* palpitations, tachycardia. *GI:* dry mouth, constipation, nausea, vomiting, **paralytic ileus**, loss of taste. *GU:* urinary hesitancy, retention. *Skin:* urticaria, pruritus, decreased sweating. *Other:* fever, allergic reaction, **anaphylaxis**

**Nursing Implications:**
*Assess:* Obtain baseline vital signs.
*Administer: PO:* Give 30 minutes before meals and at bedtime. Tablet can be crushed and capsule taken apart and mixed with small amounts of food or fluid.
*Monitor:* Treatment of infants with colic under 2 months is dangerous because of their susceptibility to toxic effects especially in high dosage; onset of symptoms can occur in minutes. Use with caution in hot and humid climates because of potential of heat stroke caused by drug. Monitor vital signs and side effects.
*Patient Teaching:* Measure drug carefully and give only in amounts and frequency prescribed. Drug can alter mental alertness, therefore, adjust activities accordingly. Do not share this medication with others.

**Storage Requirements:** Store at 15 to 30°C (59 to 86°F), protect from heat and light.

---

# □ DIGOXIN                                    (di-jox'in)

(Lanoxicaps, Lanoxin, Masoxin, Novodigoxin, SK-Digoxin)

**Classification:** cardiac glycoside

**Available Preparations:**
- 50 μg/ml elixir

- 125, 250, 500-µg tablets
- 50, 100, 200 µg capsules
- 100, 250 µg/ml vials for parenteral use

**Action and Use:** Acts on the heart to increase myocardial contractility, increase automaticity, reduce excitability, reduce conduction velocity, and prolong the refractory period. Inhibits activity of an exzyme that transports sodium across cell membranes, therefore, sodium may be retained and potassium lost from myocardium. Used in treatment of congestive heart failure and for ventricular rate control in atrial flutter and atrial fibrillation.

## Routes and Dosages:
### PO, tablets and elixir:
Digitalizing Dose:
- premature neonate: 20 to 35 µg/kg day in 2 or more doses
- neonate: 20 to 35 µg/kg day in 2 or more doses
- 1 to 24 months: 35 to 60 µg/kg day in 2 or more doses
- 2 to 5 years: 30 to 40 µg/kg day in 2 or more doses
- 5 to 10 years: 20 to 35 µg/kg in 2 or more doses
- over 10 years: Fast, 0.75 to 1.25 mg in 2 doses; slow, 1.25 mcg to 500 µg/day times 7 days

Maintenance Dose:
- premature: 1/5 to 1/3 of digitalizing dose given daily
- neonates, infants, children: 1/5 to 1/3 of digitalizing dose given daily
- 10 years and over 125 to 500 µg/day

Alternate for maintenance dose: elixir may be calculated as 17 µg/kg/daily given in divided doses

### PO, capsules:
Digitalizing Dose:
- premature neonate: 15 to 25 µg/kg in 2 or more doses
- neonate: 20 to 30 µg/kg in 2 or more doses
- 1 to 24 months: 30 to 50 µg/kg in 2 or more doses
- 2 to 5 years: 25 to 35 µg/kg in 2 or more doses
- 5 to 10 years: 15 to 30 µg/kg in 2 or more doses
- over 10 years: 8 to 12 µg/kg/day in 2 or more doses

Maintenance Dose:
- premature: 20% to 30% of digitalizing dose in 2 to 3 daily doses
- neonates, infants, children: 25% to 35% of digitalizing dose in 2 to 3 daily doses
- 10 years and over: 25% to 35% of digitalizing dose given once daily

### IV:
Digitalizing Dose:
- premature neonate: 15 to 25 µg/kg in 3 or more doses
- neonate: 20 to 30 µg/kg in 3 or more doses
- 1 to 24 months: 30 to 50 µg/kg in 3 or more doses
- 2 to 5 years: 25 to 35 µg/kg in 3 or more doses
- 5 to 10 years: 15 to 30 µg/kg in 3 or more doses
- over 10 years: 8 to 12 µg/kg in 3 or more doses

Maintenance Dose:
- premature: 20% to 30% of digitalizing dose in 2 to 3 daily doses
- neonates, infants, children: 25% to 35% of digitalizing dose in 2 to 3 daily doses
- 10 years and over: 25% to 35% of digitalizing dose given once daily

**Absorption and Fate:** About 60 to 85% of PO dose absorbed from tablets and elixir and 90% or more from capsules. 20 to 30% bound to plasma proteins. Some of drug metabolized in liver and intestine with metabolites and unchanged drug excreted mainly in urine. Onset of action after PO form is 30 to 120 minutes and after IV is 5 to 30 minutes. Peak effect is 2 to 6 hours after PO and 1 to 4 hours after IV. Duration of action is 6 hours and half-life is 32 to 48 hours. Therapeutic level is 0.5 to 2.0 ng/ml with 1.1 to 1.7 ng/ml as usual desired range.

**Contraindications and Precautions:** Pregnancy category A. Contraindicated in those hypersensitive to digitalis preparations, patients with excessive bradycardia, digitalis toxicity, ventricular fibrillation, and ventricular tachycardia not due to congestive heart failure. Usually withheld 1 to 2 days before elective cardioversion. Cautious use in prematures, hypovolemia, hypokalemia, renal dysfunction, acute glomerulonephritis, hepatic dysfunction, hypercalcemia, hypomagnesemia, severe pulmonary disease, hypertension, AV block, carotid sinus hypersensitivity, idiopathic hypertrophic subaortic stenosis, myocardial infarction, myocarditis, myxedema, PVCs, ventricular tachycardia.

**Side Effects:**
*CNS:* tiredness, weakness, headache, confusion, depression, fainting, facial neuralgia, paresthesias, hallucinations, agitation. *CV:* bradycardia, **arrhythmias**, hypotension, tachycardia (particularly in children). *GI:* anorexia, nausea, vomiting, stomach pain, diarrhea. *Sensory:* halos, blurred vision.

**Nursing Implications:**
*Assess:* Establish baseline vital signs and EKG. Check serum electrolytes, hepatic and renal function. Assess hydration status and hydrate if hypovolemic.
*Administer: PO:* Take at same times daily either with or without food to ensure equivalent bioavailability. Food will slow absorption but not decrease total amount absorbed. If giving elixir, use only calibrated dropper provided. Be certain digoxin, not digitoxin, tablets are administered. *IV:* Dilute with at least four times the volume, using sterile water, 5% dextrose, or saline and give over at least 5 minutes. Use immediately after dilution. Do not mix with other medications. Patient is moved from IV to PO form as soon as possible.
*Monitor:* Before giving any dose take apical pulse for 1 full minute. Withhold dose and notify prescriber if pulse is below normal for age group; this is often 100 beats/minute for children. EKG is monitored during IV dose. Dosage needs to be carefully individualized and the drug has a low therapeutic index; monitoring of effects is, therefore, critical. Hepatic and renal function are monitored. If creatinine clearance is 50 ml/minute or less dosage will be reduced. Serum electrolytes, particularly potassium, calcium, magnesium, are checked;

close monitoring of those also on diuretics. Serum potassium of 3.5 mEq/L or less may be a contraindication to digoxin administration; clarify with physician. Hypokalemia makes the patient more prone to digitalis toxicity. Serum digoxin levels are taken 6 to 8 hours after a dose with a level above 2 ng/ml considered potentially toxic. Early toxicity may be manifested by tachycardia in young children and stomach upset or bradycardia in older children. Monitor I & O and daily weight. When routes are changed, absorption of digoxin may be altered, therefore, close monitoring is needed. Generally tablets and elixir dosages will need to be decreased by 20 to 25% when changing to IV or capsule preparations.

***Patient Teaching:*** Teach parent and child to take pulse for 1 full minute and record. Report abnormalities to physician. Take at same time each day. If nausea or vomiting occur, withhold dose and see physician. Teach correct measurement and administration of dosage. Use only calibrated dropper provided with elixir if giving that preparation. Teach signs of congestive failure. The poisioning potential of the drug is great. Keep locked and keep syrup of ipecac and the poison control number at hand. Wear medic alert identification.

**Drug Interactions:** Drugs that cause hypokalemia increase toxicity of digoxin. Other antiarrhythmics, calcium, or sympathomimetics may increase risk of arrhythmias. Calcium-channel blocking agents and quinidine may increase digoxin levels. Increased dosage of heparin may be needed. Increased digoxin may be needed with a patient on thyroid hormone. Antacids reduce absorption of digoxin. Absorption of tablets may be decreased in those on radiation or chemotherapy.

**Food–Drug Interactions:** Food will slow but not cause a decrease in the total amount of digoxin absorbed.

**Laboratory Test Interferences:** Falsely elevated 17-ketogenic steroids.

**Storage Requirements:** Store at 15 to 30°C (59 to 86°F). Protect from light and freezing.

---

# □ DIGOXIN IMMUNE FAB

(Digibind)

**Classification:** antidote to digitalis

**Action and Use:** This drug contains fragments of antidigoxin antibodies obtained from sheep who are immunized with a preparation of digoxin and albumin. It binds digoxin and digitoxin molecules that are then excreted. Used for treatment of potentially fatal digoxin or digitoxin toxicity.

**Available Preparations:** 40-mg vial of powder for parenteral use

**Absorption and Fate:** Distributes rapidly into plasma and interstitial fluids. Begins binding rapidly (within 1 minute) with free digoxin or digitoxin. Symptoms of toxicity decrease within 15 to 30 minutes. Excreted mainly in urine. Peak level is at completion of IV infusion and half-life is 14 to 20 hours.

## Routes and Dosages:

*IV:* Dosage is established by calculating total dose of glycoside or by estimating amount of glycoside from serum level. If dose is known of digoxin tablets, elixir, or IM dose:

$$\text{digoxin immune fab (mg)} = \frac{\text{dose ingested (mg)} \times 0.8}{0.6} \times 40$$

If dose is known of digitoxin tablets, digoxin capsules, or IV form of either:

$$\text{digoxin immune fab (mg)} = \frac{\text{dose ingested (mg)}}{0.6} \times 40$$

If digoxin dose is unknown, serum levels are obtained and:

$$\text{digoxin immune fab (mg)} = \frac{\text{ng/ml} \times \text{body weight (kg)}}{100} \times 40$$

If digitoxin dose is unknown, serum levels are obtained and:

$$\text{digitoxin immune FAB (mg)} = \frac{\text{ng/ml} \times \text{body weight (kg)}}{1000} \times 40$$

**Contraindications and Precautions:** Pregnancy category C. Use with caution in lactation. Use in infants and children has been limited. Use should be limited to those with potentially fatal digoxin or digitoxin toxicity. The drug has not been used widely enough to establish safety in other circumstances. Cautious use in renal impairment is advisable.

## Side Effects:

*CV:* progression of congestive heart failure and decreased cardiac output, increased ventricular rate. *Other:* hypokalemia, sensitivity reactions have not occurred but are possible due to the preparation's source from sheep.

## Nursing Implications:

*Assess:* Serum glycoside levels should be obtained. Take vital signs, including temperature, blood pressure, pulse, serum potassium. Monitor EKG. A skin test may be performed in individuals with a history of allergies.

*Administer:* Sterile water (4 ml) is added to vial; solution will contain 10 mg/ml. Reconstituted solution is added to normal saline injections and infused IV over 15 to 30 minutes. Reconstituted solutions should be used immediately or stored up to 4 hours at 2 to 8°C (35 to 46°F). For administration of small doses (e.g., less than 3 mg) to infants, the reconstituted solution can be diluted with 36 ml of normal saline to provide a solution of 1 mg/ml. Alternatively, a loading dose followed by IV infusion for several hours may be used. Rapid IV infusion may be used in treatment of imminent cardiac arrest. If given to someone with a positive skin test, an antihistamine and corticosteroid may be given if digoxin immune fab must be used.

***Monitor:*** Serum glycoside levels are monitored. Vital signs including temperature, blood pressure, pulse, EKG are monitored. Serum potassium levels are monitored carefully as rapid, severe hypokalemia can result and will require potassium therapy.

**Drug Interactions:** The drug obviously interferes with levels of cardiac glycosides. After treatment it is advisable to wait several days for fab fragments to be eliminated from the body before redigitalizing the patient.

**Laboratory Test Interferences:** Serum glycoside levels rise upon administration of digoxin immune fab; this is the result of the high levels of fab-bound digoxin or digitoxin.

**Storage Requirements:** Refrigerate powder at 2 to 8°C (35 to 46°F).

---

## □ DIMENHYDRINATE                               (dye-men-hye'dri-nate)

(Apo-Dimenhydrinate, Dimentabs, Dipendrate, Dramaject, Dramamine, Dramamine Junior, Dymenate Gravol, Hydrate, Marmine, Nauseal, Nauseatol, Reidamine, Travamine, Wehamine)

**Classification:** antihistamine, antiemetic

### Available Preparations:
- 12.5 mg/4 ml oral solution
- 50-mg tablets
- 50 mg/ml for parenteral injection

**Action and Use:** Ethanolamine derivative whose exact mechanism of action in the prevention and treatment of motion sickness is unknown. It is felt it inhibits acetylcholine whose stimulation of vestibular and reticular systems may produce nausea and vomiting. It is most effective in the prophylaxis of motion sickness. Used to control dizziness and vertigo.

### Routes and Dosage:
***PO:***
- 5 mg/kg/day or 15 mg/m$^2$ every 6 hours;
- 2 to 6 years: do not exceed 75 mg/day;
- 6 to 12 years: do not exceed 150 mg/day
- adults: 50 to 100 mg every 4 to 6 hours

***PO, IM:*** 1.25 mg/kg or 37.5 mg/m$^2$ 4 times per day. (Maximum total daily dosage 300 mg)
***IV:*** Usage not established for children

**Absorption and Fate:** Onset of drug's action: PO, 15 to 30 minutes; IM, 20 to 30 minutes. Duration action: 3 to 6 hours. Metabolized in liver and excreted in urine.

**Contraindications and Precautions:** Pregnancy category B. Safe use during lactation not established. Contraindicated in prematures, neonates, if hypersensitivity to drug or angle closure glaucoma. Use caution in children under 2 years, and seizure disorders.

### Side Effects:
*CNS:* drowsiness, dizziness, headache (nervousness, excitation, insomnia, especially in children). *CV:* tachycardia, hypotension. *GI:* anorexia, constipation, diarrhea. *GU:* urinary frequency, dysuria. *Sensory:* dry nose,throat and respiratory tract, blurred vision. *Other:* Local: pain at IM site.

### Nursing Implications:
*Assess:* Establish baseline pulse and blood pressure.
*Administer: PO:* Give 30 minutes to 1 hour before travel. Solution contains 5% alcohol. Tablet can be crushed and mixed with small amount of food or fluid. *IM:* Injection painful. Do not mix with any other solutions or drugs in same syringe.
*Monitor:* Assess for side effects. Observe for overdosage symptoms: dilated pupils, flushing, excitability, confusion, hallucinations, disorientation, clonic seizures, coma, cardiac arrest, death. Can occur up to 2 hours after ingestion. Phenobarbital may control seizures.
*Patient Teaching:* Warn child or parent that drug may interfere with physical coordination and mental alertness. Observe for symptoms of excitation and other side effects; notify physician if these occur.

**Drug Interactions:** May potentiate depressive effects of alcohol, barbiturates, or tranquilizers. Drug may increase anticholinergic activity of anticholinergic drugs and tricyclic antidepressants. Do not give with aminoglycosides or other ototoxic drugs; may mask symptoms of ototoxicity.

**Laboratory Test Interference:** False-negative results can occur with allergy skin testing; schedule skin testing 4 days after drug is discontinued.

**Storage Requirements:** Store at 15 to 30°C (59 to 86°F) in tightly closed containers.

---

### □ DIPHENHYDRAMINE HYDROCHLORIDE (dye-fen-hye′dra-meen)

(Allerdryl, Baramine, Bax, Belix, Benachlor, Benadryl, Benahist, Bendylate, Benoject, Bentract, Benylin, Bonyl, Compoz, Diphenacen, Fenylhist, Nordryl, Rodryl, Rohydra, Span-Lanin, Surfadil, Valdrene, Wehdryl)

**Combination Products:** Diphenhydramine HCl is combined with other drugs such as: acetaminophen; pseudoephedrine hydrochloride, ammonium chloride, codeine, dexromethoraphan, calamine, camphor, and zinc oxide

**Classification:** antihistamine, antiemetic, antivertigo

## Available Preparations:
- 12.5 mg/5 ml oral elixir
- 12.5 mg/5 ml, 133.3 mg/5 ml oral solutions
- 25, 50-mg tablets
- 25-mg film-coated tablets
- 25, 50-mg capsules
- 10, 50 mg/ml for parental administration
- 2 % topical solution
- 1 % topical lotion
- 1 % topical cream

**Action and Use:** Ethanolamine-derivative antihistamine that by competing with $H_1$ receptor sites on effector cells, blocks histamine release, decreasing the allergic response. Does not reverse histamine response. Has sedation effect within 1 to 3 hours of dosage. Directly suppresses cough reflex in the medulla, has strong antiemetic and antivertigo effects, and has local anesthetic properties by prevention of initiation and transmission of nerve impulses. Used to treat symptoms of allergies, vertigo, motion sickness, as cough suppressant, temporary sleep aid, and in combination products to treat URI and colds. Topical form is used for short-term treatment of pruritus and pain from sunburn, insect bites, and minor skin irritations.

## Routes and Dosage:
*PO:*
- under 9.1 kg: 6.25 to 12.5 mg every 4 to 6 hours
- over 9.1 kg: 12.5 to 25 mg every 4 to 6 hours or

*PO, IM, IV:* 5mg/kg/day or 150 mg/m²/day divided in 3 or 4 doses. (Maximum dosage is 300 mg/day)

*Topical:* over 2 years: 1 to 2% applied to affected area 3 to 4 times/day

*Self-Medication (OTC): PO:* under 6 years of age not recommended.

Allergic Rhinitis, Rhinorrhea, Motion Sickness:
- over 12 years: 25 to 50 mg every 4 to 6 hours. (Maximum dose 300 mg/day)
- 6 to 12 years: 12.5 to 25 mg every 4 to 6 hours. (Maximum dose 150 mg/day)

Cough Suppressant:
- over 12 years: 25 mg every 4 hours. (Maximum dose 150 mg/day)
- 6 to 12 years: 12.5 mg every 4 hours. (Maximum dose 75 mg/day)

Sleep Aid: over 12 years: 50 mg 20 minutes before HS; do not use longer than 2 weeks

**Absorption and Fate:** Well absorbed from GI tract; PO onset of action in 15 minutes. Onset of action IM: 20 to 30 minutes. Peak plasma level: 1 to 4

hours. 80 to 85% bound to plasma proteins with 50 to 75% excreted in the urine.

**Contraindications and Precautions:** Pregnancy category C and do not use during lactation. Contraindicated in prematures, neonates, topical preparations in children under 2 years, combination product with codeine in children under 6 years, as nighttime sleep aid in those under 12 years, hypersensitivity to any components of drug, sulfite allergy, acute asthma attack, lower respiratory tract disease. Use with caution in children under 6 years, angle-closure glaucoma, intraocular pressure, stenosing peptic ulcer, pyloroduodenal or bladder neck obstruction, asthma, hyperthyroidism, seizures cardiovascular disease, or hypertension.

## Side Effects:
*CNS:* mild drowsiness to deep sleep, dizziness, headaches, paradoxical excitement (especially in children); restlessness, insomnia, tremors, euphoria, delirium palpitations, **seizures**. *CV:* palpitations, hypertension, hypotension can lead to **cardiovascular collapse**. *GI:* dry mouth, nausea, vomiting, diarrhea, constipation. *Resp:* thickening bronchial secretions, nasal stuffiness, wheezing. *GU:* dysuria, urinary retention. *Skin:* photosensitivity, eczema, pruritus, papular rash, contact dermatitis (topical). *Hemic:* agranulocytosis, hemolytic anemia, leukopenia, thrombocytopenia (rare). *Sensory:* diplopia

## Nursing Implications:
*Assess:* Obtain baseline vital signs, P, BP, and respirations. CBC for long-term therapy.
*Administer: PO:* Give with food to reduce GI symptoms. For motion sickness, give 30 minutes before travel. Tablet can be crushed and capsules opened and mixed with small amount of food or fluid. *IM:* Avoid inadvertent SC injection; causes irritation. *IV:* IV administration used only in emergency situations. Give slow IV push undiluted over 3 to 5 minutes (25 mg/minute maximum). Intermittent infusion, dilute to desired volume; infuse over no less than 15 minutes. Compatible with $D_5W$, $D_5W/0.2\%NS$, $D_5W/0.5\%NS$, $D_{10}W$, NS, LR, Ionosol products, dextran $6\%/D_5W$, fat emulsions 10%. Incompatible with amobarbital, amphotericin B, cephalothin sodium, dexamethasone, furosemide, hydrocortisone, methylprednisolone, pentobarbital, phenobarbital, phenytoin, thiopental. *Topical:* Cleanse area with mild soap and water; apply sparingly to affected area.
*Monitor:* Monitor during IV infusion for hypotension and arrhythmias. Assess for side effects especially CNS agitation in children. If on long-term therapy, obtain periodic CBC. Can use sugarless gum or hard candy to combat dry mouth. If topical condition worsens or area does not appear to heal in 7 days, discontinue medication.
*Patient Teaching:* Warn child or parent about CNS side effects. Although this medication comes as OTC, it can cause serious side effects especially in those under 6 years. Only use with this age group if prescribed by physician. Take or use only as directed or prescribed.

**Drug Interactions:** May potentiate depressive effects of opiates, analgesics, anticolinergics, sedatives, alcohol, barbiturates, or tranquilizers. MAO inhibitors increase effects of this drug. Diphenhydramine increases effects of oral anticoagulants.

**Laboratory Test Interference:** False-negative results can occur with allergy skin testing; schedule testing 4 days after drug is discontinued.

**Storage Requirements:** Store at 15 to 30°C (59 to 86°F), in light-resistant container and avoid freezing.

---

☐ **DIPHENOXYLATE HYDROCHLORIDE WITH ATROPINE SULFATE**    (dye-fen-ox′i-late)

(Diphenatol, Lofene, Logen, Lomanate, Lomotil, Lo-Trol, SK-Diphenoxylate)

**Classification:** antidiarrheal, controlled substance schedule V

**Available Preparations:**
- 2.5 mg/5 ml diphenoxylate hydrochloride and 0.025 mg/5ml atropine sulfate oral solution
- 2.5 mg diphenoxylate hydrochloride and 0.025 mg atropine sulfate tablets

**Action and Use:** Compound similar to meperidine but free of any analgesic action. Inhibits gastrointestinal motility and excessive propulsion. Used for the symptomatic treatment of diarrhea. Not used for diarrhea; caused by poisoning, organisms that penetrate intestinal mucosa, e.g., *Shigella, Salmonella, and E. coli,* or pseudomembranous enterocolitis secondary to broad-spectrum antibiotics.

**Routes and Dosage:** Dosage expressed in terms of diphenoxylate
*PO:*
Do not use in children under 2 years; 2 to 12 years use oral solution
- 2 to 12 years: Initial Dosage: 0.3 to 0.4 mg/kg/day in 3 to 4 divided doses
- Adults: 15 to 20 mg/day equally divided 3 to 4 times a day

**Absorption and Fate:** Well absorbed from GI tract; onset of action: about 45 minutes. Peak serum level: 2 hours; half-life, 2 to 3 hours. Rapidly metabolized and metabolites are principally excreted in feces; small amount in urine.

**Contraindications and Precautions:** Pregnancy category C. Excreted in breast milk, not recommended during lactation. Contraindicated in children under 2 years, hypersensitivity to drug, atropine sulfate, obstructive jaundice electrolyte imbalance, dehydration, and diarrhea associated with pseudomembranous enterocolitis, intestinal mucosal penetrating organisms or diarrhea from poison until toxic substances have been excreted. Use caution for patients with history of physical dependence, hepatic disease, Down's syndrome, and acute ulcerative colitis.

**Side Effects:** Greater variability of response in children.
*CNS:* headache, dizziness, excitability, drowsiness, lethargy, confusion, malaise, depression, euphoria, numbness of extremities. *CV:* tachycardia. *GI:* nausea, vomiting, abdominal cramps, paralytic ileus, distention (fluid retention in bowel), megacolon. *GU:* urinary retention. *Skin:* flushing, giant urticaria, rash, pruritus. *Sensory:* Ophthalmic: blurred vision, mydriasis. *Other:* Hypersensitivity: swelling gums, angioedema, **anaphylaxis**

**Nursing Implications:**
*Assess:* Assess for drug hypersensitivity. Assess number, color, consistency, history of onset and course of diarrhea, as well as hydration level and electrolyte balance. Obtain weight. If child is dehydrated, do not use drug.
*Administer: PO:* Tablet may be crushed, mixed, and given with a small amount of food or fluid.
*Monitor:* Observe and chart stool pattern. Assess level of hydration by I & O, frequent weights, serum electrolytes, and symptoms of hydration. If dehydration occurs, discontinue drug and inform physician. Do not exceed recommended dosage; if child does not respond to therapy in 48 hours, stop drug. As soon as diarrhea is under control, dosage should be reduced to maintenance (may be 1/4 of initial dosage). Monitor for side effects.
*Patient Teaching:* Take only as scheduled. Observe for side effects and hydration levels. Monitor and note stool patterns for physician.

**Drug Interactions:** When used with MAO inhibitors, may cause hypertensive crisis. This drug potentiates action of alcohol, barbiturates, and tranquilizers.

**Storage Requirements:** Store at 15 to 30°C (59 to 86°F) in light-resistant containers.

---

□ **DIPHTHERIATETANUS
TOXOIDS AND
PERTUSSIS VACCINE**

(dif-thee'ree-ah)
(tet'ah-nus)
(per-tuss'is)

(DTP, Tri-Immunol)

**Classification:** immunization

**Available Preparations:** 7.5 ml multiple dose vials for parenteral use

**Action and Use:** Stimulates body production of antibodies and antitoxins against the organisms and exotoxins causing diphtheria, tetanus, and pertussis. Used for initial series and booster in children under 7 years.

## Routes and Dosages:
*IM:* 0.5 ml at 2, 4, 6, 15 to 18 months, and 4 to 6 years (5 doses total). For those children not immunized in infancy, three doses are given 6 to 8 weeks apart, a fourth dose 6 to 12 months after the third, and a fifth dose at 4 to 6 years. If the fourth dose is given after 4 years of age, the fifth dose is not needed.

**Absorption and Fate:** Four doses provide immunity to 70 to 95% of vaccinees for at least 10 years.

**Contraindications and Precautions:** Pertussis vaccine is contraindicated after 7 years of age. A severe reaction to previous pertussis vaccine is a contraindication to further pertussis immunization. A severe reaction is manifested by any one or a combination of the following: encephalopathy (alterations in consciousness, continuing headache or vomiting, confusion, unusual irritability, somnolence, or focal neurological signs) within 7 days of immunization; convulsion within 3 days; persistent crying for 3 hours or a high-pitched cry within 48 hours; collapse or shocklike state within 48 hours; temperature of 40.5°C (104.9° F) or higher within 48 hours; anaphylaxis. Progressive or changing neurological disease or infantile spasms are reasons for withholding or delaying DTP. Careful evaluation of children having a seizure between doses of DTP, especially 4 to 7 days after DTP, should be carried out before further pertussis is given. Children with a history of seizures or a disease that predisposes them to seizures may have DTP deferred. A decision about whether to immunize the child with static neurological disease should be made by 1 year of age. These children may be at increased risk from pertussis disease if they are exposed to disease while nonimmunized. DTP is generally deferred during immunosuppressive therapy until 1 month after cessation of therapy. If therapy is continuous, the child may be immunized with serological testing done to evaluate antibody response. The immunization may be given to HIV-infected children when they are asymptomatic, but is not given when they are symptomatic. Febrile illness or acute infection is cause to delay immunization.

## Side Effects:
*CNS:* drowsiness and fussiness (common); encephalopathy, seizure, persistent crying, high-pitched cry (rare). *GI:* anorexia. *Skin:* redness, swelling, pain at injection site; nodule at site that may remain for several weeks. *Other:* low-grade fever (up to 101°F) is common; moderate or high fever (102 to 106°F) and anaphylaxis are rare.

## Nursing Implications:
*Assess:* Careful review of records and history should rule out those children who have a contraindication to pertussis vaccine. Question parents about reac-

tions to previous DTP injections as well as presence of neurological disease or seizures. Static neurological disease puts the child at slightly increased risk for seizures after DTP, but these are not associated with permanent brain damage. A history of seizures in siblings or parents leads to a slightly increased risk (about 3%) for neurological side effects in vaccinated children. The risk is not a reason to withhold pertussis immunization. This risk, the benefits of pertussis vaccination, and the need to seek emergency medical care for postvaccine neurological effects should be discussed with the parents and documented in the record.

*Administer:* Epinephrine 1:1000 and resuscitative equipment should be available in case of anaphylaxis. Children on immunosuppressive drugs may have a lessened immune response to the immunization, although it contains no live viruses and is not contraindicated for immunosuppressed children. If the immunosuppressive therapy is short term, it is advisable to wait until 1 month after the end of therapy to give DTP. If the drug therapy is long term, it may be desirable to immunize the child with DTP and perform testing of serum to verify adequacy of immune response. If a schedule of immunization is interrupted, it may be resumed without beginning the series again. *IM:* Shake solution well before withdrawal; solution will be cloudy. Give deep IM into deltoid of older child or anterolateral thigh of infant. The National Childhood Vaccine Injury Act requires recording of patient name, address, site, and route of administration, lot number and manufacturer of vaccine, date of immunization as well as the name, address, and title of the person who administers the vaccine. If pertussis is withheld because of prior reaction, diphtheria and tetanus toxoid for pediatric use is administered. Do not confuse this with tetanus and diphtheria toxoid for adult use, which is used for immunization of persons 7 years and older. DTP may be given on the same visit with other immunizations such as oral polio, or measles–mumps–rubella, or *Haemophilus* influenzae type b when the latter two are given by separate syringes into different sites.

*Monitor:* Observe child for 20 minutes after immunization for signs of anaphylaxis or other unfavorable reaction. Severe reactions such as those listed under contraindications for future pertussis immunization are reported to the United States Department of Health and Human Services (see Appendix J).

*Patient Teaching:* Media exposure about risks of pertussis vaccine necessitates careful explanation to parents about the risks and incidence of side effects and disease. Parents should be told of common side effects (erythema, induration at site, fussiness, low-grade fever), as well as the incidence of severe reactions (acute encephalopathy occurs in 1 per 110,000 doses and permanent neurologic impairment in 1 per 310,000 doses within 7 days of the immunization). They are informed to seek health care immediately if any of the severe neurological symptoms occur. Acetaminophen (40 mg up to 3 months, 80 mg from 4 to 11 months, and 120 mg from 1 to 2 years) may be given at the time of immunization and every 4 to 6 hours for 48 to 72 hours to lessen the risk of fever, particularly for children at higher risk of seizures. Inform parents when child is to return for next immunization in the series and remind them to bring immunization records with them. After the fifth dose at 4 to 6 years, parents can be taught that everyone should have a booster of tetanus–diphtheria (Td) every 10 years. A skin wound 5 years after previous tetanus immunization may necessitate reimmunization at that time.

**Drug Interactions:** Immunosuppressive therapy may decrease the response to the immunization. Radiation therapy may decrease the response to the immunization.

**Storage Requirements:** Store in refrigerator at 2 to 8°C (35 to 46°F). Store in body of refrigerator rather than on door where temperature variations may be greater. Do not freeze.

---

## ☐ DOBUTAMINE                                    (doe-byoo'ta-meen)

(Dobutrex)

**Classification:** catecholamine, cardiac stimulant

**Available Preparations:** 12.5 mg/ml vial for parenteral use

**Action and Use:** A synthetic sympathomimetic similar to dopamine. Stimulates β-adrenergic receptors and causes cardiac stimulation but does not cause release of norepinephrine. Increases contractility, stroke volume, and cardiac output. Decreases peripheral vascular resistance but has minimal effect on blood pressure. Used in treatment of acute cardiac failure associated with low cardiac output and increased diastolic filling pressures.

**Routes and Dosages:**
*IV:* 2 to 10 μg/kg/minute
Dosage established by clinicians rather than the manufacturer.

**Absorption and Fate:** Peak effects 10 minutes after IV infusion with duration continuing only moments after infusion stops. Metabolized in the liver. Half-life: 2 minutes. Excreted mainly in urine, with small amount in feces.

**Contraindications and Precautions:** Pregnancy category C. Safety and efficacy in children not established but it is used in this age group for emergency treatment of cardiac failure. Contraindicated in those hypersensitive to the drug, in subaortic stenosis, hypovolemia. Cautious use in hypertension, atrial fibrillation, PVCs, after myocardial infarction.

**Side Effects:**
*CNS:* headache, paresthesia. *CV:* ectopic beats, tachycardia, angina, palpitations, hypertension. *GI:* nausea. *Respiratory:* dyspnea

**Nursing Implications:**
*Assess:* Vital signs especially blood pressure, EKG, cardiac output, pulmonary wedge pressure.

*Administer:* Facilities and personnel for continuous monitoring must be available. Hypovolemia should be corrected before the drug is given. *IV:* Avoid contact with the skin or eyes and do not inhale particles of solution. Add 10 ml sterile water or 5% dextrose to vial. Further dilute solution for administration in at least 50 ml saline, 5% dextrose, or sodium lactate solution. Prepared solutions should be used within 24 hours. Incompatible with sodium bicarbonate or other alkaline solutions and with solutions containing common preservatives sodium bisulfite and ethanol. Incompatible with heparin, hydrocortisone, cefazolin, penicillin, and other antiinfectives; mixing with other drugs discouraged. A slight pink color does not indicate lack of potency. Give by slow IV infusion with an infusion pump. Often used in children in solution with dopamine. See Appendix for infusion solution combinations.

*Monitor:* BP and EKG are continually monitored during infusion. Pulmonary artery wedge pressure and cardiac output are monitored. Tachycardia, hypertension, and arrhythmias require prompt attention and reduction of dosage. Measure I & O.

*Patient Teaching:* Not applicable. Given in critical care situations in the hospital.

**Drug Interactions:** Beta-adrenergic blockers, such as propranolol, decrease drug effects. Ventricular arrhythmias may occur during halothane or cyclopropane anesthesia. Decreased hypotensive action with guanethidine. Increased cardiac output and decreased pulmonary wedge pressure with nitroprusside. MAO inhibitors and tricyclic antidepressants may increase pressor effects.

**Storage Requirements:** Store at 15 to 30°C (59 to 86°F).

---

## □ DOPAMINE
(doe′pa-meen)

(Dopastat, Intropin, Revimine)

**Classification:** adrenergic agonist, catecholamine, vasopressor

**Action and Use:** This amine is a precursor of norepinephrine. It increases myocardial contractility and stroke volume and, therefore, cardiac output by β-adrenergic action. Has vasodilating effects on renal, mesenteric, coronary, and intracerebral arteries. May increase systolic blood pressure and pulse pressure. Used as a cardiac stimulant and in cardiogenic shock, acute hypertension and congestive heart failure to increase cardiac output, blood pressure, and renal blood flow.

**Available Preparations:**
- 40, 80, 160 mg/ml ampules for parenteral use
- 0.8, 1.6, 3.2, 6.4 mg/ml in 5% dextrose

**Absorption and Fate:** Widely distributed in body but does not cross blood-brain barrier. Metabolized by liver, kidney, and in plasma. Excreted in urine. Onset of action in 2 minutes with duration of 10 minutes. Half-life: 2 minutes.

## Routes and Dosages:
*IV:*

- Shock: 1 to 20 μg/kg/minute; increase by 1 to 4 μg/kg/minute at 10 to 30-minute intervals; not to exceed 50 μg/kg/minute
- Congestive Heart Failure: 0.5 to 2 μg/kg/minute; increase gradually until urine flow increases

Dosages established by clinicians rather than manufacturers.

## Contraindications and Precautions: Pregnancy category C. Safety and efficacy in children have not been established. Contraindicated in pheochromocytoma, uncorrected ventricular fibrillation, or tachyarrhythmia. Preparation containing sulfite contraindicated in those with sulfite allergy. Use with caution in those with occlusive vascular disease, acidosis, hypercapnia, hypoxia, ischemic heart disease, and patients receiving IV phenytoin. Use dopamine preparation in 5% dextrose cautiously in diabetics.

## Side Effects:
*CNS:* headache, numbness or tingling of fingers or toes, nervousness. *CV:* chest pain, hypotension, irregular pulse, hypertension and tachycardia especially with rapid infusion; bradycardia, palpitations. *GI:* nausea, vomiting. *Respiratory:* dyspnea. *Skin:* color changes or pain with vasoconstriction in extremities; gangrene of extremities with prolonged use; tissue necrosis with extravasation.

## Nursing Implications:
*Assess:* Assess EKG, vital signs especially blood pressure, hydration status. Dopamine is most effective in patients who are not hypovolemic or before severe shock is present. Correct hypovolemia before dopamine use if possible. CVP is helpful measurement of fluid status.

*Administer: IV:* Dilute concentrated solution in saline, 5% dextrose, lactated Ringer's. For example, if 5 ml of 40 mg/ml solution is diluted in 250 ml, injection contains 800 μg/ml. Diluted solutions are stable for 24 hours at 2 to 15°C (36 to 59°F) or 6 hours at 15 to 30°C (59 to 86°F). Incompatible with alkaline solutions such as sodium bicarbonate, aminophylline, alkalizing agents, and iron salts. Give into large vein by infusion pump. If extravasation occurs, it may be treated with 10 to 15 ml 0.9% sodium chloride injection with 5 to 10 mg phentolamine infiltrated into the site.

*Monitor:* Check IV site frequently for extravasation. EKG, blood pressure, urine output, cardiac output, pulmonary wedge pressure monitoring are carried out during therapy. Monitor patients with occlusive vascular disease very carefully for decreased circulation to extremities (lowered temperature, color changes, pain, change in peripheral pulses). If increased diastolic blood pressure, decreased pulse pressure, decreased urine output, or increased pulse occur, infuse slowly and monitor closely. If hypotension occurs, rate of infusion is increased. Inform physician of above changes.

**Drug Interactions:** Effects are prolonged if given with MAO inhibitors. Dopamine doses are begun at 10% of usual doses in these patients. Cardiac effects are decreased by β-adrenergic blocking agents. Concurrent IV phenytoin can cause hypotension and bradycardia. Increased arrhythmias occur with digitalis and guanethidine. When given with halothane or cyclopropane anesthetics, ventricular arrhythmias and hypertension can result. Increased diuretic effect with diuretics. Increased effects with thyroid medication.

**Storage Requirements:** Protect from light at 15 to 30°C (59 to 86°F). Do not use solutions darker than light yellow or any other color.

---

## □ DOXORUBICIN                                        (dox-oh-roo′bi-sin)

(Adriamycin)

**Classification:** antineoplastic, antibiotic, anthracycline

**Available Preparations:** 10, 20, 50, 100, 150-mg vials for parenteral use; 2 mg/ml

**Action and Use:** Binds with DNA, thereby interfering with DNA and RNA synthesis; interferes with protein synthesis. Active throughout the cell cycle. Used in solid tumors such as osteogenic sarcoma, neuroblastoma, Wilms' tumor, Ewing's sarcoma, Hodgkin's lymphoma, non-Hodgkin's lymphoma, acute lymphoblastic, and acute myeloblastic leukemia.

**Routes and Dosages:**
*IV:* Dosage variable with diagnosis ranging from 20 to 25 mg/m² for 3 days every 4 to 6 weeks to 30 to 45 mg/m² every 3 to 6 weeks
Total cumulative lifetime dose of anthracyclines not to exceed 400 mg/m².

**Absorption and Fate:** Not absorbed from GI tract. Absorbed rapidly and widely distributed after IV administration. Does not cross blood-brain barrier. Binds to cellular components such as nucleic acids. Metabolized by the liver and excreted mainly in bile, with small amounts in feces and urine. Biphasic half-life of 30 minutes initially and 16 to 17 hours terminally.

**Contraindications and Precautions:** Pregnancy category D. Not recommended during lactation as small amounts may be present in breast milk. Use caution in children under 2 years as cardiotoxicity may be more common in that age group. Contraindicated in those with existing myelosuppression, cardiac disease, chicken pox or herpes zoster, or in those who have received maximum cumulative doses for anthracyclines (doxorubicin and daunorubicin). Use with caution and adjust dosage in those with hepatic, renal, or cardiac dysfunction, or infections.

## Side Effects:

**CV:** acute, transient EKG changes that are not serious; chronic, **dose-related toxicity** that is life threatening. The latter manifests as congestive heart failure and may occur weeks, months, or years after therapy; more common in those under 2 years. **GI:** stomatitis, esophagitis, nausea, vomiting, anorexia, diarrhea. **GU:** hyperuricemia, reddish orange urine up to 48 hours after infusion. **Skin:** alopecia, hyperpigmentation of nail beds, nail changes, erythema in postradiation patients, severe necrosis with extravasation. **Hemic: leukopenia,** thrombocytopenia, anemia with maximum effects at 10 to 14 days, normal levels at 3 weeks. **Other:** anaphylaxis

## Nursing Implications:

**Assess:** Take baseline EKG and ECHO. Ask about history of prior antineoplastic therapy or radiation, with particular attention to anthracyclines. Measure bilirubin levels. Notify physician if elevated as dose reduction may be ordered.

**Administer:** This drug has potentially severe side effects and should be given only under the supervision of a physician with training and experience in cancer chemotherapy. The drug's potential for toxic effects on health-care personnel as well as patients necessitates careful handling during preparation and administration. Generally, during preparation of chemotherapy, latex gloves, a mask, and a solid front gown are worn, and a laminar flow hood is used. Gloves and gown may also be recommended for administration. Contaminated equipment, such as needles, syringes, vials, and unused medication, is disposed of properly. Clean-up of spills is carefully performed, and accidental contact by patient or personnel receives prompt flushing and cleaning. **IV:** Given IV only, as it is irritating to tissues. Reconstitute with 5 to 25 ml saline, shake vial, and allow to dissolve. Give IV push in a minimum of 3 to 5 minutes in 10 to 20 ml of isotonic solution. Give IV continuous infusion as ordered, usually over 10 to 96 hours. A central line is recommended; must not be given into veins over joints, which are small, or in edematous extremities. Reconstituted solution is stable for 24 hours at room temperature and 48 hours if refrigerated. Solution must be protected from sunlight (includes continuous infusion that is running). Drug is incompatible with many other drugs in solution such as fluorouracil, dexamethasone, hydrocortisone, aminophylline, cephalothin, heparin; best given alone.

**Monitor:** Assure vein patency before administration and constantly monitor IV site for extravasation. If it occurs, or if patient complains of pain at IV site, stop injection, and use another site. The infiltrated site is sometimes treated with local infiltration with corticosteroid and irrigation with saline. The area should be examined and referral to plastic surgeon may be indicated. Monitor CBC with differential, platelets. Monitor vital signs and be alert for signs of infection. Watch for bruising and other signs of bleeding. EKG and ECHO performed before each course to assess for cardiac toxicity. Signs of congestive heart failure such as weight gain, edema, dyspnea, fatigue, and vital sign changes are monitored and reported promptly. Monitor hepatic and renal function with BUN, SGPT, SGOT, bilirubin, creatinine, LDH, uric acid. Monitor nausea and vomiting and administer antiemetics and IV fluids as needed. Daily weight and I & O measures.

**Patient Teaching:** Prepare for possibility of nausea and vomiting; and alopecia. Drug may turn urine red in color for 48 hours after infusion. Increase fluid intake. Avoid persons with colds, influenza, chicken pox, or other illness. Report signs of infection such as fever, sore throat, or malaise, bruising or bleeding. Encourage good oral care and nutritious diet. Return for scheduled appointments for follow-up as cardiac toxicity may occur even months or years after therapy.

**Drug Interactions:** Administration of daunorubicin may increase cardiac toxicity. Cyclophosphamide administration may have same effect. Barbiturates may increase plasma clearance of doxorubicin. Increased possibility of cystitis if given with cyclophosphamide. Increased possibility of hepatotoxicity if given with mercaptopurine. Suppresses immune response to immunization. Live virus vaccines must not be given, nor oral polio vaccine to those in close contact with the patient on this drug due to the chance of infection with a virus; these vaccines are delayed at least 3 months after chemotherapy when the patient is in remission.

**Storage Requirements:** Store in dry place, protected from sunlight, at 15 to 30°C (59 to 86°F).

---

# □ DOXYCYCLINE HYCLATE

(dox-i-sye′kleen)

(Doxy-100, Doxy-200, Doxy-Caps, Doxychel, Doxy-Lemmon, Doxy-Tabs, Vibramycin, Vibra-Tabs Vivox)

# □ DOXYCYELINE MONOHYDRATE

**Classification:** antiinfective, tetracycline

## Available Preparations:
- 25 mg/5ml, 50 mg/5ml oral suspension
- 50, 100-mg film-coated tablets
- 50, 100, 500-mg capsules
- 100-mg delayed-release capsules
- 100, 200-mg for parenteral administration

**Action and Use:** Semisynthetic tetracycline inhibits protein synthesis by blocking binding of 30S ribosomal subunit of susceptible organism. Active against a variety of gm + and gm − organisms, trachoma, rickettsiae, *Mycoplasma*, and *Chlamydia*.

## Routes and Dosage:
**Not recommended in children under 8 years.**

*PO:*
- over 8 years, under 45 kg: 4.4 mg/kg in 2 divided doses first 24 hours, then 2.2 mg/kg in 1 to 2 equally divided doses per day
- adult dose: 100 mg every 12 hours first 24 hours, then 100 mg/day in 1 or 2 doses

*IV:*
- over 8 years, under 45 kg: 4.4 mg/kg in 1 or 2 infusions first day, then 2.2 to 4.4 mg/kg/day in 1 to 2 infusions
- adult dose: 200 mg in 1 or 2 infusions first day, then 100 to 200 mg/ day in 1 to 2 infusions

**Absorption and Fate:** 90 to 100% drug absorbed from GI tract. Drug distributed to most body tissues and fluids; concentrated in bone, liver, spleen, tumors, teeth. Peak level: about 1.5 to 4 hours. Half-life: 12 to 24 hours. Excreted by feces (20 to 40%) and urine (20 to 26%).

**Contraindications and Precautions:** Pregnancy category D. Not recommended during last half of pregnancy or lactation. American Academy of Pediatrics recommends this drug only be used under unusual circumstances in children under 9 years of age. Causes skeletal retardation in infants and neonates and permanent staining (yellow gray to brown) of deciduous and permanent teeth. Contraindicated if hypersensitive to tetracyclines, or with sulfite allergies. Use caution in renal or hepatic function impairment.

**Side Effects:**
*CNS:* **increased intracranial pressure** and bulging fontanels in infants. *CV:* **pericarditis.** *GI:* nausea, vomiting, diarrhea, anorexia, epigastric distress, stomatitis, glossitis, dysphagia, black hairy tongue, esophageal ulceration, oral candidiasis enterocolitis. *GU:* vaginal candidiasis, increased BUN. *Skin:* maculopapular, erythematous rashes, urticaria, photosensitivity, onycholysis, discoloration of nails. *Hemic:* leukocytosis, neutropenia, eosinophilia. *Other:* Hypersensitivity: **anaphylaxis, anaphylactoid purpura**; Local: IV: thrombophlebitis.

**Nursing Implications:**
*Assess:* Obtain baseline renal, hepatic and hematological data if long-term therapy is anticipated. Obtain cultures before therapy.
*Administer:* Check for outdated drug; causes nephrotoxicity. *PO:* Give without regard to food. Shake suspension well. Regular tablets can be crushed and capsules taken apart, mixed with small amount of food or fluid. Give with as much water as child will take after tablets and capsules to prevent esophageal irritation. Delayed-release capsules may also be opened; administered as described above but caution child not to chew particles (destroys enteric coating). Follow immediately with fluids to wash particles from mouth. If child has reflux, do not give dosage just before bedtime to prevent esophageal irritation. Do not give within 3 hours of other medications. *IV:* Discard any solutions that are dark or cloudy. Reconstitute 100 mg with 10 ml sterile water for injection. Do not give IV push. Dilute with compatible IV solution to 0.1 to 10 mg/ml and infuse over 1 to 4 hours. Compatible with $D_5W$, $D_5W/LR$, NS, LR,

Normosol. Has many incompatibilities; avoid mixing with other drugs. Protect from direct sunlight while infusing.

*Monitor:* IV can cause thrombophlebitis, start oral therapy as soon as possible to replace IV administration. Assess hepatic, renal, and hematologic function periodically. Long-term therapy: assess serum drug levels. Assess for side effects and report immediately to physician. Superinfections may occur. Maintain fluid intake for age group.

*Patient Teaching:* Inform physician of vestibular side effects and adapt activities to prevent injuries. Maintain good oral hygiene, and inspect mouth daily for signs of superinfections. Stress importance of following dosage schedule and taking for entire duration even if symptoms dissipate. Inform physician of any side effects. Avoid exposure to sun or sunlamps. Do not take outdated medication. Do not take OTC medications without contacting physician.

**Drug Interactions:** Doxycycline readily chelate with divalent or trivalent cations, thus drugs containing aluminum, calcium, magnesium, iron, zinc (e.g., antacids, iron preparations, mineral supplements, laxatives) should not be given concurrently but 3 hours after or 2 hours before. May potentiate effects of oral anticoagulants. Corticosteroids may mask signs of superinfections. Antidiarrheal agents with kaolin, pectin, or bismuth subsalicylate impair absorption oral form of this drug. Alcohol, barbiturates, carbamezephine decrease serum half-life of doxycycline.

**Laboratory Test Interference:** False-positive urinary catecholamines may result. False negative urine glucose with Clinistix and Tes-Tape. IV doxycycline containing ascorbic acid can cause false-positive urine glucose with Benedict's and Clinitest.

**Storage Requirements:** Store at 15 to 30°C in tight, light-resistant containers. Reconstituted IV form stable for 72 hours at 2 to 8°C (36 to 46°F).

---

## ☐ DROPERIDOL                                    (droe-per′i-dole)

(Inapsine)

**Combination Products:** Innovar (with Fentanyl)

**Classification:** antipsychotic, antiemetic

**Available Preparations:**
- 2.5 mg/ml vials for parenteral use
- 2.5 mg/ml with fentanyl citrate 50 μg/ml

**Action and Use:** This butyrophenone derivative is similar in action to haloperidol and the phenothiazines. Acts on the CNS, creating sedation by effect on subcortical level. Acts as an antiemetic and produces hypotension by adrenergic blocking. Used as a preoperative medication to relieve anxiety, to decrease nausea and vomiting during procedures, and in combination with the narcotic analgesic fentanyl.

## Routes and Dosages:
*IM, IV:* Premedication, anesthesia induction, or nausea: 2 to 12 years: 0.088 to 0.165 mg/kg

## Absorption and Fate: Quickly absorbed after injection. Crosses the blood-brain barrier. Metabolized in the liver and excreted in urine and feces. Onset of action: 3 to 10 minutes; peak action: 30 minutes; duration: 2 to 4 hours for sedation and 12 hours for alteration of consciousness.

## Contraindications and Precautions: Pregnancy category C. Safety has not been established in children under 2 years. Contraindicated in those with prior hypersensitivity to the drug. Cautious use in hepatic or renal dysfunction, cardiac dysfunction, hypotension.

## Side Effects:
*CNS:* Extrapyramidal reactions such as dystonia, akathisia, tremor, upward eye rotation, flexion of arms. Anticholinergic drugs can be used for treatment of these side effects. Other CNS symptoms include restlessness, dizziness, anxiety, hyperactivity, drowsiness, hallucinations, depression. *CV:* hypotension and tachycardia are frequent, mild, transient effects. Hypertension less common and seen when droperidol is given with fentanyl. *Respiratory:* laryngospasm, bronchospasm; **respiratory depression** when given with opiate such as fentanyl

## Nursing Implications:
*Assess:* Take vital signs.
*Administer:* Generally used IM for preoperative medication. IV injection may be given slowly by 5% dextrose or lactated Ringer's. May be incompatible with some other drugs in the same IV such as barbiturates. Resuscitative drugs and equipment should be readily available when the drug is given with fentanyl.
*Monitor:* Monitor vital signs carefully. Hypotension and tachycardia are common side effects. Hypotension may indicate hypovolemia, therefore, fluid intake is often increased. Respirations are observed especially if given with fentanyl.

## Drug Interactions: Additive effects with other CNS depressants.

## Storage Requirements: Store in light-resistant containers at 15 to 30°C (59 to 86°F).

---

## □ EPINEPHRINE                                    (ep-i-nef'rin)

(Adrenalin, Ana-Kit, AsthmaHaler, Asthmanefrin, Breatheasy, Bronkaid Mist, Bronitin, Dey-Dose, EpiPen, Epifrin, Epinal, Epinephrine Dropperettes,

Epitrate, Eppy/N, Glaucon, Medihaler-Epi, MicroNefrin, Nephron Inhalant, Primatene Mist, Sus-Phrine, Vaponefrin)

## Combination Products: E-Pilo

## Classification: adrenergic agonist, sympathomimetic, mydriatic

## Action and Use: A natural catecholamine with potent α- and β-adrenergic effect. Causes vasoconstriction, bronchodilation, increased heart rate, and cardiac stimulation. Used in cardiac arrest to treat asystole. Given in acute asthma attack or anaphylaxis. Used for treatment of open-angle glaucoma and as an ophthalmic decongestant. Present in small amounts in some local anesthetics to decrease their systemic absorption. Topical preparation used to control superficial bleeding.

## Available Preparations:
- 1:200 (5 mg/ml), 1:400 (10 mg/ml) suspension for parenteral use
- 1:1000 (1 mg/ml), 1:2000 (0.5 mg/ml), 1:10000 (0.1 mg/ml) ampules for parenteral use
- 160, 200, 250-mg metered spray for inhalation
- 1.83, 2.25, 1% solution for nebulization
- 0.1, 0.25, 0.5, 1, 2% ophthalmic solution
- 1% ophthalmic solution with pilocarpine
- In combination with chlorpheniramine in chewable tablets in anaphylaxis kits

## Absorption and Fate: Oral ingestion leads to rapid metabolization in GI tract and is not a generally effective route. Well absorbed after SC or IM injection, especially if site is massaged. Absorption after inhalation is small except with large doses. Drug is metabolized by the liver and excreted mainly in urine. Peak level is 1 to 2 minutes after IV. Half-life is short, doses repeated in 3 to 5 minutes.

## Routes and Dosages: PO (rare); SC, IM, IV, Intracardiac, Inhalation, Topical (eye, skin, mucous membranes)
*IM, IV:* Anaphylaxis: 300 μg initially; repeat q15min 3 to 4 times PRN
*IV, intracardiac:* Cardiac Stimulation: 5 to 10 μg/kg or 150 to 300 μg/m²; repeat q5min PRN or follow initial dose with IV infusion of 0.1 μg/kg/minute; increase by 0.1 μg/kg/minute; not to exceed 1.5 μg/kg/minute
*SC:*
- Asthma and Anaphylaxis: 10 μg/kg (0.01 ml/kg of 1:1000 preparation) or 300 μg/m²; not to exceed 500 μg/dose. Repeat q15min 2 times PRN; then give q4h PRN
- Severe Anaphylaxis: 0.1 mg (10 ml of 1:10000) over 5 to 10 minutes initially, followed by continuous IV of 0.1 μg/kg/minute up to 1.5 μg/kg/minute if needed
- Bronchodilator with Sus-Phrine (prolonged action): 25 μg/kg or 625 μg/m²; may repeat q6h; not to exceed 750 μg in children 30 kg or less.

*Inhalation:*
- over 6 years: Metered aerosol: 160 to 250 μg or 1 inhalation; repeat once if needed; do not take again for 4 hours
- over 6 years: Hand-bulb nebulizer: 1 to 2 deep inhalations of 1% solution, repeat in 1 to 2 minutes if needed; do not take again for 4 hours
- 4 years and over: Racepinephrine hand-held nebulizer: 2 to 3 inhalation of 2.25% solution; repeat in 5 minutes PRN; given 4 to 6 times/day

**Contraindications and Precautions:** Pregnancy category C. May slow labor and increase fetal heart rate. Not used during second stage of labor. Use cautiously in infants and children as they may get syncope especially if they are asthmatics. Sulfite-containing preparations should be avoided in those with sulfite sensitivity. Contraindicated in shock other than anaphylaxis, in arrhythmia, congestive heart failure, coronary artery disease, hypertension, ischemic heart disease, CVA history, narrow-angle glaucoma. Do not give with other sympathomimetics. Cautious use in hypertension, hyperthyroidism, those with diabetes, CV disease, pheochromocytoma, sensitivity to sympathetic amines, bronchial asthma, and emphysema.

**Side Effects:**
*CNS:* anxiety, restlessness, dizziness, headache, excitability, weakness, syncope, convulsions, fever, chills. *CV:* **tachycardia**, palpitation, increased blood pressure, flushing, EKG changes, chest pain, irregular pulse; with intracardial injection coronary artery laceration, cardiac tamponade, pneumothorax. *GI:* nausea, vomiting. *Respiratory:* dyspnea, rebound bronchospasm after withdrawal of inhalation administration. *Skin:* necrosis at injection site with repeated injections; pale cold skin. *Sensory:* blurred vision, enlarged pupils. *Other:* prolonged use can lead to metabolic acidosis; stinging of tissues upon topical application.

**Nursing Implications:**
*Assess:* Establish baseline vital signs especially pulse and blood pressure. Evaluate EKG, $Pco_2$, bicarbonate, pH, CVP, urine output.
*Administer: IV:* 1 mg/ml injection (1:1000) used. Add 1 mg to 250 ml solution for 4 μg/ml solution. Given slowly or by infusion. Discard unused solution. *Intracardiac:* Diluted as described for IV use; intracardial use only for patients with other routes not accessible. *IM:* 1 mg/ml injection (1:1000) used. Avoid buttock administration. *SC:* aqueous solution can be used.
*Monitor:* Monitor vital signs, especially pulse and blood pressure. Monitor EKG, $Pco_2$, bicarbonate, pH, CVP, urine output. Close monitoring of diabetic as increased blood glucose can result.
*Patient Teaching:* Teach correct inhalation technique. Use inhalation products as directed. Do not use discolored solutions or those with precipitate. Seek care if asthma is not helped in 20 minutes with inhalation agent. Do not exceed recommended dosages. Rinse mouth with water after dose to prevent dry mouth.

**Drug Interactions:** Additive effects with other sympathomimetics. Cardiac and respiratory effects lessened if given with β-adrenergic blockers. Severe hypotension and tachycardia possible if given with rapid-acting vasodilators. Decreased effects of antihypertensives. Increased hypotension with guanethidine. Increased cardiac effect observed if given with some general anesthetics (cyclopropane, hydrogenated hydrocarbons) and may be contraindicated with them. Decreases antianginal effects of nitrates. Cardiac glycosides, tricyclic antidepressants, antihistamines, and thyroid increase the cardiac effects of epinephrine; EKG monitoring needed with digitalis. Additive CNS effects with other CNS stimulants and xanthines (such as theophylline). Increase adrenergic and thyroid effect with thyroid medications. It can increase serum glucose, therefore, increased insulin may be needed in diabetics.

**Laboratory Test Interferences:** Increased blood glucose and lactic acid.

**Storage Requirements:** Store in tightly closed, light-resistant containers at below 40°C (104°F). Avoid freezing. Sus-Phrine (suspension form), keep at 2 to 8°C (35 to 46°F). Do not use discolored solution.

---

## ☐ ERYTHROMYCIN

(Akne-Mycin, A-Mycin, E-Mycin, ERYC, Erycette, Erygel, Ery-Tab, Erythromid, Ethril 500, Ilotycin, Novorythro, Robimycin, Staticin, Wyamtycin)

## ☐ ERYTHROMYCIN ESTOLATE

(Ilosone, Novorthro)

## ☐ ERYTHROMYCIN ETHYLSUCCINATE

(E.E.S., EryPed, Erythrocin, Pediamycin, Wyamycin)

## ☐ ERYTHROMYCIN GLUCEPTATE

(Ilotycin)

# ☐ ERYTHROMYCIN LACTOBIONATE

(Erythrocin Lactobionate-IV)

# ☐ ERYTHROMYCIN STERATE

(E-Biotic, Eramycin, Erypar, Erythrocin, Ethril, Novorthro, SK-Erythromycin, Wyamycin)

**Combination Products:** 200 mg erythromycin ethylsuccinate with 600 mg sulfisoxazole acetyl/5ml (Eryzole Pediazole)

**Classification:** antibiotic, antiinfective

**Available Preparations:**
- 100 mg/5ml, 125 mg/5ml, 200 mg/5ml, 250 mg/5ml, 400 mg/5ml oral suspension
- 500-mg tablets
- 250, 400, 500-mg film-coated tablets
- 250, 333, 500-mg delayed-release tablets
- 125, 200, 250-mg chewable tablets
- 250-mg capsules
- 125, 250-mg delayed-release capsules
- 250, 500 mg, 1 g for parenteral administration
- 0.5% ophthalmic ointment
- 1.5, 2% solution, 2% ointment, 2% gel, 2% pledgets, topical administration

**Action and Use:** Inhibits protein synthesis by binding to 50S ribosomal subunit inhibiting peptide formation. Active against most gram-positive bacteria including most strains of penicillin-resistant *Staphylococcus* and certain gram-negative coccobacilli, such as *Haemophilus influenzae, Bordetella pertussis, Borrelia burgdorferi, Chlamydia trachomatis*, and species of *Neisseria*. It is the drug of choice for *Mycoplasma pneumoniae*. Used to treat infections of upper, lower respiratory tract, skin, soft tissue, otitis media, and Lyme disease (drug of choice for children under 9 years). Ophthalmic ointment used for prophylaxis of ophthalmia neonatorum and of neonatal conjunctivitis and ocular infections. Topical form used to treat acne vulgaris and superficial wounds.

**Routes and Dosage:**
*PO:*
- 30 to 50 mg/kg/day in equally divided doses every 6 to 8 hours
- Prophylaxis Rheumatic Fever: 500 mg/day divided every 12 hours

*IV:* 10 to 20 mg/kg/day in equally divided doses every 6 hours
*Ophthalmic:*
- Prophylaxis Neonatal Gonococcal Ophthalmia, Ointment: instill 0.5 to 2-cm strip into conjunctival sac within 1 hour after delivery
- Ocular Infections, Ointment: instill 0.5 to 2-cm strip into conjunctival sac 2 to 4 times per day

*Topical:* Solution, Ointment, Pledgets: apply to skin, 2 times a day, morning and evening

*Combination Form:* Pediazole: over 2 months of age: 50 mg erythromycin and 150 mg sulfisoxazole /kg/day in equally divided dose every 6 hours

**Absorption and Fate:** Oral absorption of drug occurs in duodenum; it is effected by formulation, food, and gastric emptying time. Peak levels: PO, 1 to 2 hours; IV, at end of infusion. Widely distributed to most body fluids and tissues, only small concentrations in CSF. Half-life: 1.5 to 2 hours. Partly metabolized by liver and excreted mainly unchanged in urine.

**Contraindications and Precautions:** Pregnancy category B. Distributed into breast milk, use caution during lactation. Contraindicated if hypersensitivity to drug, hepatic dysfunction, or liver disease (erythromycin estolate). Use caution in impaired hepatic function or impaired biliary excretion.

**Side Effects:** Erythromycin estolate most toxic.
*GI:* abdominal pain and cramping, nausea, vomiting, diarrhea, stomatitis, anorexia, melena, pruritus ani. *Hepatic:* reversible cholestatic hepatitis with erythromycin estolate (rare in children under 12 years). *Skin:* Topical: dryness, erythema, burning, peeling (ointment). *Sensory:* tinnitus, vertigo, **ototoxicity**: reversible bilateral hearing loss (seen rarely with lactobionate, stearate, ethylsuccinate). *Other:* Hypersensitivity: urticaria, skin eruptions, rash, **anaphylaxis**; Local: IV: venous irritation, **thrombophlebitis**, IM causes severe pain.

**Nursing Implications:**
*Assess:* Assess previous allergy to this drug and hepatic function. Obtain cultures and sensitivity before treatment, but can start treatment before results. Observe and record appearance of skin or eye if used topically.
*Administer: PO:* Erthromycin base acid labile. Give erythromycin and stearate on empty stomach (1 hour before or 2 hours after meals); estolate can be given without regard to meals. Ethylsuccinate in those under 2 years: Give on empty stomach and with those over 2 years give without regard to meals. Shake suspension well. Regular tablets can be crushed and capsules taken apart and mixed with small amount of food or fluid. Do not crush film-coated or enteric-coated tablets; must be swallowed whole. Delayed-release capsules can be taken apart, given as contents of other capsules but particles must not be chewed. Give with small amount of water after to ensure particles are swallowed. Chewable tablets must be chewed. *IV:* Reconstitute according to package insert with sterile water for injection. Do not give IV push. Gluceptate intermittent infusion: dilute to 1 to 25 mg/ml and infused over 20 to 60 minutes. Lactobionate intermittent infusion: dilute to 1 mg/ml infused over 20

to 60 minutes. Compatible with $D_5W$, $D_5W/NS$, NS, LR, and Gluceptate is also compatible in amino acid 4.25%/D25%. Drug unstable in acid solutions (<pH 5.5); do not add other drugs unless chemical compatibility confirmed. Sodium bicarbonate buffer may be needed if pH below 5.5. *Ophthalmic:* See Part I for instillation of drops or ointments. After given for prophylaxis ophthalmia neonatorum, do not flush medication from eye, excess may be wiped away. Use new tube or single unit for each neonate. *Topical:* Apply sparingly as thin film to cleansed skin.

*Monitor:* IV solution is irritating and slower infusion rates will decrease pain; observe for irritation and thrombophlebitis. Start oral therapy as soon as possible to replace IV administration. Assess hepatic function if on therapy over 10 days. Assess for symptoms of hearing loss on those high doses of lactobionate, stearate, or ethylsuccinate. Symptoms can occur within few days up to 3 weeks of initiation of therapy. Superinfections may occur. Maintain fluid I & O for age group. If given for β-hemolytic streptococcal infection, 10-day course needed to prevent risk of acute rheumatic fever or glomerulonephritis.

*Patient Teaching:* Teach proper administration, instillation, and application of prescribed preparations. Importance of following dosage schedule and taking for full amount of time even if symptoms dissipate. Inform physician of any side effects.

**Drug Interactions:** Avoid giving with clindamycin, antagonistic action may occur. Concomitant use with carbamazepine, cyclosporine, theophylline, and digoxin increases action of these drugs resulting in their potential toxicity. Monitor prothrombin time when used with oral anticoagulants, it may increase its effects.

**Laboratory Test Interference:** False elevations SGOT, SGPT, urinary steroids, and catecholamines.

**Storage Requirements:** Store tablets, capsules, ophthalmic, topical, at 15 to 30°C (59 to 86°F) in tight containers. Reconstituted solutions: store according to package inserts. Store suspensions according to manufacturer's directions.

---

## ☐ ETHAMBUTOL HYDROCHLORIDE

(e-tham′byoo-tole)

(Etibi, Myambutol)

**Available Preparations:** Antitubercular
- 100-mg tablets
- 400-mg film-coated tablets

**Action and Use:** Exact mechanism of action unknown but it appears to inhibit RNA synthesis in *Mycobacterium* organism during cell division; arresting tubercle bacilli multiplication. Used in combination treatment of tuberculosis.

## Routes and Dosage:
*PO:*
- under 13 years: not recommended
- over 13 years: 15 to 25 mg/kg/day as single dose

**Absorption and Fate:** Well absorbed from GI tract (75 to 80%). Peak levels: 2 to 4 hours. Well distributed to body tissues, fluids, low concentrations CSF. Half-life: 3 to 4 hours. Metabolized by liver; drug and its metabolites excreted in urine (65%) and feces (20%).

**Contraindications and Precautions:** Pregnancy category B. Small amounts of drug excreted in breast milk. Contraindicated in children under 13 by manufacturer, (however, drug has been reported safely used in children over 6 years), if hypersensitivity to drug or optic neuritis. Use caution in renal function impairment (reduced dosages required), ocular defects such as cataracts, ocular inflammatory conditions, and diabetic retinopathy.

## Side Effects:
*CNS:* headache, dizziness, malaise, confusion, disorientation, hallucinations, peripheral neuritis. *GI:* abdominal pain, nausea, vomiting, anorexia. *GU:* increased serum uric acid concentrations. *Hepatic:* transient rise in liver function tests. *Sensory:* Eye: **optic neuritis** resulting in visual losses of acuity, visual fields, peripheral scotomas, loss of red–green color discrimination. *Other:* Hypersensitivity: **anaphylactoid reactions**, fever, joint pain, bloody sputum, dermatitis, pruritus

## Nursing Implications:
*Assess:* Obtain diagnostic cultures. Obtain baseline liver function studies, renal and hematopoietic status studies. Baseline ophthalmic tests (bilateral) of visual acuity and color discrimination.
*Administer: PO:* May give with meals if GI irritation. Tablets can be crushed and mixed with food or fluid. This drug usually given concurrently with at least one other antitubercular medication.
*Monitor:* Assess for side effects. Periodic hepatic, renal, and hematopoietic examinations should be obtained. Ophthalmologic examinations with tests for visual fields, acuity, and red–green discrimination should be done monthly. If any change in visual ability occurs, stop medication and notify physician. Visual changes may occur 1 to 7 months after therapy is initiated. Should symptoms occur, they are usually reversible in 2 to 3 months after drug is discontinued, depending on amount of damage incurred.
*Patient Teaching:* Report any symptoms of side effects especially visual symptoms. Medication must be taken as prescribed. Drug therapy may continue from months to years. Its important to have close medical follow-up. Do not take any OTC drugs without consulting physician.

**Drug Interactions:** Neurotoxic medications, e.g., aminoglycosides, penicillins, anticonvulsants, and other drugs may increase potential for optic and peripheral neuritis when used concurrently with this drug.

**Storage Requirements:** Store at 15 to 30°C (59 to 86°F); protect from light, air, and excessive heat. Solutions should be used within 24 hours.

---

## □ ETHOSUXIMIDE

(eth-oh-sux′i-mide)

(Zarontin)

**Classification:** anticonvulsant, succinimide

### Available Preparations:
- 250-mg capsules
- 250 mg/5 ml solution

**Action and Use:** Raises seizure threshold in the cortex and basal ganglia and reduces synaptic response to low frequency, repetitive stimulation. Used in treatment of absence (petit mal), psychomotor, and tonic-clonic (grand mal) seizures.

### Routes and Dosages:
*PO:*
- 3 to 6 years: 250 mg/day in one dose initially
- 6 years and over: 500 mg/day in 2 to 3 doses initially

Dosage can be increased 250 mg q4–7d PRN; not to exceed 1 g/day if under 6 years, 1.5 g/day if over 6 years. Usual maintenance dose is 20 mg/kg/day or 1.2 g/m$^2$/day

**Absorption and Fate:** Well absorbed from GI tract. Negligible protein plasma binding and distributed widely in body tissues. Partially metabolized and excreted mainly in urine. Peak level in serum, 4 hours; in CSF, 1 to 2 hours. Half-life is 30 to 36 hours. Therapeutic level is 40 to 100 μg/ml.

**Contraindications and Precautions:** Pregnancy category C. Contraindicated in those with known hypersensitivity to succinimides, those with severe liver or kidney disease. Cautious use as sole therapy in mixed seizure disorders, in blood dyscrasias.

### Side Effects:
*CNS:* drowsiness, fatigue, lethargy, headache, dizziness, ataxia, hyperactivity, irritability. *GI:* anorexia, weight loss, cramps, GI pain, diarrhea, nausea, vomiting, growth of gums. *Skin:* rash, urticaria, hirsutism. *Hemic:* leukopenia, aplastic anemia, eosinophilia, agranulocytosis, pancytopenia, systemic lupus erythematosus. *Other:* myopia, vaginal bleeding.

## Nursing Implications:

*Assess:* Establish baseline weight. CBC, liver function tests and UA are done.

*Administer:* Doses are given orally usually 2 to 3 times daily

*Monitor:* Weigh children regularly and record as drug can cause anorexia and weight loss. CBC, liver, and renal function tests, and UA are done regularly and abnormalities are reported. Monitor and record seizure activity.

*Patient Teaching:* Eat a nutritious diet and report weight loss. Avoid driving and operating machinery. Do not take other medications, including OTC drugs before checking with prescriber. See prescriber on a regular basis. Wear bracelet noting person has seizures and is on anticonvulsant medication.

## Drug Interactions: Additive CNS sedative effect with other CNS drugs. Lowers level of oral contraceptives; alternative birth control should be used. Phenothiazines and antipsychotics can decrease anticonvulsant effects. Levels of both drugs may be decreased when carbamazepine given concurrently. May decrease haloperidol level. Increased need for folic acid.

## Laboratory Test Interferences: Can produce positive direct Coombs' test.

## Storage Requirements: Keep capsules tightly covered at 15 to 30° C (59 to 86°F). Keep solution tightly closed in light-resistant container at 15 to 30°C (59 to 86°F); avoid freezing.

---

## ☐ ETOPOSIDE                    (e-toe-poe'side)

(VePesid, VP-16)

## Classification: antineoplastic

## Available Preparations:
- 50-mg capsules
- 20 mg/ml concentrate in vial for parenteral use

## Action and Use: This semisynthetic derivative of the May apple plant (mandrake) produces DNA breaks. Exact mechanism of action is unknown but it interferes with DNA synthesis at the premitotic stage. Arrests mitosis at metaphase; maximum effect at S and G2 phases of cell division. It is used in children in treatment of lymphoma and Hodgkin's disease and for acute myelogenous leukemia. Although not labeled for such uses by the FDA, the drug has also been used for acute lymphocytic leukemia, neuroblastoma, Ewing's sarcoma, rhabdomyosarcoma, Wilms' tumor, brain tumors, and for use in bone marrow transplantation.

## Routes and Dosages:
*PO:* dosage not established; not routinely used in children

*IV:* dosage not established for children by manufacturer. Clinicians use 100 to 150 mg/m² q3–4wk

**Absorption and Fate:** PO form absorbed with variability. IV form absorbed quickly and rapidly distributed in tissues. Pattern of distribution in tissues is not yet established although it is evident that therapeutic levels are not reached in cerebral spinal fluid. Highly bound to plasma proteins. Metabolized and excreted mainly in urine in its metabolized and unchanged forms. Peak level after PO is variable with a range of 45 minutes to 4 hours; most within 1 to 1 1/2 hours. After IV, at end of infusion. Peak serum levels range from 17 to 88 μg/ml in children. Biphasic half-life with 0.6 to 1.4 hours initially and 3 to 5.8 hours in terminal phase in children.

**Contraindications and Precautions:** Pregnancy category D. The drug is to be used in pregnancy only if clearly needed as there is potential of fetal harm. Use during lactation is discouraged. Safety of the drug in children has not been established and is used investigationally in this age group. Contraindicated in those who have shown hypersensitivity to the drug, those with chicken pox or herpes zoster infection. Discontinue if anaphylactic reaction occurs, or if hypotension occurs during administration. Dosage adjustment occurs if platelet count falls below 50,000/mm³ or the neutrophil count falls below 500/mm³. The drug is used with caution in renal or hepatic disease, infection.

**Side Effects:**
*CNS:* peripheral neuropathy, fatigue, somnolence, headache. *CV:* hypotension, especially if given rapidly IV. *GI:* nausea, vomiting, anorexia, diarrhea, abdominal pain, stomatitis. *GU:* hyperuricemia. *Skin:* alopecia, rash, pruritus, hyperpigmentation. *Hemic:* **leukopenia** (particularly granulocytopenia), thrombocytopenia, anemia. Leukocyte and platelet counts are lowest between 1 and 2 weeks, with recovery 3 weeks after treatment. Myelosuppression more pronounced in those with prior chemotherapy or radiation treatment. *Other:* **anaphylaxis** with fever, chills, bronchospasm, hypotension.

**Nursing Implications:**
*Assess:* Establish baseline vital signs, especially blood pressure. Take CBC, SGOT, SGPT, bilirubin, LDH, BUN, creatinine before therapy.
*Administer:* This drug has potentially severe toxic effects and should be given only under the supervision of a physician with training and experience in cancer chemotherapy. The drug's potential for toxic effects on health-care personnel as well as patients necessitates careful handling during preparation and administration. Generally, during preparation of antineoplastics, latex gloves, a mask, and a solid front gown are worn, and a laminar flow is used. Gloves and gown are recommended for administration. Contaminated equipment, such as needles, syringes, vials and unused medication, is disposed of properly. Clean-up of spills is carefully performed and accidental contact by patient or personnel receives prompt flushing and cleaning. *IV:* Dilute IV concentrate with saline or 5% dextrose to 0.2 or 0.4 mg/ml. The 0.2-mg/ml solution is

stable for 96 hours, the 0.4-mg/ml solution stable for 48 hours at room temperature with normal lighting or in plastic containers. Use syringes with Luer-Loks to avoid displacement and leaking of solution. Give IV over at least 30 to 60 minutes. The drug should never be given by rapid IV infusion. Low WBC or platelet counts may necessitate alteration of dosage, protective isolation and avoidance of invasive procedures.

*Monitor:* Observe patient during infusion for signs of anaphylaxis such as chills, fever, bronchospasm, hypotension. Emergency drugs and equipment should be readily available. If anaphylaxis or hypotension occurs, discontinue infusion and notify physician immediately. Monitor IV site to avoid extravasation; sodium chloride infiltration may be used if extravasation occurs. CBC should be done at least twice weekly during therapy and before further courses of treatment. Platelet count below 50,000/mm³ or neutrophil count below 500/mm³ may necessitate alteration of dosages. Monitor I & O. Observe for nausea and vomiting. Take blood pressure every 15 minutes during infusions. Take vital signs several times daily. Watch for signs of infection such as fever, sore throat, malaise, and for bleeding. Monitor hepatic and renal function with BUN, SGPT, SGOT, bilirubin, creatinine, LDH, uric acid.

*Patient Teaching:* Prepare for possibility of alopecia. Instruct to avoid sources of infections such as persons with colds. Encourage nutritious diet. Plan meals to minimize nausea. Encourage additional fluid intake. Teach patient to report signs of infection such as fever, malaise, sore throat, and signs of bleeding or bruising. Perform good oral hygiene to avoid stomatitis. Return for follow-up care as instructed.

**Drug Interactions:** Increased bone marrow effects with other myelosuppressive drugs or radiation. Suppresses immune response to immunizations. Live virus vaccines must not be given, nor oral polio vaccine to close contacts of the patient on this drug due to the chance of infection with a virus; these vaccines are delayed until at least 3 months after therapy when the patient is in remission.

**Laboratory Test Interferences:** May increase serum bilirubin, SGOT, alkaline phosphatase, uric acid levels.

**Storage Requirements:** Refrigerate capsules at 2 to 8°C (35 to 46°F). Store parenteral solution at room temperature of 15 to 30°C (59 to 86°F). Reconstituted solution is unstable; follow directions for reconstitution and discard at recommended times.

# □ FACTOR IX COMPLEX

(Konyne, Profilnine, Proplex)

**Classification:** hemostatic

**Available Preparations:** powder for parenteral use

**Action and Use:** A concentrate of blood coagulation factors II, VII, IX, and X. Prepared from plasma of multiple donors. Used in treatment of factor IX deficiency such as hemophilia B (Christmas disease) and to reverse effects of excess anticoagulant therapy.

**Routes and Dosages:**
*IV:* Dosage highly individualized; depending on degree of factor deficiency, child's weight, and amount of bleeding. Usually 1 U/kg will increase factor IX level by about 1%. Minimal level to control severe bleeding is 25% of normal level. Reversal of anticoagulant overdose: 15 U/kg

**Absorption and Fate:** Rapidly cleared from serum. Half-life is likely biphasic with 4 to 6 hours initially and 22 to 29 hours terminally.

**Contraindications and Precautions:** Pregnancy category C. Contraindicated in those with disseminated intravascular coagulation or fibrinolysis, in conjunction with elective surgery especially in those at risk of thrombosis. Cautious use in those with liver dysfunction.

**Side Effects:**
*CNS:* **Infusion reaction,** headache, flushing, fever, chills, tingling. *CV:* disseminated intravascular coagulation; changes in pulse and blood pressure especially with rapid administration. *Other:* risk of hepatitis B and HIV infection.

**Nursing Implications:**
*Assess:* coagulation studies such as bleeding time, PTT, levels of factors. Type and cross-match blood.
*Administer:* Warm diluent to room temperature, add to powder, rotate gently until dissolved. Given through filter needle by slow IV injection at about 100 U/minute; not to exceed 3 ml/minute. Give within 3 hours of reconstitution; do not refrigerate.
*Monitor:* Monitor vital signs during injection and be alert for fever, chills, tingling, and flushing. If these occur, slow rate of injection. Stop infusion in case of anaphylaxis. Be alert for signs of transfusion reaction as small amounts of A and B antibodies may be present; reaction most common in those with A, B, AB blood types. Monitor I & O. Coagulation studies are regularly performed.
*Patient Teaching:* Self- or parental administration of factor may be done.

**Drug Interactions:** Increased hemostatic effect with other anticoagulants.

**Storage Requirements:** Store powder and diluent at 2 to 8°C (35 to 46° F). Do not freeze.

# ☐ FENTANYL CITRATE                                    (fen'ta-nil)

(Sublimaze)

**Combination Products:** Innovar

**Classification:** opiate agonist, general anesthetic

**Available Preparations:** 50 µg/ml vials for parenteral use
Also available in 50 mg/ml with 2.5 mg/ml Droperidol

**Action and Use:** Affects the CNS by alteration of release of neurotransmitters. Acts as a general anesthetic in higher doses and an analgesic in lower doses. Produces effects on other body organs such as depressed respirations, increased growth hormone and other hormone levels, decreased GI movement, hypotension, bradycardia. Used as a general anesthetic and for moderate to severe pain treatment.

## Routes and Dosages:
*IM:* Analgesia: over 12 years: 0.001 mg/kg/dose
*IV:* used by anesthetist and anesthesiologist; nurses do not administer this route

**Absorption and Fate:** Rapidly distributed in body and crosses blood-brain barrier. Highly (80 to 90%) protein bound. Metabolized by the liver and excreted in the urine. Onset of action for analgesia is 7 to 15 minutes after IV administration, with duration of 1 to 2 hours. Peak level in 20 to 30 minutes. Half-life is triphasic with 2 minutes, 13 minutes, and 3.6 hours in terminal phase.

**Contraindications and Precautions:** Pregnancy category C. Not administered to pregnant women unless benefits outweigh risks. Not used in children under 2 years. Contraindicated in those with prior hypersensitivity to the drug. Cautious use in lactation, respiratory depression, increased intracranial pressure, hepatic or renal dysfunction, bradycardia, GI problems, urinary tract surgery, and hypothyroidism.

## Side Effects:
*CNS:* dizziness, sedation, weakness, fainting, restlessness, seizures, insomnia. *CV:* sweating, flushing, **bradycardia, hypotension**. *GI:* nausea, vomiting, abdominal cramps, constipation. *Respiratory:* respiratory depression, atelectasis, dyspnea. *GU:* oliguria, retention. *Skin:* rash, itching, hives, cool clammy skin.

## Nursing Implications:
*Assess:* Establish baseline vital signs.
*Administer:* Classified as a Schedule II drug under Federal Controlled Substances Act.

*Monitor:* Vital signs especially depth, rate, and quality of repirations are carefully observed.

*Patient Teaching:* Encourage deep breathing and coughing and movement in patient who has received this drug to minimize chance of respiratory complications. Instruct to stay in bed with side rails up.

**Drug Interactions:** Increased CNS and respiratory depression with other drugs having same action. Increased hypotensive effect with antihypertensives. Preoperative use of benzodiazepines may increase amount of fentanyl needed. Potential excitement, hypertension, and other effects when given within 14 days of MAO inhibitors; such use is discouraged. Phenothiazines may decrease the analgesic effect in addition to causing some increase in CNS depression.

**Diagnostic Test Interferences:** Increased serum amylase and lipase. Increased CSF pressure.

**Storage Requirements:** Store at 15 to 30°C (59 to 86°F) and protect from light.

---

# □ FLUCYTOSINE    (floo-sye'toe-seen)

(Ancobon, Ancotil, 5-FC, 5-Fluorocytosine)

**Classification:** antifungal

**Available Preparations:** 250, 500-mg capsules

**Action and Use:** Acts as an antimetabolite in fungal cells; effective in treating candidiasis, cryptococcosis, chromomycosis, and torulopsosis. Owing to the high frequency of drug resistance arising during therapy, it is used in combination with other antifungal agents such as amphotericin B.

**Routes and Dosage:**
*PO:* 50 to 150 mg/kg/day divided every 6 hours or 1.5 to 4.5 g/m²/day for children under 50 kg

**Absorption and Fate:** 75 to 90% well absorbed from GI tract. Marked intersubject variation for peak level from 2 to 6 hours. Widely distributed to body tissues; CSF is 60 to 90% of serum concentrations. Half-life: 0.5 to 2 hours. 80 to 90% excreted unchanged in urine. Therapeutic level 25 μg/ml.

**Contraindications and Precautions:** Pregnancy category C. Safe use during lactation not established. Contraindicated if hypersensitivity to drug. Use with caution in bone marrow depression, impaired renal function, hematologic disorders, radiation therapy, or with myelosuppressive drugs.

## Side Effects:

*CNS:* confusion, hallucinations, headache, sedation, vertigo. *GI:* nausea, vomiting, anorexia, abdominal bloating, diarrhea, **bowel perforation**. *Hepatic:* elevations in serum alkaline phosphatase, SGOT, SGPT, **hepatomegaly.** *GU:* increased BUN and serum creatinine. *Skin:* rash. *Hemic:* hypoplasia of bone marrow: anemia, leukopenia, thrombocytopenia pancytopenia, eosinophilia, **agranulocytosis** (rare), **aplastic anemia**

## Nursing Implications:

*Assess:* Obtain baseline hematological, renal, and liver function tests. Culture and sensitivities should be obtained before therapy.

*Administer: PO:* **Do not confuse this drug with 5-FU**. Capsules can be taken apart and mixed with small amounts of food or fluid. Nausea and vomiting incidence may be decreased by giving capsules over a time span of 15 minutes. Lower dosages are used with children with impaired renal function.

*Monitor:* Frequent hematological, renal, and liver function tests should be preformed during therapy. Monitor I & O and weights. Observe for side effects and report to physician. Therapeutic blood levels will also help indicate if toxicity occurs, especially if child has renal impairment. Drug usually used in combination with amphotericin B; effects may be synergistic.

*Patient Teaching:* Therapy requires close monitoring by physician. Report any side effects immediately. Therapy may be 4 to 6 weeks, but it can take several months.

## Storage Requirements: Store at 15 to 30°C (59 to 86°F) in light-resistant containers.

---

# □ FLUDROCORTISONE ACETATE                          (floo-droe-kor′ti-sone)

(Florinef)

## Classification: mineralocorticoid

## Available Preparations: 0.1 mg-tablet

## Action and Use: Mineralocorticoid that has moderate levels of glucocorticoid activity. It acts on the nephron's distal convoluted tubule to increase sodium reabsorption and potassium and hydrogen excretion, as well as water retention. Used to treat salt-losing adrenogenital syndrome and adrenocortical insufficiency.

## Routes and Dosage:
*PO:* 0.1 mg/day or 0.1 mg 3 times a week

## Absorption and Fate: Bound to plasma proteins; metabolized by kidney

and liver. Plasma half-life, 30 minutes. Excreted by the kidney. Duration of action: 1 to 2 hours.

**Contraindications and Precautions:** Pregnancy category C. Drug crosses into breast milk and can cause growth suppression in the fetus. Contraindicated in cardiac disease, congestive heart failure, hypertension, and renal and hepatic function impairment. Use with caution in Addison's disease.

**Side Effects:**
*CNS:* dizziness, headaches. *CV:* **hypertension**, sodium retention and edema, unusual weakness in arms or legs (low serum potassium), **cardiac hypertrophy.** *Other:* unusual weight gain

**Nursing Implications:**
*Assess:* Obtain baseline weight, blood pressure, and serum electrolytes.
*Administer: PO:* Can crush tablets and mix with small amounts of food or fluids.
*Monitor:* Monitor drug's response. Dosage determined more by severity of the condition and child's response to drug than by age or body weight. Treatment may require using a glucocorticoid, such as hydrocortisone or cortisone, to achieve a desired clinical response. When dosage first used, blood pressure should be taken every 1 to 6 hours. Monitor I & O, obtain daily weights, and monitor serum electrolytes. Observe for symptoms of overdose; weight gain, edema, congestive heart failure, ravenous appetite, elevation of blood pressure, psychosis, and severe insomnia. Observe for side effects of medication, hypokalemia, and child's response to medication (underdosage). If child is NPO for more than 4 to 6 hours while on this drug, he could develop hypoglycemia symptoms.
*Patient Teaching:* Dosing schedule must be understood and the importance of taking medication as prescribed. Regular physician visits to monitor clinical response to medication. Observe for signs and symptoms of medication overdosage, underdosage, and hypokalemia. Report any variations to physician. If on long-term therapy, child should wear identification jewelry or carry medication alert card information. Inform dentists, other physicians, and any one who gives care to child that he is on this medication.
**Drug Interactions:** Amphotericin B and carbonic anhydrase inhibitors may result in severe hypokalemia when used with this drug. Anabolic steroids and androgens may increase risk of edema with fludrocortisone. This drug used with digitalis glycosides increases possibility of cardiac arrhythmias; sodium- and potassium-depleting diuretics may cause hypokalemia. Nondepolarizing neuromuscular blocking agents may cause prolonged respiratory depression or apnea if serum potassium has been lowered by mineralocorticoids. Thyroid dosages may require adjustment with this drug.

**Food–Drug Interactions:** Increasing diet intake of salt may increase potassium loss. Salt intake needs to be individualized to child's drug response. Diet rich in potassium and protein is recommended.

**Laboratory Test Interferences:** Serum potassium may be decreased and serum sodium concentrations may be increased while on drug.

**Storage Requirements:** Store between 15 and 30°C (59 and 86°F) in light-resistant containers.

---

## ☐ FLUNISOLIDE                                    (floo-niss'oh-lide)

(AeroBid, Nasalide, Rhinalar)

**Classification:** corticosteroid

**Available Preparations:** 250 μg (0.25 mg) per metered spray, in 100 metered spray canisters for inhalation

**Action and Use:** Has potent antiinflammatory activity. Used to control symptoms of bronchial asthma and seasonal or perennial rhinitis (cases poorly responsive to conventional treatments).

**Routes and Dosage:**
- under 6 years: dosage has not been established.
- over 6 to 15 years: 2 inhalations twice a day (total daily dose 1000 mg)

**Absorption and Fate:** Absorbed through nasal mucosa and gastric tissues if inadvertently swallowed. Bound to plasm proteins; half-life approximately 1.8 hours. Metabolized by liver; excreted by the kidneys (50%) and feces (40%).

**Contraindications and Precautions:** Pregnancy category C and use caution during lactation. Insufficient data available for use in children under 6 years. Contraindicated if hypersensitivity to any ingredients in preparation (propellant is fluorocarbon), primary treatment of status asthmaticus, or acute episodes of asthma. Not indicated for relief of bronchospasm, or until nasal surgery, nasal injury, or nasal ulcers healed. Use with caution in systemic, viral, bacterial, or fungal infections.

**Side Effects:**
*CNS:* headache, dizziness, irritability, nervousness, shakiness *GI:* nausea, vomiting, unpleasant taste, GI upset, diarrhea *Resp:* sore throat, upper respiratory infections, cold symptoms, irritation and burning nasal mucosa, *Candida albicans* infection of nose and pharynx, ulceration, bloody mucus or unexplained nose bleeds, nasal septum perforation, shortness of breath, troubled breathing, tightness in chest, wheezing. *Other:* Hypersensitivity: urticaria, angioedema, rash, bronchospasm

## Nursing Implications:

**Assess:** Assess for acute asthma attack, nasal irritation, or URI before administration; do not give if these are present. Asthma condition should be reasonably stable before treatment with this drug.

**Administer: Inhaler:** Shake before use. Follow package instructions for proper administration. Inform child he may experience some local burning or stinging of nasal tissues after usage. Administer only amount prescribed. Rinse mouth after use of oral inhalers to prevent further drug absorption. After usage detach inhaler mouth or nose piece from canister; rinse in warm water and dry. If used in conjunction with a bronchodilator inhalation, use it 5 minutes before adrenocorticoid inhalation to prevent toxicity from fluorocarbons contained in both aerosols.

**Monitor:** Observe for side effects and symptoms of infections. Good oral hygiene may delay or prevent oral dryness, hoarseness, or candidiasis. Inspect oral membranes daily for symptoms of *Candida* infections. If child has been on systemic adrenocorticoid therapy, observe for signs of withdrawal (abdominal or back pain, dizziness or fainting, fever, muscle or joint pain, nausea or vomiting, prolonged loss of appetite, shortness of breath, unusual tiredness, weakness, or unusal weight loss.) If systemic corticosteroids are discontinued, the use of flunisolide inhaler will not prevent signs of adrenal insufficiency especially when child is exposed to trauma, surgery, infections, or other stresses. A number of months may be required for recovery of hypothalamic–pituitary–adrenal function. If child has an asthma attack, contact physician immediately so that systemic corticosteroid may be started. Monitor child's height at a regular interval.

**Patient Teaching:** Usage and care for inhaler. Use inhaler only as prescribed. It may take several days or 1 to 2 weeks to see benefits of drug. Overusage will increase the incidence of side effects. If symptoms do not improve after 3 weeks of proper usage, contact physician. Do not use during an asthma attack. Contact physician before using any other nasal medication.

**Storage Requirements:** Store at 2 to 30°C (36 to 86°F). Do not store near heat, flame, or exposure to temperatures over 120°F; may cause bursting. Do not puncture contents under pressure.

---

# □ FLUORIDE                                        (flor'ide)

(Fluoritab, Fluorodex, Flura, Karidium, Luride, Pediaflor)

**Classification:** nutritional supplement, mineral

## Available Preparations:
- 0.5, 1.0-mg tablets
- 0.25, 0.5, 1.0-mg chewable tablets
- 1.1, 4.4, 5.5, 8.8, 11, 13.75 mg/ml oral solution
- topical gel, paste, rinsing solution

**Action and Use:** This mineral becomes part of teeth and bones, adding to their integrity. It has both systemic effects during tooth formation and eruption and topical effects on already erupted teeth. Used as a dietary supplement when the natural water does not contain adequate amounts of fluoride. Topical preparations used for periodic dental prophylaxis. Some use in prevention or treatment of osteoporosis in older adults is under study.

**Routes and Dosages:** oral, topical (to teeth)

*PO:* When water supply contains under 0.3 ppm fluoride:
- birth-2 years: 0.25 mg/day
- 2 to 3 years: 0.5 mg/day
- 3 to 13 years: 1.0 mg/day

When water supply contains 0.3 to 0.7 ppm fluoride:
- birth to 2 years: none
- 2 to 3 years: 0.25 mg/day
- 3 to 13 years: 0.5 mg/day

When water supply contains over 0.7 ppm fluoride: no supplement needed

*Topical:* Sodium Fluoride:
- 6 to 12 years: 5 ml of 0.2% or 10 ml of 0.05% mouth rinse solution QD or weekly
- Over 12 years: 10 ml of 0.2% or 0.05% mouth rinse solution QD or weekly

Acidulated Phosphate: 6 years and over: 5 to 10 ml of 0.02% mouth rinse solution QD

Other topical preparations are used by dental care providers.

**Absorption and Fate:** Well absorbed from GI tract. Stored in bone and teeth. Crosses placenta and appears in breast milk. Excreted mainly in urine. Normal serum fluoride is 0.14 to 0.19 µg/ml.

**Contraindications and Precautions:** Not generally given as a nutritional supplement during pregnancy as its efficacy for tooth formation in the fetus is not proven; a prenatal multivitamin with fluoride is available for those who wish to use that. Contraindicated when the water supply contains over 0.7 ppm fluoride and in those with hypersensitivity to fluoride.

**Side Effects:**
*CNS:* weakness, tremor, excitement with overdose. *GI:* stomatitis, anorexia, constipation, nausea, vomiting, black stools. *Skin:* urticaria, dermatitis with hypersensitivity. *Respiratory:* dyspnea with hypersensitivity. *Other:* fluorosis (white flecks to brownish discoloration of enamel) with excess intake.

**Nursing Implications:**
*Assess:* Obtain information about the fluoride content of the available water supply. Assess other forms of fluoride that the child may be receiving such as a rinse in school.
*Administer: PO:* The chewable tablet is chewed and then swallowed to provide both systemic and topical effects. Best time for administration is after

brushing teeth in evening. Avoid food and fluid for 15 minutes after taking. PO solution may be given in small amount of fluid or food. **Topical:** Some solutions are rinsed around teeth and then swallowed; others are expectorated. Read directions for proper method. Generally not used under 6 years as rinsing properly would be difficult at younger ages. The topical form is most commonly used in school administration of fluoride. Nurses obtain signed permission forms from parents for these programs and provide information about proper fluoride use and intake for the famlies.

**Monitor:** Evaluate intake of fluoride during health-care visits with children. Monitor tooth eruption and color; recommend dental care as appropriate.

**Patient Teaching:** Teach proper dose and administration. Caution against overdosing due to potential for fluorosis. When products are given in school, do not repeat at home on the same days. Encourage regular dental care for children from 2 1/2 to 3 years onward. Keep out of reach of children as acute overdose can result in death.

**Storage Requirements:** Store tightly covered at 15 to 30°C (59 to 86°F); protect solution from freezing.

---

# □ FLUOROURACIL OR 5-FU                    (flure-oh-yoor′a-sill)

(Adrucil, Efudex, Fluorplex, Fluorocil)

**Classification:** antineoplastic, antimetabolite

## Available Preparations:
- 50 mg/ml vials for parenteral use
- 1%, 5% topical cream
- 1%, 2%, 5% topical solution

**Action and Use:** This pyrimidine antagonist inhibits DNA synthesis, inhibits RNA synthesis, and becomes incorporated into body RNA. Cell cycle specific for S phase of cell division. Used in treatment of solid tumors not amenable to surgery such as carcinomas of GI tract, pancreas, breast, hepatoblastoma. Topical forms are used to treat multiple actinic keratosis and basal cell carcinoma.

## Routes and Dosages:
*IV:* 7 to 12 mg/kg in one dose daily for 4 days; or 6 mg/kg may be given on days 6, 8, 10, and 12; or 6 to 10 mg q3–4d for 2 weeks total unless toxicity is evident. Alternatively, clinicians may use a loading dose regime of 400 to 500 mg/m$^2$ or 12 mg/kg/day for 4 days; or 500 mg/m$^2$/week twice then repeat in 30 days; dose not to exceed 800 mg/day.

***Topical:*** 1%, 2% solutions for multiple actinic keratosis BID; 5% solution for basal cell carcinoma BID for at least 3 to 6 weeks

## Absorption and Fate:
Distributes well into tumor tissue and crosses blood-brain barrier. Metabolized mainly by the liver and excreted by respiration and in the urine. Half-life is biphasic with 10 to 20 minutes initially and 20 hours in terminal phase. No drug in plasma after 3 hours.

## Contraindications and Precautions:
Pregnancy category C. Avoid during lactation. Safety of the drug in children has not been established, but it is used in this age group with no evidence of specific age-related complications. The drug must be adjusted or discontinued if the toxic effects of intractable vomiting, stomatitis, diarrhea, hemorrhage, GI bleeding, leukocyte count below 2000/mm³, or platelet count below 100,000/mm³ occur. Contraindicated in those with depressed bone marrow, during chicken pox or herpes zoster infection, in poor nutritional states, those who have serious infections, or have had major surgery in past month, who have had previous cancer treatment or radiation, or who have bone marrow metastases, or who have kidney or renal malfunction.

## Side Effects:
***CNS:*** disorientation, headache, weakness, cerebellar syndrome. ***CV:*** angina (rare). ***GI:*** anorexia, nausea, vomiting are common within first week of therapy, decreasing 2 to 3 days after therapy; stomatitis and diarrhea are common early signs of toxicity; GI ulceration and bleeding. ***Skin:*** alopecia is common, nail loss less common; maculopapular rash, dry skin, erythema; skin reactions increase with exposure to ultraviolet light; topical preparations may cause erythema, vesiculation, necrosis. ***Hemic:*** **leukopenia** (begins in 9 to 14 days, nadir 21 to 25 days, recovery 30 days), thrombocytopenia, anemia are common; blood counts are usually normal again by 30 days after therapy. ***Sensory:*** visual changes. ***Other:*** **hypersensitivity reaction**, fever.

## Nursing Implications:
***Assess:*** Establish baseline vital signs and blood counts.
***Administer:*** This drug has potentially severe toxic effects and should be given only under the supervision of a physician with training and experience in cancer chemotherapy. The drug's potential for toxic effects on health-care personnel as well as patients necessitates careful handling during preparation and administration. Generally, during preparation of chemotherapy drugs, latex gloves, a mask, and a solid front gown are worn, and a laminar flow hood is used. Gloves and gown may also be recommended for administration. Contaminated equipment, such as needles, syringes, vials, and unused medication, is disposed of properly. Clean-up of spills is carefully performed and accidental contact by patient or personnel receives prompt flushing and cleaning. ***IV:*** The solution may be used as supplied or mixed with normal saline or 5% dextrose solution. Precipitate must be redissolved by heating the drug, shaking vigorously, and allowing to recool before administration. Drug in an opened vial must be used within 1 hour or discarded. A 25-gauge needle is used for IV

infusion. Avoid extravasation. **Topical:** preparations are applied with applicator or gloved fingers. Do not use occlusive dressings over medicated area

**Monitor:** Observe for side effects and toxic effects of the drug. Leukocyte and platelet counts must be done before administering each dose to watch for toxic effects. A WBC count below 2000/mm³ necessitates protective isolation as well as discontinuance of the drug. Topical administration is discontinued when skin ulceration or necrosis occur.

**Patient Teaching:** Patient should avoid persons with colds, chicken pox, and other infections. Teach patient to recognize signs of side effects and toxicity and to promptly report these, e.g., stomatitis, diarrhea, vomiting, GI or other bleeding, fever, sore throat. Caution patient to avoid sun and ultraviolet exposure, whether on IV or topical preparations. Increase fluid intake. Plan for adequate nutrition and use antiemetics as needed. If topical preparation is applied, wash fingers well if used for application. Use caution if applied around eyes and mouth to avoid systemic effects. The 5% solution should never be used on the head for this reason. Inform patient of length of therapy if applying topical preparation at home. Patient must realize the importance of follow-up as this drug is usually used only for those with inoperable carcinoma.

**Drug Interactions:** Cancer chemotherapy and radiation can increase incidence of toxic effects of this drug. Suppresses immune response to immunization. Live virus vaccines must not be given, nor oral polio vaccine to those in close contact with the patient on this drug due to the chance of infection with the virus; these vaccines are delayed until at least 3 months after chemotherapy when the patient is in remission.

**Storage Requirements:** Store at 15 to 30°C (59 to 86°F). Avoid freezing and exposure to light. Discard unused drug in vial within 1 hour. The solution is colorless or faint yellowish.

---

# ☐ FLUROMETHOLONE                    (flure-oh-meth'oh-lone)

(Fluor-Op, FML, FML Forte, FML Liquifilm)

**Classification:** corticosteroid, ophthalmic

## Available Preparations:
- 0.1%, 0.25% drops for ophthalmic administration
- 0.1% ointment for ophthalmic administration

**Action and Use:** Adrenocorticoid with antiinflammatory effects that decrease infiltration of leukocytes to the site. Used to treat adrenocorticoid responsive inflammatory and allergic conditions of the conjunctiva, cornea, and anterior segment of the globe. Drug preferred in long-term therapy because of its lower incidence of causing increased intraocular pressure.

## Routes and Dosage:
*Ophthalmic:*
- Drops: instill 1 to 2 drops of 0.1 or .25% solution in conjunctival sac 2 to 4 times a day
- Ointment: instill 1/2 inch strip of 1% preparation into conjunctival sac 2 to 3 times a day

**Contraindications and Precautions:** Pregnancy category C. Caution should be used in children under 2 years due to increased risk of systemic effects. Usage should be limited to 5 days or less if child is under 2 years. Contraindicated in vaccinia, varicella, fungal, bacterial, or viral infections of the eye, ocular tuberculosis, herpes simplex keratitis. Use caution in corneal abrasions, cataracts, glaucoma, and diabetes mellitus.

## Side Effects:
*Sensory:* blurred vision, burning, lacrimation, eye pain, headache; long-term use: halos around lights, cataracts, glaucoma, diminished visual fields, optic nerve damage. *Other:* Systemic effects: symptoms of adrenal suppression especially with long-term therapy

## Nursing Implications:
*Assess:* Carefully observe and record the amount and appearance of inflammation.
*Administer: Ophthalmic:* Consult physician if contact lenses should be removed before drug instillation and if child should wear them during therapy. They may become a source of infection. For administration see Part I *Drops:* Shake solution well before withdrawal of drop. Apply finger on lacrimal sac using light pressure for 1 to 2 minutes after instillation to minimize systemic absorption. Very carefully blot up excess eye drops. *Ointment:* For administration see Part I. Inform child that vision will be blurred for several minutes after instillation.
*Monitor:* Observe for symptoms of side effects or adrenal suppression. Tonometry measurements are usually taken every 2 to 3 weeks with long-term therapy. Assess and chart response to treatment. Contact physician in 5 to 7 days to see if child is to remain on therapy.
*Patient Teaching:* Instruct parents on proper instillation of eye medication. Importance of giving drug only as prescribed. Vision may be blurred after installation of ointment. Observe for side effects. Close ophthalmic supervision necessary. Inform any care providers and dentists that child is on this drug before treatment or surgery.

**Storage Requirement:** Store at 15 to 30°C (59 to 86°F) in tightly closed container. Protect from freezing and light.

## ☐ FOLIC ACID
   ## OR FOLACIN

(Folvite)

**Classification:** nutritional supplement

## Available Preparations:
■ 0.1, 0.4, 0.8, 1 mg
■ 5 mg/ml, 10 mg/ml vials for parenteral use

**Action and Use:** This water-soluble vitamin is needed for erythropoiesis and nucleoprotein synthesis. Deficiency manifested by megaloblastic anemia, abnormal growth, and glossitis. Used in treatment of folic acid deficiency, such as in sprue, various anemias, pregnancy.

## Routes and Dosages:
*PO:* Nutritional Supplement:
■ Infant on goat milk formula: 50 μg/day
■ Infant: up to 100 mg/day
■ 1 to 4 years: 300 μg/day
■ over 4 years: 400 μg/day
■ OR: children: 100 μg/day, up to 500 to 1000 μg/day with increased requirement states

*IM, SC, IV:* Deficiency: 250 to 1000 μg/day until improved. Dose never to exceed 1 mg/day.

**Absorption and Fate:** Nearly completely absorbed from proximal small intestine with transport across mucosa enhanced by glucose. Distributed in body and stored in liver. Highly bound to plasma proteins. Metabolized by the liver and excreted in the urine. Serum levels range from 0.005 to 0.015 μg/ml with those below 0.002 indicating megaloblastic anemia and those below 0.005 indicating folate deficiency.

**Contraindications and Precautions:** Pregnancy category A. Injection solution with benzyl alcohol contraindicated in newborns. Contraindicated when pernicious anemia is present.

## Side Effects:
*Skin:* rash, flushing. *GU:* yellow urine. *Other:* (rare) fever and hypersensitivity.

## Nursing Implications:
*Assess:* Obtain diet history. Pernicious anemia should be ruled out before therapy as folic acid will correct the hematologic abnormalities but the neurologic damage caused by vitamin $B_{12}$ deficiency will continue. Pernicious anemia requires treatment with vitamin $B_{12}$. A folic acid dose of 100 to 200 μg/

day × 10 days in conjunction with a low folate and vitamin $B_{12}$ diet may be used to assess presence of folic acid deficiency. After 10 days, reticulocytosis, normoblastic hematopoiesis, and normal hemoglobin indicates folic acid deficiency.
RDAs of folacin are:

- 0 to 6 months: 30 μg
- 6 to 12 months: 45 μg
- 1 to 3 years: 100 μg
- 4 to 6 years: 200 μg
- 7 to 10 years: 300 μg
- over 10 years: 400 μg
- pregnancy: 800 μg
- lactation: 500 μg

*Administer:* Usually given PO unless patient cannot eat. *IM, SC, IV:* Incompatible with oxidizing or reducing agents and heavy metals; decomposes with riboflavin.

*Monitor:* Repeated blood studies. Record nutritional intake.

*Patient Teaching:* Take as directed. Dietary teaching includes lists of foods high in folic acid such as yeast, whole grains, organ meats, dried beans and lentils, green leafy vegetables, asparagus, broccoli. Because it is heat sensitive, raw foods are best source.

**Drug Interactions:** Increased folic acid needs in those taking adrenocorticosteroids, analgesics, anticonvulsants, estrogen. Most antibiotics cause false low serum folic acid levels. Methotrexate, triamterene, and trimethoprim are folate antagonists. Sulfonamides interfere with folic acid absorption. Folic acid decreases phenytoin levels. Chloramphenicol may antagonize hematopoietic effect.

**Laboratory Test Interferences:** Antibiotics such as tetracycline falsely lower serum folate levels. Folic acid lowers vitamin $B_{12}$ levels.

**Storage Requirements:** Store at 15 to 30°C (59 to 86°F) in tightly closed container. Protect injection solution from light and freezing.

---

## □ FURAZOLIDONE                    (fur-a-zoe′li-done)

(Furoxone)

**Classification:** antibacterial, antiprotozoal

## Available Preparations:
- 16.7 mg/5ml oral suspension
- 100-mg tablets

**Action and Use:** Interferes with the bacterial enzyme systems. Drug has monoamine oxidase inhibitor activities. Used in the treatment of bacterial and protozoal diarrhea. It is not always drug of choice for diarrhea. Drug used for enteritis treatment caused by *Giardia lamblia* and in treatment of cholera.

## Routes and Dosage:
*PO:*
- 1 to 12 months: 8 to 17 mg 4 times a day
- 1 to 4 years: 7 to 25 mg 4 times a day
- over 5 years: 25 to 50 mg 4 times a day

(Maximum dosage 8.8 mg/kg/day)

**Absorption and Fate:** Poorly absorbed from GI tract; inactivated by intestine.

**Contraindications and Precautions:** Pregnancy category C. Safe usage during lactation not established. Contraindicated in infants under 1 month, hypersensitivity to drug. Use with caution in glucose-6-phosphate dehydrogenase, with other MAO inhibitors, tyramine-containing foods, indirectly acts on sympathomimetic amines.

## Side Effects:
*CNS:* headache, malaise; dizziness and partial deafness (rare). *GI:* nausea, vomiting, abdominal pain, diarrhea. *Other:* Hypersensitivity: hypotension, angioedema, fever, arthralgia, urticaria, vesicular or morbilliform rash, erythema multiforme.

## Nursing Implications:
*Assess:* Obtain history of diarrhea, assess dehydration status and fluid and electrolyte balance, and home and sanitation history. Diagnosis confirmed by stool cultures; obtain according to agency policy.

*Administer: PO:* Light causes drug to darken. Tablet may be crushed, mixed with small amount of food or fluid.

*Monitor:* If nausea and vomiting occurs, it may be reduced by decreasing dosage. Observe for side effects. Assessment of diarrhea (amount, quantity, characteristics of stools), dehydration status, fluid and electrolyte balance.

*Patient Teaching:* Do not take more often or in larger doses than prescribed. Parent should keep flow chart denoting number of stools, appearance, and amount for drug evaluation. Teach parent assessment for dehydration. If diarrhea persists or worsens, nausea, vomiting or other symptoms occur, inform physician. If no significant improvement in diarrhea in 7 days, drug should be discontinued. Inform family that child should not ingest alcohol for at least 4 days after furazolidone is stopped. Drug may cause urine to have brown color. Patient should avoid foods high in tyramine. Do not take OTC without consulting pharmacist or physician.

**Drug Interactions:** Causes a disulfiram-like reaction with alcohol. Use cautiously with MAO inhibitors, narcotics, sedatives, indirect-acting sympathomimetic amines; they can cause hypertensive reactions when combined with this drug.

**Food Interactions:** Avoid foods high in tyramine, e.g., yeast extracts, beer, wine, chicken livers, strong unpasteurized cheese, pickled herring, fermented products, broad beans.

**Laboratory Test Interference:** False-positive for urinary glucose with Benedict's test and Clinitest.

**Storage Requirements:** Store at 15 to 30°C (59 to 86°F) in light-resistant container.

---

## ☐ FUROSEMIDE                                    (fur-oh′se-mide)

(Furomide, Lasix)

**Classification:** loop diuretic, antihypertensive

## Available Preparations:
- 20, 40, 80-mg tablets
- 40 mg/5 ml, 10 mg/ml oral solution
- 10 mg/ml vials for parenteral use

**Action and Use:** This rapid-acting diuretic inhibits reabsorption of sodium in the ascending Henle's loop. Increases potassium excretion in distal tubule and may effect electrolyte transfer in proximal tubule as well. Used in treatment of edema from renal failure, congestive heart failure, cerebral edema, pulmonary edema, congenital heart disease, and nephrotic syndrome. Used without FDA approval in treatment of hypercalcemia.

## Routes and Dosages:
*PO:*
- Diuretic: 2 mg/kg initially; increase by 1 to 2 mg/kg q6–8h PRN; not to exceed 6 mg/kg/day

*IM, IV:*
- Diuretic: 1 mg/kg initially; increase by 1 mg/kg q2h PRN; not to exceed 6 mg/kg/day
- Hypercalcemia: 25 to 50 mg q4h PRN; dosage established by clinicians rather than manufacturer

**Absorption and Fate:** Rapidly absorbed from IV, IM, and PO routes. Food may slow PO absorption. Highly bound to plasma proteins. Metabolized by liver and metabolites and unchanged drug eliminated in urine and bile. Onset of action for PO form is 30 to 60 minutes, with peak effect in 1 to 2 hours and duration of action 6 to 8 hours. Onset of action for IV form is 5 minutes, with peak effect in 20 to 60 minutes and duration of action 2 hours. Half-life variable depending on study with ranges from under 1 hour to nearly 10 hours.

## Contraindications and Precautions:

Pregnancy category C. May cause hydronephrosis in laboratory animals. Excreted in breast milk, therefore, not advised during lactation. Cautious use in neonates due to long half-life. Contraindicated in those with hypersensitivity to the drug, in anuria, increasing azotemia, hypotension, dehydration with hyponatremia, metabolic alkalosis with hypokalemia. Cautious use in cirrhosis, diabetes, hyperuricemia, hepatic and renal dysfunction, hearing problem, lupus, pancreatitis, myocardial infarction.

## Side Effects:

*CNS:* vertigo, tinnitus, headache, confusion, fatigue. *CV:* orthostatic hypotension, irregular pulse, weak pulse. *GI:* nausea, vomiting, dry mouth, thirst, stomach pain, diarrhea, anorexia. *Hepatic:* jaundice, hepatic dysfunction, elevated liver enzymes. *GU:* profound diuresis. *Metabolic:* **hypokalemia**, hyponatremia, hypochloremic alkalosis. *Sensory:* tinnitus, deafness (may be permanent), vision changes, photosensitivity. *Hemic:* thrombocytopenia, neutropenia, anemia, leukopenia, aplastic anemia, agranulocytosis. *Other:* local pain, irritation, and thrombophlebitis with IV use, allergy with skin rash, urticaria, purpura, dermatitis.

## Nursing Implications:

*Assess:* Baseline vital signs, particularly blood pressure. Check hydration status and serum electrolytes. Check weight and hepatic and renal function.

*Administer: PO:* Administer with food to decrease GI irritation. Give no later than 3 PM to avoid nocturia. Solution contains alcohol. *IV:* Added to saline, 5 % dextrose, or lactated Ringer's solutions. IV solution given slowly over 1 to 2 minutes. If high dose is used, it may be given in solution with infusion pump and membrane filter. Do not mix with acidic solutions or drugs such as ascorbic acid, epinephrine, tetracycline.

*Monitor:* Monitor BP constantly during IV use; regularly during PO use. Monitor regularly BUN, $CO_2$, CBC, creatinine, hepatic and renal function, serum electrolytes, glucose. Perform hearing tests. Weigh daily. Measure I & O. Diabetics need close monitoring due to possible hyperglycemia.

*Patient Teaching:* Take at same time each day with food; take no later than 3 PM. Do not discontinue unless instructed by physician. Caution against rapid position changes to avoid postural hypotension. Avoid hot tubs, excessive exercise, hot weather, and alcohol. Diet teaching and sodium restriction may need to be discussed. Report signs of electrolyte imbalance such as weakness, thirst, anorexia, fatigue, muscle cramps. GI symptoms may signal need for dosage adjustment. Eat potassium-containing foods such as orange juice, tomatoes, apricots, figs, prunes, avocados, raisins, bananas, meat, potatoes.

## Drug Interactions:

Increased risk of ototoxicity with other ototoxic drugs

such as aminoglycosides and amphotericin B. Increased diuretic and antihypertensive effects with indomethacin. Increased potential for digitalis toxicity due to hypokalemia. Additive effects with other diuretics. Prolongs blocking action of neuromuscular blockers. Hyperglycemia in those on insulin. Decreased lithium clearance. Probenecid decreases the drug's urinary excretion. Decreased effects of anticoagulants. Reduced antihypertensive effects with sympathomimetics.

**Laboratory Test Interferences:** Increased blood and urine glucose. Increased BUN, uric acid. Decreased serum calcium, chloride, magnesium, potassium, sodium.

**Storage Requirements:** Store all preparations tightly closed in light-resistant containers from 15 to 30°C (59 to 86°F). Protect solutions from freezing.

---

## □ GENTAMICIN (jen-ta-mye′sin)

(Apogen, Alcomicin, Cidomycin, Garamycin, Jenamicin)

**Classification:** aminoglycoside

**Available Preparations:**
- 10, 40 mg/ml for parenteral administration
- 2 mg/ml intrathecal or intraventricular administration
- 0.3% ophthalmic drops and ointment
- 0.1% topical cream and ointment

**Action and Use:** Inhibits protein synthesis by binding irreversibly to bacterial ribosomes. Active against wide range of both gram-positive and gram-negative bacteria, e.g., staphylococci, enterococci, *Escherichia coli, Proteus, Klebsiella, Enterobacter, Serratia, and Pseudomonas.* Combined with other antibiotics in treating severe gram-negative infections. Treats infections of bone, skin, urinary, and GI tract, and infections such as neonatal and bacterial septicemias and meningitis. Ophthalmic preparations used for topical infections of external eye and its adnexa. Topical form used for primary and secondary skin infections.

**Routes and Dosage:**
*IM, IV:*
- premature, ≤7 days, < 28 weeks: 2.5 mg/kg every 24 hours
- premature, ≤7 days, 28 to 34 weeks: 2.5 mg/kg every 18 hours
- premature > 7 days, < 28 weeks: 2.5 mg/kg every 18 hours
- premature > 7 days, 28 to 34 weeks: 2.5 mg/kg every 12 hours
- full-term neonates, birth to 7 days: 2.5 mg/kg every 12 hours
- full-term neonates, 7 days to 1 year: 2.5 mg/kg every 8 hours

- over 1 year: 2 to 2.5 mg/kg every 8 hours
- children: 6 to 7.5 mg/kg/day in equally divided doses every 8 hours

Note: Dosages based on normal renal function. Treatment should be limited to 7 to 10 days.

### Intrathecal (IT):

- under 3 months: dosage not established
- over 3 months: 1 to 2 mg once a day

### Ophthalmic:

- Drops: instill 1 drop of 0.3% solution into conjunctival sac every 4 to 8 hours
- Ointment: instill 1 cm strip of 0.3% ointment into conjunctival sac every 6 to 12 hours

### Topical:

- Cream or Ointment: apply 0.1% sparingly to effected area 3 to 4 times a day

**Absorption and Fate:** IM absorption rapid, complete. Distributed in extracellular fluids, CSF (slight increase when meninges are inflamed). Topical only absorbed through broken skin tissue. Topical cream more rapidly and completely absorbed than ointment. Peak level: IM, 30 to 60 minutes, immediately following to 30 minutes of IV. Half-life: 2 to 3 hours normal renal function, 40 to 50 hours with impaired renal function; 3 to 11.5 hours in neonates; intrathecal: 5.5 hours. Protein binding low; 50 to 93% excreted unchanged in urine.

**Contraindications and Precautions:** Pregnancy category C. Safety during lactation not established. Use caution in premature infants and neonates due to renal immaturity. Contraindicated in hypersensitivity to this drug or other aminoglycosides and in renal failure. Use with caution in renal function impairment, botulism, hypocalcemia, hypomagnesemia, hypokalemia, dehydration, or eighth cranial nerve impairment.

### Side Effects:

**CNS:** **neurotoxicity**: numbness, tingling, muscle twitching, seizures; **neuromuscular blockade**: muscle weakness, respiratory depression, lethargy, headache. **GI:** nausea, vomiting, loss of appetite. **GU:** **nephrotoxicity**: blood or casts in urine, **oliguria**, increased thirst, proteinuria, increased BUN and serum creatinine, decreased urine creatinine clearance and specific gravity, **renal failure**. **Skin:** itching, redness, edema. **Hemic:** eosinophilia, anemia, leukopenia, agranulocytosis, thrombocytopenia. **Sensory:** ophthalmic: burning, stinging, blurred vision, photosensitivity; **ototoxicity**: eight cranial nerve damage causing hearing loss, vertigo, loss of balance, tinnitus; cochlear damage: high frequency hearing loss detected only at first by audiometric testing

### Nursing Implications:

**Assess:** Obtain cultures and sensitivity before treatment, but can start treatment before results. Obtain baseline weights, BUN, creatinine levels, and hearing tests before therapy. Assess and record appearance of skin lesions and eye irritation.

*Administer:* If solution has precipitate do not use. Occasional report of pain at injection site. *IV:* Do not give IV push. Prepared solutions are 10 or 100 mg/ml. Intermittent infusion, dilute with normal saline or 5% dextrose to 1 mg/ml concentration and infuse over 30 to 120 minutes. Compatible in $D_5W$, $D_5W/0.2\%NS$, $D_5W/0.45\%NS$, NS, LR, Ionosol products. Inactivated by penicillins. Do not premix with other medications and infuse separately, then flush line with normal saline or 5% dextrose in water. Piggyback injection only for IV use; contains no preservatives, use immediately after seal broken. Unit contains 1 mg/ml. Follow package insert for dosage adjustment. *IT:* Use preparation for intrathecal use only, does not contain preservatives; discard unused portion. Prepare for sterile injection in 5 to 10 ml sterile syringe. After lumbar puncture, physician will usually further dilute gentamicin with CSF, then inject over 3 to 5 minutes. If spinal fluid grossly purulent, gentamicin can be diluted instead with sterile normal saline. *Ophthalmic:* For administration, see Part I. Ointment will blurr vision for several minutes. *Topical:* Do not apply to large denuded areas; increased possibility of systemic absorption. Treatment of impetigo contagiosa: gently clean crusted area with soap and water before applying gentamicin. Use clean technique to prevent spread of infection. Area treated with this drug can be left open or covered with gauze dressings. Cream is drug of choice for wet oozing wounds, whereas ointment is more effective for treatment of dry eczematous areas.

*Monitor:* Observe for signs of respiratory depression with IV infusion. Peak blood levels can be drawn 1 hour after IM dosage and 30 minutes to 1 hour after infusion ends. Desirable peak concentrations should be 4 to 10 μg/ml and maximum trough concentrations (drawn just before next dose) should not exceed 1–2 μg/ml. Measurements above these levels are associated with increased incidence of toxicity. Maintain daily hydration for child's age group. If no response in 3 to 5 days, therapy should be discontinued. Monitor child's hearing levels daily. Renal function assessed by I & O, daily weights, urine specific gravity, urinalysis, creatinine levels, and BUN. Report any side effects immediately to physician. Observe for superinfections. If therapy continues beyond 10 days, daily renal function tests and weekly audiograms should be obtained. If using two forms of gentamicin concurrently (systemic and ophthalmic or topical), monitor serum levels.

*Patient Teaching:* Encourage parents to aid in daily hearing assessments of child. Teach parents proper instillation techniques. If no improvement in 3 to 5 days, notify physician. Observe for superinfections. When using for eye infections do not share towels, wash cloths, or pillow cases with other family members.

**Drug Interactions:** Increased chance for ototoxicity and nephrotoxicity when used concurrently with amphotericin B, salicylates, bacitracin (parenteral), bumetanide (parenteral), carmustine, cephalothin, cisplatin, cyclosporine, ethacrynic acid, furosemide, paromomycin, streptozocin, and vancomycin when used concurrently with gentamicin. Masked symptoms of ototoxicity can occur when used with dimenhydrinate. Gentamicin used in combination with aminoglycosides or capreomycin may increase ototoxicity. Decreased renal clearance occurs with neonates when given indomethacin and this drug. Nephrotoxicity and neuromuscular blockade increase with use of methoxyflurane or polymyxins with this drug. Neuromuscular blockade possible with halogenated hydrocarbon inhalation anesthetic, citrate-anticoagulated blood transfusion, and neuromuscular blocking agents combined with gentamicin. This drug may increase respiratory depressant effects of opioids and analgesics. Parenteral carbenicillin and ticarcillin inactivates gentamicin.

**Laboratory Test Interference:** Increased LDH and decreased serum sodium.

**Storage Requirements:** Store at 15 to 30°C (59 to 86°F) and protect from freezing. Discard parenteral forms without preservatives immediately after opening.

---

## □ GLUCAGON                                    (gloo'ka-gon)

**Classification:** antihypoglycemic

**Available Preparations:** 1, 10 units for parenteral administration

**Action & Use:** Hormone derived from beef or pork pancreas; enables hepatic glycogenolysis and gluconeogenesis through a complicated enzymatic activity. Causes increase in plasma glucose, relaxing of smooth musculature and inotropic myocardial effects; however, glucagon will only increase glucose levels if hepatic stores are available. It will not be of help in chronic hypoglycemia, starvation states, or adrenal insufficiency. Used for emergency treatment of severe hypoglycemia in patients with diabetes mellitus.

**Routes and Dosage:**
*SC, IM, IV:* Antihypoglycemic: 0.025 mg/kg/dose if child does not awaken within 5 to 20 minutes; 1 or 2 additional doses may be given

**Absorption and Fate:** Metabolized by the liver (primarily) but also by kidneys, plasma, and other body tissues. Half-Life: 3 to 10 minutes.

**Contraindications and Precautions:** Pregnancy category B; does not appear to effect nursing mothers. Contraindicated with hypersensitivity to drug, in birth asphyxia, infants with intrauterine growth retardation, hypoglycemia in premature infants, and hypersensitivity to protein compounds. Use with caution in insulinoma and pheochromocytoma.

## Side Effects:
*CV:* hypotension. *GI:* nausea, vomiting. *Other:* allergic reaction: dizziness, light-headedness, skin rash, difficulty breathing.

## Nursing Implications:
*Assess:* Observe for hypoglycemia symptoms; anxious or nervous feeling, behavior change, headache, difficulty in concentration, tiredness, shakiness, chills, cool, pale skin, hunger, nausea, weakness, unconsciousness, and coma. Most likely used with child who is unconscious. Obtain history of what precipitated this attack: increased exercise, illness, diet history, and what type of insulin was given and time of last injection.

*Administer: IM, SC:* Check expiration date prior to usage. Use only diluent supplied to reconstitute, because glucagon may precipitate in saline solutions or those solutions having pH of 3 to 9.5. Date and label bottle after reconstitution; Stable for 3 months if refrigerated. Response should occur (child awakens) within 5 to 20 minutes. If no response after 20 minutes, dosage can be repeated. **Have IV glucose available if child does not respond to therapy.** Many juvenile diabetics will not respond to glucagon and will need 10% to 50% glucose IV. *IV:* Dilute with diluent provided by manufacture and give IV push. In IV drip infusions, glucagon is compatible with dextrose solution but will precipitate in saline solutions. Incompatible with pH of 3.0 to 9.5. 1 unit equals 1 mg.

*Monitor:* If child unconscious after dosage, turn child on side to prevent aspiration if vomiting occurs. Vomiting may occur upon awakening, so have an emesis basin nearby and emergency suction. Have PO form of glucose or sucrose ready after child is alert and responding to prevent secondary hypoglycemia. Each child tends to develop a symptom response pattern to hypoglycemia. If child has had hypoglycemic reaction previously, document the pattern. This information is important if child is hospitalized and needs to appear on his care plan.

*Patient Teaching:* Always check expiration date on vial before administration. Teach proper mixing, preparation, and administration of injection. Make sure parents have supply of needles and syringes to give drug. An insulin syringe can be used but give at a 90° angle. This is not the syringe of choice as the medication is absorbed quicker from IM site and the insulin syringe may not be large enough for dosage necessary, especially in older child. If no response in 20 minutes, can repeat dosage and seek immediate medical assistance. Child may vomit, parent needs to know how to prevent aspiration. Give child PO sugar after recovery and inform physician of incident. Evaluation of insulin dosage necessary. Reconstituted medication should be labeled, refrigerated, and discarded after 3 months. Replace medication as necessary.

**Laboratory Test Interferences:** May decrease serum cholesterol levels and increase or decrease serum potassium levels.

**Storage Requirements:** Store at 15 to 30°C (59 to 86°F), protect from heat and light. After reconstitution store in refrigerator 2 to 8°C (36 to 46°F); solution retains potency for about 3 months.

---

□ **GRISEOFULVIN**                                    (gri-see-oh-ful'vin)
**MICROSIZE**

(Fulvicin-U/F, Grifulvin V, Grisactin, Grisovin-FP)

□ **GRISEOFULVIN**
**ULTRAMICROSIZE**

(Fulvicin P/G, Grisactin Ultra, Gris-PEG)

**Classification:** antifungal

**Available Preparations:**
- 125 mg/5 ml oral suspension (microsize)
- 250, 500-mg tablets (microsize)
- 125, 165, 250, 330-mg tablets (ultramicrosize)
- 125, 250-mg film-coated tablet (ultramicrosize)
- 125, 250-mg capsules (microsize)

**Action and Use:** Mechanism is unknown; believed to arrest cell division. Effective against infections caused by most species of *Trichophyton*, *Epidermophyton*, and *Microsporum*.

**Routes and Dosage:**
*PO:*
- over 2 years (ultramicrosize): 7.3 mg/kg/day given daily
- children (microsize): 10 to 11 mg/kg/day given daily or 300 mg/m²/day
- adults: 500 to 1000 mg/day given daily

**Absorption and Fate:** Principally adsorbed from duodenum; absorption of ultramicrosize is almost complete but absorption of microsize may range from 25 to 70%. Peak level: 4 to 8 hours. Concentrates in skin, hair, nails, liver, fat, and skeletal muscles. Half-life: 9 to 24 hours. Excreted in urine, feces, and perspiration. Therapeutic level: 0.15 to 0.5 μg/ml in vitro.

**Contraindications and Precautions:** Pregnancy category C. Safe use of ultramicrosize in those under 2 years not established. Contraindicated in hypersensitivity to drug, porphyria, hepatocellular failure. Use caution if penicillin sensitivity exists; drug is penicillin derivative, however patients with hypersensitivity have been treated with this drug without reactions.

## Side Effects:

*CNS:* headache early in therapy, fatigue, dizziness, insomnia; rarely transient decrease in hearing, paresthesia in hands and feet, mental confusion, impairment of routine activity performance, **psychotic symptoms**. *GI:* nausea, vomiting, epigastric distress, polydipsia, flatulence, diarrhea, oral thrush. *GU:* **protcinuria** (rare). *Skin:* photosensitivity, urticaria, rashes, angioedema, serumlike sickness. *Hemic:* leukopenia, **granulocytopenia** (rare). *Other:* estrogenlike effects, **lupus erythematosus** or **lupuslike syndromes**.

## Nursing Implications:

*Assess:* Confirm infection by laboratory identification. Before long-term therapy, obtain CBC, renal, and hepatic tests.

*Administer: PO:* Giving with food or meals may decrease GI distress. Shake suspension well. Tablets can be crushed and capsules taken apart, mixed with small amounts of food or fluids. Microsize preparation adsorption may be increased by giving with fatty meal; consult with physician.

*Monitor:* Headache common side effect that may disappear with continuation of drug therapy. Frequent hematological, renal, and liver function tests should be performed during long-term therapy. Observe for side effects and report to physician (if granulocytopenia occurs, discontinue drug). Treatment continues until negative cultures (2 to 3 consecutive weekly cultures) and time necessary for infected skin, hair, or nails to be replaced. For example: tinea corporis, 2 to 4 weeks; tinea pedis, 4 to 8 weeks; tinea capitis, 4 to 6 weeks; and infected fingernails, 3 to 6 months and toenails 6 months.

*Patient Teaching:* Therapy requires close monitoring by physician. Report any side effects immediately. Therapy may be 4 to 6 weeks, but it can take several months. Avoid exposure to sunlight or sunlamps due to potential photosensitivity.

**Drug Interactions:** Concurrent ingestion of alcohol and this drug causes flushing and tachycardia. Phenobarbital decreases drug concentrations. Patients stabilized on warfarin who then receive this drug may note a decrease in prothrombin time. With oral contraceptives, griseofulvin may cause breakthrough bleeding.

**Food Interactions:** Microsize griseofulvin is enhanced when given with high fat meal.

**Storage Requirements:** Store at 15 to 30°C (59 to 86°F) in tight containers.

---

## □ HAEMOPHILUS INFLUENZAE B VACCINE

(hah-moff'i-lus)

(Hib-Immune, b-CAPSA I, ProHIBiT)

**Classification:** immunization

## Available Preparations:
- single dose vials with diluent for parenteral use
- 10-dose vials with diluent for parenteral use
- 1, 5, 10-dose vials for parenteral use

There are two polysaccharide vaccines (Hib-Immune and b-CAPSA I) and one conjugate vaccine (ProHIBiT).

**Action and Use:** Stimulates body production of antibodies against *Haemophilus influenzae* type b, which can cause a variety of illnesses in children such as meningitis, epiglottis, sepsis, osteomyelitis, and pneumonia. Used for immunization of children from 18 months to 5 years.

## Routes and Dosages:
*IM, SC:* 0.5 ml one time dose (children immunized from 18 to 24 months with the polysaccharide vaccine need reimmunization after 24 months).

**Absorption and Fate:** One dose of polysaccharide vaccine given to children from 15 to 24 months produces immunity in less than 50% of recipients; conjugate vaccine produces 90% immunity in this age group. Response rate increases after 24 months of age. Immune levels are adequate 2 to 3 weeks after immunization. Eliminated at least partially in urine.

**Contraindications and Precautions:** Not recommended during pregnancy or lactation. Not generally given to persons older than 5 years. Not to be used for immunization before 18 months as the vaccine's effectiveness in the younger age group is not yet established. Studies are being conducted to learn if a 3-dose administration of conjugate will be effective in infants. Hypersensitivity to any vaccine component, including thimerosal (a mercury derivative used as preservative) or diphtheria toxoid (the latter found only in the conjugate vaccine) is contraindication for the vaccine. A febrile illness or acute infection is cause for delaying vaccination. The conjugate vaccine is **not** contraindicated, and is recommended, for HIV-infected children, whether symptomatic or asymptomatic.

## Side Effects:
*Skin:* erythema, tenderness, warmth, edema, induration at injection site.
*Other:* fever, anaphylaxis (extremely rate).

## Nursing Implications:
*Assess:* Gather history to find those children at high risk of *Haemophilus influenzae* b disease so they can be targeted for immunization. They include children who are Eskimos, American Indians, who have sickle cell disease, asplenia, antibody deficiency disease, or who attend day-care centers. History is taken to rule out contraindications.
*Administer:* Read package insert to verify route (IM or SC) for the specific

preparation. Reconstitute with diluent provided. Shake gently. Hib-Immune is stable for 8 hours if refrigerated after reconstitution; b-CAPSA I for 30 days if refrigerated. *Haempohlus influenzae* b conjugate (ProHIBiT) is recommended for use at 18 months as it appears to create an adequate immune response at that age. The other *Haemophilus* b vaccines (polysaccharide) should be repeated after age 24 months, if used in children 18 to 24 months of age. Studies are now being conducted to ascertain the lasting qualities of the vaccine. If the conjugate vaccine is used, all children are immunized at 18 months. If the polysaccharide vaccine is used, children in high-risk groups (those attending day-care centers or with chronic illness such as asplenia, sickle cell disease, malignancies associated with immunosuppression) should receive the vaccine at 18 months. Other children should be immunized one time at 24 months or up to 5 years of age. The conjugate vaccine is the preparation of choice as it has greatest efficacy in younger children. Although the conjugate vaccine contains diphtheria toxoid, it does not replace the need for immunization with DTP or other preparations of diphtheria.

Children who have a *Haemophilus influenzae* b disease before 24 months of age should receive the immunization after they are well and old enough for immunization as they do not have an adequate immune response when the disease is contracted in the first 2 years of life.

The vaccine may be given on the same visit with other immunizations, such as DTP, when given by separate syringes into different sites. It may be given on the same visit with oral polio vaccine or measles–mumps–rubella vaccine if the patient may not return for future immunization.

Because immune response is not immediate the vaccine should not be used as prophylaxis for children exposed to *Haemophilus* infection. Rifampin prophylaxis, in addition to the vaccine in children over 18 months, is needed in such cases. Children with malignancies or who are on immunosuppressive therapy may have a lessened immune response to the vaccine. Epinephrine 1:1000 and resuscitative equipment should be available in case of anaphylaxis.

*IM:* Give into lateral thigh or into deltoid of older children with sufficient deltoid muscle.

*Patient Teaching:* Inform of side effects and need for repeat immunization if child is under 24 months of age.

**Drug Interactions:** Immunosuppressive therapy may lessen immune response.

**Storage Requirements:** Store in refrigerator at 2 to 8°C (35 to 46°F). Reconstituted solutions must be refrigerated if not immediately used. Store in body of refrigerator rather than on door where temperature variations may be greater.

---

# □ HALOPERIDOL                                          (ha-loe-per'i-dole)

(Haldol)

**Classification:** antipsychotic

## Available Preparations:
- 0.5, 1, 2, 5, 10, 20-mg tablets
- 0.5, 1, 2, 5-mg film-coated tablets
- 2 mg/ml oral concentrate solution
- 50 mg/ml haloperidol decanoate vials for parenteral use
- 5 mg/ml haloperidol lactate vials for parenteral use

**Action and Use:** A butyrophenone derivative with effects like those of the phenothiazines. Depresses several areas in the CNS and interferences with use of neurotransmitters such as dopamine. Suppresses motor activity, acts as an antiemetic. Has weak anticholinergic effect and can cause extrapyramidal effects. Used in treatment of tics, Tourette's disorder, for children with severe disorders and hyperexcitable behavior, and for short-term treatment of attention-deficit disorder. Although not approved by the FDA for this purpose, it is used for control of nausea and vomiting in cancer chemotherapy patients.

**Routes and Dosages:** PO (haloperidol and haloperidol lactate); IM (haloperidol lactate and haloperidol decanoate)
*PO:*
- Psychosis: 3 to 12 years (15 to 40 kg): 0.5 mg/day in 2 to 3 doses initially; increased by 0.5 mg at 5 to 7-day intervals PRN: usual dose is 0.05 to 0.15 mg/kg/day
- Behavior Problems and Tourette's Disorder: 3 to 12 years: 0.05 to 0.15 mg/kg/day in 2 to 3 doses; not recommended to exceed 6 mg/day

*IM:* Use not approved for children

**Absorption and Fate:** Well absorbed from GI tract. About 90% bound to plasma proteins. Metabolized in the liver and excreted in urine and feces. Peak action: 2 to 6 hours after PO administration. Duration of action several days; half-life: 12 to 38 hours after PO. Therapeutic level: 3 to 10 mg/ml.

**Contraindications and Precautions:** Pregnancy category C. Safety of the drug in children under 3 years is not established; safety of haloperidol decanoate injection in children of any age is not established. Contraindicated during lactation, CNS depression, coma, hypersensitivity, and the 1, 5, and 10-mg tablets are contraindicated in those with tartrazine (yellow dye #5) hypersensitivity. Cautious use in seizure disorders, those on anticonvulsants, cardiovascular disorders, thyrotoxicosis, history of drug allergies, and glaucoma.

## Side Effects:
*CNS:* extrapyramidal reactions: drowsiness and lethargy, motor restlessness, dystonic reaction manifested by neck spasm, torticollis, opisthotonus, tongue spasm, difficult swallowing; symptoms generally improve with reduction in dosage or anticholinergics. Other CNS effects include tardive dyskinesia, neuropletic malignant syndrome, insomnia, headache, seizures, vertigo. *CV:*

hypotension, tachycardia, hypertension, EKG changes. *GI:* dry mouth, hyper-salivation, constipation, nausea, vomiting, diarrhea. *Respiratory:* laryngo-spasm, bronchospasm, pneumonia. *Hepatic:* jaundice, liver dysfunction. *GU:* urinary retention. *Skin:* rash, photosensitivity, urticaria, dermatitis, alopecia. *Hemic:* mild and temporary leukopenia and leukocytosis; anemia, decreased RBC. *Endocrine:* gynecomastia, lactation, hyperglycemia or hypoglycemia. *Sensory:* visual changes, cataracts, retinopathy. *Other:* hyperpyrexia, heat stroke.

## Nursing Implications:
*Assess:* Establish baseline vital signs. CBC and liver function tests are done before therapy.
*Administer: PO:* May give with food or fluid to decrease GI upset. Do not crush film-coated tablets. *IM:* IM form rarely used in children. Haloperidol decanoate injection incompatible with sterile water for injection or normal saline; it is recommended that haloperidol lactate injection not be mixed with other drugs.
*Monitor:* Vital sign checks, especially blood pressure and temperature. Peri-odic CBC and liver function tests. Monitor toxic effects of antineoplastic drugs if patient is on concurrent therapy with drugs whose toxicity is manifested by nausea and vomiting, as above effects may be masked by haloperidol.
*Patient Teaching:* Drug can alter mental alertness; therefore, avoid driving and adjust activities accordingly. Take drug as directed. Avoid OTC drugs or alcohol. Return for scheduled health-care visits. Encourage good oral hygiene, adequate fluids, and nutritious food.

**Drug Interactions:** Additive or potentiating effects of other CNS depres-sants. Acute encephalopathy infrequently occurs with patient also on lithium.

**Laboratory Test Interferences:** hyponatremia, increased serum prolac-tin

**Storage Requirements:** Store tightly covered in light-resistant containers at 15 to 30°C (50 to 86°F).

---

## □ HEPARIN                                        (hep′a-rin)

(Calciparine, Hepulean, Hep-Lock of IV flush, Lipo-Hepin, Liquaemin Sodium, Panheprin)

**Combination Product:** Embolex

**Classification:** anticoagulant

## Available Preparations:
- 1000, 2500, 5000, 7500, 10,000, 15,000, 20,000, 40,000 U/ml heparin sodium vials for parenteral use

- 25,000 U/ml heparin calcium vials for parenteral use
- 40, 50, 100 U/ml in 5% dextrose
- 2, 50, 100 U/ml in saline
- 10, 100 U/ml heparin flush solution
- 5000 U/0.7 ml with dihydroergotamine 0.5 mg/0.7 ml

**Action and Use:** A substance originated from cow or pig protein that binds with antithrombin III, a plasma protein, thereby inhibiting thrombin formation from prothrombin and fibrin formation from fibrinogen. Blocks activity of clotting factors VII, IX, X, XI, and XII. It increases whole blood clotting time, thrombin time, partial thromboplastin time, and prothrombin time; bleeding time is usually unaffected. Both calcium and sodium heparin solutions are available. Used to prevent additional fibrin deposition or established thrombi (it will not dissolve clots that are present); used to treat deep vein thrombosis and pulmonary emboli.

**Routes and Dosages:**
*IV:*

- Continuous Infusion: 50 U/kg initially, then 100 U/kg over every 4 hours or 50 U/kg initially, then 20,000 U/m²/24 hours
- Intermittent Infusion: 100 U/kg initially, then 50 to 100 U/kg q4h
- DIC: 25 to 50 U/kg q4h by continuous or intermittent infusion
- Heart and Blood Vessel Surgery: 150 U/kg or up to 300 U/kg for lengthy procedures; dose regulated with results of coagulation studies

*SC:* Dosage not provided by manufacturers for pediatrics.
Dosage decreased in liver or renal dysfunction.

**Absorption and Fate:** Highly protein bound. Metabolized by liver and eliminated in metabolized and unchanged forms in urine. Peak level immediate after IV with duration of action 2 to 6 hours. Peak level under 1 hour for SC, with duration of 8 to 12 hours. Half-life is 52 to 80 minutes in patients with pulmonary emboli; 93 to 106 minutes in patients with thrombophlebitis; half-life increases with additional doses and renal or hepatic dysfunction and obesity. Therapeutic level: 0.25 to 0.5 U/ml; rarely used to monitor clinical response; therapeutic goal is to prolong PTT to 1½ to 2½ times control.

**Contraindications and Precautions:** Pregnancy category C. Does not cross placenta. Not excreted in breast milk, but if given during lactation, can lead to severe osteoporosis and vertebral collapse. Contraindicated with hypersensitivity to the drug, in patients who are bleeding or have tendency to bleed (e.g., hemophiliacs), recent surgery, other open wounds, in abortions, CVA, aneurysm, hemorrhage, severe hypertension, active tuberculosis. Use with caution in patients with allergy history, during menstruation, in blood dyscrasia, and when procedures with potential for bleeding are performed. Cautious use in kidney and hepatic dysfunction. Use heparin preparation preserved with benzyl alcohol with caution in neonates and monitor for signs of toxicity. Use with caution to maintain patency or umbilical artery catheter in low birthweight neonates.

## Side Effects:

*CNS:* neuropathy, chills, fever. *CV:* **bleeding**, thrombocytopenia, chest pain; blue and painful legs and arms. *Respiratory:* dyspnea, rhinitis. *Skin:* pain, itching, ecchymosis at injection site, rash, hives. *Other:* hypersensitivity and **anaphylaxis** (rare).

## Nursing Implications:

*Assess:* Baseline blood coagulation studies and hematocrit are needed.

*Administer:* Dose should be checked by another nurse. Potential for error is great due to variable concentrations available and calculation required. Heparin is designed in U for international units of activity rather than in mg. *SC:* This route is used for low-dose prophylaxis. Do not aspirate before injecting. Do not massage site before or after injection. Apply gently pressure after injection. Inject into abdomen or above iliac crest. Change needle after drawing up and before injecting heparin. Do not pinch tissue but bunch up a roll of tissue and inject at 90-degree angle with a 25- or 26-gauge ½ or ⅝-inch needle. Withdraw needle rapidly while simultaneously releasing tissue roll. Apply gentle pressure for 5 to 10 seconds. *IM:* Avoid this route because of risk of hematoma formation. *IV:* Invert container at least six times to ensure adequate mixing when added to IV solution. Avoid mixing in same IV solution with other drugs. A monitoring device must be used to prevent inadvertent rapid infusion. Have protamine sulfate available as an antidote for heparin. Give within 30 minutes after excess heparin dose. See protamine for dosage and other information. Heparin flush is used to maintain open line when a lock is used. Precede infusion with 1 to 2 ml of normal saline to check patency of line and prevent incompatibility of drugs; administer ordered IV infusion; flush with 1 to 2 ml normal saline; administer heparin lock solution slowly. The flush solution should be used only for IV flushing.

*Monitor:* Continuous blood studies are needed. Activated PTT between 1½ and 2½ times control and activated coagulation time (ACT) 2 to 3 times control are the therapeutic levels desired. Blood for tests is drawn 30 minutes before scheduled doses or every 4 hours for patients on continual infusion. Monitor patient for bleeding: injection sites, urine, stools, oral mucosa, vomitus, ecchymosis, petechiae, pain, headache, dizziness. Discontinue drug immediately if hemorrhage occurs and notify physician. Platelet counts, hematocrit, and stool blood tests should be done regularly during therapy. Monitor I & O and vital signs. When therapy is discontinued, heparin dose is generally tapered over 3 to 5 days while oral anticoagulant therapy begins. When changing to PO dose, wait 4 to 6 hours after last IV dose or 12 to 24 hours after last SC dose to draw blood for PTT.

*Patient Teaching:* Inform all care providers about heparin intake. Report any signs of bleeding such as dark urine, red vomitus, dark stools, bleeding mouth, chest pain, dizziness, or other unusual symptoms. Avoid OTC drugs unless instructed by physician.

**Drug Interactions:** Other drugs that affect coagulation, such as aspirin and indomethacin, should be avoided as the risk of hemorrhage increases. Drugs that cause GI ulceration may lead to GI bleeding. Other anticoagulants, such as coumarin, increase potential for bleeding. Antihistamines, digitalis, tetracyclines decrease effect of heparin. Drugs that inhibit platelet formation, such as carbencillin, valproic acid, increase bleeding tendency. Drugs, such as cefamandole, which lead to hypoprothrombinemia can increase bleeding tendency. Probenicid increases effects of heparin.

**Laboratory Test Interferences:** False-negative I-fibrinogen uptake test; false-positive BSP. Increased one stage prothrombin time test, SGOT, SGPT, thyroxine, free fatty acid. Decreased triglyceride, cholesterol.

**Storage Requirements:** Store at room temperature of 15 to 30°C (59 to 86°F). Do not freeze.

---

## □ HEPATITIS B VACCINE

(hep-a'tah-vax)

(Hepatavax, Heptavax B, Hevac B, Recombivax HB)

**Classification:** immunization

**Available Preparations:** 0.5-ml single dose (pediatric) and 3-ml multiple dose vials for parenteral use
A plasma-derived vaccine and recombinant vaccine (produced from yeast using recombinant DNA technology) are available.

**Action and Use:** Contains hepatitis B surface antigen and induces antibody formation against hepatitis B virus. Used to immunize susceptible individuals.

**Routes and Dosages:** IM, SC (in those with hemophilia or other bleeding disorders)
*IM:*
Plasma Derived:
- neonates to 10 years: 10 μg/dose (0.5 ml)
- over 10 years: 20 μg/dose (1.0 ml)
Recombinant:
- neonates to 10 years: 5 μg/dose (0.5 ml)
- over 10 years: 10 μg/dose (1.0 ml)
Three doses are given with the second 1 month after the first and the third dose 6 months later. Larger doses (2.0 ml) may be given to those who are immunosuppressed or on hemodialysis.

**Absorption and Fate:** 77% of recipients are immune after two injections; approximately 90% are immune after three injections. Nearly all young children appear to become immune with response rate decreasing with increasing age. Antibodies appear 2 weeks after injection. Peak level occurs in 6 months. Therapeutic level is a serum titer of 10 mIU/ml or above. Levels may decrease within 5 years of the last dose. Titer may be tested at that time and a booster dose given if under 10 mIU/ml.

## Contraindications and Precautions:
Use in pregnancy only if clearly needed. Avoid use in lactation. Contraindicated if prior hypersensitivity to the vaccine occurred. Recombinant preparation not used in those hypersensitive to yeast or in the immunosuppressed. Both vaccines use thimerosal, a mercury derivative, as a preservative and are contraindicated in those allergic to this substance. Delay administration in those with active infection. Cautious use in those with cardiopulmonary disease and bleeding disorder.

## Side Effects:
*CNS:* headache. *GI:* nausea. *Skin:* pain, erythema at injection site. *Sensory:* uveitis, blurred vision, photophobia (may require stopping course of vaccine). *Other:* fever, fatigue, hypersensitivity.

## Nursing Implications:
*Assess:* The vaccine is recommended for those at high and moderate risk for hepatitis B disease. The children in these groups include immigrants from areas where hepatitis B is endemic (eastern Asia and sub-Saharan Africa), those in institutions for the mentally retarded, hemodialysis patients, and recipients of certain blood products. Hemodialysis patients and other immunosuppressed persons should receive the plasma-derived vaccine (Hepatavax) rather than the recombinant vaccine (Recombivax HB). Take a careful history to rule out hypersensitive individuals.

It is now recommended that all pregnant women be tested for hepatitis B during pregnancy. The infants of mothers who are hepatitis B carriers should get a first dose of vaccine within 12 hours of birth with concomitant administration of hepatitis B immune globulin (0.5 ml) IM given at a second site at the same time. The second and third doses of vaccine are given at the usual times and the infant is tested for the disease at 12 to 15 months.

*Administer:* As with all vaccines, epinephrine 1:1000 and resuscitative equipment should be readily available in case of anaphylaxis. The schedule for booster doses has not yet been established; however, hemodialysis patients should have antibody testing twice yearly and receive a booster dose when antibody levels fall below 10 mIU/ml. Likewise others should be tested after 5 years and receive a booster dose if levels indicate low immunity. *IM:* Shake vial well before withdrawal. Administer to infants in anterolateral thigh; to older children in the deltoid. Other sites lead to a lower response rate. Avoid intravenous administration. *SC:* Administration may be used in those with bleeding disorders to decrease risk of bleeding.

*Monitor:* Observe child for 20 minutes after injection for unfavorable reactions.

*Patient Teaching:* Teach patient when to return for next dose.

## Storage Requirements:
Refrigerate at 2 to 8°C (35 to 46°F) in body of refrigerator rather than on the door where temperature variations may be greater. Avoid freezing. Shake well; vaccine will appear cloudy white.

# □ HOMATROPINE HYDROBROMIDE

(hoe-ma'troe-peen)

(Ak Homatropine, I-Homatrine, Isopto Homatropine, Minims, Homatropine)

**Classification:** cycloplegic, mydriatics

## Available Preparations:
- 2%, 5% drops for ophthalmic administration

**Action and Use:** Anticholinergic that blocks the response caused by acetylcholine. This causes sphincter muscle of the iris to dilate (mydriasis) and paralysis of accommodation of the ciliary body (cycloplegia). Used in refraction, diagnostic ophthalmic procedures, and treatment of uveitis.

## Routes and Dosage:
*Ophthalmic:*
- Cycloplegic Refraction: instill 1 drop of 2% solution every 10 minutes for 3 to 5 doses just before procedure
- Uveitis: instill 1 drop of a 2% solution 2 to 3 times a day

**Absorption and Fate:** Shorter acting than atropine. Peak action: mydriatic effect in 10 to 30 minutes and maximum cycloplegic effect is 30 to 90 minutes. Residual effects may persist for 24 to 72 hours after instillation.

**Contraindications and Precautions:** Pregnancy category C. Use with caution in infants and younger children because of increased susceptibility to drug's systemic effects. Contraindicated if hypersensitivity to this drug or to atropine and in narrow-angle glaucoma. Use caution in infants and young children with spastic paralysis or brain damage, Down's syndrome, or blond, blue eyed children, hypertension, diabetes, or cardiac disease.

## Side Effects:
*Skin:* contact dermatitis. *Sensory:* burning upon instillation, blurred vision, photophobia, conjunctivitis, ocular congestion, increased intraocular pressure. *Other:* Systemic Effects: clumsiness or unsteadiness, confusion, disorientation and unusual behavior, failure to recognize people, drowsiness, weakness, tachycardia, fever, urinary retention, flushing of face, dry mouth, slurred speech, distended abdomen in infants, hallucinations, seizures.

## Nursing Implications:
*Assess:* Tonometric examinations are recommended before drug usage.
*Administer: Ophthalmic:* Remove contact lenses before drug instillation. Wash hands before and after administration, drug may cause contact dermatitis.
*Drops:* Warn child that the drug causes burning just before giving. Do not place drop on colored portion of the eye because it causes discomfort, stimulat-

ing tearing or blinking. Apply pressure to lacrimal sac for 1 to 2 minutes to reduce systemic absorption. Brown or hazel eyes may require more medication because dark eyes seem to be less responsive to this drug.

*Monitor:* Observe for symptoms of systemic effects; these occur more frequently in children on long-term therapy. If blurring of vision or photosensitivity lasts longer than 72 hours, contact physician.

*Patient Teaching:* Instruct child not to rub eyes. Wear sunglasses to decrease photophobic discomfort. Do not perform hazardous tasks until drug has worn off.

**Drug Interactions:** Ophthalmic preparations of carbachol, pilocarpine, and cholinesterase inhibitors interfere with this drug's action.

**Storage Requirement:** Store at 15 to 30°C (59 to 86°F) in tightly closed container. Prevent freezing.

---

## □ HYDRALAZINE                              (hye-dral'a-zeen)

(Apresoline, Dralzine)

**Combination Products:** Apresazide, Apresodex, Apresoline-Esidrex, Cherapas, Hydral, Hydralazine-Thiazide, Hydrazide, Ser-A-Gen, Serpasil-Apresoline, Ser-Ap-Es, Serathide, Tri-Hydroserpine, Unipres

**Classification:** antihypertensive

## Available Preparations:
- 10, 25, 50, 100-mg tablets
- 25, 50, 100-mg capsules with hydrochlorothiazide
- 25, 50-mg tablets with hydrochlorothiazide
- 25-mg tablets with reserpine and hydrochlorothiazide
- 20 mg/ml ampule for parenteral use

**Action and Use:** Acts on vascular smooth muscle to reduce vascular wall tension and create vasodilation. Peripheral resistance and increased cerebral blood flow result, leading to increased stroke volume and cardiac output. Used for hypertensive crisis and moderate to servere chronic hypertension, and sometimes in congestive heart failure, although the latter use is not approved by the FDA.

## Routes and Dosages:
*PO:* 0.75 to 1 mg/kg/day or 25 mg/m²/day in 2 to 4 doses. Initial dose not to

exceed 25 mg. Adjust upward for clinical response up to 7.5 mg/kg/day or 300 mg/day.

**IM, IV:** 1.7 to 3.5 mg/kg/day or 50 to 100 mg/m²/day in 4 to 6 doses. Initial dose not to exceed 20 mg.

Doses established by clinicians rather than manufacturer.

**Absorption and Fate:** Rapidly and well absorbed from GI tract. 85% protein bound. Metabolized by GI mucosa and liver. Some people slowly metabolize the drug and may develop hydralazine-induced systemic lupus erythematosus.Metabolites eliminated mainly in urine. Onset of action after IV 5 to 20 minutes with peak action at 10 to 80 minutes and duration 3 to 8 hours. Onset of action after IM 10 to 60 minutes with peak action in 1 hour and duration 2 to 6 hours. Onset of action after PO 20 to 30 minutes but 3 to 4 days of therapy may be needed to reach maximal therapeutic response. Half-life is 2 to 4 hours; longer in renal failure.

**Contraindications and Precautions:** Pregnancy category C. Is teratogenic in some laboratory animals. Contraindicated in mitral valve, rheumatic heart disease, tachycardia, lupus erythematosus. Some preparations contain tartrazine (yellow dye #5) and others contain sulfite; such preparations should not be given to patients with those allergies. Use with caution in renal disease, CVA, aortic aneurysm, CHF, coronary artery disease, rheumatic heart disease. Generally not given to those who develop hydralazine-induced systemic lupus erythematosus.

**Side Effects:**

**CNS:** headache, dizziness, paresthesia. **CV:** flushing, tachycardia, increased cardiac output, palpitation, orthostatic hypotension, arrhythmia, chest pain. **GI:** anorexia, nausea, vomiting, diarrhea, constipation. **Other:** sodium and water retention without concomitant diuretic use, edema, weight gain; hydralazine-induced systemic lupus erythematosus manifested by arthralgia, fever, rash, chest pain.

**Nursing Implications:**

**Assess:** Collect baseline data of CBC, LE cell preparation, antinuclear antibody titer determination, vital signs, especially BP. Check on allergy to yellow dye #5, ASA, bronchial asthma, or sulfite allergy if preparations are used with the dye or sulfite.

**Administer: PO:** Food enhances absorption, therefore, medication should be taken at the same time each day with or without food. Withdraw slowly when discontinued. **IV:** The solution is stable for 8 to 12 hours in IV solutions if kept at 30°C (86°F) or lower, even if color change has occurred. Give slowly and monitor BP every 5 minutes until stable, then every 15 minutes. Usually transferred to PO form in 24 to 48 hours.

**Monitor:** Monitor I & O, blood pressure, weight, edema, CBC, electrolyte status. Repeat LE cell preparation test and antinuclear antibody titer if arthralgia, fever, malaise, or rash occur.

*Patient Teaching:* Take at same times each day. Diet teaching with sodium restriction may be appropriate. Avoid quick position change. Avoid OTC drugs, such as cold and allergy medicines, unless prescribed by physician. Drug can alter mental alertness; therefore, avoid driving and adjust activities accordingly.

**Drug Interactions:** When given with other antihypertensives or diuretics additive or potentiation of antihypertensive effects can be observed. Decreased antihypertensive effect with nonsteroidal antiinflammatories, estrogen, sympathomimetics. Use MAO inhibitors cautiously, as there may be a synergistic effect of lowering blood pressure.

**Laboratory Test Interferences:** Positive direct Coombs' test.

**Storage Requirements:** Store at 15 to 30°C (59 to 86°F) in light-resistant containers. Avoid freezing. Injection for parenteral use may change color in IV solutions.

---

## □ HYDROCHLOROTHIAZIDE    (hye-droe-klor-oh-thye'a-zide)

(Aquazide-H, Diaqua, Esidrex, Hydro-Chlor, Hydro-Z-50, HydroDIURIL, Hydromal, Oretic)

**Combination Products:** Aldoril, Aldactazide, Apresazide, Apresodex, Capozide, Cherapas, Diazide, Esimil, Hydralazine Plus, Hydralazine-Thiazide, Hydrazide, Hydropres, Hydro-Reserpine, Hydroserp, Hydroserpine, Hydrotensin, Interide, Lopressor HCT, Mallopres, Maxzide, Moduretic, Normozide, Oreticyl, Ser-A-Gen, Ser-Ap-Es, Serathide, Serpasil-Esidrex, Spironazide, Timolide, Triamterene and Hydrochlorothiazide, Tri-Hydroserpine, Unipres, Vaseretic

**Classification:** thiazide diuretic, antihypertensive

**Available Preparations:**
- 25, 50, 100-mg tablets
- 50 mg/5 ml oral solution

Also available in tablets and capsules in combination with amiloride, propranolol, hydralazine, triamterene, captopril, deserpidine, enalapril, guanethidine, metoprolol, reserpine, spironolactone, timolol, mythyldopa, and labetalol

**Action and Use:** this short-acting thiazide diuretic interferes with sodium reabsorption and promotes potassium secretion in the distal convoluted tubules, thus reducing plasma and extracellular fluid volume. Also decreases excretion of calcium. Used to treat hypertension and in conjunction with digitalis, to treat congestive heart failure. Use not approved by the FDA: prevention of calcium renal stones.

## Routes and Dosages:
*PO:*

- under 6 months: 1 to 3.3 mg/kg/day in 2 divided doses.
- over 6 months: 1 to 2.2 mg/kg/day or 30 to 60 mg/m$^2$/day given in 1 to 2 daily doses

Daily dose range for children under 2 years is 12.5 to 37.5 mg/day and for children 2 to 12 years is 37.5 to 100 mg/day.

## Absorption and Fate: Rapidly absorbed from PO route. Crosses the placenta and present in breast milk. Excreted primarily in urine in unchanged form. Onset of action is within 2 hours; peak effect in 6 hours; and duration of action is up to 24 hours, more commonly 6 to 12 hours. Therapeutic effect: best after 3 to 4 days of therapy. Half-life is 15 hours.

## Contraindications and Precautions: Pregnancy category B. No known teratogenesis in animals. Present in breast milk so not advised during lactation. Contraindicated in those with allergy to thiazides or sulfonamide derivatives, in anuric patients. Cautious use in infants with jaundice, electrolyte imbalance, renal dysfunction, hepatic dysfunction, diabetes, hyperuricemia, hypercalcemia, lupus, pancreatitis.

## Side Effects:
*CNS:* fatigue, headache, weakness, mood change. *CV:* orthostatic hypotension, irregular pulse. *GI:* nausea, vomiting, anorexia, abdominal cramping, dry mouth, thirst. *Hepatic:* dysfunction, yellowish eye sclera and skin. *Metabolic:* **hypokalemia** and **hyponatremia** manifested by fatigue, lethargy, muscle weakness, anorexia, constipation; hypochloremic alkalosis, hyperuricemia, hypercalcemia, hypophosphatemia, hyperglycemia, glycosuria in diabetics. *Hemic:* thrombocytopenia leading to bruising, eosinophilia leading to fever and sore throat. *Other:* hypersensitivity manifested by urticaria, purpura, photosensitivity, rash, fever, anaphylaxis.

## Nursing Implications:
*Assess:* Establish baseline CBC, serum electrolytes, blood glucose, uric acid, weight, and vital signs, particularly blood pressure.
*Administer: PO:* Schedule early in day (before 3 PM) and after eating to avoid nocturia and stomach upset.
*Monitor:* Monitor CBC, serum potassium and sodium, other serum electrolytes, daily weight, vital signs, I & O, and check hydration status. Evaluate BUN and uric acid periodically. Monitor blood glucose and status of the diabetic patient carefully as hyperglycemia may occur and necessitate insulin adjustment. Watch for signs of hypokalemia such as confusion, weakness, muscle cramps, dry mouth, and anorexia.

## Patient Teaching: Take at same time each day; early in day to avoid nocturia; may take with food. Eat potassium-rich foods such as orange juice, tomatoes, apricots, figs, prunes, avocados, raisins, bananas, meat, potatoes.

Diet with sodium restriction may be ordered. Teach to get up slowly to avoid orthostatic hypotension. Avoid OTC medications unless recommended by physician; many contain sodium. Weigh and report changes to physician. Continue to take as directed; do not discontinue unless instructed. Avoid exposure to sun. Watch for and report nausea, vomiting, diarrhea. Careful blood glucose monitoring for diabetic patients.

**Drug Interactions:** Hypokalemia such as that resulting from this drug increases susceptibility to digitalis toxicity and increases blocking effect of neuromuscular blocking agents. Additive effect of hypokalemia with other drugs that lower potassium such as corticosteroids, amphotericin B. Reduced lithium clearance. Caution when given to patient on insulin due to hyperglycemia. Increased antihypertensive effect with other antihypertensives. Probenecid decreases uric acid retention. Alkalinization of urine caused by the drug may lead to decreased excretion of some amine drugs such as quindine and amphetamine. Other drugs that cause orthostatic hypotension, such as alcohol and barbiturates, may lead to additive effect. Cholestyramine and colestipol may bind thiazides and decrease their absorption, therefore, should be given at least 1 hour later. Increased diuresis with other diuretics. Hypercalcemia when given with calcium-containing medications. Increased potential for renal dysfunction if given with nonsteroidal antiinflammatories.

**Laboratory Test Interferences:** Increased serum amylase. False decreased urinary estrogen. False-negative tyramine and phentolamine tests and histamine test for pheochromocytoma. Decreased urinary corticosteriod. Invalidates bentiromide test. Increases serum and urine glucose in diabetics. Increased serum cholesterol, triglyceride, low-density lipoprotein, bilirubin, uric acid, magnesium, and potassium. May decrease serum PBI, sodium. Decreases urinary calcium.

**Storage Requirements:** Store tightly closed at 15 to 30°C (59 to 86°F). Do not freeze oral solution.

---

☐ **HYDROCODONE BITARTRATE**                                    (hye-droe-koe′done)

**Combination Products:** Hydrocodone bitartrate used in combination with other drugs such as: acetaminophen, aspirin, phenylpropanolamine HCl, guaifenesin, pseudoephedrine HCl; potassium guaiacolsulfonate, homatropine methylbromide, phenindamine tartrate, pheniramine maleate, pyrilamine maleate, chlorpheniramine maleate, and caffeine.

**Classification:** opiate agonist, antitussive; narcotic agonist, analgesic; CIII

## Available Preparations:
- 5 mg/5ml oral syrup (only available in Canada)
- 5 mg tablet (only available in Canada)
- oral solutions, tablets, and capsules available in U.S. as combination products

**Action and Use:** Hydrogenated ketone, codeine derivative, cough suppressant that acts through direct suppression of cough reflex center in medulla. Has a drying effect that increases viscosity of mucous secretions. This narcotic drug is used to treat nonproductive cough and as an analgesic. More sedating than codeine and should not be used indiscriminately.

## Routes and Dosage:
*PO:* 0.6 mg/kg/day or 20 mg/m²/day given in 3 to 4 equally divided doses PRN in intervals not less than every 4 hours apart. Maximum dosage: under 2 years: 1.25 mg/day; 2 to 12 years: 5mg/day; over 12 years: 10 mg/day

**Absorption and Fate:** Onset of action: 10 to 30 minutes; duration: 4 to 6 hours. Peak level: 1.3 hours; half-life: 3.8 hours. Metabolized in liver; excreted in urine.

**Contraindications and Precautions:** Pregnancy category C. Use caution during lactation and in those under 1 year. Contraindicated in hypersensitivity to drug or sulfites, debilitated patients, head injuries, intracranial lesions, increased intracranial pressure, patients who have undergone thoracotomies or laparotomies.

## Side Effects:
*CNS:* light-headedness dizziness, sedation, euphoria, dysphoria. *GI:* nausea, vomiting, constipation. *Skin:* rash, pruritus.

## Nursing Implications:
*Assess:* Cough: type, characteristics, and frequency.
*Administer: PO:* Can be given with food to prevent GI distress. Schedule III drug.
*Monitor:* This drug should not be used when coughing is necessary to remove sputum from lungs as immediately postoperatively or for infrequent coughs. Monitor response to medication and assess respiratory status. Maintain hydration for age group.
*Patient Teaching:* Take drug only as prescribed; this is a narcotic and can cause physical dependence. CNS symptoms may alter child's ability to ride bike, skate board, or do other hazardous activities. Do not consume alcohol while on this drug.

**Drug Interactions:** May enhance CNS effects of other opiates, anesthetics, tranquilizers, sedatives, alcohol, MAO inhibitors.

**Storage Requirements:** Store at 15 to 30°C (59 to 86°F), in light-resistant containers.

# ☐ HYDROCORTISONE
(hye-droe-kor′ti-sone)

(Aeroseb-HC, Cetacort, CaldeCORT, Cort-Dome, Cortef, Cortenema, Cortizone, DermiCort, Dermolate, Ecosone, Hydro-tex, Hydrocortone, Hytone, Proctocort, Synacort, Unicort and others)

# ☐ HYDROCORTISONE ACETATE

(Biosone, CaldeCort, Carmol-HC, Cortef Acetate, Cortaid, Cortifoam, Cremesone, Epifoam, Hydrocortone Acetate, and others)

# ☐ HYDROCORTISONE CYPIONATE

(Cortef Fluid)

# ☐ HYDROCORTISONE SODIUM PHOSPHATE

(Efcortesol, Hydrocortone Phosphate)

# ☐ HYDROCORTISONE SODIUM SUCCINATE

(A-hydroCort, Soluble, S-Cortilean, Solu-Cortef)

# ☐ HYDROCORTISONE VALERATE

(Westcort)

**Combination Products:** Hydrocortisone with neomycin sulfate (Neo-Cort-Dome); hydrocortisone with bacitracin zinc, neomycin sulfate, polymyxin B sulfate (Cortisporin); hydrocortisone acetate with pramoxine HCl (Proctofoam-HC, Parmosone); Available in topical combinations with antihistamines, astringents, local anesthetics and others.

**Classification:** corticosteroid, glucocorticoid, mineralocorticoid

## Available Preparations:
- 10 mg/5 ml oral suspension
- 5, 10, 20 mg tablets
- 25 mg/ml, 50 mg/ml for parenteral administration

- 50 mg/ml for parenteral administration (sodium phosphate)
- 100, 250, 500 mg, 1 g parenteral administration (sodium succinate)
- suspensions, creams, ointments, aerosols for rectal administration
- 0.25%, 0.5%, 1.0%, 2.5% topical lotions
- 0.1% 0.2%, 0.25%, 0.5%, 1.0%, 2.5% topical creams
- 0.1%, 0.2%, 0.5%, 1%, 2.5% topical ointment
- 1% topical gel and 0.5%, 1% topical aerosol

**Action and Use:** Natural or synthetic, short-acting glucocorticoid that has strong antiinflammatory, immunosuppressant, and metabolic actions. Used to treat several diseases such as collagen, dermatologic, allergy, acute leukemia, fetal respiratory distress syndrome, and others. Its salt-retaining properties are used as replacement therapy in adrenocortical deficiencies.

## Routes and Dosage:
*PO:*

- Cypionate: 0.56 to 8 mg/kg/day or 16 to 240 mg/m²/day in 3 to 4 divided doses

*IM:*

- Sodium Phosphate: 0.16 to 1 mg/kg/day or 6 to 30 mg/m²/day in 1 to 2 equally divided doses

*IM, IV:*

- Sodium Succinate: 0.16 to 1 mg/kg/day or 6 to 30 mg/m²/day in 1 to 2 equally divided doses
- Acute Adrenal Insufficiency: 1 to 2 mg/kg per IV dosage times 1 dose then; infants: 25 to 150 mg/day or children: 150 to 250 mg/day given in divided doses. (Cortisone acetate is also usually started at this time to allow for gradual tapering of IV hydrocortisone doses)
- Status Asthmaticus: Loading: 4 to 8 mg/kg, then 8 mg/kg/day in equally divided dose every 6 hours

Note: Dosage determined by severity of condition and child's response. Long-term therapy for chronic adrenocortical insufficiency, it is recommended that the drug be timed to stimulate the endogenous corticosteroid secretion by giving 2/3 daily dose in AM and 1/3 dose in PM. For adrenogenital syndrome suppression of corticotropin to decrease hypersecretion of adrenal androgens; give as above, or 1/3 daily dose 3 times a day in evenly spaced intervals.

*Topical:*

- Lotions: apply 0.25%, 0.5%, 1% sparingly to affected area 1 to 2 times a day; 2.5% once a day
- Cream: apply 0.1%, 0.25%, 0.5%, 1% as thin film 1 to 2 times a day; 0.2% daily (valerate)
- Ointment: apply 0.1%, 0.5%, 1% as thin film 1 to 2 times a day; 0.2%, 2.5% daily.

**Absorption and Fate:** Absorption: PO, rapid, complete; IM sodium phosphate or succinate, rapid; IM acetate, slow but complete; topical, increased in inflamed or diseased skin or use of occlusive dressings. Peak level: PO, 1 hour; IM sodium phosphate or succinate, 1 hour. Half-life: 0.5 hour. Duration: PO, 1.25 to 1.5 days; IM, variable. Metabolized by liver; excreted in urine.

**Contraindications and Precautions:** Pregnancy category C and drug is not recommended during lactation. Intraarticular, intrabursal, tendon-sheath, intralesional, or rectal forms dosages not established in children. Use caution in children; possible growth suppression. Contraindicated in hypersensitivity to drug or its components (sulfites), sensitivity to corticosteroids, varicella, systemic fungal infections, latent amebiasis, acquired immune deficiency syndrome (AIDS), fetal respiratory distress syndrome; do not use if delivery is imminent, immunizations with live virus vaccines and oral polio virus vaccine or contact with those who have had the vaccine. Use with caution in renal disease, hypertension, congestive heart failure, diabetes, ulcerative colitis, gastrointestinal ulceration, hyperthyroidism, impaired hepatic function, osteoporosis, vaccinia, exanthema, Cushing's syndrome, seizures, myasthenia gravis, tuberculosis, ocular herpes simplex, hypoalbuminemia, emotional or psychotic tendencies.

**Side Effects:** Usually dependent on dosage and duration of treatment.
*CNS:* headache, vertigo, euphoria, insomnia, **increased intracranial pressure** (papilledema), **psychotic behavior, seizures.** *CV:* edema, **hypertension, congestive heart failure.** *GI:* nausea, vomiting, change in appetite, GI irritation, abdominal distention, pancreatitis, ulcerative esophagitis, peptic ulcer. *Skin:* impaired wound healing, thin fragile skin, petechia, ecchymosis, acne, facial erythema, increased sweating, may mask infections; Topical: burning, itching, irritation, dryness, folliculitis, hypertrichosis, hypopigmentation, allergic contact dermatitis, maceration of the skin, secondary infection, **skin atrophy, striae, miliaria.** *Hemic:* **thrombocytopenia.** *Endocrine:* **HPA-axis suppression,** menstrual irregularities, Cushing's states, **secondary adrenocortical, pituitary unresponsiveness.** *Musculoskeletal:* **suppression of bone growth, osteoporosis,** muscle weakness, **aseptic necrosis of femoral and humeral heads.** *Sensory:* Ophthalmic: **posterior subcapsular cataracts, increased intraocular pressure.** *Other:* sodium retention, potassium loss, **negative nitrogen balance, hypokalemia, hyperglycemia,** susceptibility to infections; Withdrawal Symptoms: rebound inflammation, fatigue, weakness, fever, arthralgia, dizziness, lethargy, depression, fainting, orthostatic hypotension, dyspnea, anorexia, hypoglycemia, nausea and vomiting, shortness of breath, unusual weight loss.

**Nursing Implications:**
*Assess:* Obtain baseline weight, height; before-long term therapy: ECG, chest and spinal x-rays, glucose tolerance test, evaluation of HPA-axis function, and BP before therapy. Topical: observe, record appearance of involved area for baseline information.
*Administer:* Best to calculate drug dosage on $mg/m^2$; reduces overdosage possibilities in very short or heavy children. *PO:* Take with food or milk to reduce GI irritation. Best to give daily dosage prior to 9 AM. It suppresses adrenal cortex activity less, this may reduce risk of HPA axis suppression.

Alternate-day therapy recommended to reduce growth retarding effects. Tablet can be crushed, mixed with small amount of food or fluid. *IM:* Shake well (hydrocortisone, acetate) before withdrawal. Do not use deltoid muscle; drug may produce subcutaneous abscesses. *IV:* Hydrocortisone sodium phosphate or succinate are the forms of drug used IV. Sodium phosphate is commercially diluted but can be further diluted with sodium chloride and 5% dextrose. Sodium succinate can be diluted with bacteriostatic water, but not the Mix-0-Vial formulation; sodium succinate contains benzyl alcohol as a preservative. Use with caution in neonates. Do not mix with other drugs in same syringe as hydrocortisone. Can give IV push slowly, 30 seconds to several minutes. Intermittent infusion rate 1 mg/ml over at least 30 minutes. Preferred compatible solutions $D_5W$, $D_5W/NS$, NS; consult pharmacist for others. Sodium succinate incompatible with aminophylline and other drugs, thus consult pharmacist before usage of either form. *Topical:* Cleanse with water before application or as physician prescribes. Cleaning prevents cumulative depot effect that may increase systemic absorption, duration of drug's action, and side effects. Apply thin coat, gently rubbing into area, avoiding eye area and mucous membranes. Do not cover with occlusive dressing unless directed by physician. If used occlusive dressing, it should not remain in place for more than 16 hours; increases incidence of side effects. Disposable diapers or plastic pants act as an occlusive dressing if covering medicated groin area.

*Monitor:* Monitor BP during infusion. Carefully assess child's response to drug; necessary for dosage adjustments. Observe for side effects, especially hypocalcemia, signs of adrenal insufficiency, symptoms of infections, or worsening of condition. Children more prone to musculoskeletal side effects; note any pain or gait changes and report to physician immediately. Monitor BP and daily weights, report any sudden weight gain to physician. With long-term usage, monitor serum electrolytes and height. Encourage well-balanced diet low in sodium, rich in potassium, calcium, vitamin K and D. Observe for ulcer development; in long-term therapy, prophylactic antacids may be used. Encourage good hygiene and dental care (possible oral fungal infections). Tonometry (eye) examinations every 6 weeks. Diabetics may need increase in insulin due to steroid-induced hyperglycemia. Discontinuing of drug dosage should be reduced gradually, especially after long-term usage so it does not cause acute life-threatening adrenal insufficiency. After discontinuation of short-term therapy (up to 5 days) with high dosage, adrenal recovery may occur within 1 week. After prolonged high-dose therapy, complete recovery of adrenal function may require up to 1 year. Topical: assess wound site with every new application of medication and record. Notify physician of any variations. If infection occurs, discontinue drug and inform physician. With long-term therapy (over 2 weeks) or medicated over large body surface area (15% of body surface), the following laboratory tests may be helpful in evaluating the HPA-axis suppression: urinary free cortisol test and ACTH stimulation test. Itching can lead to scratching and introduction of infections. Younger children may need restraining especially during naps or at night; keep nails short and clean. Contact physician if itching persists.

**Patient Teaching:** Do not alter dosage or stop drug abruptly, it could cause very serious side effects, even death. Gradual tapering of dosage is necessary. Increasing amount of medication will not hasten healing process. Demonstrate how to apply topical medication or dosing schedule for oral form. Monitor signs and symptoms of medication, symptoms of adrenal insufficiency or worsening of condition and report to physician. Obtain daily weights; report any sudden weight gains to physician. Importance of close medical supervision and follow-up. Regular ophthalmic examinations if on long-term therapy. Caution about receiving skin tests, vaccinations or other immunizations, or coming in contact with persons receiving oral polio virus vaccine. Inform any health-care provider, including dentists, surgeons, or emergency care personal that child is on this medication. Child should carry a medical identification card. Observe for symptoms of infections. Do not use OTC medications without contacting health-care provider. Topical: Do not use medication on other areas than those prescribed by physician.

**Drug Interactions:** This drug in combination with high dosage of acetaminophen may increase risk of hepatotoxicity. With analgesics and antiinflammatory drugs, it may increase the risk of gastric ulceration. Amphotericin B and potassium-depleting diuretics increase risk of hypokalemia. Use with anabolic steroids may increase the risk of edema and acne. Drug in combination with anticoagulants may decrease anticoagulant effect. This drug used with anticonvulsants (phenytoin) may lower seizure threshold. Use with vaccines, live virus, or other immunizations may potentiate replication of the vaccine virus, increasing chance of developing the viral disease.

**Laboratory Test Interference:** May increase serum cholesterol, sodium, and blood glucose. May decrease serum calcium, potassium, $T_4$, $^{131}I$ uptake, urine 17-hydroxysteroid and 17-ketosteroids. Tends to suppress skin tests; may give a false-negative result with nitroblue-tetrazolium for bacterial infection. Adrenal function assessed by ACTH stimulation or plasma cortisol may be decreased.

**Storage Requirements:** Store at 15 to 30°C (59 to 86°F). Protect from light and freezing. Do not puncture or dispose of aerosol preparations into fire or incinerator. Consult package inserts for storage of parenteral forms.

---

☐ **HYDROXYCHLOROQUINE SULFATE**    (hye-drox-ee-klor'oh-kwin)

(Plaquenil Sulfate)

**Classification:** antimalarial

**Available Preparations:** 155-mg tablets

**Action and Use:** Exact mechanism of action unknown, but appears to bind and alter the properties of DNA. This blood schizonticidal agent is active against asexual forms of *Plasmodium malariae, P. ovale, P. vivax*, and *P. falciparum*. Preerythrocytic or exoerythrocytic forms of *Plasmodium* are not affected by this drug and it is gametocyticidal for only *P. malariae* and *P. vivax*. Used in suppression and treatment of the above forms of malaria.

## Routes and Dosage:
### PO:
- Uncomplicated Attacks of Malaria (caused by *P. malariae, P. ovale, P. vivax*, and certain strains of *P. falciparum*: 10 mg/kg initial dosage, then 5 mg/kg 6 hours later, then 5 mg/kg 18 hours after second dose, 5mg/kg 24 hours after third dose
- Suppression or Chemoprophylaxis of Malaria: 5 mg/kg once weekly. (Maximum 310 mg/day regardless of weight)

**Contraindications and Precautions:** Pregnancy category C. Safe use during lactation not established. Contraindicated for prolonged therapy in children, in hypersensitivity to drug, retinal or visual field changes, porphyria, psoriasis. Use with caution in those with hepatic disease, alcoholism, other hepatotoxic drugs, G-6-PD deficiency.

**Side Effects:** Effects are usually mild and reversible when used for malaria. *CNS:* irritability, nightmares, ataxia, **convulsions**, tinnitus, nystagmus, lassitude, fatigue, hypoactive deep-tendon reflexes, **confusion**, vertigo. *GI:* anorexia, nausea, vomiting, epigastric pain, weight loss. *Skin:* bleaching or loss of hair, blue-black skin discoloration, lichen planuslike eruptions, eczema, **exfoliative dermatitis**. *Hemic:* **agranulocytosis, thrombocytopenia, aplastic anemia**. *Sensory:* blurred vision, difficulty focusing, corneal changes, retinal changes, **optic atrophy**, patchy retinal pigmentation, **ototoxicity with tinnitus, labyrinthitis**. *Other:* Hypersensitivity: flushing, intense, generalized pruritus, fever, urticarial or papular rash, facial edema, hemoglobinuria, **asthma** (rare)

## Nursing Implications:
*Assess:* History of travel or exposure. Obtain blood studies to identify organism.
*Administer: PO:* For prophylaxis, give drug on same day of each week. Centers for Disease Control (CDC) recommend that treatment should start 1 to 2 weeks before travel to endemic area and for 6 weeks after leaving area. Take with meals to decrease gastric distress. Tablet can be crushed; mix with small amount of food or fluid.
*Monitor:* Observe for any side effects and monitor closely. This drug should not be used for long-term therapy in children as they are very susceptible to side effects. Discontinue drug immediately if any visual or hearing alterations occur and contact physician. Obtain CBC, liver function tests, ophthalmologic examinations, audiometric tests before and during long-term therapy with adults. Periodic blood samples should be obtained to check on progression of disease.
*Patient Teaching:* Importance of taking drug only as directed and not omitting doses. Observe for any signs and symptoms of side effects and contact

physician immediately if they occur. Take precautions for mosquito control while in infested areas. Fatalities have occurred with accidental ingestion of just 3 to 4 tablets; keep drug out of reach of children.

**Drug Interactions:** Products containing magnesium, kaolin, aluminum decrease action of this drug.

**Storage Requirements:** Store at 15 to 30°C (59 to 86°F) in tight containers.

---

# □ HYDROXYUREA                    (hye-drox′ee-yoo-ree-ah)

(Hydrea)

**Classification:** antineoplastic

**Available Preparations:** 500-mg capsules

**Action and Use:** A urea derivative that interferes with DNA synthesis by blocking incorporation of thymidine into DNA structure. It has no effect on RNA or protein synthesis and is cell cycle specific for the S phase of cell division. Used in treatment of ovarian cancer, malignant melanoma, and chronic myelocytic leukemia. Used experimentally in psoriasis and hypereosinophilic syndrome, although not approved by the FDA for these uses.

## Routes and Dosages:
*PO:* Pediatric dosages have not been established by the manufacturer. Adult dose is 20 to 30 mg/kg/day. Clinicians have used 10 to 20 mg/kg/day for children with dosage adjusted in relation to blastocyte count.

**Absorption and Fate:** Well absorbed from GI tract. Crosses blood-brain barrier. Metabolized by the liver and excreted in urine and through respirations. Peak level is 2 hours in circulation; 3 hours in CSF. Half-life is 3 to 4 hours.

**Contraindications and Precautions:** Pregnancy category D. Contraindicated in pregnancy or in women of childbearing age. Not to be given if WBC count is less than 2500/mm³ or platelet count is less than 100,000/mm³. Contraindicated in chicken pox or herpes zoster infection. Cautious use in those with previous chemotherapy or radiation, those with renal dysfunction.

## Side Effects:
*CNS:* headache, dizziness, disorientation, seizures, hallucinations, dizziness. *GI:* stomatitis, nausea, vomiting, constipation, diarrhea; GI complaints are more common if hydroxyurea is used in conjunction with radiation. *Skin:* rash, erythema, pruritus, alopecia. *GU:* hyperuricemia, renal dysfunction, dysuria. *Hemic:* **leukopenia**, thrombocytopenia, anemia

## Nursing Implications:

*Assess:* Obtain history of prior chemotherapy or radiation. Obtain renal function studies. Obtain CBC and bone marrow study before treatment.

*Administer:* This drug has potentially severe toxic effects and should be given only under the supervision of a physician with training and experience in cancer chemotherapy. The drug's potential for toxic effects on health-care personnel as well as patients necessitates careful handling during preparation and administration. *PO:* Daily dose is given qd or BID to achieve highest serum level.

*Monitor:* CBC counts with platelet levels, leukocytes, and hemoglogin are done at least weekly. Anemia is treated with blood transfusions. WBC count of less than 2500/mm³ or platelet count of less than 100,000/mm³ necessitates stopping or adjusting drug until levels are normal. If drug is stopped CBC counts are done within 3 days; counts improve rapidly, therefore, drug can usually be restarted soon. Monitor vital signs and report signs of infection promptly. Monitor dietary intake and provide nutritious diet. Hepatic and renal function may be monitored with BUN, SGPT, SGOT, bilirubin, creatinine, LDH, uric acid.

*Patient Teaching:* Avoid persons with infections such as colds, influenza, chicken pox. Report promptly signs of infection such as fever, sore throat, cough, watch for signs of bleeding and bruising. Return for scheduled follow-up visits. Perform good oral hygiene. Increase fluid intake. Encourage nutritious diet.

## Drug Interactions:
Suppresses immune response to immunization. Live virus vaccines must not be given, nor oral polio vaccine to those in close contact with the patient on this drug due to the chance of infection with a virus: these vaccines are delayed for at least 3 months after chemotherapy when the patient is in remisssion.

## Laboratory Test Interferences:
Elevated serum creatinine, BUN, uric acid. Retention of bromosulphalein.

## Storage Requirements:
Store tightly covered at 15 to 30°C (59 to 86°F). Avoid excessive heat.

---

## □ HYDROXYZINE     (hye-drox'i-zeen)

(Anxanil, Atarax, Atozine, Durrax, E-Vista, Hy-Pam, Hydroxacen, Hyzine-50, Neucalm, Orgatrax, Quiess, Vamate, Vistacon-50, Vistaject-25, Vistaject-50, Vistaril, Vistaquel, Vistazine)

**Classification:** antihistamine, sedative, analgesic, anxiolytic

## Available Preparations:
- 10 mg/5 ml syrup

- 25 mg/5 ml suspension
- 10, 25, 50, 100-mg tablets
- 25, 50, 100-mg capsules
- 25 mg/ml, 50 mg/ml solution for parenteral use

**Action and Use:** Acts at the subcortical level by depressing the hypothalamus and the reticular system in the brainstem. Effects include those of an antihistamine, sedative, antiemetic, antispasmodic, anticholinergic, local anesthetic. Used for control of anxiety such as preoperatively, to treat allergic pruritus, to treat nausea and vomiting of surgery and motion sickness, and in conjunction with opiates for analgesia.

**Routes and Dosages:**
*PO:*
- Anxiety and Pruritus: under 6 years: 50 mg/day in 4 doses
- 6 years and over: 50 to 100 mg/day in 4 doses
- Preoperative and Postoperative Sedation: 0.6 mg/kg

*IM:*
- Nausea and Vomiting: 1.1 mg/kg or 30 mg/m$^2$
- Preoperative and Postoperative Sedation: 1.1 mg/kg or 30 mg/m$^2$

**Absorption and Fate:** Rapidly absorbed from GI tract. Distribution unknown. Metabolized in liver and excreted mainly in feces. Peak level reached in 15 to 30 minutes after PO administration. Sedation lasts 4 to 6 hours; antihistamine effect lasts 4 days.

**Contraindications and Precautions:** Pregnancy category C. Unknown if drug crosses placenta or enters breast milk; not used in early pregnancy as it is teratogenic in animals. Not recommended in lactation and contraindicated in those hypersensitive to the drug.

**Side Effects:**
*CNS:* drowsiness, dizziness, weakness, headache, agitation, seizures. *GI:* dry mouth, nausea, bitter taste. *Respiratory:* wheezing. *Skin:* toxic to tissues causing abscess and necrosis; digital gangrene and thrombosis with intraarterial injection; rash

**Nursing Implications:**
*Assess:* Establish baseline vital signs. Obtain history of other medications.
*Administer: PO:* Tablet may be crushed or capsule opened for administration, although liquid forms (suspension and syrup) are available. Shake suspension well before giving. *IM:* Give deep into muscle using Z track technique; aspirate carefully. The lateral thigh is preferred site in young children. Avoid IV, SC, intraarterial injection, which may cause severe tissue damage. IM injection is painful. Rotate injection sites and chart sites carefully.
*Monitor:* Observe injection sites and report signs of tissue damage.
*Patient Teaching:* Patient on oral drug should be encouraged to perform good oral care daily. Measures to treat dry mouth, such as hard candy and ice

chips, can be suggested. Avoid alcohol, driving, or any hazardous activities.

**Drug Interactions:** Additive or potentiation effects with other CNS depressants such as analgesics, barbiturates, sedatives. Additive anticholinergic effects with other anticholinergics. Inhibits vasopressor effect of epinephrine so norepinephrine or metaraminol should be used instead.

**Laboratory Test Interferences:** Elevates results of urinary 17-hydroxycorticosteroid tests. May cause false-negative skin tests; decrease drug 72 hours or more before test.

**Storage Requirements:** Store at 15 to 30°C (59 to 86°F). Keep tightly closed in light-resistant containers.

---

## □ HYOSCYAMINE SULFATE

(hye-oh-sye'a-meen)

(Anaspaz, Bellaspaz, Cystospaz, Levsin, Levsinex, Neoquess, Seatone)

**Classification:** anticholinergic, antispasmodic

**Available Preparations:**
- 0.125 mg/5 ml oral elixir
- 0.125 mg/ml oral solution
- 0.125, 0.15-mg tablets
- 0.375-mg extended-release capsules
- 0.5 mg/ml for parenteral administration
- 0.25 mg released over 72 hours in transderm patches

**Action and Use:** Antimuscarinic that is one of the principal belladonna components. Through its parasympatholytic action, it relaxes smooth muscle spasms of lower urinary tract; reduces GI motility. Used for hypermotility of GI tract, infant colic, symptomatic relief of hypermotility of lower urinary tract. Because of its atropine effect (twice as potent as atropine), it has been used as a drying agent in acute rhinitis and preoperative medication to inhibit salivation and control excessive secretions of URT.

**Routes and Dosage:**
*PO:* Weighing (2.3 to 3.3 kg): 0.0125 mg; (3.4 to 4.4 kg): 0.0156 mg; (4.5 to 6.7): 0.0188 mg; (6.8 to 9 kg): 0.025mg; (9.1 to 13.5 kg): 0.0313 mg; (13.6 to 22.6 kg): 0.063 mg; (22.7 to 33 kg): 0.94 to 0.125 mg; (34 to 36 kg): 0.125 to 0.187 mg; all given every 4 hours if needed, titrated to child's response
Over 12 years: 0.125 to 0.25 mg 3 to 4 times per day
*IM, SC, IV:* Preoperatively: over 2 years: 0.005 mg/kg 30 to 60 minutes preoperatively

**Absorption and Fate:** Well absorbed orally. Onset of action: PO, 20 to 30 minutes; IV, 2 to 3 minutes. Duration of action: 4 to 6 hours. Well distributed to body tissues and drug crosses blood-brain barrier. Excreted in urine.

**Contraindications and Precautions:** Pregnancy category C and safety during lactation not established. Contraindicated in hypersensitivity to drug and sulfites, obstruction of bladder or GI tract, paralytic ileus, intestinal atony, cardiospasms, toxic megacolon, and narrow-angle glaucoma. Use caution with autonomic neurophathy, hepatic or renal impairment, ulcerative colitis, hyperthyroidism, coronary heart disease, congestive heart failure, hypertension, cardiac arrhythmias, hiatal hernia, or biliary tract disease.

### Side Effects:
**CNS:** drowsiness, headache, dizziness, weakness, insomnia, confusion. **CV:** palpitations, tachycardia. **GI:** dry mouth, constipation, nausea, vomiting, **paralytic ileus**, loss of taste, dysphagia. **GU:** urinary hesitancy, retention. **Skin:** urticaria, pruritus, decreased sweating, photophobia. **Sensory:** EENT: blurred vision, photophobia, mydriasis. **Other:** fever, allergic reaction, **anaphylaxis**

### Nursing Implications:
**Assess:** Obtain baseline vital signs.
**Administer: PO:** Give 30 minutes before meals and at bedtime at least 2 hours after meal. Tablet can be crushed and capsule taken apart (sustained-release particles are not to be chewed) and mixed with small amounts of food or fluid. Give small amount of water after sustained-release particles to prevent chewing of particles.
**Monitor:** Use with caution in hot and humid climates because of potential of heat stroke caused by drug. Monitor vital signs and side effects. If dizziness, tachycardia, or blurred vision occur, stop drug and notify physician. First symptoms of overdosage: dry hot, flushed skin, hyperpyrexia, difficulty in speech and dilated pupils.
**Patient Teaching:** Measure drug carefully and give only in amounts and frequency prescribed. Drug can cause blurred vision or alter mental alertness, so adjust activities accordingly. Sugarless candy or gum may relieve dry mouth symptoms. Sunglasses may help with photophobia when in sunlight.

**Storage Requirements:** Store at 15 to 30°C (59 to 86°F) protect from heat and light.

---

□ **IBUPROFEN**                                    (eye-byoo-proe-fen)

(Aches-N-Pain, Advil, Cap-Profen, Children's Advil, Genpril, Haltran, Ibuprin, Ifen, Menadol, Medipren, Midol 200, Motrin, Nuprin, Pamprin-IB, PediaProfen, Rufen, Tab-Profen, Trendar, Uni-Pro)

**Classification:** nonsteroidal antiiflammatory, analgesic, antipyretic, antirheumatic

## Available Preparations:
- 100 mg/5ml suspension
- 200, 300, 400, 600, 800-mg tablets
- 200, 300, 400, 600, 800-mg film-coated tablets

**Action and Use:** Interferes with action of prostaglandins, has an effect on the hypothalamus, and acts to block peripheral nerve transfer. Interferes with platelet aggregation, thereby prolonging bleeding time. Used for its nonnarcotic analgesic action to provide pain relief for mild to moderate pain and for discomfort of menstruation. Its antiinflammatory action makes it useful in rheumatoid arthritis. The 200-mg dose is used for treatment of fever due to its antipyretic effect.

## Routes and Dosages:
*PO:*
- Juvenile Rheumatoid Arthritis: up to 20 kg: 400 mg/day maximum; 20 to 30 kg: 600 mg/day maximum; 30 to 40 kg: 800 mg/day maximum; doses established by clinicians rather than manufacturers
- Menstrual Pain: 200 to 400 mg q4–6h PRN
- Fever: 5 to 10 mg/kg q6–8h

**Absorption and Fate:** Fairly well (80%) absorbed from GI tract with amount and speed of absorption decreased by food. Highly protein bound with distribution in the body unknown. Metabolized by the liver and mainly excreted in the urine. Peak level reached in 1 to 2 hours. Onset of analgesic action in 30 minutes but antiinflammatory effect not evident for up to 2 weeks. Duration of analgesic action 4 to 6 hours. Half-life: 2 to 4 hours.

**Contraindications and Precautions:** Pregnancy category B. Safe use during pregnancy has not been proven by study. Animal studies suggest the possibility of premature closure of the ductus arteriosus in the fetus and prolonged pregnancy due to uterine prostaglandin inhibition, therefore, use in the second half of pregnancy is not recommended. Has not been noted in breast milk but is not recommended during lactation due to the possibility of prostaglandin inhibition in the infant. Safety and efficacy in children have not been demonstrated, therefore, the drug is not recommended for OTC use; its use when indicated should be supervised by a health-care provider. Contraindicated in those with allergy to this drug, aspirin, or other nonsteroidal antiinflammatories. Cautious use in GI disease such as ulcers, coagulation disorder, cardiac dysfunction, renal dysfunction, hypertension, hepatic dysfunction, asthma, congestive heart failure, systemic lupus erythematosus.

## Side Effects:
*CNS:* dizziness, headache, fatigue, confusion, fever, mood changes and de-

pression, aseptic meningitis more common with systemic lupus erythematosus. **CV:** fluid retention and congestive heart failure, hypertension, palpitation, arrhythmias, anaphylaxis. **GI:** heartburn, nausea, vomiting, pain, constipation, diarrhea, peptic ulcer, GI bleeding, dry mouth, gingivitis. **Respiratory:** bronchospasm, dyspnea, and anaphylaxis as allergic response. **Hepatic:** jaundice, hepatitis, altered liver enzymes. **GU:** polyuria, hematuria, renal failure. **Skin:** rash, urticaria, alopecia, Stevens-Johnson syndrome. **Hemic:** inhibited platelet action and prolonged bleeding time, neutropenia, agranulocytosis, aplastic anemia, thrombocytopenia, anemia. **Sensory:** blurred or disturbed vision, amblyopia, cataracts, tinnitus

## Nursing Implications:

**Assess:** History of prior allergy to this drug, aspirin, or other nonsteroidal antiiflammatories is taken. Patient with asthma is at higher risk for allergy. Visual disturbances and coagulation disorders need to be noted.

**Administer:** Administration with food may help decrease GI discomfort although this may also interfere with drug absorption. Tablets may be crushed and given in food if necessary.

**Monitor:** BUN, creatinine, SGOT, SGPT, serum potassium dose in those with hepatic or renal dysfunction. Bleeding time monitored in those with coagulation disorder. If visual changes occur, an eye examination should be performed. Upper GI tests may be done if GI symptoms occur; stool for guaiac regularly performed. UA done periodically. Periodic physical assessments are useful, as symptoms of illness may be masked.

**Patient Teaching:** The OTC (200-mg) dose not intended for home management of minor discomfort for children. The drug is usually used only in diseases such as juvenile rheumatoid arthritis in the pediatric population and its use is monitored by a health-care provider. For long-term use the drug is taken with food to decrease GI discomfort. Take as directed; improvement may not be seen for about 2 weeks. Avoid alcohol and OTC drugs (such as acetaminophen) unless directed by prescriber. Report drug to other health-care providers such as dentists or surgeons. Report skin rash and flulike symptoms immediately as this may be an allergic reaction. Report visual changes and yellowing skin.

**Drug Interactions:** Increased risk of renal side effects with other drugs having similar effects such as acetaminophen, diuretics. Increased risk of GI side effects with other drugs having similar effects such as corticosteroids, potassium, aspirin. Potentiation of anticoagulant effects with drugs such as aspirin, heparin, and coumarin. Hypoglycemia with insulin. Decreased effect of antihypertensive medications. Increased risk of hemic side effects with other drugs with same effect or with radiation. Increased serum lithium levels. Potential for decreased serum levels when given with aspirin; not recommended to be given with any other nonsteroidal antiinflammatory drug.

**Laboratory Test Intereferences:** Prolongs bleeding time for about 1

day; no effect on prothrombin time or whole blood clotting time. Increased SGOT, SGPT, alkaline phosphatase, LDH, transaminase, BUN, creatinine, potassium, urine glucose, urine protein. Decreased blood glucose. Potenaial decreased urine output and uric acid.

**Storage Requirements:** Store at 15 to 30°C (59 to 86°F) in tightly closed, light-resistant containers.

---

# □ IDOXURIDINE (IDU)                          (eye-dox-yoor′i-deen)

(Dendrid, Herplex, Herplex Liquifilm, Stoxil)

**Classification:** antiviral ophthalmic

## Available Preparations:
- 0.1% solution for ophthalmic administration
- 0.5% ointment for ophthalmic administration

**Action and Use:** Drug closely resembles thymidine (metabolite essential for DNA synthesis) and during viral replication drug is used in place of thymidine resulting in faulty viral DNA that is unable to infect, destroy tissue, or reproduce itself. Treats keratitis and keratoconjunctivitis caused by herpes simplex virus but does not prevent accumulated scarring, vascularization, or progressive loss of vision. Not effective against HSV-2 virus.

## Routes and Dosage:
*Ophthalmic:*
- Drops: Instill 1 drop 0.1% solution in conjunctival sac every hour during day and every 2 hours at night initially until improvement; then 1 drop every 2 hours during day and every 4 hours during night.
- Ointment: Instill 1 cm strip of 0.5% preparation in conjunctival sac every 4 hours 5 times per day (late dosage at bedtime) until improvement

**Absorption and Fate:** Increasing drug concentrations or amount applied does not increase drug's effectiveness. Slowly degraded, which allows for adequate contact for antiviral activity.

**Contraindications and Precautions:** Pregnancy category C. Contraindicated in hypersensitivity to drug, iodine, iodine-containing preparations, deep eye ulcerations.

## Side Effects:
*Sensory:* blurred vision, pruritus, irritation, pain, burning, redness, mild edema of eyelid or cornea, lacrimation, photosensitivity, small punctuate de-

fects in corneal epithelium, corneal ulceration; slowed corneal wound healing with ointment

## Nursing Implications:

*Assess:* Note and record appearance of eye.

*Administer: Ophthalmic:* Do not use old solutions, may be toxic, can cause burning upon instillation and antiviral action lost. See Part I for instillation. Do not use with other ophthalmic medications.

*Monitor:* Improvement of affected tissue can be evaluated by loss of fluorescein staining. If no signs of improvement in 7 to 8 days reevaluation of therapy required. Duration of therapy is usually not longer than 21 days.

*Patient Teaching:* Proper instillation of ointment. Do not use more frequently than prescribed. Close ophthalmic supervision necessary. Warn child drug will blur vision for several minutes after instillation. If side effects occur, contact physician. Use sunglasses if photosensitivity occurs. Use good handwashing technique to prevent spread of infection (liquid soap preferred). Child should have separate towels and washcloths. Do not share eye make-up. Encourage child to keep hands away from eyes. Do not use OTC eye preparations.

## Drug Interactions: Precipitate may form if used with boric acid.

## Storage Requirements: Store at 8 to 15°C (36 to 46°F) in tight, light-resistant container. Some brands of ointment do not require refrigeration.

---

## ☐ IMIPRAMINE                                    (im-ip'ra-meen)

(Janimine, Filmtab, Tofranil)

## Classification: tricyclic antidepressant

## Available Preparations:
- 10, 25, 50-mg tablets
- 10, 25, 50-mg film-coated tablets
- 75, 100, 125, 150-mg capsules
- 12.5 mg/ml vial for parenteral use

## Action and Use: This drug inhibits the reuptake and metabolism of endogenous catecholamines in the CNS, thus potentiating effects of norepinephrine and serotonin. It is used for treatment of endogenous depression and depressive states of other psychiatric disorders. It is used without FDA approval for some children with attention-deficit disorder. It is the only tricyclic antidepressant used in treatment of enuresis. Its mechanism of action in these cases is not clear but it may increase bladder capacity in susceptible children and its anticholinergic effects may cause urinary retention.

## Routes and Dosages:
*PO:*

- Depression: 1.5 mg/kg/day; increase by 1 mg/kg q3–4d PRN; not to exceed 5 mg/kg/day
- Enuresis: 25 mg/day, 1 hour before bedtime. Increase to 50 mg/day after 1 week PRN if under 12 years or 75 mg/day after 1 week PRN if over 12 years. Total dose not to exceed 2.5 mg/kg/day.

**Absorption and Fate:** Well absorbed from GI tract. Distributed in body organs and crosses blood-brain barrier. Highly bound to plasma proteins. Metabolized in the liver and excreted mainly in the urine with smaller amounts in bile and feces. Peak levels reached after 30 minutes with IM administration and 1 to 2 hours with oral forms. Full antidepressant effect may not occur for 2 to 4 weeks. Half-life is 8 to 16 hours. Therapeutic level is 200 to 350 µg/ml.

**Contraindications and Precautions:** Pregnancy category C. Used during pregnancy only if clearly needed as there is teratogenic potential. Drug is not approved for use in children under 12 years for depression and under 6 years for enuresis. Contraindicated after myocardial infarction, hypersensitivity to any tricyclic antidepressant, those with untreated glaucoma, and during lactation. The film-coated tablets and some capsules contain yellow dye #5 or tartrazine that has caused allergy, such as asthma, in hypersensitive persons. These preparations should not be used in those with a known allergy to the dye. Use with caution in children, adolescents, treated glaucoma, respiratory and cardiovascular disease, those with seizures, those with ASA allergy.

## Side Effects:
*CNS:* drowsiness, lethargy, fatigue are common; agitation, sleep disturbance, confusion, anxiety, mood changes, worsening of psychosis, fine motor tremor, ataxia, dysphagia, dysarthria, incoordination; seizures particularly in those with seizure history when doses are increased in large increments. *CV:* EKG changes, particularly in children with AV dissociation (prolonged PR intervals, widening of QRS); postural hypotension, arryhthmia, thrombosis, congestive heart failure, hypertension, tachycardia, ventricular flutter and fibrillation, heart block. *GI:* anorexia, nausea, vomiting, diarrhea, GI distress, dry mouth, constipation. *Hepatic:* jaundice, hepatitis, altered liver function tests. *GU:* urinary retention (common), renal damage (uncommon). *Skin:* **allergic reaction** with rash, erythema, petechiae, edema of face and tongue, photosensitivity. *Hemic:* agranulocytosis, eosinophilia, leukopenia and thrombocytopenia (rare). *Endocrine:* breast engorgement, testicular edema, increase or decrease in blood glucose.

## Nursing Implications:
*Assess:* Careful history to identify cardiac, blood, and other diseases. Ask about drug and yellow dye allergies. Take baseline vital signs. EKG plus CBC taken before therapy begins.
*Administer: PO:* May give with food to lessen GI irritation. If 50 mg or

more is given for enuresis, 25 mg may be given at bedtime and 25 mg in late afternoon, particularly if child wets bed early in night; otherwise entire dose is given 1 hour before bedtime. If given for depression, be sure drug is taken. Only small amount of drug is dispensed for home use. Drug is withdrawn before surgery but should be tapered slowly rather than quickly withdrawn. **IM:** This route is rarely used. If used for depression treatment when patient is NPO, PO administration is used as soon as possible.

**Monitor:** Monitor vital signs especially pulse and supine and standing blood pressure. EKG and CBC are periodically done. Measure weight regularly and observe food and fluid intake, and bowel and bladder elimination. Watch patient for side effects of drug especially if a history of seizures, allergies, or cardiac disease is present. Therapeutic level in serum may be obtained. Record night wettings if used as treatment for enuresis and mood if used as treatment for depression. If sore throat or fever occur, CBC should be done as hemic side effects may be present. If jaundice occurs, liver function tests should be done.

**Patient Teaching:** Take drug as directed. Do not discontinue quickly or without prescriber instructions. Return for follow-up visits as recommended. Report excess fatigue, mood changes, weight change, enuresis episodes. Do not drive cars and avoid hazardous activities. Good oral care may help symptoms of dry mouth. Do not use OTC drugs without consulting prescriber. Instruct to change position slowly especially when rising. If drug is successful for enuresis, it is usually used for about 3 months. If enuresis occurs after drug is discontinued, it may be restarted but is not always successful.

**Drug Interactions:** Increased side effects of both drugs if used with monoamine oxidase inhibitors with hyperpyrexia, hypertension, tachycardia, seizures. Additive effects with other CNS depresssant drugs, including alcohol. Potentiation of imipramine side effects with barbiturates. Increased imipramine levels with phenothiazines. Increased sympathetic activity with other sympathomimetics. May decrease the activity of antihypertensives. Can increase activity of dicumarol and warfarin. Increases gastric emptying time so may slow absorption and cause inactivation of some drugs in the stomach.

**Laboratory Test Interferences:** May increase or decrease blood glucose. Elevates serum bilirubin, alkaline phosphatase, transaminase. Increase urinary catecholamines.

**Storage Requirements:** Store tightly closed at 15 to 30°C (59 to 86°F). Avoid freezing parenteral solution. Slight discoloration of solution does not preclude use but marked yellow or red solution should not be used. Preparations have expiration dates 3 to 5 years after manufacture.

## □ INDOMETHACIN

(in-doe-meth'a-sin)

(Indameth, Indocin, Indo-Lemmon)

**Classification:** nonsteroidal antiinflammatory, antirheumatic

**Available Preparations:**
- 25 mg/5 ml oral suspension
- 25, 50-mg tablets
- 75-mg extended-release capsules
- 50 mg rectal suppositories
- vials for parenteral use

**Action and Use:** Interferes with action of prostaglandins, has an effect on the hypothalamus, and acts to block peripheral nerve transfer. Interferes with platelet aggregation, thereby prolonging bleeding time. Its potential toxic effects negate its use for analgesia or antipyresis or when another nonsteroidal antiinflammatory drug is therapeutic. Its antiinflammatory action makes it useful in rheumatoid arthritis; also used for osteoarthritis and ankylosing spondylitis. Used rather than surgery for treatment of patent ductus arteriosus, particularly in prematures.

**Routes and Dosages:**
*PO, PR:* Juvenile Rheumatoid Arthritis: 2 to 14 years: 1.5 to 2.5 mg/kg/day in 3 to 4 doses; not to exceed 4 mg/kg/day or 150 to 200 mg/day
*IV:* Patent Ductus Arteriosus: 0.2 mg/kg for first dose; second dose is administered in 12 to 24 hours and is 0.1 mg/kg if premature was under 48 hours at time of first dose; 0.2 mg/kg if 2 to 7 days of age at time of first dose; and 0.25 mg/kg if over 7 days of age at time of first dose; third dose is administered in 12 to 24 hours after second and same dose as second is used. Another course of 1 to 3 doses may be used if the ductus arteriosus reopens.

**Absorption and Fate:** Well (90%) absorbed from GI tract with amount and speed of absorption decreased by food. Poor absorption of PO form by neonates. Highly protein bound with distribution throughout the body. Crosses blood-brain barrier and placenta and is present in breast milk. Absorption and bioavailability after rectal application similar to that of PO forms. Metabolized by the liver and mainly excreted in the urine and stool by bile. Peak level reached in 30 minutes to 2 hours with tablets and 2 to 4 hours with extended-release capsules. Half-life: 2 to 11 hours. A therapeutic range of 0.5 to 3 μg/ml may be needed for antiinflammatory action. When IV form used in prematures, a serum level of more than 0.25 μg/ml appears to be needed to achieve closure of the patent ductus arteriosus.

**Contraindications and Precautions:** Pregnancy category B; D in third trimester. Safe use during pregnancy has not been proven by study. Animal studies suggest the possibility of premature closure of the ductus arteriosus in the fetus and prolonged pregnancy due to uterine prostaglandin inhibition, therefore, use in the second half of pregnancy is not recommended. Is present in breast milk and has been known to cause seizures in a breast-fed infant. Safety and efficacy in children have not been demonstrated; its use when indicated for children 2 to 14 years should be supervised by a health-care provider. Capsules are not recommended for use in children. Contraindicated in those with allergy to this drug, aspirin, or other nonsteroidal antiinflammatories. Cautious use in GI disease such as ulcers, coagulation disorder, cardiac dysfunction, renal dysfunction, hypertension, hepatic dysfunction, asthma, congestive heart failure, mental depression, systemic lupus erythematosus. Cautious use of rectal form in those with history of rectal lesions or bleeding.

## Side Effects:
*CNS:* dizziness, headache, fatigue, confusion, fever, mood changes and depression, potential **intracranial hemorrhage** with neonates receiving IV form. *CV:* fluid retention and congestive heart failure, hypertension, palpitation, arrhythmias, **anaphylaxis**. *GI:* heartburn, nausea, vomiting, pain, constipation, diarrhea, peptic ulcer, GI bleeding, dry mouth, gingivitis. *Respiratory:* bronchospasm, dyspnea, and **anaphylaxis** as allergic response. *Hepatic:* jaundice, hepatitis, altered liver enzymes. *GU:* polyuria, hematuria, proteinuria, **oliguria**. *Skin:* rash, urticaria, alopecia, Stevens-Johnson syndrome. *Hemic:* inhibited platelet action and prolonged bleeding time, neutropenia, agranulocytosis, aplastic anemia, thrombocytopenia, anemia. *Sensory:* blurred or disturbed vision, amblyopia, cataracts, tinnitus

## Nursing Implications:
*Assess:* History of prior allergy to this drug, aspirin, or other nonsteroidal antiinflammatories is taken. Patient with asthma is at higher risk for allergy. Visual disturbances and coagulation disorders need to be noted.
*Administer: PO:* Administration with food may help decrease GI discomfort although this may also interfere with drug absorption. Tablet may be crushed and given in food if necessary althrough a suspension form is available. Suspension should not be given with antacid or liquid. *PR:* Suppository should remain in rectum for 1 hour after administration. *IV:* Reconstitute powder with 1 to 2 ml sterile water or normal saline. Give over 5 to 10 seconds; do not add to IV fluid. Do not administer discolored medication or if particulates are present. Use immediately after reconstitution and discard unused portion.
*Monitor:* IV line is monitored for that route with care to avoid extravasation. BUN, creatinine, SGOT, SGPT, serum potassium done in those with hepatic or renal dysfunction. Bleeding time monitored in neonates and those with coagulation disorder. If visual changes occur, an eye examination should be performed. Upper GI tests may be done if GI symptoms occur; stool for guaiac regularly performed. UA done periodically. Periodic physical assessments are useful as symptoms of illness may be masked. If neonate has anuria or oliguria of under 0.6 ml/kg/hr, subsequent doses are held until renal studies indicate normal renal function.
*Patient Teaching:* Not intended for management of minor discomfort; usually used only in diseases such as juvenile rheumatoid arthritis in the pediatric population and its use is monitored by a health-care provider. For long-term use, the drug is taken with food to decrease GI discomfort. Take as directed; improvement may not be seen for about 2 weeks. Avoid alcohol and OTC drugs (such as acetaminophen) unless directed by prescriber. Report drug to other health-care providers such as dentists or surgeons. Report skin rash and flulike symptoms immediately as this may be an allergic reaction. Report visual changes and yellowing skin.

**Drug Interactions:** Increased risk of renal side effects with other drugs having similar effects such as acetaminophen and diuretics. Increased risk of GI side effects with other drugs having similar effects such as corticosteroids, potassium, and aspirin. Potentiation of anticoagulant effects with drugs such as aspirin, heparin, and coumarin. Hypogylcemia with insulin. Decreased effect of antihypertensive medications such as hydralazine, furosemide, β blockers. Increased risk of hemic side effects with other drugs with same effect or with radiation. Increased serum lithium levels. Potential for decreased serum levels when given with aspirin; not recommended to be given with any other nonsteroidal antiinflammatory drugs. Can increase serum levels of digoxin, an effect important to consider in the premature receiving the IV form who is on digoxin. Increased hyperkalemia with other drugs having the same effect such as potassium-sparing diuretics. Increased level and potentially toxic effects of methotrexate when given with this drug. Increased levels of aminoglycosides in prematures.

**Labortory Test Interferences:** Prolongs bleeding time for about 1 day; no effect on prothrombin time or whole blood clotting time. Increased SGOT, SGPT, alkaline phosphatase, LDH, transaminase, BUN, creatinine, potassium, urine glucose, urine protein. Decreased blood glucose, plasma renin activity. Potentially decreased urine output and uric acid.

**Storage Requirements:** Store at 15 to 30°C (59 to 86°F) in tightly closed, light-resistant containers. Do not freeze suspension.

---

## □ INFLUENZA VIRUS VACCINE

(in-floo-en'zah)

(Flu-Immune, Fluogen, Fluzone, Subvirion; year is listed, e.g. 1988–1989)

**Classification:** immunization

**Available Preparations:**
- ready to use tubex
- multiple dose vial for parenteral use

**Action and Use:** Contains inactivated influenza virus to induce antibody formation against influenza virus strains contained in the vaccine. Used for children over 6 months who have chronic illness.

**Routes and Dosages:**
*IM:*
- 6 to 35 months: two 0.25-ml doses of subvirion preparation (split virus) at least 4 weeks apart

- 3 to 12 years: two 0.5-ml doses of subvirion preparation (split virus) at least 4 weeks apart
- over 12 years: one 0.5-ml dose of whole or subvirion preparation (split virus)

**Absorption and Fate:** Approximately 75% of recipients produce an adequate immune response within 2 weeks after vaccination. Response is greatest in young adults and less in young children and the elderly.

**Contraindications and Precautions:** Use in pregnancy only if clearly needed; defer until after first trimester. Contraindicated in infants under 6 months. Contraindicated in those allergic to eggs or other vaccine components, or who have shown previous hypersensitivity to an influenza vaccine. Febrile illness or acute infection are cause to delay immunization.

**Side Effects:**
*Skin:* redness, pain, induration at injection site. *Musculoskeletal:* myalgia. *Other:* fever, malaise, **anaphylaxis** (rare)

**Nursing Implications:**
*Assess:* Identify target groups for immunization. The vaccine is not necessary for all children. It is recommended for children over 6 months who have chronic diseases that required follow-up or hospitalization within the previous year. Examples include diabetes, renal dysfunction, anemia, immunosuppression, severe asthma or other pulmonary system disease, and children on long-term aspirin therapy. It is recommended for HIV-infected children who are symptomatic but not for those asymptomatic. Take history to rule out those at risk of hypersensitivity reactions. Some preparations contain thimerosal, a mercury derivative used as preservative, gentamycin, as well as eggs. Read package insert to identify specific components in each particular vaccine.
*Administer:* Only subvirion (split virus) vaccine is used in children under 12 years due to its lower potential for causing fever. The vaccine needs to be readministered annually for protection against that year's influenza. Administration each autumn, preferably November, is recommended. As with all vaccines, epinephrine 1:1000 and resuscitative equipment should be readily available in case of anaphylaxis. *IM:* Give into lateral thigh of infants and young children and deltoid muscle of older children. May be administered on the same day as another vaccine given at a separate site.
*Monitor:* Observe child for 20 minutes after immunization for signs of anaphylaxis.
*Patient Teaching:* Instruct about side effects.

**Drug Interactions:** The vaccine may have an effect on clearance of warfarin and theophylline, thereby increasing serum levels of those drugs. Concurrent administration of immunosuppressants can lessen antibody response to the vaccine.

**Storage Requirements:** Refrigerate at 2 to 8°C (35 to 46°F) in the refrigerator rather than on the door where temperature variations may be greater. Avoid freezing. Discard vaccine not labeled for the present season.

---

# □ INSULIN

(in'su-lin)

(Humulin R, Iletin Regular, Novolin R, Regular Iletin I, Regular Iletin II, Regular Pork Insulin, Velosulin, Velosulin Human (Concentrated Iletin II, U-500)

## □ ISOPHANE INSULIN SUSPENSION

(NPH) (Beef NPH Iletin II, Humulin N, Iletin NPH, Insulatard NPH, Insulatard NPH Human, NPH, NPH Iletin I, Pork NPH Iletin II, Protaphane NPH, Novolin N)

## □ ISOPHANE INSULIN SUSPENSION AND INSULIN

(Initard, Mixtard)

## □ ISOPHANE INSULIN HUMAN, SUSPENSION AND INSULIN HUMAN

(Novolin 70/30)

## □ INSULIN ZINC SUSPENSION (LENTE)

(Beef Lente Iletin II, Humulin L, Lente Iletin I, Lente Insulin, Pork Lente Iletin II, Lentard, Monotard, Novolin L)

## □ EXTENDED INSULIN ZINC SUSPENSION (ULTRALENTE INSULIN)

(Ultralente, Ultralente Iletin I, Ultralente purified Beef)

## ☐ PROMPT
## INSULIN ZINC
## (SEMILENTE)

(Semilente, Semilente Iletin I, Semilente purified Pork)

## ☐ PROTAMINE
## ZINC INSULIN
## (PZI)

(Beef Portamine Zinc and Iletin II, Pork Protamine Zinc and Iletin II, Protamine Zinc and Iletin I, PZI)

**Classification:** antidiabetic, hypoglycemic

## Available Preparations:
- 40, 100, 500 U/ml (Regular) for parenteral administration
- 40 U/ml, 100 U/ml (NPH), (Lente), (Ultralente), (Semilente), (PZI) for parenteral administration
- 100 U 70% isophane to 30% insulin (Isophane and Insulin) for parenteral administration

**Action and Use:** An endogenous hormone, secreted by the β cells of the pancreas that facilitates the transport of glucose to body tissues. Other physiologic functions of insulin include:(1) stimulation of glycogen synthesis by the liver; (2) inhibition of lipolysis, the breakdown of triglycerides to fatty acid and glycerol; and (3) stimulation of protein synthesis by facilitating storage of ingested amino acids. Used as a replacement for physiological production of endogenous insulin in juvenile-onset diabetes and as IV diagnostic tool to evaluate pituitary growth hormone. Insulin for injection is obtained from β cells of beef or pork. Insulin human injection is derived by enzyme modification of pork pancreas or from microbial synthesis.

**Routes and Dosage:** Dose is individualized. Factors, such as stress, activity, dietary intake, and status of health, cause variations in the insulin dose. Following recommendations can be used for initiating therapy:
*SC, IM, IV:* (regular) Diabetic Ketoacidosis (DKA): IV: 0.1 U/kg bolus, then 0.1 U/kg/hour or SC: 0.25 to 2 U/kg/dose, may repeat every 4 to 6 hours depending on glucose levels, degree of acidosis, and patient's clinical condition;
*SC:* (Lente or NPH) Maintenance: 0.5 U/kg in early AM; additional regular insulin 0.25 U/kg in the afternoon, depending on urine results. Dose of the long-acting insulin should be increased in the morning if additional doses of regular insulin were needed in previous 24 hour or reduced if urine glucose is negative for two mornings in a row.

**Absorption and Fate:** Absorbed into blood; circulated as free hormone. Metabolized primarily by the liver (see below).

## SUBCUTANEOUS INJECTION (HOURS)

| TYPE | STRENGTH SOURCE | ONSET | PEAK | DURATION | COMPATIBLE |
|---|---|---|---|---|---|
| Insulin (regular) | U-40, mixed U-100, mixed beef and pork, purified, biosynthetic, semisynthetic human | 1/2–1 | 2–4 | 5–7 | NPH, Lente, PZI purified |
| Semilente | U-40, mixed U-100, mixed purified pork and beef | 1–3 | 2–8 | 12–16 | Lente preparation |
| NPH | U-40, mixed U-100, mixed beef, purified beef and pork biosynthetic, semisynthetic human | 3–4 | 6–12 | 18–28 | Regular |
| Isophane Insulin 30–70% | U-100 purified pork semisynthetic human | 1/2 | 4–8 | 24 | |
| Lente | U-40, mixed U-100, mixed beef, purified beef and pork, biosynthetic semisynthetic human | 1–3 | 8–12 | 18–28 | Regular and Semilente |
| Ultralente | U-40 U-100 mixed beef, purified beef | 4–6 | 18–24 | 36 | Regular and Semilente |
| PZI | U-40, mixed U-100, mixed purified beef | 4–6 | 14–24 | 36 | Regular |

Regular, IV Push: Onset: 10 to 30 minutes; Peak: 15 to 30 minutes; Duration: 30 to 60 minutes.

**Contraindications and Precautions:** Contraindicated in sensitivity to drug or its components. Intolerance to beef insulin is more common than to pork insulin. Intolerance often reduced by use of purified pork insulin, biosynthetic human insulin, or semisynthetic human insulin.

## Side Effects:

*Skin:* three types of local cutaneous reactions: (1) hivelike or urticarial reaction associated with systemic manifestations including itching, GI complaints, and (rarely) hypotension; (2) local wheal or firm red, indurated area that begins to form 20 to 40 minutes after injection and reaches peak size (1 to 5 cm) around injection site within 2 to 6 hours; may require 7 to 10 days to subside or may persist 2 to 3 months; and (3) insulin **lipodystrophy**, dimpling or atrophy of fat tissue; common in children. *Endocrine:* Hypoglycemia: (rapid, frequent in occurrence) anxious or nervous feelings, blurred vision, chills, cool pale skin, sweating, confusion or difficulty concentrating, drowsiness, headache, hunger, **tachycardia**, nausea, shakiness, irritability, **ataxia**, **coma**, **convulsions**, **death**. Symptoms usually occur when blood sugar drops to 50 mg/dl or when fall in blood sugar is sudden and rapid. Reaction tends to correspond to insulin's peak action time. Somogyi effect: occurs when child receives too large a dose of insulin over long time causing rebound hyperglycemia. They do not react to increasing insulin dose, blood glucose levels tend to be low in the evening but morning readings indicate hyperglycemia. Hyperglycemia: (slower onset) drowsiness, dry mouth, flushed dry skin, fruitlike breath odor, polyuria, polydipsia, loss of appetite, nausea or vomiting, tiredness, **hypotension**, **weak rapid pulse**, **Kussmaul's respirations**, **coma**. *Other:* allergic reaction, urticaria, itching, stinging, warmth at IM site.

## Nursing Implications:

*Assess:* For symptoms of hyperglycemia or hypoglycemia, including urine and blood glucose levels. History of events leading to onset of symptoms, time and amount of last insulin dosage, illness, exercise, stress or dietary intake. Assess child's level of growth and development, attitude and understanding of disease and treatment, and family dynamics and interactions. If newly diagnosed, assess diabetic family and child's level of acceptance, willingness to learn, and ability to grasp large amount of information.

*Administer:* All insulins available over the counter (OTC) except concentrated iletin II, U-500 that requires a prescription. Never store U-500 with other insulins to avoid accidentally injecting; when giving this drug, use U-100 syringe to prepare and administer. Use only insulin ordered and carefully read label to prevent giving incorrect insulin. Do not switch brands, strengths, type (regular, PZI, or etc.), species (beef, pork, human) or purity because it may affect dosage adjustment. Use correct syringe for correct strength: red top, U-40; orange top, U-100. Changing syringe brands may effect dosage. There is about 0.1 ml dead space in disposable syringes without the needle, however, there is no dead space in syringes with needle, thus eliminating air space. Giving of cold insulin increases likelihood of lipodystrophy. First dose of insulin is given early AM about 30 minutes before breakfast. Rotate sites using subcutaneous tissue of upper arms, thighs, upper buttocks, and stomach; avoiding 2-inch area around naval. Follow your hospital protocol; but best to keep 1 inch between injection sites for 6 to 8 weeks. Always record location of injection site. When cleaning injection site with alcohol swab; allow to dry before injecting to prevent insulin from being precipitated by alcohol. (REGU-

LAR INSULIN) This insulin is clear in appearance and should not be cloudy or have precipitate; if it does, discard. This form can be given IM, SC, and **regular is the only form that can be given IV. Exception: do not use concentrated U-500 IV.** *IV:* Regular can be given as a bolus or by constant infusion. Give IV push slowly over 1 to 5 minutes. When given by constant infusion, a pump is recommended to deliver O.1 U/kg/hour. Plastic infusion bags and tubing absorb 20 to 80% of drug. Salt-poor albumin may be added to bind the insulin for infusion or tubing can be primed with insulin solution to saturate insulin binding sites, thereby reducing amount lost. Because this phenomenon cannot be accurately controlled, monitor child closely by blood and urine glucose levels. Insulin is compatible with the following solutions: $D_5W$, $D_5/0.5\%S$, $D_5NS$, $D_{10}W$, NS. Do not mix with these drugs: aminophylline, amobarbital, chlorothiazide, dobutamine, methylprednisolone sodium succinate, nitrofurantoin, pentobarbital, phenobarbital, phenytoin, secobarbital, sodium bicarbonate, sulfisoxazole, and thiopental. Regular insulin is the only insulin given during a ketoacidosis crisis; once it is under control a combination of intermediate and short-acting insulins can be used usually at a 2 to 1 ratio. As child is regulated, insulin dosage is based on previous day's insulin effects. Most newly diagnosed juvenile diabetics are now receiving the synthetic human insulin. (NPH INSULIN) Given SC: this form is cloudy and to disperse evenly, gently roll vial between palms. Never shake solution because it causes bubbles to form that interfere with measurement of dosage. If precipitate remains, or solution is clear after rolling, discard vial. NPH can be mixed with regular insulin but not with lente. **When mixing insulin, always remember to prepare clear to cloudy**. For example: if dosage is 2U Regular and 4U NPH, using aseptic technique, first inject 4U air into NPH vial, then inject 2U air into regular vial and withdraw regular insulin, remove excess air and bubbles, insert needle below fluid level of NPH and withdraw 4U NPH without injecting anything into the vial. This method prevents contamination of regular insulin by NPH, which would alter its action. Inject insulin SC immediately to prevent binding. (LENTE) This is an intermediate-acting insulin that is cloudy in appearance. Do not shake, but roll between palms to mix. Can be mixed with Regular, Semilente, and Ultralente, but do not mix with other modified insulins. (ULTRALENTE INSULIN) Given SC: insulin is cloudy and must be gently rolled to mix. Can be mixed with lente and semilente but not with other modified insulin. (SEMILENTE) Is a short-acting cloudy insulin. Roll vial gently between palms to mix. This form is not used for ketoacidosis. Can be mixed with Lente and Ultralente only. (PZI) This is long-acting insulin that is cloudy in appearance. Mix insulin by gently rolling between palms. PZI can be mixed with regular insulin but not with lente.

***Monitor:*** Monitor child for symptoms of hypoglycemia, hyperglycemia, and Somogyi reactions. Insulin (regular) is rapid acting, peaks in 2 to 4 hours, and this is when hypoglycemia attack could occur. NPH is an intermediate-acting insulin; peaks will be midafternoon and dinner time, this is time child could experience hypoglycemia. Plan snacks and mealtime accordingly. Ultralente hypoglycemic attacks most likely to occur during night and early morning. Observe child closely for clammy skin and restlessness. Give child sucrose or glucose PO and check blood level immediately. Urine glucose may not indicate true hypoglycemic state because urine has been pooling in bladder all night. Blood glucose monitoring is performed several times daily. With lente insulin, symptoms of hypoglycemia are most likely to occur at midafternoon, or dinner time; child is most likely to present with symptom of fatigue. Also when child is first placed on this form of insulin he may experience nocturnal hypoglycemia; monitor for clammy skin and restlessness. With semilente hypoglycemia will occur before lunch. PZI is a long-acting insulin, therefore, monitor child at night and early morning for hypoglycemia. Remember when short-acting insulin and intermediate-acting insulins are combined hypoglycemic attacks can occur with peak action of both insulins. In diabetic ketoacidosis monitor fluid balance and potassium levels as well as symptoms of acidosis.

**Patient Teaching:** It is best if one nurse coordinates and does teaching care plan for family. Approach family and child on their level of understanding because they must understand the disease process and how to care for its symptoms. Help parents deal with their emotions and amount of guilt and allow them to express feelings at all times. The most important thing parents must master is that the child has to be treated as a normal child. Discipline and family dynamics toward child should remain the same; they need a good communication system with child. The care of this child, urine and blood glucoses, and injections should become as routine as brushing teeth. A child no matter how young needs to be involved in his own care from the beginning. As soon as child is diagnosed or out of coma he can begin by learning to do urine sugars and acetone checks. Let child teach parents this. Parent and child have to understand importance of urine and blood testing, recording, and interpretation. Urine tests are usually done upon awaking, lunch, late afternoon (4 to 5 PM) and before bed. Test is usually taken after having child void, discard, and then 15 minutes later checking second voiding. When child is in school, urine usually is not checked unless child is very brittle. For hard to manage diabetics, capillary blood glucose test kits are available. Acetone is measured as physician directs. Some states require that patient have prescription for needles and syringes. Insulin injections, how to prepare, sterile technique, how to use syringe, and how to administer and recording of site rotations must be mastered. Children usually can give own injections into thighs and abdomen. Upper arm injections can be done by pressing upper arm against wall or chair to roll tissue forward providing subcutaneous tissue for injection. Parents should decide which type of syringe (disposable or reusable) they wish to use along with proper care and usage. Once a type of syringe is used, it is best to stay with that brand because it could effect dosage due to difference in syringes. Understanding of insulin action, peak time, and side effects of hypoglycemia are required. Two adults should know how to administer insulin. The child, once able to count, manipulate syringe, and understand how to inject medication should give his own injections. Most 6 to 7-year-olds can comprehend this information. Parents should always have extra syringes, needles, and an extra vial of insulin available. Properly dispose of used needles and syringes and keep out of reach of young children. Parents need to know how to adjust insulin to urine test results, exercise, diet, stress, illness, and daily schedules. This is done at first by physician and then family makes these decisions when they understand disease but they always need 24-hour access to a physician or health professional. They must understand the importance of a balanced diet, low in concentrated sugar, with adequate calories for growth. It is usually composed of 50 to 55% carbohydrates, 30 to 35% fat, and 15 to 20% protein. Food intake should be divided into three meals (1/4 of calories/ meal) and 2 snacks (1/8 calories) predominantly carbohydrate in the afternoon, and protein/fat before bedtime. Teach how exercise, stress, and illness effects insulin control. Understand the cause, symptoms and treatment of hyperglycemia and hypoglycemia. Good hygiene, foot care, dental care, treatment, and prevention of infections and regular eye examinations are necessary. Discuss cautious use of OTC medications and how alcohol, drugs, and smoking affect diabetes. Child should wear medical alert jewelry; teachers and other caretakers need to know child's diagnosis and symptoms of hyperglycemia. Children should always have some form of carbohydrate (sugar) with them. Inform any health professionals and dentist that child is a diabetic. Importance of close medical follow-up; this disease can be managed but insulin does not cure diabetes. When children become adolescents, diabetes may be hard to manage because of adolescent rebellion. Parents need to know this will probably happen and to seek help. Child may respond better to another adult than to parent. American diabetic association provides support, information, and camps for children.

**Drug Interactions:** These medications taken concurrently with insulin: adrenocorticoids, glucocorticoid, amphetamines, contraceptives, corticotropin, dextrothyroxine, diuretics (thiazide or thiazide-related), epinephrine, ethacrynic acid, furosemide, glucagon, phenytoin, or thyroid hormone, all may increase blood glucose levels. Anabolic steroids, androgens, disopyramide, guanethidine imipramine, large doses of salicylates, may enhance hypoglycemic effects. Antiinflammatory analgesics, nonsteroidal may increase hypoglycemic effects. Beta-andrenergic blocking agents may increase risk of hypoglycemia or hypoglycemia and carbonic anhydrase inhibitors may decrease hypoglycemic response. Diazoxide reverse the hyperglycemia effects of diazoxide and alcohol enhances the hypoglycemic effects. Smoking decreases the amount of insulin absorbed; smoking of marijuana may increase insulin requirements.

**Food Interactions:** Avoid concentrated sugars in any form, saturated fats, cholesterol, and salt.

**Laboratory Test Interference:** May cause alteration in thyroid function tests, liver function tests, decrease serum potassium and serum calcium levels.

**Storage Requirements:** Refrigerate all forms and avoid freezing. Insulin is usually stable if refrigerated for 24 months from date of manufacture. Vials can be kept at room temperature and will retain potency for 12 months.

# ☐ **IODOQUINOL**                    (eye-oh-do-kwin'ole)

(Diiodohydroxyquin, Diodoquin, Diquinol, Inserfem, Moebiquin, Yodoxin)

**Classification:** amebicide

## Available Preparations:
210, 650-mg tablet

**Action and Use:** Halogenated 8-hydroxyquinoline, whose action is limited to intestinal lumen, where it acts against protozoa, both trophozoites and cyst forms. Especially effective against *Entamoeba histolytica*. Used in combination with tissue amebicides.

## Routes and Dosage:
*PO:* Intestinal Amebiasis: 30 to 40 mg/kg/day in 2 or 3 divided doses for 5 to 20 days. (Maximum 650 mg/dose)

**Absorption and Fate:** Poorly absorbed from GI tract. Excreted primarily in feces.

**Contraindications and Precautions:** Pregnancy category C. Safety in lactation not established. Contraindicated in hypersensitivity to 8-hydroxyquinoline or iodine preparations, renal or hepatic disease, preexisting optic neuropathy, or severe thyroid disease. Use with caution in thyroid disease.

## Side Effects:
*CNS:* headache, vertigo, dysesthesia, weakness malaise, agitation, ataxia, retrograde amnesia, **peripheral neuropathy.** *GI:* anorexia, nausea, vomiting, abdominal cramps, diarrhea, increased motility, epigastric burning and pain, gastritis, constipation, anal itching and irritation. *Skin:* pruritus, urticaria, papular and pustular acneiform, bullae, vegetating or tuberous iododerma, discoloration nails and hair. *Hemic:* **agranulocytosis** (rare). *Other:* fever, chills, hair loss (rare). *EENT:* **optic neuritis, atrophy and peripheral neuropathy frequent in children (permanent vision loss may occur)**

## Nursing Implications:
*Assess:* Obtain stool cultures according to agency policy (stool must be warm for detection of parasitic movement). Inspect and record appearance of stool. All family members need stool cultures. Obtain family history of home and sanitation conditions and presence of pets. Obtain baseline ophthalmic examination.
*Administer: PO:* Give with meals. Tablets may be crushed and mixed with food.
*Monitor:* Stool cultures obtained weekly, then 1, 3, and 6 months after ther-

apy has stopped. Obtain stool cultures according to agency policy. Record number, frequency, and characteristics of stools. If not potty trained, keep tight-fitting diapers or training pants on to prevent child from handling own fecal matter. Change diapers immediately after stools; properly dispose and use good handwashing technique. Ophthalmic examinations should be done during therapy. Discontinue drug and report immediately to physician ophthalmic symptoms of blurred vision or eye pain, and skin rashes. Observe for overgrowth nonsusceptible organisms especially *Monilia*.

**Patient Teaching:** Stress that all family members use good handwashing techniques both before meals and after defecations. Use liquid soap; bar soap can harbor organisms for 48 hours. Discuss how disease is transmitted and preventive measures, and proper food preparation and handling. If child is in diapers, discuss how to dispose of fecal matter. Observe for overgrowth of nonsusceptible organisms, symptoms of ophthalmic side effects or skin symptoms, report to physician immediately. How to collect stool specimens properly. Importance of follow-up medical care.

**Laboratory Test Interferences:** Increased protein bound serum iodine concentrations, decreased iodine-131 uptake, false-positive PKU. These may persist for 6 months.

**Storage Requirements:** Store at 15 to 30°C (59 to 86°F) in light-resistant container.

---

## □ IPECAC SYRUP

(ip′e-kak)

**Classification:** emetic

**Available Preparations:**
  30 ml of oral syrup

**Action and Use:** Produces emesis by stimulation of chemoreceptor trigger zone in medulla and by local irritation of gastric mucosa. Effective as emetic in accidental poisoning; also used as expectorant in cough preparations.

**Routes and Dosage:**
*PO:*
- 6 month to 1 year: 5 ml/dose
- 1 to 5 years under 25 lbs: 10 to 15 ml/dose
- over 5 to 12 years over 25 lbs: 15 ml/dose
- over 12 years: 30 ml/dose

**Absorption and Fate:** Onset of action: 15 to 30 minutes; duration of action: 45 to 60 minutes.

**Contraindications and Precautions:** Pregnancy category C. Use with caution if nursing. Contraindicated in those who are not fully conscious, impending or experiencing seizures, inebriated, in shock, those with depressed gag reflex, those who have ingested strychnine, petroleum distillates (depending on amount, toxicity of substance), alkali, strong acids, volatile oils, rapid acting CNS depressants. Use caution after overdosage of digitalis glycosides.

**Side Effects:** Usually only if drug is not vomited but systemically absorbed. Toxicity also occurs with eating disorders where drug is chronically used as emetic. Drug is slowly eliminated; chronic dosages may cause cumulative effects. *CNS:* lethargy, tremors, **convulsions**, coma. *CV:* tachycardia, arrhythmias, **atrial fibrillation**, **cardiomypathy**, **cardiotoxicity**. *GI:* bloody diarrhea, protracted vomiting

**Nursing Implications:**
*Assess:* Assess what child ingested, time of ingestion, how much ingested, did parents give anything for treatment. Assess level of consciousness and if any contraindications conditions present; notify poison control center. Obtain vital signs and start flow chart.

*Administer:* **Do not confuse ipecac syrup with ipecac fluid-extract which is 14 times more potent and can lead to death.** *PO:* Measure with calibrated measuring device. Give 120 to 240 ml of clear fluids or carbonated beverages; either before or after ipecac. Do not use milk as it delays action of ipecac; however, if child will not take any other fluid, then give milk after medication. Gently bouncing a young child may also induce vomiting. Do not give activated charcoal concurrently, it nulls ipeccac's effect.

*Monitor:* Emesis should occur within 20 to 30 minutes of dosage. Child may vomit more than once; vomiting should subside within 2 or 3 hours; if it does not, inform physician. Can repeat same dosage once; follow second dosage with fluids. If no vomiting occurs, notify physician at once and have gastric lavage equipment and activated charcoal available.

*Patient Teaching:* This nonprescription drug is widely available. Keep locked up with other medications. Always check expiration date before usage. Call poison control center before inducing emesis. Explain how to give; how to monitor child's condition. Review how to prevent poisonings, what to do if incident occurs (e.g., determine what child took, try to assess how much consumed, time of ingestion, and if bringing child to emergency room bring container with them).

**Drug Interactions:** Activated charcoal used with drug neutralizes its emetic effect. Give charcoal after emesis has occurred.

**Food Interactions:** Milk delays onset of emesis.

**Storage Requirements:** Store at 15 to 30°C (59 to 86°F).

## ☐ IRON, FERROUS FUMARATE

(Femiron, Feostat, Fumasorb, Fumerin, Hemocyte, Ircon, Palmiron, Span-FF)

## ☐ FERROUS GLUCONATE

(FeG Iron, Fergon, Ferralet, Simron)

## ☐ FERROUS SULFATE

(Feosol, Fer-In-Sol, Fer-Iron, Fero-Gradumet, Ferralyn, Ferra-TD, Mol-Iron, Slow Fe)

## ☐ POLYSACCHARIDE IRON

(Hytinic, Niferex, Nu-Iron)

## ☐ IRON DEXTRAN

(Feronim, Hematran, Hydextran, Imfergen, Imferon, Irodex, Nor-Feron, Proferdex)

**Combination Products:** Difuleron, Fermalox, Ferroctyl, Ferro-DSS, Ferro-Dox TR, Fer-Regules, Ferro-Sequels, Ferrous-DS. Also available in numerous multivitamin and mineral preparations.

**Classification:** nutritional supplement

## Available Preparations:
*Ferrous fumarate:*
- 45 mg/0.6 ml and 100 mg/5 ml oral suspension
- 60, 195, 200, 300, 324, 325-mg tablets
- 100-mg chewable tablets
- 300-mg extended-release tablets

- Also available in combination with docusate sodium.

***Ferrous gluconate:***
- 300 mg/5 ml oral solution
- 300, 320, 325-mg tablets
- 300-mg film-coated tablets
- 435 extended-release tablets
- 86, 325-mg capsules

***Ferrous sulfate:***
- 195, 300, 325-mg tablets
- 300-mg film-coated tablets
- 325-mg enteric-coated tablets
- 525-mg extended-release tablets
- 150, 225, 250, 390-mg extended-release capsules
- 75 mg/0.6 ml, 90 mg/5 ml, 125 mg/ml, 220 mg/5 ml oral solution

***Ferrous sulfate dried:***
- 200-mg tablets
- 160-mg extended-release tablets
- 190-mg capsules
- 150, 159, 167-mg extended-release capsules
- Also available in combination with aluminum and magnesium hydroxide

***Polysaccharide iron:***
- 100 mg/5 ml oral solution
- 50-mg tablets
- 150-mg capsules

***Iron Dextran:***
- 50 mg/ml vials for parenteral use

**Action and Use:** Iron is a necessary component of hemoglobin and is, therefore, essential in the oxygen transfer carried out by red blood cells. Used in microcytic and hypochromic anemia, which results from iron deficiency. Frequent supplement used during pregnancy when intake often does not meet iron needs, and in infants with decreased iron stores such as small for gestational age and premature infants.

**Routes and Dosages:**
*PO:*
- Ferrous Fumarate: Supplement: 3 mg/kg/day; Deficiency: 3 to 6 mg/kg TID
- Ferrous Gluconate: Supplement: over 2 years: 8 mg/kg/day; Deficiency: over 2 years: 16 mg/kg TID
- Ferrous Sulfate: Supplement: 5 mg/kg/day; Deficiency: 10 mg/kg TID
- Ferrous Sulfate, Dried: 160 mg/day
- Polysaccharide Iron: Supplement: 1.5 mg/kg/day

*IM:*
- Iron Dextran: under 5 kg: not to exceed 25 mg/day; 5 to 10 kg: not to exceed 50 mg/day; over 10 kg: not to exceed 100 mg/day

**Absorption and Fate:** Absorbed mainly from duodenum and jejunum with 3 to 30% absorbed from GI route. Absorption is increased with an empty stomach and in iron deficient patients; ferrous form most readily absorbed. Highly (90%) protein bound. Very small amounts are lost daily in urine, sweat, skin, and other body products; women lose iron in menstrual flow. Most iron available from red blood cell breakdown is recaptured and used. Stored in liver, spleen, bone marrow. Iron can accumulate to toxic amounts.

**Contraindications and Precautions:** Pregnancy category A for oral forms and category B for iron dextran. iron dextran not given under 4 months of age. Contraindicated in hemochromatosis, anemia other than iron deficiency, and in patients with repeated blood transfusions. Oral forms contraindicated in GI ulcer or colitis. Oral and parenteral forms not used concomitantly. Parenteral form not used with history of hypersensitivity reaction to the drug. Cautious use of parenteral form in allergic and asthmatic patients due to increased hypersensitivity; in rheumatoid arthritis. Caution with hepatic or renal dysfunction, pancreatitis.

**Side Effects:**
*CNS:* fever, chills, dizziness as delayed reaction to parenteral form. *CV:* hypotension, **cardiac arrest** as hypersensitivity reaction after parenteral form. *GI:* nausea, vomiting, epigastric pain, diarrhea, constipation, black stools common with oral forms; GI bleeding. *Respiratory:* dyspnea in hypersensitivity reaction to parenteral form. *Skin:* skin rash, hives, redness at IV injection site; pain, inflammation, necrosis, and permanent staining of skin at site of IM injection. *Hemic:* hemosiderosis with overdosage or use of iron in those with anemia not due to iron deficiency such as thalessemia. *Other:* **anaphylaxis** to parenteral form may occur; 1 to 2-day delayed sensitivity reactions manifest by fever, dizziness, arthralgia, nausea, and vomiting.

**Nursing Implications:**
*Assess:* Obtain diet history. Be alert for elements that can decrease iron absorption such as low calcium or high phosphate diet, infection, or decreased GI acid. Watch for signs of deficiency in infants after 4 to 6 months of age when maternal iron stores are depleted (earlier in prematures). A CBC, including hematocrit, hemoglobin, and reticulocytes, is done to establish iron deficiency anemia. Before administering parenteral iron, a test dose of 0.5 ml is given.
RDAs for iron are:
- 0 to 6 months: 10 mg
- 6 to 12 months: 15 mg
- 1 to 3 years: 15 mg
- 4 to 10 years: 10 mg
- 11 to 18 years: 18 mg
- Pregnancy: 30 to 60 mg supplement daily
- Lactation: 30 to 60 mg supplement for 2 to 3 months after delivery

***Administer: PO:*** The mg doses of various forms of iron are not equivalent; rather the amount of elemental iron in various preparations is important. Ferrous fumarate = 330 mg elemental iron/g; ferrous gluconate = 120 mg elemental iron/g; ferrous sulfate = 200 mg elemental iron/g; ferrous sulfate dried = 300 mg elemental iron/g. Polysaccharide iron (ferric) contains variable amounts of elemental iron according to brand and may not be absorbed as well as ferrous forms.

Giving with snack decreases absorption but is often recommended as GI irritation will be lessened. Accompanying with vitamin C may enhance iron absorption. Liquid preparations should be given with fluid, such as juice, and by a dropper or straw as they can stain teeth. ***IM:*** Do not mix with other medications. Given into upper outer buttock, therefore, this form is used only in older children. Change needle after drawing up iron. Use long needle and 2 track injection technique. Permanent tissue staining can occur if not given deep IM. Aspirate after inserting needle and inject slowly. ***IV:*** Do not mix with other medications and do not use the multidose vial (latter only for IM injection). Give at rate slower than 1 ml/minute.

***Monitor:*** Have epinephrine 1:1000 available during parenteral administration especially with test dose. Monitor for signs of hypersensitivity. Keep supine after IV dose and monitor blood pressure and pulse. Delayed reaction may occur up to 2 days after injection. Observe IV injection site for redness, prior IM sites for inflammation, necrosis, or staining. Hemoglobin, hematocrit, and reticulocytes are monitored at least every 3 weeks. Total iron binding, serum iron and ferritin, and transferring are performed regularly.

***Patient Teaching:*** Teach to take oral preparation between meals unless GI distress occurs, then with food; do not take with dairy products, eggs, whole grains, coffee, or tea. Take liquid forms with generous amount of fluid and straw to avoid staining teeth. Dietary teaching may be necessary; good sources of iron include meats, seafood, eggs, beans, dried fruits, enriched baby cereals and formulas.

## Drug Interactions:
Decreased absorption of both drugs when oral form given with tetracycline. Vitamin C increases iron absorption. Antacids decrease absorption and should not be given simultaneously. Decreases effects of chloramphenicol and penicillamine. In infants with vitamin E deficiency, iron can cause red blood cell hemolysis and hemolytic anemia.

## Food–Drug Interactions:
Dairy products, eggs, whole grains, tea, and coffee decrease iron absorption.

## Laboratory Test Interferences:
False-positive orthotoluidine. False elevated bilirubin. False decrease in calcium. False-negative glucose oxidase with ferrous sulfate. Altered PTT with injectable iron forms. Blackens stool and interferes with stool for guaiac results.

## Storage Requirements:
Store tightly covered at 15 to 30°C (59 to 86°F). Protect solutions from freezing.

# □ ISONIAZID (INH)                              (eye-soe-nye′a-zid)

(Hyzyd Isotamine Laniazid, Nydrazid, PMS-Isoniazid, Rimifon, Rolazid, Teebaconin)

**Combination Products:** 150-mg isoniazid with 300 mg rifampin

**Classification:** antitubercular

## Available Preparations:
- 50 mg/5ml oral solution
- 50, 100, 300-mg tablets
- 100 mg/ml for parenteral administration

**Action and Use:** Exact mechanism of action is unknown but appears that drug causes disruption of cell wall in *Mycobacterium* undergoing cell division; occurs primarily by inhibition of mycolic acid synthesis. Used in treatment of tuberculosis with at least one other antituberculosis drug. This drug is used alone to prevent tuberculosis in household members or other close contacts of person recently diagnosed with tuberculosis, those with significant reaction to Mantoux skin test for tuberculosis, and those who fall into other priorities of the US Centers for Disease Control.

## Routes and Dosage:
*PO, IM:* Therapeutic: 10 to 20 mg/kg/day as single dose or every 12 hours. (Maximum dosage 300 to 500 mg/day)
*PO:* Prophylaxis: 10 mg/kg/day as single dose or every 12 hours for 12 months. (Maximum dosage 300 mg/day)

**Absorption and Fate:** Well absorbed from GI tract and IM site. Peak level: oral, 1 to 2 hours. Well distributed to body tissues and fluids including CSF. Half-life: 0.5 to 1.6 hours (fast acetylators), 2 to 5 hours (slow acetylators). Inactivated by liver mainly by acetylation and dehydrazination. Acetylation rate is metabolic process that inactivates the drug. This determines and thus effects plasma drug concentration, slow acetylation increases plasma level, possibly increasing side effects. Fast acetylators have increased chance of drug-induced hepatitis and drug may be less effective. Genetically determined with high percentage of Egyptian, Israeli, Scandinavian, and about 50% of whites and blacks are slow acetylators. 80% of Eskimos, Japanese, Chinese, and American Indians are rapid acetylators. This may correlate with drug-induced hepatotoxicity. Excreted primarily by urine.

**Contraindications and Precautions:** Pregnancy category C. Drug excreted in breast milk; nursing infants should be closely observed for drug side effects. Contraindicated in hypersensitivity to drug, acute liver disease, or previous isoniazid hepatic injury. Use caution with chronic liver disease, alcoholism, seizure disorders, or severe renal impairment.

## Side Effects:

*CNS:* **peripheral neuritis** (usually preceded by paresthesia of hands and feet, especially in malnourished, alcoholics, diabetics); **seizures**, ataxia, stupor, memory impairment, loss of self control. *GI:* nausea, epigastric distress, vomiting, dry mouth. *Hepatic:* transient rise in SGPT, SGOT, bilirubin, **hepatitis** (rare). *GU:* urinary retention. *Hemic:* agranulocytosis, **thrombocytopenia**, eosinophilia, **aplastic anemia**, leukopenia, **hemolytic anemia**. *Musculoskeletal:* rheumatic syndrome with arthralgia. *Endocrine:* hyperglycemia, metabolic acidosis. *Other:* Hypersensitivity: fever, morbilliform, purpuric, maculopapular or exfoliative rashes, lymphadenopathy, vasculitis (rare, occurs in 3 to 7 weeks), systemic lupus erythematosus-like syndrome, gynecomastia in males; Local: IM irritation at site.

## Nursing Implications:

*Assess:* Obtain diagnostic cultures and x-rays. Obtain baseline liver function studies: SGPT, SGOT, bilirubin, and weight. Ophthalmologic and hematopoietic status should also be obtained.

*Administer: PO:* Give 1 hour before meals or 2 hours after, absorption decreased with food. If GI irritation occurs, take with food. Tablet can be crushed and mixed with food. Drug usually given concurrently with at least one other antitubercular drug for tuberculous treatment; therapy length varies from 6 to 9 months. Usually given alone for preventive therapy for about 6 to 12 months. *IM:* Crystallization of parenteral form may occur at low temperatures, warm to room temperature to redissolve crystals. Usually only given for several dosages when oral form is not tolerated. Give deep IM. Injection may be painful, massaging site after injection may relieve pain.

*Monitor:* Assess for symptoms of hepatotoxicity (anorexia, fatigue, fever, malaise, nausea, vomiting, diarrhea, weight loss), by the time other side effects occur (dark urine and jaundice) child may have hepatitis (more likely to occur in those over 35 years). Periodic hepatic tests and patient assessment should be done monthly. Symptoms of drug induced hepatitis usually occur 3 to 6 months after therapy, but may occur at any time. Obtain periodic hematopoietic and ophthalmologic examinations. In the malnourished, diabetic, or predisposed to neuropathy, pyridoxine may be given to decrease neurological effects.

*Patient Teaching:* Report any symptoms of side effects, especially hepatic symptoms, immediately to physician. Medication must be taken as prescribed. Importance for close medical follow-up. Do not take any OTC medications without consulting physician.

**Drug Interactions:** Alcohol causes increased risk for hepatotoxicity. This drug interferes with hepatic matabolism of phenytoin causing increased levels of phenytoin and possible toxicity. Other antitubercular agents, cycloserine or ethionamide, may have additive effect with isoniazid causing adverse neurological effects. Aluminum hydroxide gel decreases adsorption of this drug, give 1 hour apart. Disulfiram and this drug have resulted in coordination problems and psychotic episodes. BCG vaccine may not be reliable because isoniazide inhibits multiplication of BCG.

**Food Interactions:** Tyramine-containing foods: aged cheeses, smoked fish, beef or chicken livers, yeast vitamin supplements, broad bean pods, could cause palpitations, flushing, and hypertension. Histamine containing foods: tuna, sauerkraut, skipjack fish, yeast extracts, may cause headache, rash, palpitations, hypotension, flushing, and diarrhea.

**Laboratory Test Interference:** False-positive for urine glucose with Benedict's reagent and Clinitest.

**Storage Requirements:** Store at 15 to 30°C (59 to 86°F); protect from light, air, and excessive heat.

---

## □ ISOPROTERENOL  (eye-soe-proe-ter′e-nole)

(Aerolone, Dey-Dose, Dispos-A-Med, Medihaler-Iso, Norisodrine, Isuprel, Vapo-Iso)

**Combination Products:** Duo-Medihaler

**Classification:** beta-adrenergic agonist, sympathomimetic, bronchodilator

**Action and Use:** This β-adrenergic stimulant reduces peripheral resistance and increases the force of cardiac contraction without producing vasoconstriction. Relaxes bronchial smooth muscle and creates peripheral vasodilation. Used to relieve bronchospasm, especially in asthmatics and during some general anesthesia. Used as a cardiac stimulant during cardiac arrest and some forms of shock.

**Available Preparations:**
- 10, 15-mg sublingual tablets
- 0.02 mg/ml, 0.2 mg/ml ampules for parenteral use
- 80 μg (0.2%), 120 μg (0.25%), 131 μg (0.25%) metered spray
- 160-μg metered spray with phenylephrine

Also in some oral combination products for treatment of asthma.

**Absorption and Fate:** Absorption after parenteral or inhalation routes is rapid. Sublingual tablets have unreliable absorption. The oral drug is rapidly metabolized in GI tract. After being metabolized, the drug is excreted primarily in the urine. Children may metabolize the drug more quickly than adults. Peak level is immediate for IV and inhalation routes. After IV administration, effects last only minutes and after SL, effects last 2 hours.

**Routes and Dosages:** Sublingual (SL tablets also given PR), IV, Inhalation.
*SL:*
- Cardiac Stimulant: 5 mg; adjust according to patient response

- Bronchospasm: 5 to 10 mg TID; not to exceed 30 mg/day

*IV:*

- Cardiac Arrest or Arrhythmia: 2.5 μg/minute or 0.1 μg/kg/minute initially; adjust according to patient response
- Bradycardia in Advanced Life Support: 0.1 mg/kg/minute initially; increased as needed; not to exceed 1 μg/kg/minute
- Complete Heart Block after VSD Closure: IV bolus of 0.01 to 0.03 mg (0.5 to 1.5 ml of 1:50,000) in infants
- Status Asthmaticus: 0.08 to 1.7 μg/kg/minute; investigational use

IV dosages established by clinicians rather than manufacturers.

*Inhalation:*

- Asthma: metered spray: 120 to 262 μg (1 to 2 inhalations of 0.2 or 0.25 % solution); repeat in 1 to 5 minutes if needed. Not to exceed 4 to 6 treatments/24 hours. For maintenance treatments, 4 to 6 treatments/day
- Hand-Bulb Nebulizer: 5 to 15 deep inhalations 0.5% solution; repeat 5 to 10 minutes if needed. Not to exceed 5 treatments/day
- IPPB: 2.5 ml of 0.05% solution up to 5 times/day given over 10 to 15 minutes. Not to exceed 2 doses in any hour
- Nebulizer Solution: 6 to 12 inhalation of 0.025%; repeat 15 minutes, no more than 3 treatments at once; not to exceed 8 treatment/24 hours

**Contraindications and Precautions:** Pregnancy category C. Cautious use in pregnancy and lactation as effects are unknown. Contraindicated for use with tachycardia caused by cardiac glycoside toxicity. Use in cardiac arrest only in temporary control of atropine-resistant bradycardia. Not used in shock if peripheral vascular bed is already vasodilated. Not to be given with epinephrine or other sympathomimetic bronchodilators. Preparations with sulfite contraindicated in those allergic to this substance. Use with caution in diabetes, those with cardiovascular or renal disease, in hyperthyroidism, pheochromocytoma, or those hypersensitive to sympathomimetic amines. Use cautiously or not at all in patients receiving cyclopropane or halogenated hydrocarbon general anesthetic.

**Side Effects:**

*CNS:* nervousness, weakness, anxiety, insomnia, dizziness, headache. *CV:* **tachycardia**, chest pain, **palpitation**, **decreased blood pressure** after slight increase in blood pressure, irregular pulse. *GI:* nausea, vomiting, ulcerations, teeth damage (from SL tablets), dry mouth, parotid swelling, pinkish red saliva with SL product. *Skin:* pale cold skin, increased sweating.

**Nursing Implications:**

*Assess:* Baseline vital signs especially pulse and blood pressure. Assess EKG, $PCO_2$, bicarbonate, pH, CVP, urine output.

*Administer:* **SL:** Oral care to avoid mucosal irritation and tooth damage. *IV:* Generally diluted to 1 to 2 μg/ml by diluting 1 to 10 ml of 0.2 mg/ml solution with 500 ml 5% dextrose; solution contains 0.4 to 4 μg/ml. Compatible with most IV fluids. If mixed in solution with other drugs, use immediately if resulting pH is above 6 (isoproterenol has greater stability in alkaline, less stability in acidic solutions). Physician orders infusion rate; infusion control device used.

*Monitor:* For IV form monitor EKG, CVP, vital signs, urine output constantly. Blood pH and $Pco_2$ are monitored.

*Patient Teaching:* For SL or inhalation, teach side effects as systemic absorption may occur. These effects should be reported immediately. See care provider if more than 3 aerosol treatments/ day are needed. Perform oral care after SL tablet or inhalation. Saliva may appear pinkish red after inhalation or SL doses; this is a harmless effect. Tolerance and rebound bronchospasm result from frequent use. Product will need to be withdrawn for a time if this occurs; not given in ever greater doses.

**Drug Interactions:** Effects of isoproterenol are decreased by propranolol and other β-adrenergic blockers. Can cause arrhythmias if given to those receiving cyclopropane or hydrogenated hydrocarbon general anesthesia. Additive cardiac effects with epinephrine and other sympathomimetics. Potential cardiotoxic effects with theophylline.

**Storage Requirements:** Store at 15 to 30°C (59 to 86°F) in light-resistant containers, tightly covered. Do not use if discolored or if a precipitate is present.

---

## □ KANAMYCIN                                    (kan-a-mye'sin)

(Anamid, Kantrex, Klebcil)

**Classification:** aminoglycoside

## Available Preparations:
- 500-mg capsules
- 37.5 mg, 250 mg, 333 mg/ml for parenteral administration

**Action and Use:** Derived from *Streptomyces kanamyceticus*, inhibits protein synthesis by binding irreversibly to bacterial ribosomes. Its bactericidal spectrum of activity is somewhat narrower because it has no activity at all against *Pseudomonas* species, but it is active against *Escherichia coli, Proteus, Klebsiella, Enterobacter*, and *Serratia*. Used to treat infections of bone, skin, urinary tract, GI tract. Oral preparation used as preoperative agent for bowel surgery.

## Routes and Dosage:
*PO IM, IV:*
- birth to 7 days, ≤ 2000 g: 7.5 mg/kg every 12 hours
- birth to 7 days, > 2000 g: 7.5 mg/kg every 8 to 12 hours

- 1 to 4 weeks, ≤ 2000 g: 10 mg/kg every 12 hours
- 1 to 4 weeks, > 2000 g: 10 mg/kg every 8 hours
- over 4 weeks: 15 to 30 mg/kg/day in equally divided doses every 8 to 12 hours

Note: Dosages are based on normal renal function. Treatment duration should be limited to 7 to 10 days.

**Absorption and Fate:** Absorption: about 1% orally, IM rapid and complete. Distributed mainly to extracellular fluids and CSF concentrations may be increased 50% when meninges are inflamed. Peak levels: in minutes of IM injection and at end of IV infusion. Half-life: 2 to 4 hours with normal renal function, about 28 to 80 hours impaired renal function, neonates 6 to 18 hours. Protein binding low; drug is primarily excreted in urine and minimal amount in feces.

**Contraindications and Precautions:** Pregnancy category D and safety during lactation not established. Use caution in premature infants and neonates due to renal immaturity. Contraindicated in hypersensitivity to this drug or other aminoglycosides; oral route in intestinal obstruction and systemic infections, or in renal failure. Use caution in renal function impairment, botulism, hypocalcemia, hypomagnesemia, hypokalemia, dehydration, or eighth cranial nerve impairment.

**Side Effects:**
*CNS:* **neurotoxicity**: numbness, tingling, muscle twitching, seizures **neuromuscular blockade**: muscle weakness, respiratory depression, lethargy, headache. *GI:* nausea, vomiting, loss of appetite, **malabsorption syndrome** (long-term oral therapy). *GU:* **nephrotoxicity**: blood or casts in urine, oliguria, increased thirst, proteinuria, increased BUN, increased serum creatinine, decreased urine creatinine clearance, decreased specific gravity, **renal failure**. *Skin:* itching, redness, edema. *Hemic:* eosinophilia, anemia, leukopenia, agranulocytosis, thrombocytopenia. *Sensory:* ophthalmic: burning, stinging, blurred vision, photosensitivity; **ototoxicity**: eighth cranial nerve damage: hearing loss, vertigo, loss of balance, tinnitus; **cochlear damage** causing high frequency hearing loss detected only at first by audiometric testing. *Other:* Local: pain at site of injection.

**Nursing Implications:**
*Assess:* Obtain cultures and sensitivity before treatment, but can start treatment before results. Obtain baseline weights, BUN, creatinine levels, and hearing tests before therapy.
*Administer: PO:* Use as preparation preoperatively for bowel surgery; dosage used is that for adults. May take without regard to meals. Capsules may be taken apart and contents mixed with small amount of food or fluid. *IM, IV:* Solution may darken with age; this does not indicate loss of potency. *IM:* Injection may be painful. *IV:* Do not give IV push because of possible neuromuscular blockade. Recommended concentration for continuous infusion is 25

mg/10 ml and infuse not more than 7.5 mg/minute, usually over 30 to 60 minutes. Check with pharmacists for infusion concentrations for infants. Compatible in the following solutions for injection: $D_5W$, $D_5W/0.2\%$ NS, $D_5W/0.45\%$ NS, NS, LR, amino acids 4.25%/$D_{25}\%$. Do not premix with other medications and infuse separately. After infusion, flush line with normal saline or 5% dextrose in water.

***Monitor:*** Observe for signs of respiratory depression with IV infusion. Peak blood levels can be drawn 1 hour after IM dosage and 30 minutes to 1 hour after infusion ends. Desirable peak concentrations should be 15 to 30 μg/ml and maximum trough concentrations (drawn just before next dose) should be 5 μg/ml. Measurements should not exceed 5 to 10 μg/ml and levels above 30 to 35 μg/ml are associated with increased incidence of toxicity. Maintain daily hydration level for child's age. If no response in 3 to 5 days, therapy should be discontinued. Monitor child's hearing levels daily (can use ticking watch). Renal function assessed by I & O, daily weights, urine specific gravity, urinalysis, creatinine levels, and BUN. Report any side effects immediately to physician. Observe for superinfections. If therapy continues for more than 10 days, daily renal function tests and weekly audiograms should be obtained.

**Drug Interactions:** Increased chance for ototoxicity and nephrotoxicity with amphotericin B, salicylates, bacitracin (parenteral), bumetanide (parenteral), carmustine, cephalothin, cisplatin, cyclosporine, (potent diuretics such as ethacrynic acid, furosemide, mannitol, sodium mercaptomerin), paromomycin, streptozocin, and vancomycin when used concurrently with kanamycin. Masked symptoms of ototoxicity can occur when used with dimenhydrinate. Kanamycin used in combination with aminoglycosides or capreomycin increases chance for ototoxicity. Decreased renal clearance occurs with neonates when given indomethacin and this drug. Nephrotoxicity and neuromuscular blockade increase with use of methoxyflurane or polymyxins. Neuromuscular blockade possible with halogenated hydrocarbon inhalation anesthetic, citrate-anticoagulated blood transfusion, and neuromuscular blocking agents combined with kanamycin. This drug may increased respiratory depressant effects of opioid and analgesics. Parenteral penicillin, carbenicillin, and ticarcillin inactivates kanamycin.

**Laboratory Test Interference:** LDH may be increased and serum sodium decreased.

**Storage Requirements:** Store at 15 to 30°C (59 to 86°F), protect from freezing.

---

## □ KETOCONAZOLE (ke-to-con′a-zol)

(Nizoral)

**Classification:** antiinfective, antifungal

## Available Preparations:
- 100 mg/5 ml
- 200-mg tablets
- 2% cream for topical application

**Action and Use:** Appears to alter cellular membrane increasing fungal cell wall permeability, causing loss of essential intracellular elements. It interferes with cell enzyme synthesis. It also appears to inhibit testicular testosterone synthesis for 2 to 12 hours in normal dosages. Used to treat candidiasis, mucocandidiasis, candiduria, histoplasmosis, paracoccidioidomycosis.

## Routes and Dosage:
**PO:** over 2 years: 3.3 to 6.6 mg/kg/day as single dose
**Topical:** Safe use has not been established in children. Some clinicians have used this drug in limited numbers of children without ill effects. Dosage: Apply sufficient amount to affected areas once daily.

**Absorption and Fate:** Rapidly and well absorbed from GI tract; however, bioavailability depends on pH of gastric contents; an increase in pH may cause decrease in drug adsorption. Peak levels: 1 to 2 hours. Drug distributed to bile, urine, saliva, synovial fluid, cerumen; CNS penetration is minimal and unpredictable. 84 to 99% bound to plasma proteins; biphasic half-life, first phase 2 hours, terminal phase 8 hours. Excreted primarily in feces and about 13% in urine.

**Contraindications and Precautions:** Pregnancy category C. Contraindicated in breast-feeding, those under 2 years, hypersensitivity to drug, and fungal meningitis. Use only when necessary in children. Use caution in achlorhydria, alcoholism, reduced hepatic function.

## Side Effects:
**CNS:** headache, dizziness, lethargy, nervousness, weakness, paresthesia, **bulging fontanelles**, tinnitus. **GI:** nausea, vomiting, abdominal pain, diarrhea, constipation. **Hepatic:** increased SCOT, SGPT, alkaline phosphatase, **hepatotoxicity. Skin:** rash, dermatitis, purpura, urticaria, photophobia; topical. irritation, pruritus, stinging. **Hemic:** thrombocytopenia, leukopenia, **hemolytic anemia. Musuloskeletal:** arthralgia. **Other:** bilateral gynecomastia in men.

## Nursing Implications:
**Assess:** Organism should be identified but therapy may be started before results. Before therapy, obtain hepatic function tests.
**Administer: PO:** Giving with food or meals may decrease GI distress. Tablets can be crushed and capsules taken apart, mixed with small amounts of food or fluid. In those with achlorhydria, better absorption of drug will occur by dissolving tablet in 4 ml of 0.2 N hydrochloric acid. Further dilute with 30 to 60 ml of fruit juice and have child take through straw. Follow with water and swish in mouth, swallow.

*Monitor:* Observe for side effects of hepatotoxicity, pale stools, dark urine, nausea, anorexia, jaundice, weight loss; report to physician immediately. Frequent (usually every month) liver function tests should be obtained during long therapy. Treatment continues until negative cultures and may vary 1 to 4 weeks to 6 to 12 months depending on infecting organism.

*Patient Teaching:* Therapy requires close monitoring by physician. Report any side effects immediately. Avoid exposure to sunlight or sunlamps due to potential photosensitivity. Do not take antacid, OTC medications for gastric distress, or other OTC drugs without consulting physician.

**Drug Interactions:** Concurrent ingestion of alcohol and this drug causes flushing and tachycardia. Antacids, cimetidine, antimuscarinics, or other drugs that decrease gastric acid should be given 2 hours after this drug. Concurrent administration of other hepatotoxic drugs should be used with extreme caution. Do not give rifampin or isoniazid with this drug because it decreases serum levels of ketoconazole. Patients stabilized on coumarin who then receive this drug may note a decrease in prothrombin time. With phenytoin, mutual antagonism can occur. When given with theophylline, it may lower theophylline levels.

**Storage Requirements:** Store at 15 to 30°C (59 to 86°F) in tight containers.

---

## □ LACTULOSE                                          (lak'tyoo-lose)

(Cephulac, Chronulac)

**Classification:** ammonia detoxicant, laxative

**Available Preparations:** 3.33 g/5 ml oral or rectal solution

**Action and Use:** Cathartic that also inhibits ammonia production by changing fecal flora and acidifying the colon. Used as laxative or to lower serum ammonia in patient with hepatic encephalopathy.

## Routes and Dosage:
**PO:**
- Laxative: over 12 years: 15 to 30 ml daily. (Maximum dosage 60 ml/day)
- Hepatic Encephalopathy: under 2 years: 2.5 to 10 ml/day in divided doses; over 2 years: 40 to 90 ml/day in divided doses

**Absorption and Fate:** Onset action 24 to 48 hours. Less than 3% adsorbed.

**Contraindications and Precautions:** Pregnancy category C. Use caution during lactation. Safe use for chronic constipation in children not established. Contraindicated in hypersensitivity to drug or on low galactose diet. Use caution in diabetes mellitus, those undergoing proctoscopy or colonoscopy (need cleansing enemas before taking drug as it causes an accumulation of hydrogen gas in the bowel).

## Side Effects:
*GI:* gaseous distention, abdominal cramping, anorexia, belching, diarrhea, flatulence. *Other:* **hypokalemia and dehydration** (in infants), **hypernatremia**

## Nursing Implications:
*Assess:* Assess blood ammonia level and serum electrolytes.
*Administer: PO:* Syrup: measure with calibrated measuring device. Syrup base contains lactose, galactose, and other sugars; it should be diluted with fruit juice because of its very sweet taste. Safe to use with diabetics because not systemically absorbed. Syrup darkens with exposure to light; discard cloudy or very dark solutions. Chilling increases viscosity. *Rectal:* Efficacy of retention enema is questionable; give orally rather than rectally for best results.
*Monitor:* Dosage reduced if diarrhea occurs. Assess for dehydration and hypernatremia. Maintain normal hydration level for child's age. Obtain periodic serum potassium if on long-term therapy. If given for ammonia elimination, fecal pH should be 5; this usually occurs if bowel pattern is about 3 soft stools per day while on drug. Response to medication positive when mental state clears, EEG patterns improve, and blood ammonia levels are reduced.
*Patient Teaching:* Slow onset of laxative effect; action occurs in colon. Do not use any other laxative. Report any symptoms of diarrhea, sign of overdosage. For ammonia, excretion should have 2 to 3 soft stools per day.

**Drug Interactions:** Do not use other laxatives that may interfere with therapeutic evaluation. Neomycin and other antiinfective agents may decrease colonic bacteria necessary to metabolize lactulose; monitor usage of drugs closely.

**Food Interactions:** Do not use with low-galactose diet.

**Storage Requirements:** Store at 15 to 30°C (59 to 86°F).

---

## □ LEUCOVORIN                      (loo-koe-vor'in)

(Citrovorum Factor, Folinic Acid, Wellcovorin)

**Classification:** folic acid antagonist antidote, antianemic

## Available Preparations:
- 5, 10, 15, 25-mg tablets
- 3 mg/ml, 5 mg/ml vials for parenteral use
- 25, 50, 100, 350-mg vials for parenteral use

**Action and Use:** This reduced form of folic acid protects normal cells from action of antineoplastics such as methotrexate. Used to treat methotrexate, trimethoprim, and pyremethamine toxicity and for treatment of megaloblastic anemia of sprue and in infancy.

**Routes and Dosages:**
**PO, IM, IV:** Folic Acid Antagonist Antidote: 10 mg/m² parenterally within 24 hours of methotrexate; then 10 mg/m² PO q6h × 72 hours or until methotrexate serum level is below $5 \times 10^{-8}$ M. If, 24 hours after methotrexate dose, serum creatine is 50% above baseline or if methotrexate serum level is over $5 \times 10^{-6}$ M, dosage of leucovarin is increased to 100 mg/m² q3h until methotrexate serum level is below $5 \times 10^{-8}$ M.
**IM:** Trimethoprim and Pyrimethamine Antidote: 400 μg–5 mg with each drug dose prophylaxis or 5 to 15 mg/day for treatment.
**IM:** Megaloblastic Anemia: 1 mg/day

**Absorption and Fate:** Well absorbed from GI tract. Concentrated in CSF and liver. Metabolized in intestine and liver. Excreted in urine. Peak level after PO form about 1 3/4 hours and after IM 3/4 hour. Onset of action is up to 20 minutes for IM and PO, 5 minutes for IV. Duration of action: 3 to 6 hours. Half-life: 6.2 hours. Normal folate level is 0.005 to 0.015 μg/ml.

**Contraindications and Precautions:** Pregnancy category C. Drug is used for megaloblastic anemia in pregnancy. Contraindicated in pernicious anemia of vitamin $B_{12}$ deficiency. Cautious use in children on seizure medication, renal dysfunction, dehydration, aciduria

**Side Effects:**
**Skin:** rash, hives, **allergic response**. **Respiratory:** wheezing as allergic response. **Hemic:** thrombocytopenia

**Nursing Implications:**
**Assess:** Serum creatinine, creatinine clearance, urine pH.
**Administer:** Check preparation carefully; this is folinic acid and should not be confused with folic acid. **PO:** Powder for oral solution is reconstituted with aromatic elixir and solution is 1 mg/ml. **IM, IV:** Parenteral solutions used when dosage is over 25 mg or when nausea and vomiting or other GI complications are present. Reconstitute powder for injection with 5 ml sterile or bacteriostatic water; solution is 10 mg/ml. Maximum IV infusion rate is 16 ml (160 mg)/minute. Reconstituted solution stable of 14 days if refrigerated at 2 to 8°C (35 to 46°F) or for 7 days at 15 to 30°C (59 to 86°F). For methotrexate rescue, treatment must begin within 24 hours and preferably 4 hours of methotrexate therapy. It is given at least 1 hour after methotrexate. High-dose methotrexate therapy is not instituted without leucovorin readily available. Patient is kept well hydrated by IV.
**Monitor:** I & O. Serum creatinine and creatinine clearance q12h. Serum methotrexate levels q12h. Leucovorin blood level should be equal or greater than methotrexate blood level. Urinary pH q6h at least. Drug usually only given in hospital setting.

**Drug Interactions:** Leukovorin can interfere with action of anticonvulsants, such as barbiturates, primidone, phenytoin, therefore, should be used cautiously in child on these drugs for seizure control; serum levels of anticonvulsants monitored closely. Increased CNS depression with oral solution and other CNS depressants due to high alcohol levels in the drug.

**Storage Requirements:** Store at 15 to 30°C (59 to 86°F) in tightly closed, light-resistant container.

---

## □ LEVOTHYROXINE SODIUM

(lee-voe-thye-rox'een)

(Eltroxin, Levoid, Levothroid, Levoxine, L-Thyroxine, Noroxine, Synthroid, $T_4$)

**Classification:** hormone, thyroid

**Available Preparations:**
- 12.5, 25, 50, 75, 100, 112, 125, 150, 175, 200, 300-μg tablet
- 200, 500 μg for parenteral administration

**Action and Use:** Synthetic hormone used as replacement therapy for hypothyroidism. It increases metabolic rate of body tissues and is concerned with growth and differentiation of tissues. Lack of hormone not only causes retardation of growth, but retards the development of the brain and failure of ossification of epiphyses does not allow the skeletal systems to mature. Levothyroxine is preferred thyroid hormone because of its standardized hormonal content.

**Routes and Dosage:**
*PO:*
- premature infants, < 2kg or infants at risk for cardiac failure: starting dose of 25 μg/day; may be increased to 50 μg/day in 4 to 6 weeks
- birth to 6 months: 25 to 50 μg/day or 8 to 10 μg/kg daily
- 6 to 12 months: 50 to 75 μg/day or 6 to 8 μg/kg daily
- 1 to 5 years: 75 to 100 μg/day or 5 to 6 μg/kg daily
- 6 to 12 years: 100 to 150 μg/day or 4 to 5 μg/kg daily
- over 12 years: over 150 μg/day or 2 to 3 μg/kg daily until the adult dose is reached (150 to 200 μg/day)

*IM, IV:* Replacement therapy is 1/2 to 3/4 child's normal dosage.

**Absorption and Fate:** Absorption of PO form incomplete, variable when taken with food (50 to 70%). Bound to plasma proteins and deiodinated in peripheral tissues with small amounts metabolized in liver. Half-life: 6 to 7 days. Time to peak therapeutic level 3 to 4 weeks.

**Contraindications and Precautions:** Pregnancy category A and minimal amounts of exogenous thyroid excreted in breast milk. Contraindicated in untreated thyrotoxicosis, acute myocardial infarction, uncorrected adrenal insufficiency, sensitivity to lactose or dye tartrazine (Levoxine and Synthroid 100, 200, 300-g tablets). Use caution with cardiovascular disease, hypertension, diabetes mellitus or insipidus, adrenal cortical insufficiency.

**Side Effects:** Dose-related. **CNS:** nervousness, headache, insomnia, clumsiness, hand tremors, irritability, severe headache (rare, pseudotumor cerebri). **CV:** palpitations, tachycardia, arrhythmias, hypertension, angina pectoris. **Resp:** shortness of breath. **GI:** change in appetite, vomiting, weight loss or gain, diarrhea, constipation. **GU:** menstrual irregularities. **Skin:** dry puffy, rash or hives (allergic reaction), partial loss of hair during first few months of therapy, usually transient. **Musculoskeletal:** muscle aches, leg cramps, excessive doses can result in craniosynostosis in infants. **Other:** fever, sensitivity to heat, sweating, coldness, weakness

## Nursing Implications:

**Assess:** Tests (serum $T_4$ and TSH) should be obtained as soon after birth as possible if congenital hypothyroidism is suspected to prevent development deficiency. Establish baseline for bone age, growth, psychomotor development before treatment. Obtain infant's head circumference and note size of fontanels.

**Administer: PO:** Take on an empty stomach in early AM to increase absorption and decrease insomnia. Tablet can be crushed, and mixed with small amount of food or fluid (infant's formula can be used). **IM, IV:** Drug can be given IM this route usually not used because of erratic absorption. Reconstitute 0.9% sodium chloride (without preservatives) for injection; do not use bacteriostatic sodium chloride. Shake to dissolve contents and use immediately; discard unused portion. Initial dilution is 100 mg/ml given IV push over 30 to 60 seconds. Do not infuse through IV fluids or mix with any other drugs.

**Monitor:** Monitor BP and P in child taking this medication for cretinism. Regular evaluations of bone age, growth, psychomotor, and development levels, TSH, $T_4$, $T_3$, free thyroxine index levels should be done to monitor child's response to drug. Obtain infant's head circumference and check fontanel closure with each health visit or as physician directs. Observe for signs of overdosage: headache, insomnia, nervousness, tremors, tachycardia, palpitations, arrhythmias, angina pectoris, hypertension, change in appetite, nausea, diarrhea, leg cramps, weight loss, sweating, heat intolerance, fever. Do not switch brands of levothyroxine because of potential difference between brands. If switching from levothyroxine to liothyronine, discontinue levothyroxine first before starting with liothyronine; start with small dose and increase in small increments until residual effects from levothyroxine have subsided. If switching from liothyronine to levothyroxine, start with levothyroxine several days before discontinuing liothyronine.

**Patient Teaching:** Take medication only as prescribed. Take on empty stomach the same time of day to keep blood level of drug constant. Usually needed for lifelong treatment; do not stop taking medication without consulting physician, it could be life threatening. Do not switch brands after stabilized on medication; trade drugs do not all have same bioequivalents. Do not use generic levothyroxine. Teach signs of side effects. Partial loss of hair may occur but normal hair growth will usually return in several months. Do not take any OTC or other medications without consulting physician. Close medical follow-up to monitor thyroid levels, growth and development is necessary. Inform dentists, other physicians, or health-care providers child is on this medication before any treatments.

**Drug Interactions:** May require an increased need for insulin with diabetics using this drug. With anticoagulants, coumadin dosages may need to be lowered while on thyroid; base dosage on prothrombin time. Use of this drug and ketamine may produced marked hypertension and tachycardia. Phenytoin used with thyroid may cause a release of free thyroid resulting in tachycardia. Use with somatrem or somatropin may accelerate epiphyseal maturation. Cholestyramine resin impairs this drug's absorption, administer 4 hours apart. Those with coronary artery disease who receive this drug and sympathomimetic agents may precipitate episode of coronary insufficiency.

**Laboratory Test Interference:** Radio-iodine uptake tests while on this medication produces low uptake values that may not reflect a true decrease in hormone synthesis. Discontinue drug for 4 weeks for a true reading.

**Storage Requirements:** Store at 15 to 30°C (59 to 86°F) in a tight, light-resistant container.

---

## ☐ LIDOCAINE                                    (lye'doe-kane)

(Anestacon, Dilocaine, L-Caine, Lida-Mantle, Lidoject, LidoPen, Nervocaine, Nulicaine, Octocaine, Ultracaine, Xylocaine, Xylocard)

**Classification:** local anesthetic, antiarrhythmic (class IB)

**Available Preparations:**
- 10, 20, 40, 100, 200 mg/ml vials for parenteral use
- 2, 4, 8 mg/ml with 5% dextrose vials for parenteral use
- 0.5%, 1%, 1.5%, 2%, 4% vials (local anesthetic)
- 1.5%, 5% with 7.5% dextrose (local anesthetic)
- 0.5%, 1%, 1.5%, 2% with epinephrine (local anesthetic)
- Aerosol, jelly, ointment, cream, oral and topical solution; all for topical anesthetic effect

**Action and Use:** Depresses myocardial activity by acting on the tissue to suppress automaticity, delay conduction, and decrease depolarization and excitability. Depresses the CNS, creating anticonvulsant, sedative, antitussive, and analgesic effects. Used to treat ventricular cardiac arrhythmias during cardiac surgery, cardiac catheterization, and digitalis toxicity. Used for anesthetic by local infiltration, spinal, or topical application such as is dental work, esophagus, throat, and other areas. Used to treat nonresponsive status epilepticus, although not approved by the FDA for this purpose.

**Routes and Dosages:** IM, IV, infiltration, nerve block, epidural, caudal, spinal, saddle block, topical
*IV:*
- Antiarrhythmic: 0.5 to 1 mg/kg bolus; repeat PRN in 5 to 10 minutes. Maintenance Infusion: 10 to 50 μg/kg/minute may be started if needed; not to exceed 4 mg/minute. If solution for direct IV infusion is used, loading dose is 1 mg/kg at rate of 25 to 50 mg/minute; repeat in 5 minutes PRN: total dose not to exceed 3 mg/kg.
- Advanced Life Support: 1 mg/kg bolus; if not corrected, an additional bolus of 1 mg/kg is given followed by maintenance infusion of 20 to 50 μg/kg/minute.
- Status Epilepticus: 1 mg/kg bolus; 0.5 mg/kg 2 minutes after completion of first injection PRN; maintenance infusion of 30 μg/kg/minute.

Doses are established by clinicians rather than manufacturers.
*IM:* pediatric dosage not established

***Anesthetic Use:*** 0.5 to 2% depending on type of anesthetic. Generally 0.25 to 1% is maximum strength used for children. Doses of IV regional for children should not exceed 3 mg/kg. Only preservative-free solutions are used for epidural and caudal injection; a test dose of 2 to 5 ml is given 5 minutes before the dose.
***Topical:*** 2.5 to 5%

**Absorption and Fate:** Rapid absorption. Metabolized by the liver and excreted in the urine. 60 to 80% protein bound. Peak level is reached soon after bolus IV infusion; a continuous infusion is then generally started. Duration: 10 to 20 minutes after IV. Distribution half-life is 8 minutes; elimination half-life is 100 minutes. After local application peak levels are reached in 2 to 5 minutes. Therapeutic serum level for suppression of ventricular arrhythmia is 1.5 to 5 μg/ml (take serum level sample 5 to 6 hours after infusion has begun). Level exceeding 5 μg/ml is toxic.

**Contraindications and Precautions:** Pregnancy category B. Crosses placenta but no known hazards associated with use in pregnancy or lactation. Safe use in children has not been established. Use of LidoPen Auto-Injector is not recommended in children weighing less than 50 kg. Contraindicated with history of hypersensitivity to amide type local anesthetics, in Adams-Stokes syndrome, severe heart block. Use with caution in patients with severe renal disease, liver disease, bradycardia, congestive heart failure, heart block, hypoxia, respiratory depression, shock, hypovolemia. Dosage is lowered in congestive heart failure or hepatic dysfunction.

**Side Effects:**
***CNS:*** drowsiness, dizziness, confusion, impaired vision, paresthesia, tremors, **seizures, coma.** ***CV:*** **bradycardia, hypotension,** thrombophlebitis at IV site. ***GI:*** nausea, vomiting. ***Respiratory:*** **respiratory arrest.** ***Sensory:*** tinnitus,

visual disturbance. *Other:* **hypersensitivity** reaction. Overdose: 6 to 8 µg/ml in serum: blurred vision, nausea and vomiting, tinnitus, tremors; over 8 µg/ml: dyspnea, dizziness, seizures, bradycardia, agitation, irritability, combativeness, delirium

## Nursing Implications:

*Assess:* Baseline vital signs should be taken.

*Administer:* Resuscitative drugs and equipment must be readily available. *IM:* This route not generally used in children. If used for older children, deltoid is preferred site; aspirate carefully. *IV:* Only lidocaine hydrochloride without epinephrine should be used IV. Read labels carefully and use only a preparation labeled for IV use. Usually 1 g is added to 1 L of 5% dextrose for a solution of 1 mg/ml. The syringes and single-dose vials of 40 or 200 mg/ml are to be used for preparation of infusion, not administered without added solution. The prepared solution is stable for 24 hours. Although lidocaine is compatible with some other additives, such as epinephrine, dopamine, isoproterenol, these other drugs may be changed by the pH of the solution, therefore, the solutions should be given directly after administration; consult package inserts. *Anesthetic:* Solution with preservative should not be used for epidural and caudal injection. Read labels carefully if handling bottles to be used to an anesthetist. Vials containing solutions without preservative should be discarded after use. Systemic effects may result from anesthetic use if inadvertent intravascular infusion occurs. A test dose may be used to evaluate proper placement of anesthetics. *Topical:* Apply to mouth with cotton swab or swish or gargle; solution is not to be swallowed. Use only in child old enough to follow these directions. Do not inhale. Do not spray throat unless prescribed. *Monitor:* Monitor patient carefully for CNS and CV side effects. Constant EKG and BP monitoring should be performed during IV infusion. Prolonged PR interval and QRS complex or arrhythmias necessitates stopping infusion. Serum electrolyte and lidocaine levels are measured.

*Patient Teaching:* Oral topical use of lidocaine may diminish gag reflex for up to 60 minutes. Caution against ingesting food, candy, or chewing gum for that time to avoid aspiration and oral trauma. For temporary use, only for toothache.

## Drug Interactions: Phenytoin and propranolol and other antiarrhythmics may increase cardiac depressant effect. Phenytoin may increase hepatic metabolism of the drug. Barbiturates may decrease the effects of lidocaine. Increased neuromuscular blocking effects with succinylcholine. Cimetidine and propranolol can reduce hepatic clearance of lidocaine, resulting in lidocaine toxicity; lidocaine levels must be monitored closely.

## Laboratory Test Interferences: Increased serum creatine kinase (CK), creatine phosphokinase (CPK).

## Storage Requirements: Store at 15 to 30°C (59 to 86°F). Avoid freezing and exposure to light.

☐ **LINCOMYCIN** (lin-koe-mye'sin)
**HYDROCHLORIDE**

(Lincocin)

**Classification:** antibiotic, antiinfective

**Available Preparations:**
- 250, 500-mg capsules
- 300 mg/ml for parenteral administration

**Action and Use:** Obtained from cultures of *Streptomyces lincolnensis* that inhibits protein synthesis by binding to 50S ribosomal subunit, inhibiting peptide formation. Active against many gm + organisms (staphylococci, pneumococci, and streptococci), anaerobes (such as *Bacteroides*), but is relatively inactive against gm − bacteria. Less active against susceptible organisms than clindamycin.

**Routes and Dosage:**
*PO:* over 1 month: 30 to 60 mg/kg/day every 6 to 8 hours
*IM:* over 1 month: 10 mg/kg every 12 to 24 hours
*IV:* over 1 month: 10 to 20 mg/kg/day in equally divided doses every 8 to 12 hours

**Absorption and Fate:** 30% of PO dose rapidly absorbed from GI tract. Peak levels: PO, 2 to 4 hour; IM, 30 minutes; and IV, at end of infusion. Distributed to body tissues and fluids with minimal amounts in CSF, even if meninges are inflamed. Half-life: 4 to 6.4 hours. Excreted in urine and feces.

**Contraindications and Precautions:** Pregnancy category B. Use during lactation not recommended. Do not use with neonates. Contraindicated in hypersensitivity to this drug, clindamycin, or liver disease. Use with caution with history of GI disease, especially colitis or renal impairment.

**Side Effects:**
*CNS:* headache, vertigo. *GI:* nausea, vomiting, abdominal pain, diarrhea, tenesmus, stomatitis, glossitis, pruritus ani, **pseudomembranous colitis**. *Hepatic:* transient increase SGOT, serum bilirubin, alkaline phosphatase *GU:* azotemia, **oliguria, proteinuria** (rare and relationship to drug not established). *Hemic:* transient leukopenia, **neutropenia, thrombocytopenia**, eosinophilia, **agranulocytosis, thrombocytopenic purpura** (rare). *Other:* Hypersensitivity: rash, urticaria, pruritus, exfoliative dermatitis, erythema multiforme resembling Stevens-Johnson syndrome (rare); Local: IM pain, induration sterile abscess; IV pain, swelling, erythema, thrombophlebitis, **hypotension** and **cardiac arrest** if infused too rapidly

## Nursing Implications:

*Assess:* Assess previous allergy to this drug or clindamycin. Obtain cultures and sensitivity before treatment, but can start treatment before results. Obtain baseline hematological, renal, and hepatic data before long-term therapy.

*Administer: PO:* Give on empty stomach 1 hour before or 2 hours after meal. Capsules may be taken apart and mixed with a small amount of food or fluid. Give oral forms with as much fluid as child will take to decrease possibility of esophageal irritation. *IM:* Injection is painful. *IV:* Do not give IV push. May dilute medication further with compatible IV solution to dilution of 10 mg/ml and infuse over 1 hour or longer. Too rapid infusion can cause syncope, hypotension, and cardiac arrest. Compatible with $D_5W$, $D_{10}W$, $D_5W/$ NS, $D_{10}W$, NS, Ringer's solution, sodium lactate 1/6 molar, travert 10%, dextran 6% NS. Do not premix with kanamycin, novobiocin, phenytoin, ampicillin, or carbenicillin.

*Monitor:* Observe IM site for induration and abscess; IV site for extravasation and thrombophlebitis. During long-term therapy, assess CBC, liver, and renal function. If symptoms of severe diarrhea, abdominal cramps, and passage of blood or mucus occur, notify physician and discontinue drug until assessment of pseudomembranous colitis is obtained. Symptoms of colitis develop 2 to 9 days after therapy is initiated or can start several weeks after drug is stopped. Watch for symptoms of superinfections, primarily yeasts. Maintain fluid I & O for age group.

*Patient Teaching:* Take medication as prescribed and for duration of therapy. Inform physician of any side effects, especially diarrhea. If diarrhea occurs, do not take OTC, as it may interfere with this drug.

**Drug Interactions:** Lincomycin may enhance neuromuscular blocking properties of nondepolarizing muscle relaxants such as ether, tubocurarine, pancuronium, and atracurium. Kaolin reduces the absorption of lincomycin by as much as 90% in the GI tract. If given concurrently, give kaolin 2 hours before lincomycin dosage.

**Laboratory Test Interference:** Creatinine phosphokinase increased after IM.

**Storage Requirements:** Store capsules, parenteral at 15 to 30°C (59 to 86°F). Parenteral solution stable for 24 hours when diluted in above listed compatible fluids.

---

## □ LINDANE                                                                    (lin'dane)

(gBh, G-Well, Kwell, Kwelleda, Kwildane, Scabene)

**Classification:** scabicide, pediculocide

## Available Preparations:
- 1% topical lotion
- 1% topical cream
- 1% shampoo

## Action and Use:
A cyclic chlorinated hydrocarbon that is used to eradicate *Sarcoptes scabiei* (scabies), *Pediculus capitis* (head louse), *Pediculus corporis* (body louse), and *Phthirus pubis* (crab louse). When drug is adsorbed through arthropod's chitinous exoskeleton, it stimulates the nervous system causing seizures and death.

## Routes and Dosage:
*Topical:*
- Scabies and Body Louse: Apply thin layer of 1% preparation to all body parts from chin downward to feet. Wash off in 6 to 8 hours.
- Head Louse: Shampoo hair with 15 to 30 ml shampoo, leave on 4 to 10 minutes, rinse. May reapply in 7 days if necessary
- Crab Louse: Lather pubic area for 4 minutes rinse and dry (see Administration on how to apply)

## Absorption and Fate:
Absorbed slowly through intact skin, especially face, scalp, axillae, neck, scrotum, damaged or occluded skin. Absorption may also occur if inhaled, or inadvertently swallowed. Collected in body fat, metabolized by liver; excreted in feces and urine.

## Contraindications and Precautions:
Pregnancy category C. Use caution during lactation. Use caution in those under 10 years. Contraindicated in prematures and neonates, in hypersensitivity to drug or its components; in acutely inflamed, raw, or weeping skin surfaces. Use caution in seizures.

## Side Effects:
Low toxicity when applied appropriately; however, inhalation of vapors (especially chronic) may produce symptoms. *CNS:* headache, dizziness, clumsiness, restless, irritability, **seizures** (especially if ingested). *Resp:* inhalation of vapors: nausea, vomiting, irritation of nose throat and eyes. *Skin:* local irritation, rash, eczematous eruptions. *Other:* chronic vapor exposure: **fatal aplastic anemia, hematologic disorders**

## Nursing Implications:
*Assess:* Carefully inspect and note extent and amount of infestation. Scabies diagnosis confirmed by examining material from burrow track area. Pediculosis confirmed by finding lice or eggs (nits).

*Administer: Topical:* Use gloves to apply. Scabies and body louse: Bathe child with soap and water gently removing scales and crusts; towel dry. Apply very thin layer of medication (massaging in) from chin downward making sure that all skin surfaces are covered, e.g., folds of skin, hands, fingers, feet including toes and soles of feet. Do not apply to face, eyes, mucous membranes, or urethral meatus. Bathe child in 6 to 8 hours to remove medication.

Usually one dosage effective but can repeat in 1 week if reinfestations develop. Shampoo: Do not shampoo child's hair in bath tub or shower because of risk of getting shampoo in eyes and increasing systemic absorption. If hair has oil-based dressings, it should be washed with regular shampoo first, rinsed, towel dried. Apply about 15 to 30 ml shampoo to wet hair making sure entire scalp and hair covered; use just enough water to form lather. Take care not to get shampoo in eyes or other mucous membranes. Leave on for 4 to 10 minutes. Rinse hair well (cup or glass prevents shampoo from getting into eyes or ears); a rinsing solution of ½ water and ½ white vinegar may aid in nit removal. Using fine toothed comb, carefully comb hair to remove nits. Pay particular attention to nape of neck and area behind ears. Shampoo or topical preparations can be used to treat crab louse. If eyelashes are involved in louse infestation, use petroleum gel as ordered; do not use drug. Lindane can be repeated in 7 days if necessary. With all infestations fresh bedding should be placed on bed; then all bedding, personal clothes, and towels that child used should be washed in hot water and dried on hot dryer setting. Combs and hair care items can be washed in solution of drug. Items that cannot be washed should be dry cleaned (stuffed animals, etc.) or placed in dryer for 20 minutes on hot setting. For scabies, if child sleeps with another child, he too should be treated. Some clinicians believe the entire household should be treated. For pediculosis, all family members should be treated.

*Monitor:* If child hospitalized during this infestation, take proper isolation precautions used by agency. Assess skin for healing and notify physician if condition does not improve or worsens. Recheck child in 1 week for symptoms of disease. Notify schools, nursery schools, or day-care centers.

*Patient Teaching:* Parent and child should understand that this is a contagious condition and why it has to be treated. Head lice is a result of contact with someone with disease and not indicative of poor hygiene. Explain how to apply medicine and how to prevent reinfestations or spreading of scabies or pediculosis. Thick applications will not hasten healing and may cause irritation. School, day-care center, or child's preschool should be informed of infestation to prevent spread to other children. If child (with scabies or crab louse) is sexually active, sexual partner also needs treatment. Can cause fatal aplastic anemia if ingested.

**Storage Requirements:** Store at 15 to 30°C (59 to 86°F) in light-resistant containers.

---

## □ LOMUSTINE
(loe-mus'teen)

(CeeNU, CCNU)

**Classification:** antineoplastic, nitrosurea, alkylating agent

**Available Preparations:** 10, 40, 100-mg capsules

**Action and Use:** This nitrosurea derivative most likely works as an alkylating agent to inhibit DNA and RNA synthesis. It is cell-phase nonspecific. Used to treat brain tumors and disseminated Hodgkin's disease. Has been used experimentally in other carcinomas and topically in treatment of psoriasis and mycosis fungoides, although not approved for these uses by the FDA.

## Routes and Dosages:
*PO:* single dose of 75 to 130 mg/m², repeated at 6-week intervals if platelet and leukocyte levels are normal. Dosage reduced if given with other antineoplastics or if patient has bone marrow suppression, former chemotherapy, or radiation therapy.

**Absorption and Fate:** Rapidly absorbed from GI tract and distributed widely to body tissues. Crosses the blood-brain barrier and is present at 15 to 30% higher levels in CSF than in plasma. Metabolized and excreted mainly in urine. Peak level in 1 to 6 hours. Nearly all of dose metabolized in 1 hour. Half-life of metabolites is biphasic with 6 hours initially; 1 to 2 days terminally.

**Contraindications and Precautions:** Pregnancy category D. Safety in pregnancy has not been established and has been teratogenic in animals. Present in breast milk, therefore, women should not take the drug during lactation. Contraindicated in those with prior hypersensitivity to the drug or with chicken pox or herpes zoster infection. Use with caution in those with prior chemotherapy or radiation therapy, hepatic or renal dysfunction, myelosuppression, infections.

## Side Effects:
*CNS:* disorientation, lethargy, ataxia. *GI:* nausea, vomiting are frequent 45 minutes to 6 hours after dose; persist up to 36 hours; anorexia may follow for 2 to 3 days, stomatitis. *Respiratory:* pulmonary infiltrates and fibrosis with 600 to 1040-mg cumulative doses. *Hepatic:* hepatotoxicity with transient liver function test elevations. *GU:* azotemia, renal failure. *Skin:* alopecia; experimental topical administration can result in dermatitis, hyperpigmentation, pruritus, and can cause systemic myelosuppressive effects. *Hemic:* Delayed **leukopenia** 6 weeks after dose, lasting 1 to 2 weeks; thrombocytopenia 4 weeks after dose, lasting 1 to 2 weeks; decreased hematocrit

## Nursing Implications:
*Assess:* Obtain history of previous chemotherapy or radiation therapy. Obtain baseline CBC, hepatic, and renal function tests.
*Administer:* This drug has potentially severe toxic effects and should be given only under the supervision of a physician with training and experience in cancer chemotherapy. The drug's potential for toxic effects on health-care personnel as well as patients necessitates careful handling during preparation and administration. Before administration of subsequent doses, be sure leukocyte and platelet levels are adequate (see Monitor).

*Monitor:* WBC and platelet counts must be done before each dose. Dosage reductions will be done per protocols of particular institution with possible following examples: If WBC count is 4000/mm³ and platelets are 100,000/mm³, dose is generally given. If WBC count is 3000 to 3900/mm³ and platelets 75,000 to 99,999/mm³, 75% of normal dose is generally given. If WBC count is 2000 to 2900/mm³ and platelets are 25,000 to 74,999/mm³, 50% of normal dose is generally given. If WBC count is under 2000/mm³ and platelets under 25,000/mm³, the dose is generally withheld. Monitor hepatic and renal function before subsequent doses by BUN, SGPT, SGOT, bilirubin, creatinine, LDH, uric acid. Monitor I & O. Watch for nausea and vomiting.

*Patient Teaching:* Take dose as ordered. Increase fluid intake. Take anti-emetics as needed if ordered for nausea and vomiting; vomiting usually improves in 24 hours. Prepare for possibility of alopecia, although this side effect is not as common with this drug as with many other antineoplastics. Prepare for darkening of skin. Avoid persons with infections such as colds, influenza, chicken pox for 2 to 4 weeks after a dose. Report signs of infection such as fever, sore throat, cough, malaise. Perform good oral hygiene.

**Drug Interactions:** Myelosuppressive effects may be greater if prior courses of lomustine or other antineoplastics or radiation therapy have been given. Suppresses immune response to immunization. Live virus vaccines must not be given, nor oral polio vaccine to those in close contact with the patient on this drug due to the chance of infection with a virus; these vaccines are delayed until at least 3 months after chemotherapy when the patient is in remission.

**Storage Requirements:** Keep in tightly closed containers at 15 to 30°C (59 to 86°F).

---

# □ LOPERAMIDE

(loe-per'a-mide)

(Imodium)

**Classification:** antidiarrheal, Controlled Substance Schedule V

## Available Preparations:
- 1 mg/5 ml oral solution
- 2-mg capsules

**Action and Use:** Synthetic piperidine-derivative that inhibits intestinal motility by direct effect on GI mucosa and musculature through interaction with the autonomic system. Used for the symptomatic treatment of acute nonspecific diarrhea and chronic diarrhea.

## Routes and Dosage:
*PO:* Dosage first 24 hours: 2 to 6 years (13 to 20 kg): 1 mg 3 times /day; 6 to

8 years (20 to 30 kg): 2 mg 2 times /day; 8 to 12 years (over 30 kg): 2 mg 3 times /day. Second 24 hours 0.1 mg/kg only after each unformed stool. Do not exceed total daily dosage for age of first day.

Chronic Diarrhea: Although dosage has not been established due to limited use for chronic diarrhea; some clinicians recommend: 0.08 to 0.24 mg/kg/day in 2 or 3 divided doses

**Absorption and Fate:** Peak plasma levels in 2.5 to 4 hours. Half-life is 7 to 15 hours. Excreted 30% in feces and 2% in urine.

**Contraindications and Precautions:** Pregnancy category B. Use with caution during lactation. Safe use in children under 2 years not established. Contraindicated in hypersensitivity to drug, in those in whom constipation should be avoided, and diarrhea associated with pseudomembranous enterocolitis, intestinal mucosal penetrating organisms. Use caution with hepatic disease, dehydration and electrolyte balance, and acute ulcerative colitis.

**Side Effects:**
*CNS:* drowsiness, fatigue, dizziness more frequent in children. *GI:* abdominal cramps or pain, dry mouth, nausea, vomiting, abdominal distention, constipation, megacolon in ulcerative colitis. *Skin:* rash.

**Nursing Implications:**
*Assess:* Assess for drug hypersensitivity. Assess number, color, consistency, history of onset and course of diarrhea, as well as hydration level and electrolyte balance. Obtain weight. If child is dehydrated, use cautiously.
*Administer: PO:* Do not mix solution with other solutions or fluids. Capsule may be taken apart, mixed, and given with a small amount of food or fluid.
*Monitor:* Observe and chart stool pattern. Assess level of hydration by I & O, frequent weights, serum electrolytes, and symptoms of dehydration. If dehydration occurs, discontinue medication and inform physician. Do not exceed recommended dosage; if child does not respond to therapy in 48 hours, stop drug. Do not used beyond 7 days in acute diarrhea. Monitor for side effects.
*Patient Teaching:* Take only as prescribed. Observe for side effects and hydration levels. Monitor and note stool patterns for physician.

**Storage Requirements:** Store at 15 to 30°C in well-closed containers.

---

## □ MAFENIDE ACETATE                                    (ma'fe-nide)

(Sulfamylon)

**Classification:** antiinfective, sulfonamide derivative

**Available Preparations:** 8.5% cream for topical administration

**Action and Use:** Exact mechanism of drug unknown; appears to interfere with bacterial cell-wall synthesis. Used topically for treatment of second and third-degree burns to prevent infection and septicemia caused by gm − or gm + organisms especially *Pseudomonas aeruginosa.*

## Routes and Dosage:
*Topical:* Apply 16-mm (1/16 inch) thickness to entire debrided burn area 1 to 2 times a day

## Absorption and Fate: Absorbed from site; rapidly metabolized to *p*-carboxybenzenesulfonamide. This metabolite is excreted in urine.

## Contraindications and Precautions: Pregnancy category C. Excreted in breast milk; safety in nursing not established. Contraindicated in allergy to drug or any of its components, sodium bisulfite, or asthmatic. Use caution in acute renal failure, renal impairment, and with pulmonary dysfunction.

## Side Effects:
*Resp:* **hyperventilation, tachypnea, decrease in arterial** $P_{CO_2}$. *Skin:* pain and burning after application, delay in eschar separation, excoriation of new skin, bleeding after application. *Other:* rash, pruritus, facial edema, swelling, urticaria, hives, erythema, eosinophilia; **acidosis**, increase in serum chloride.

## Nursing Implications:
*Assess:* Accurate assessment and recording of appearance of wound site. Obtain baseline information on vital signs, weight, mental status, and renal function and respiratory status.
*Administer: Topical:* Apply aseptically with sterile gloves to wound in 1/16-inch thickness. Wound should be cleaned according to orders but can use bath, shower, or whirlpool (preferred) before application. Maintain room temperature when dressing is changed. Keep wound covered with medication at all times. Treated area usually left open but if dressing used, only thin layer is necessary. During eschar separation (16 to 20 days), dressings may be applied to expedite separation.
*Monitor:* Accurate observation and recording of wound progression. Assess for symptoms of superinfections and septicemia. Observe for side effects of medication, hypersensitivity reactions can occur 10 to 14 days into treatment. If this occurs contact physician immediately and stop application. Monitor for systemic acidosis. If large-burn area, use flow charts to monitor vital signs, weight, I & O, mental status, and laboratory information. Use of therapeutic play can help child handle dressing changes. May need analgesic before dressing change and drug application. Duration of therapy is until wound healed or site ready for grafting.
*Patient Teaching:* If parents caring for child at home, how to apply and not to use more medication than prescribed. To observe for symptoms of infections and importance of close medical follow-up.

## Storage Requirements: Store in tight, light-resistant containers avoiding excessive heat.

# ☐ MAGALDRATE

(Aluminum Magnesium Complex, Lowsium, Riopan, Riopan Plus)

**Combination Products:** Magaldrate with simethicone (Lowsium Plus, Magaldrate Plus)

**Classification:** antacid

## Available Preparations:
- 540 mg/5ml oral suspension
- 480-mg tablets
- 480-mg chewable tablets

**Action and Use:** Formulation of aluminum and magnesium hydroxides that neutralizes gastric acids by increasing pH; lowers esophageal sphincter pressure. Used in relief of symptoms of peptic ulcer, gastritis, hyperacidity, and hiatal hernia. Sodium content low, varies from 0.1 to 4.83 mg; check with pharmacist for specific dosage amount.

## Routes and Dosage:
*PO:* Peptic Ulcer: 5 to 15 ml/dose every 3 to 6 hours or 1 to 3 hour after meals and at bedtime
Maintain gastric pH below 5. Dosage variable, depends on indication and reaction in child

**Absorption and Fate:** Onset of action is intermediate and duration prolonged. Excreted in urine and feces.

**Contraindications and Precautions:** Pregnancy category C. Can be used during lactation. Not for use with children unless prescribed by physician. Contraindicated in hypersensitivity to this drug, aluminum products, or in renal failure. Use caution in renal impairment, dehydration, decreased GI motility, and sodium restrictions.

## Side Effects:
*GI:* constipation or diarrhea. *Other:* hypermagnesemia.

## Nursing Implications:
*Administer: PO:* Shake suspension well. Give with small amount of water. Masticate chewable tablet well for maximum absorption. If giving by nasogastric tube, check for patency and proper tube placement. After dosage flush tube with enough water to clear tube and ensure medication is in stomach.
*Monitor:* Monitor stool consistency and pattern; notify physician if constipation or diarrhea occurs. Assess for hypermagnesemia especially if renal output is decreased. Maintain fluid intake for age level.

***Patient Teaching:*** Take only as scheduled, in prescribed amount, and do not increase dosage. Observe for constipation or diarrhea and maintain fluid intake for age group. Do not take OTC without consulting pharmacist or physician.

**Drug Interactions:** This drug interferes with absorption of tetracyclines, digoxin, phenytoin, isoniazid, iron, or chlorpromazine; space doses 2 to 3 hours apart.

**Storage Requirements:** Store at 15 to 30°C (59 to 86°F) and protect from freezing.

---

## □ MAGNESIUM SULFATE

(mag-nee′see-um)

(Epsom salts)

**Classification:** saline laxative, anticonvulsant, electrolyte

### Available Preparations:
- 10%, 12.5%, 50% vials for parenteral use
- crystals and powder

**Action and Use:** In high IV doses, depresses the CNS and blocks nerve transmission. Reduces release of acetylcholine at myoneural junction. Used as an anticonvulsant especially in preeclampsia and eclampsia; also used for seizures in nephritis, during hypertension, and in encephalopathy. Used in treatment of barium poisoning and to prevent magnesium deficiency in total parenteral nutrition. Used as a saline laxative.

### Routes and Dosages: IV, PO
***PO:*** Laxative: 2 to 5 years: 2.5 to 5 g/day; 6 to 11 years: 5 to 10 g/day; over 12 years: 10 to 30 g/day
***IM:***
- Anticonvulsant: 20 to 40 mg/kg (0.1–0.2 ml/kg, of 20% solution) prn
- Hypertension, Encephalopathy, Seizures with Nephritis: 100 mg/kg (0.2 ml/kg of 50% solution) q4–6h prn
***IV:***
- Anticonvulsant: 100 to 200 mg/kg in 1 to 3% solution with one-half dose given in 15 to 20 minutes and total dose in 60 minutes
- Hyperalimentation: 0.5 to 3 g/day. Infants: 0.25–1.25 g/day.

**Absorption and Fate:** 15 to 30% of oral form absorbed. Affects bowel movements within 3 to 6 hours. Crosses placenta and is present in milk. Excreted by the kidneys. Onset of action is immediate after IV administration with duration of 30 minutes. Onset after IM administration is 60 minutes with 3 to 4-hour duration.

**Contraindications and Precautions:** Pregnancy category B. Usually not administered to the pregnant woman in last 2 hours of labor because of potential effects of hypotonia and respiratory depression in the newborn. Contraindicated in heart block, myocardial damage, renal failure. Cautious use in renal dysfunction, respiratory dysfunction.

## Side Effects:
***CNS:*** hypotonia, depressed reflexes, flushing, sweating, flaccid paralysis, hypothermia, **CNS depression**. ***CV:*** **hypotension, cardiac depression**, bradycardia, increased PR, increased QRS interval. ***GI:*** bitter taste, GI discomfort, and electrolyte disturbance with prolonged use of laxative form. ***Respiratory:*** **respiratory arrest** with high levels.

## Nursing Implications:
***Assess:*** Baseline vital signs and sometimes EKG are taken.
***Administer: PO:*** Give in orange or lemon juice with ice to disguise bitter taste. Give early in day to allow time for elimination while awake. Give extra fluid during the day. **IM, IV:** Have resuscitative drugs and equipment readily available. IV dose given over 1 hour.
***Monitor:*** For PO dose, record number and amount of bowel movements. Record intake to ensure adequate fluid level. Hypermagnesemia manifests as thirst, warmth, sedation, confusion, depressed deep tendon reflexes, such as patellar, and hypotonia or weakness. For parenteral doses, EKG and renal function studies may be done. Vital signs are monitored constantly during infusion and respiratory rate must be within norm for age group before administering next dose. Patellar reflex is checked often and if diminished or absent, dose is not given. Serum magnesium is measured and should be 1.5 to 2.5 mEq/L; serum calcium and phosphorus are monitored also. I & O are carefully measured and urinary output must be normal for age in 4 hours preceding dose for next dose to be given.

**Drug Interactions:** Additive neuromuscular blocking with other drugs with that action. Additive CNS depression with other CNS depressants. Calcium is used to treat overdose of magnesium as it decreases its effects. Decreases toxic effects of barium. May lead to changes in heart conduction; caution with digitalis.

**Laboratory Test Interferences:** Alters reticuloendothelial cell imaging.

**Storage Requirements:** Store at 15 to 30°C (59 to 86°F); avoid freezing.

---

## □ MANNITOL                                        (man'i-tole)

(Osmitrol)

**Classification:** osmotic diuretic

## Available Preparations:
- 5, 10, 15, 20, 25% vials for parenteral use
- 5% urogenital irrigating solution
- Also available in urogenital irrigating solution with sorbitol

**Action and Use:** This diuretic increases osmolality of plasma, thereby increasing water loss from tissues, including brain and cerebrospinal fluid and the eye. Facilitates excretion of water and toxic substances from the kidneys. Used in treatment of edema in acute renal failure, in cerebral edema, pulmonary edema, to reduce intraocular pressure, to facilitate excretion and prevent renal damage of toxic substances such as overdose of salicylates, barbiturates, and lithium. May be used to promote uric acid excretion during antineoplastic therapy. Irrigating solution used in prostatic surgery for adult men.

## Routes and Dosages:
*IV:*
- Diuretic: 2 g/kg or 60 g/m$^2$ in 15 to 20% solution over 2 to 6 hours
- Cerebral Edema, Elevated Intracranial Pressure, Glaucoma: 1 to 2 g/kg or 30 to 60 g/m$^2$ in 15 to 20% solution over 30 to 60 minutes
- Toxic Substance Treatment: up to 2 g/kg or 60 g/m$^2$ in 5 to 10% solution

Dosages established by clinicians rather than manufacturers.

**Absorption and Fate:** Remains in extracellular component. Metabolized minimally. Excreted by the kidneys. Onset of diuretic effect in 1 to 3 hours. Onset of intraocular pressure reduction in 30 to 60 minutes, with duration of 4 to 8 hours. Onset of CSF pressure reduction in 15 minutes, with duration of 3 to 8 hours. Half-life is 100 minutes or longer in renal failure.

**Contraindications and Precautions:** Pregnancy category C. Contraindicated in anuria caused by renal failure that does not respond to a test dose, in severe pulmonary congestion or pulmonary edema, severe congestive heart failure, severe dehydration, intracranial bleeding. Cautious use in cardiac or pulmonary dysfunction, hypovolemia, hyperkalemia, renal dysfunction.

## Side Effects:
*CNS:* confusion paresthesia, weakness, headache, dizziness, blurred vision, **seizures**. *CV:* chest pain, **tachycardia**. *GI:* nausea, vomiting, thirst. *Respiratory:* dyspnea, wheezing, coughing. *GU:* increased urination, urinary retention, **renal failure** with large doses. *Skin:* rash, hives, edema and necrosis with extravasation. *Metabolic:* hypovolemia, hyponatremia, hyperkalemia.

## Nursing Implications:
*Assess:* Measure serum electrolytes and vital signs. Weigh patient. Assess hydration status.
*Administer:* A test dose of 0.2 g/kg or 6 g/m$^2$ is given in oliguria or anuria to measure response; if drug is effective, then therapeutic dose is given. Solu-

tion administered over ordered time by infusion pump. Do not add to whole blood.

***Monitor:*** Frequent vital signs, especially blood pressure and pulse, weight, and serum electrolytes are performed. I & O are carefully measured and report oliguria immediately as therapy will likely be discontinued. CVP is measured. Be alert for signs of hypovolemia or electrolyte imbalance. Avoid extravasation and check IV site frequently; discontinue immediately if edema, redness, or other unusual signs occur. Rebound increase in intracranial and intraocular pressure can occur about 12 hours after therapy ends, so monitor for signs of these.

**Drug Interactions:** Potentiation of diuretic effects with other diuretics. Resultant hypokalemia can increase chance of digitalis toxicity. Increased excretion of lithium.

**Storage Requirements:** Store at 15 to 30°C (59 to 86°F); do not freeze. If crystallization occurs upon exposure to cold temperature, place in hot water and shake vigorously. Use only if all crystals are dissolved. Cool to body temperature before administering.

---

## ☐ MEASLES-MUMPS-RUBELLA VACCINES

(mees'els muhmps roo-bell'ah)

(MMR)

**Classification:** immunization

## Available Preparations:
■ single dose vials with diluent for parenteral use

Each of the vaccines is also available separately, as well as measles and rubella combination and rubella and mumps combination.

**Action and Use:** A preparation of live attenuated virus that stimulates body production of antibodies against measles, mumps, and rubella (German measles). These live virus vaccines are used primarily for immunization of children with a one-time dose.

## Routes and Dosages:
***SC:*** 0.5 ml (entire contents of reconstituted single-dose vial) at 15 months of age; to be repeated 1 time during middle childhood. Recent epidemiologic evidence of increased measles disease may necessitate a second immunization in young children in some parts of the country.

**Absorption and Fate:** One dose produces immunity in 95% of recipients in 2 to 3 weeks. Immune response rate is lower and considered inadequate in children under 12 months.

**Contraindications and Precautions:** The vaccines are contraindicated in pregnant women, those allergic to neomycin, patients with an immune deficiency disease, or who are receiving steroids or other immunosuppressant drugs. Children who have received blood products or immune serum globulin in the last 90 days and children with a fever or acute illness should have immunization delayed. Mild upper respiratory illness without fever is not contraindication to immunization with MMR. Mumps vaccine is not routinely advised for those over 21 years, unless seronegative. Separate preparations of measles and rubella are available without mumps, particularly for use in adult-age groups. Children with egg allergy should be vaccinated with extreme caution, only with resuscitative equipment, drugs, and personnel available.

**Side Effects:**
*CNS:* (rare) encephalitis or encephalopathy, (rare) febrile seizure. *Skin:* measles-like noncontagious rash approximately 7 days after immunization. *Musculoskeletal:* joint pain. *Other:* fever, anaphylaxis (rare).

**Nursing Implications:**
*Assess:* Check records of all children for immunity to measles, mumps, and rubella. Inquire about allergy to eggs or neomycin. Immunize before puberty if possible; however, do not avoid immunization of adolescents not immune to these diseases, as they are at high risk of contracting them. Unprotected children exposed to measles disease may receive immune serum globulin followed by the vaccine 3 months later. Children with leukemia in remission may receive MMR if their chemotherapy was completed. Although it was initially recommended that HIV-infected children not be immunized with these live virus vaccines, the Centers for Disease Control have recently changed their recommendation based on the data that several HIV-infected children have died from complications of measles disease in the past few years. At present, asymptomatic HIV-infected children should receive MMR, and the vaccine should be considered for symptomatic children.
A dead measles vaccine was used in the United States from 1963 through 1967. Persons who received this vaccine should be reimmunized with the present live virus vaccine as they may be infected with a type of atypical measles.
*Administer:* Epinephrine 1:1000 and resuscitative equipment should be available in case of anaphylaxis. The National Childhood Vaccine Injury Act requires recording of patient name, address, route and site of administration, lot number and manufacturer of vaccine, date of immunization, as well as the name, address, and title of the person who administered the vaccine.
Separate preparations of each vaccine component are available, although the combination MMR is generally used. There is no contraindication or increased risk to use of MMR even if a child has had a previous case of, or immunization for, one of the diseases. In case of measles outbreak, infants as young as 6 months may receive the separate preparation of measles vaccine. These children should be immunized with MMR after 12 months of age. Children immunized with any of the components before 12 months of age should be reimmunized after that age to ensure adequate response. MMR can be given concurrently with other immunizations, such as DTP and polio, when each injection is given with a separate syringe at a different site. *SC:* Add content of reconstitution

vial or syringe (approximately 0.5 ml) to vial powder. Withdraw entire amount into syringe for administration. If not used immediately the vaccine must be kept refrigerated and out of light; reconstituted solution must be discarded if not used within 8 hours. Give into upper outer arm. Avoid intravenous administration.

**Monitor:** Observe child for 20 minutes after immunization for signs of anaphylaxis. Severe reactions, such as anaphylaxis, encephalopathy, encephalitis, or seizures, are reported to the US Department of Health and Human Services.

**Patient Teaching:** Teach adolescent females with childbearing potential to avoid pregnancy for 3 months after vaccine; however, if a woman who receives the vaccine later learns she was pregnant at the time, she can be reassured that there have been no known cases of congenital rubella syndrome acquired from the immunization. There is no need to avoid the vaccine for children whose mothers, teachers, or close contacts are pregnant.

Inform parents of children with personal or family history of seizures that the child has a slight increased risk of seizures after vaccination. The benefits of immunization outweigh this slight risk.

**Drug Interactions:** May temporarily suppress reaction to tuberculin skin test. Do skin test at same visit when MMR is given or delay for 4 to 6 weeks. Immune globulins and blood products received within preceding 90 days may suppress response to vaccine.

**Storage Requirements:** Store vials of vaccine in refrigerator and out of light, at 2 to 8°C (35 to 46°F). Reconstituted vaccine should be kept out of light and under refrigeration until use. Reconstituted vaccine must be discarded if not used within 8 hours. Store in body of refrigerator rather than on door where temperature variation may be greater.

---

# □ MEBENDAZOLE                                    (me-ben'da-zole)

(Vermox)

## Classification: anthelmintic

## Available Preparations:
- 100-mg chewable tablet

**Action and Use:** Inhibits glucose uptake in the parasites and is useful against hookworm (ancylostome), roundworm (*Ascaris lumbricoides*), pinworm (*Enterobius vermicularis*), whipworm (*Trichuris trichiura*), and in mixed infestations.

## Routes and Dosage:
*PO:*
- Pinworms: 100 mg times one dosage, repeat in 2 weeks
- Hookworms, Roundworms, Whipworms: 100 mg twice daily for 3 days

**Absorption and Fate:** Minimal absorption from GI tract. Peak serum levels: 0.5 to 7 hours. Highly bound to plasma proteins. Half-life: 2.8 to 9 hours. Excreted mainly in feces as unchanged drug and metabolites.

**Contraindications and Precautions:** Pregnancy category C. Use with caution during lactation. Safe usage in children under 2 years has not been established. Contraindicated in hypersensitivity to drug.

**Side Effects:**
*GI:* occasional abdominal pain, diarrhea, nausea, vomiting with massive infestations. *Other:* Rare: alopecia, rash, pruritus, flushing, hiccups, cough, hypotension, increased liver function tests.

**Nursing Implications:**
*Assess:* Obtain pinworm test during night or when child is sleeping when worms migrate to perianal area to deposit their eggs. Commercial test kit available or can use Scotch tape with sticky side to outside of tongue blade. Obtain test by carefully exposing buttocks and pressing tape to anal area. Wash hands well after test. Diagnosis of other parasites through stool samples; follow your agency procedure for collection.
*Administer:* Tablet chewed or can be crushed and mixed with small amount of food to administer, but do not swallow tablet whole. Can be given without regard to meals.
*Monitor and Patient Teaching:* Pinworms: Highly contagious, female can deposit 17,000 eggs a night, then dies; ova mature within 3 to 8 hours. All members of family should be treated. All bed linen, towels, and personal clothes should be washed. Carpets should be vacuumed, floors damp mopped, toilets disinfected daily. Infected child should sleep alone with tight fitting underwear or diapers. Cut nails and keep clean. Change linens bedclothes, and underwear daily. This disease does not indicate family has unclean home; however, good hand washing is important to prevent spread of disease. Hookworm: Avoid going barefoot. Pica may contribute to this disease. Proper disposal of human sewage. Roundworm: Common where human waste is used as fertilizer. Occasionally worm may migrate to mouth, nose, or rectum. Whipworm: Infestation from contaminated ground. Good hand washing and washing raw vegetables and fruits. With all infestations teach parent how to obtain stool culture.

**Storage Requirements:** Store at 15 to 30°C (50 to 86°F) in tight container.

---

□ **MECHLORETHAMINE HYDROCHLORIDE**          (me-klor-eth'a-meen)

(Mustargen, Nitrogen Mustard)

**Classification:** antineoplastic, alkylating agent

## Available Preparations:

- 10-mg vial for parenteral use. A topical ointment and solution are not available in U.S. or licensed for use here.

**Action and Use:** This alkylating agent interferes with replication of DNA and RNA synthesis. Powerful action at all stages of the cell reproductive cycle and has some immunosuppressive ability. Used for Hodgkin's disease and lymphoma.

**Routes and Dosages:** IV, intrapleural, intraperitoneal, intrapericardial
*IV:* 0.4 mg/kg in 1 dose or doses divided into 2 to 4 days; repeated in 3 to 6 weeks
Advanced Hodgkin's: 6 mg/m$^2$ days 1 and 8; repeated to give a total of 6 cycles during 28-day therapy
*Intracavitary:* 0.2 mg/kg (10 to 20 mg) to 0.4 mg/kg with the lower dose used intrapericardially.

**Absorption and Fate:** Very rapid metabolism of the drug by the body after IV administration. Onset in a few seconds to minutes. Eliminated mainly in urine.

**Contraindications and Precautions:** Pregnancy category D. Not recommended during pregnancy or lactation. Contraindicated during infections particularly chicken pox or herpes zoster, suppurative inflammation. Allow time after other chemotherapy or radiation for recovery of bone marrow. Use with caution in chronic lymphocytic leukemia.

## Side Effects:

*CNS:* **neurotoxicity** especially if given intraarterially or by regional perfusion or to persons who have received procarbazine or cyclophosphamide; headache, drowsiness, vertigo, tinnitus, seizures, paresthesia. *GI:* nausea and vomiting are common, usually 1 to 3 hours after dose and lasting 8 to 24 hours; antiemetics may help; anorexia, diarrhea, ulcers. *GU:* hyperuricemia. *Skin:* inflammation and induration if extravasation occurs; maculopapular skin rash, erythema, hyperpigmentation, alopecia (rare). *Hemic:* **severe leukopenia**, anemia, thrombocytopenia, especially if dose is greater than 0.4 mg/kg in one course; leukopenia occurs 24 hours after dose; thrombus and thrombophlebitis, as well as hyperpigmentation in the vein, with injection. *Other:* systemic effects may occur after intracavitary administration, although they are usually less than with IV administration; intrapericardial administration may cause cardiac irregularities.

## Nursing Implications:

*Assess:* Take history of prior chemotherapy and radiation. Obtain baseline vital signs and CBC.

***Administer:*** This drug has potentially severe toxic effects and should be given only under the supervision of a physician with training and experience in cancer chemotherapy. The drug's potential for toxic effects on health-care personnel as well as patients necessitates careful handling during preparation and administration. Generally, during preparation of antineoplastics latex gloves, a mask, and a solid front gown are worn, and a laminar flow hood is used. Gloves and gown are recommended for administration. Contaminated equipment, such as needles, syringes, vials, and unused medication, is disposed of properly. Clean-up of spills is carefully performed and accidental contact by patient or personnel receives prompt flushing and cleaning. ***IV:*** Reconstitute powder with 10 ml sterile water or saline. Shake vial without removing needle from rubber top. Solution will contain 1 mg/ml. Must give immediately after mixing. Give into tubing or sidearm of freely running IV over a few minutes. Flush infusion after administration with 5 to 10 ml saline. Discard unused medication. Equipment used for administration and the vials should be soaked for 45 minutes in 5% sodium thiosulfate and 5% sodium bicarbonate in equal parts. Avoid extravasation. If extravasation occurs during IV administration, aspirate as much drug as possible, then infiltrate area with isotonic sodium thiosulfate injection and apply cold packs.

***Monitor:*** Monitor I & O and weight. Replace fluids lost by vomiting. Blood studies are done frequently. Dose is reduced to 50% of normal if WBC count is 3000 to 4000/mm$^3$; reduced to 25% of normal if WBC count is 1000 to 3000/mm$^3$ or platelet count is 50,000 to 100,000/mm$^3$; discontinued if WBC count is below 1000/mm$^3$ or platelet count is below 50,000/mm$^3$. Monitor vital signs and watch for signs of infection. Observe for signs of bleeding and bruising. Observe for CNS effects especially in the patient on high dosage.

***Patient Teaching:*** Avoid persons with infections such as colds, influenza, chicken pox. Report immediately signs of infection such as fever, sore throat, cough, and signs of bleeding or bruising. Encourage use of antiemetic with dose to prevent nausea and vomiting. Encourage nutritious diet. Increase fluid intake. Teach good oral hygiene. Report missed or prolonged and heavy menstrual periods, yellowing skin and eyes.

## Drug Interactions:
Increased myelosuppressive effect with other antineoplastics with same effect. Suppresses immune response to immunization. Live virus vaccines must not be given, nor oral polio vaccine to those in close contact with the patient on this drug due to the chance of infection with a virus; these vaccines are delayed until at least 3 months after chemotherapy when the patient is in remission.

## Laboratory Test Interferences:
Increased uric acid levels. Decrease serum cholinesterase.

## Storage Requirements:
Store powder at 15 to 30°C (59 to 86°F). Prepare solution immediately before administration and discard any unused drug. Not to be used if droplets of water are seen in the solution or if it is not colorless.

---

# □ MEDRYSONE

(med-rye′sone)

(HMS Liquifilm)

**Classification:** corticosteroid, ophthalmic

## Available Preparations:
- 1% drops for ophthalmic administration

**Action and Use:** Adrenocorticoid with antiinflammatory effects that decreases infiltration of leukocytes to the site. Used to treat adrenocorticoid responsive allergic and vernal conjunctivitis, episcleritis, and ocular epinephrine sensitivity.

## Routes and Dosage:
**Ophthalmic:** instill 1 drop of 1% solution in conjunctival sac 2 to 4 times per day

**Contraindications and Precautions:** Pregnancy category C. Use caution in those under 2 years due to increased risk of systemic effects. Contraindicated in vaccinia, varicella, fungal, bacterial or viral infections of the eye, ocular tuberculosis, herpes simplex keratitis, iritis, and uveitis. Use with caution in corneal abrasions, cataracts, glaucoma, and diabetes mellitus.

## Side Effects:
**Sensory:** blurred vision, burning, lacrimation, eye pain, headache; long-term usage: halos around lights, cataracts, glaucoma, diminished visual fields, optic nerve damage. **Other:** Systemic Effects: Symptoms of adrenal suppression especially with long-term therapy.

## Nursing Implications:
**Assess:** Carefully observe and record amount and appearance of eye inflammation.
**Administer: Ophthalmic:** Consult physician if contact lenses should be removed before drug instillation and if child should wear them during therapy. They may become source of infection. For administration see Part I. Drops: Shake solution well before withdrawal of drop. Apply finger to lacrimal sac using light pressure for 1 to 2 minutes after instillation to minimize systemic absorption.
**Monitor:** Observe for symptoms of side effects or adrenal suppression. Tonometry measurements are usually obtained every 2 to 3 weeks on chronic therapy. Assess and chart response to treatment. Consult physician in 5 to 7 days if child is to remain on therapy. After long-term therapy, drug should not be discontinued abruptly, but gradually tapered to prevent reoccurrence of disease.
**Patient Teaching:** Instruct parents on proper instillation of eye medication. Use medication only as prescribed. Observe for side effects. Close medical

supervision necessary. Do not reuse this drug for new eye inflammation. Inform any care providers or dentists that child is taking this drug before treatment or surgery.

**Storage Requirements:** Store at 15 to 30°C (59 to 86°F) in tightly closed container. Protect from freezing and light.

---

## ☐ MEPERIDINE                    (me-per'i-deen)

(Demerol, Mepergan)

**Combination Products:** APAP with Demerol, Atropine and Demerol, Mepergan Fortis

**Classification:** narcotic analgesic, opiate agonist

**Available Preparations:**
- 50 mg/5 ml oral solution
- 50, 100-mg tablets
- 25, 50, 75, 100-mg vials for parenteral use
- 10 mg/ml injection for use with IV infusion device

Also available in capsules with promethazine, tablets with acetaminophen, parenteral injection with promethazine and atropine.

**Action and Use:** A synthetic phenylpiperidine derivative of opium. Acts on CNS by influencing neurotransmitters, thereby inducing analgesia. Used in relief of moderate to severe pain and as a preoperative medication; not effective as an antitussive except in large doses. A combination of meperidine, promethazine, and chlorpromazine (called DPT) may be given 45 minutes before procedures.

**Routes and Dosages:** PO, IM, SC, IV (IV form generally used during surgery)
*PO, IM, SC:* Pain: 1.1 to 1.8 mg/kg q3–4h PRN or 175 mg/m$^2$/day in 6 doses; single dose not to exceed 100 mg
*IM, SC:* Peoperative medication: 1 to 2.2 mg/kg 30 to 90 minutes before surgery; not to exceed 100 mg

**Absorption and Fate:** Well absorbed after injection; one-half as effective in PO form. Distributed throughout body including breast milk. Metabolized in the liver and excreted in urine. Onset of action after IM, SC is 10 minutes, and after PO, 15 minutes. Peak level after injection is 30 to 60 minutes, after PO, 60 minutes. Half-life is 2.4 to 4 hours; duration, 2 to 4 hours.

**Contraindications and Precautions:** Pregnancy category B; category

D during labor. Contraindicated in those with hypersensitivity to the drug, preparations with metabisulfite are contraindicated in those with sulfite hypersensitivity, avoid in patients with respiratory depression, comatose, elevated CSF pressure. Cautious use in asthma, hepatic or renal dysfunction, atrial flutter, tachycardia, colitis, hypothyroidism, neonates, those who have taken MAO inhibitors in last 14 days.

## Side Effects:
*CNS:* sedation, dizziness, depression, coma, euphoria, restlessness, insomnia. *CV:* **circulatory depression** is potentially life threatening; orthostatic hypotension, palpitation, bradycardia, tachycardia (more common than with other opiates). *GI:* nausea, vomiting, constipation. ***Respiratory:*** **respiratory depression** is a serious side effect. ***Hepatic:*** biliary spasm, increased serum amylase and lipase. *GU:* urinary retention, oliguria, stimulates release of vasopressin; impotence. ***Skin:*** rash, erythema, urticaria, pruritus, facial flushing indicates hypersensitivity reaction.

## Nursing Implications:
***Assess:*** Assess type and degree of pain; use other pain control methods in addition to analgesic. Take baseline vital signs.
***Administer:*** Meperidine is a Schedule II drug under the Federal Controlled Substances Act. Meperidine (60 to 80 mg) is approximately equivalent to 10 mg morphine sulfate in analgesic potency. Check time of last dose carefully before giving as well as currency of order. *PO:* Give syrup in 120 ml of water. *IM, SC:* SC route rarely used due to discomfort to tissue. Incompatible with aminophylline, heparin, methicillin, nitrofurantoin, phenobarbital, sodium bicarbonate, and some other drugs. Consult references or pharmacologist before placing in other solutions. *IV:* Use reserved for anesthesia as tachycardia and syncope can occur. Smaller doses used for patient-controlled analgesia by pump (PCA).
***Monitor:*** Monitor vital signs every 15 to 30 minutes after administration. If hypotension occurs, or patients feel nausea or dizziness, have them lie down. After parenteral forms, patient is generally left in bed with side rails up. Evaluate pain in 30 minutes and record results.
***Patient Teaching:*** Take drug only as directed and only for patient prescribed. Drug alters mental alertness; therefore, avoid driving and adjust activities accordingly. Encourage adequate fluid intake, coughing, and deep breathing to avoid respiratory stasis. Prolonged use can be habit forming and the drug has been abused by health-care personnel. Teach patient using the drug by PCA pump the correct use of the drug and infusion device.

**Drug Interactions:** Additive CNS effects with alcohol and other CNS depressants. Phenothiazines may antagonize action. Increased effects if given with dextroamphetamine, may increase effects of neuromuscular-blocking agents. May decrease effects of diuretics in congestive heart failure. When given with MAO inhibitors, may cause coma, respiratory depression, hypotension; these drugs are not to be given within 14 days of each other.

**Diagnostic Test Interferences:** Increases serum amylase and lipase; delay drawing blood for these tests for 24 hours after the drug. Decreased serum and urine 17-ketosteroids, 17-hydroxysteroids.

**Storage Requirements:** Store in tightly covered, light-resistant containers at 15 to 30°C (59 to 86°F). Avoid freezing solutions.

---

## □ MERCAPTOPURINE                    (mer-kap-toe-pyoor'een)

(6-Mercaptopurine, 6-MP, Purinethol)

**Classification:** antineoplastic, antimetabolite

## Available Preparations:
- 50-mg tablets

**Action and Use:** This antimetabolite is converted to a ribonucleotide in the body, which acts as a purine inhibitor, thereby interfering with DNA and RNA synthesis. It is cell-phase specific for the S phase of cell division. It also acts as a potent immunosuppressant. Used in induction and maintenance therapy of leukemias, especially acute lymphoblastic leukemia and chronic myelocytic leukemia. Has been used experimentally in treatment to prevent graft rejection and to treat several autoimmune diseases when other therapy fails, e.g., nephrotic syndrome, lupus erythematosus. Such use is not approved by the FDA.

## Routes and Dosages:
*PO:*
- Induction: 2.5 mg/kg/day or 70 to 75 mg/m²/day
- Maintenance: 1.5 to 2.5 mg/kg/day or 40 to 50 mg/m²/day
- Experimental Treatment of Acute Myeloblastic Leukemia: IV: 500 mg/m²/day with other drugs.

If mercaptopurine is given with allopurinol, mercaptopurine dose should be reduced 25 to 33%.

**Absorption and Fate:** About 50% is absorbed from GI tract. It is distributed widely in body water. It does not cross the blood-brain barrier in amounts large enough to treat meningeal leukemia. Metabolized by the liver and excreted in the urine. Peak level reached in 2 hours. Triphasic half-life with 45 minutes initially, then 2.5 hours, and terminally 10 hours.

**Contraindications and Precautions:** Pregnancy category D. Not used in pregnancy unless clearly needed; to be avoided especially in first trimester. Not recommended during lactation because of potential harm to the baby. Contraindicated if prior treatment with the drug was ineffective for the patient, and during chicken pox or herpes zoster infection. Used with caution in those with hepatic disease, infection.

## Side Effects:

*GI:* nausea, vomiting, anorexia, diarrhea, GI pain, **GI ulceration**, oral lesions. *Hepatic:* jaundice, cholestasis, ascites, abnormal hepatic enzyme levels; hepatic injury is a greater risk with large doses of the drug; jaundice usually occurs 1 to 2 months after therapy begins but may appear earlier or years later. *GU:* hyperuricemia, oliguria (rare). *Skin:* pigmentation, rash, itching. *Hemic:* **leukopenia**, thrombocytopenia, anemia are frequent occurrences about 5 to 6 days after therapy begins, persisting until 7 days after therapy ends; agranulocytosis and pancytopenia are less common.

## Nursing Implications:

*Assess:* Establish baseline vital signs and CBC. Establish baseline liver function studies; serum transaminase, alkaline phosphatase, bilirubin.
*Administer:* This drug has potentially severe toxic effects and should be given only under the supervision of a physician with training and experience in cancer chemotherapy. The drug's potential for toxic effects necessitates careful handling during preparation and administration. *PO:* The PO dose is given once daily.
*Monitor:* Increase fluid intake. Monitor vital signs daily. Monitor hemic status, such as hemoglobin and hematocrit, leukocyte count, platelet count, differential, at least weekly. A large or rapid decrease in leukocytes necessitates holding drug. Bone marrow biopsy may be done to watch for bone marrow suppression. Hepatic studies, such as serum transaminase, alkaline phosphatase, BUN, and bilirubin, must be done weekly. Hepatic toxicity necessitates holding drug. Other tests such as SGOT, SGPT, creatinine, LDH, and uric acid may be done. Monitor carefully for signs of side or toxic effects. Watch for signs of infection such as fever, sore throat as immunosuppression can lead to serious infection. Measure I & O and look for signs of decreased urine output.
*Patient Teaching:* Have patient report signs of infection promptly such as sore throat, fever, malaise. Watch mouth for signs of side effect (a white thrush-like patch). Good oral hygiene may lessen side effects in mouth. Avoid contact with those who have colds, chicken pox, or other infections. Watch for bleeding such as bruises, black tarry stools. Be alert for and report yellowing of skin and eyes. Increase fluid intake. Avoid alcoholic beverages. Return for scheduled appointments for follow-up. Do not alter maintenance therapy unless instructed by physician.

**Drug Interactions:** Allopurinol inhibits mercaptopurine metabolism so the latter must be reduced in dosage by 25 to 33% if given concurrently. Increased hepatic toxicity may occur if given with other hepatotoxic drugs and alcohol. Increased chance of infection when given with other immunosuppressants. May potentiate or diminish effects of warfarin. Suppresses immune response to immunizations. Live virus vaccines must not be given, nor oral polio vaccine to those in close contact with the patient on this drug due to the chance of infection with a virus; these vaccines are delayed until at least 3 months after chemotherapy when the patient is in remission.

**Laboratory Test Interferences:** Causes elevated glucose and uric acid levels when measured by SMA (sequential multiple analyzer).

**Storage Requirements:** Store in tightly closed containers at 15 to 30°C (59 to 86°F).

---

## ☐ METAPROTERENOL SULFATE

(met-a-proe-ter′e-nole)

(Alupent, Dey-bute Metaprel)

**Classification:** adrenergic, bronchodilator

### Available Preparations:
- 10 mg/5 ml solution
- 10, 20-mg tablets
- 0.65 mg/metered spray aerosol, oral inhalation
- 0.4%, 0.6%, 5% solution for nebulization

**Action and Use:** A synthetic sympathomimetic amine that increases production of cyclic AMP through enzyme activation, which results in bronchodilation; used as a bronchodilator in management of asthma, prevention of exercise-induced asthma, or enhancement of therapeutic effect of theophylline.

### Routes and Dosage:
*PO:* under 6 years: Dosage experience limited; some clinicians recommend 1.3 to 2.6 mg/kg/day in divided doses; 6 to 9 years (less than 27.3 kg): 10 mg 3 to 4 times per day; over 9 years: 20 mg 3 to 4 times per day
*Inhalation:* over 12 years:
- Aerosol: 2 to 3 inhalations (1.3 to 1.95 mg) every 3 to 4 hours (Maximum dosage 7.8 mg or 12 inhalations per day)
- Nebulizer Solution: over 12 years: dilute 0.2 to 0.3 ml of 5% solution in 2.5 ml of NS or use 2.5 ml of 0.6% solution every 4 to 6 hours

**Absorption and Fate:** 40% absorbed systemically from GI tract. Onset action: PO, 15 minutes; aerosol, 1 minute; nebulization, 5 to 30 minutes. Peak effect: all forms about 1 hour. Duration of action: PO, 4 hours; inhalation, 1.5 hours. Excreted unchanged in urine principally as glucuronic acid conjugates.

**Contraindications and Precautions:** Pregnancy category C. Use with caution during lactation. Safe use in those under 12 years for inhalation therapy and in those under 6 years for oral therapy not established. Contraindicated in hypersensitivity to drug or its ingredients, tachycardia, arrhythmias associated with tachycardia. Use with caution in sensitivity to other sympathomimetic drugs, diabetes mellitus, hypertension, hyperthyroidism, coronary artery disease.

## Side Effects:

*CNS:* nervousness, tremors, dizziness, headache, drowsiness. *CV:* tachycardia, palpitations, **hypertension, cardiac arrest** (overdosage). *GI:* nausea, vomiting, bad taste. *Other:* muscle cramps in extremities, hypersensitivity (rare).

## Nursing Implications:

*Assess:* Assess respiratory status and obtain baseline pulse.
*Administer: PO:* Do not crush tablets. May be taken without regard to food. Side effects more common with oral form. *Inhalations:* For administration, see Part I. Shake container well. If second inhalation is prescribed, manufacturer recommends that 2 minutes elapse between doses. For administration by nebulization with IPPB apparatus, follow agency policy for operation.
*Monitor:* Monitor respiratory response to medication. Maintain hydration for weight. Tablet and areosol can be used concurrently.
*Patient Teaching:* Proper usage and care of inhaler should be taught. It is beneficial to have child demonstrate inhaler usage. Inhaler should not be used more frequently than prescribed; if symptoms worsen, contact physician. If paradoxical bronchospasm occurs, discontinue immediately. Do not use any inhalers other than those ordered by physician. Tolerance can develop with long-term therapy.

## Drug Interactions:
Avoid usage with other sympathomimetic amines because of additive effects. Effects of β-adrenergic blocking agents antagonize bronchodilation effects of this drug.

## Storage Requirements:
Store at 15 to 30°C (59 to 86°F), in light-resistant containers. Do not store aerosol at temperatures above 25°C and avoid placing near heat or in direct sunlight.

---

# □ METHICILLIN SODIUM                              (meth-i-sill'in)

(Staphcillin)

## Classification: antibiotic, penicillinase-resistant

## Available Preparations: 1, 4, 6, 10 g for parenteral administration

## Action and Use:
Similar to penicillin in action, but resistant to inactivation by penicillinase. Primarily use in penicillinase-producing *Staphylococcus aureus* and *S. epidermidis* infections. Each gram of drug contains about 2.6 to 3.1 mEq sodium.

## Routes and Dosage:

*IM, IV:* Manufacturer has not established dosage for neonates; however, some clinicians recommend:

- birth to 14 days, < 2000 gm: 50 mg/kg/day equally divided doses every 12 hours; > 2000 gm: 75 mg/kg/day equally divided every 8 hours
- 14 days to 1 month, < 2000 gm: 75 mg/kg/day equally divided doses every 8 hours; > 2000 gm: 100 mg/kg/day equally divided every 6 hours
- over 1 month: 100 to 400 mg/kg/day equally divided doses every 4 to 6 hours
- adult: 4 to 12 g/day equally divided doses every 4 to 6 hours

**Absorption and Fate:** Rapidly absorbed from IM site. Distributed in synovial, pericardial, ascitic, and pleural fluids, bone, bile. Peak level: IM is 30 minutes, IV at end of infusion. Half-life: 2 to 16-year-old children, 0.8 to 1.6 hours; neonates, 0.9 to 3.9 hours. Therapeutic level: 0.81 to 6.3 μg/ml. 30 to 60% bound to serum proteins. Excreted unchanged in urine.

**Contraindications and Precautions:** Pregnancy category B. Use caution during lactation. Manufacturer states safe use in neonates not established. Contraindicated in hypersensitivity to drug, penicillins, cephalosporins, or cephamycins. Use caution with allergies, asthma, family history of allergies, or renal impairment.

## Side Effects:

*GI:* Hairy tongue, oral lesions glossitis, stomatitis. *GU:* **Acute interstitial nephritis:** rash, macroscopic or microscopic hematuria, azotemia, dysuria, oliguria, proteinuria; onset symptoms 5 days to 5 weeks after therapy started. Usually reversible but may deteriorate causing **renal failure, death** (4 to 8% IV, doses 170 to 380 mg/kg/day), hemorrhagic cystitis. *Hepatic:* transient rise SGOT, SGPT, alkaline phosphatase. *Skin:* morbilliform, maculopapular, urticarial, or erythematous, rashes, pruritus (hypersensitivity). *Hemic:* **eosinophilia, anemia, neutropenia, thrombocytopenia, leukopenia, agranulocytosis.** *Other:* hypersensitivity: drug fever, **anaphylaxis** (rare); Local: IM: painful, sterile abscesses; IV: phlebitis, thrombophlebitis

## Nursing Implications:

*Assess:* Assess previous allergy to drug, penicillins, cephalosporins, other drugs, asthma, or family history of allergies. Obtain cultures and sensitivity before treatment, but can start treatment before results. Obtain baseline renal, hepatic, and hematologic data before therapy.

*Administer: IM, IV:* Reconstituted solutions may darken to deep orange and have hydrogen sulfide odor after being at room temperature for several days; discard. *IM:* Reconstitute according to package inserts with either sterile water or 0.9% sodium chloride for injection. Give injection slowly to reduce pain and deep into large muscle mass. *IV:* Reconstitute according to package insert with sterile water or 0.9% sodium chloride for injection. Can give IV push very slowly; dilute solution to 500 mg/25 ml and infuse at 10 ml/minute. Intermittent infusion dilute to 1 g/50 ml, minimum infusion time 200 mg/minute. Compatible with $D_5W$, $D_5W/0.5\%NS$, $D_5W/NS$, $D_{10}W$, NS, LR. Do not mix with any other drug or other solutions than those listed. Give at least 1 hour before bacteriostatic antibiotics. Do not administer through same tubing as this drug. Incompatible with aminophylline, ascorbic acid, aminoglycosides, chlorpromazine, codeine, hydrocortisone (Solu-Cortef), levorphanol, lincomycin, metaraminol, methohexital, morphine, oxytetracycline, promethazine, sodium bicarbonate tetracycline, vancomycin, vitamin B.

**Monitor:** IM site may develop sterile abscesses. Observe IV site for vein irritation and thrombophlebitis, change site every 48 hours. Monitor child for hypersensitivity (especially in first 20 minutes of first dosage), rash (onset and characteristics), and side effects. Watch for symptoms of superinfections or interstitial nephritis and hematuria. Drug's sodium content may effect patients on sodium restrictions. Assess renal and hepatic functions periodically during therapy. Hematological functions should be done 1 to 3 times per week and observe for any symptoms of bleeding. Maintain fluid intake for age group especially to prevent hemorrhagic cystitis. Therapy course varies and depends on severity and type of infection.

**Drug Interactions:** Erythromycin, tetracycline, chloramphenical may decrease the antibacterial effects of methicillin.

**Laboratory Test Interference:** False-positive direct Coombs' test. Use uricase and phosphotungstate tests for serum uric acid, other tests give false-positive results.

**Storage Requirements:** Reconstituted IM solutions, stable at room temperature for 24 hours and if refrigerated stable for 4 days. IV reconstituted solutions, stable at room temperature; 2 mg/ml for 4 hours and 10 to 30 mg/ml for 8 hours. Label solution at time of reconstitution with date and time.

---

## □ METHOTREXATE or AMETHOPTERIN or MTS

(meth-oh-trex'ate)

(Abitrexate, Folex, Mexate)

**Classification:** antineoplastic, antimetabolite

**Available Preparations:**
- 2.5-mg tablets
- 2.5, 20, 25, 50, 100, 250 mg/ml vials for parenteral use

**Action and Use:** As a folic acid antagonist this drug inhibits dihydrofolate reductase resulting in depletion of purine and pyrimidine, essential components in DNA synthesis. Acts on S phase of cell division. Used in leukemias, especially acute lymphoblastic and lymphocytic leukemia. Useful in lymphosarcomas, and some solid tumors such as osteogenic sarcoma. Used in severe untreatable psoriasis. Used experimentally in treatment of some autoimmune diseases.

## Routes and Dosages: PO, IM, IV, IT, intraarterial

Individualized doses according to disease and concomitant therapy.
*PO:*

- Psoriasis: 2.5 mg daily for 3 to 5 days; increased as needed; not above 25 to 30 mg/week
- Acute Leukemia Maintenance: 20 to 30 mg/m$^2$/week

*IM, IV:* 10 to 30 mg/m$^2$/week. High-dose therapy may be 100 mg/m$^2$ to 12 g/m$^2$ q1–3wk, followed by leukovorin therapy
*IT:* 3 months or under: 3 mg; 4 to 11 months: 6 mg; 1 to 2 years: 8 mg; 2 years: 10 mg; 3 years and over: 12 mg or 12 mg/m$^2$

## Absorption and Fate: Completely absorbed from GI tract. Widely distributed in body tissues but does not reach therapeutic levels in CNS unless given intrathecally. About 50% bound to plasma proteins. Excreted mainly by kidneys. Peak level after PO 1 to 5 hours, after IM and IV 30 minutes to 2 hours; after IT, 2 hours. Distribution half-life is 1 hour. Elimination half-life is biphasic with 2 to 3 hours initially and 8 to 10 hours terminally. Half-life increases with lower dosage of drug. Some is retained for weeks in the liver and kidney. Therapeutic level is 10$^{-5}$ to 10$^{-6}$ (low dose); 10$^{-3}$ (high dose).

## Contraindications and Precautions: Pregnancy category D. Pregnancy should be avoided and men should not father children for at least 12 weeks after the end of therapy. Generally contraindicated in those with hepatic or renal malfunction; if used in these cases, dose must be reduced. Contraindicated in chicken pox or herpes zoster infections. Use with caution in those in malnutrition states, with infections, those with GI lesions, with bone marrow suppression.

## Side Effects:

*CNS:* headache, drowsiness, dizziness. After IT administration, headache, back pain, fever, paresis, seizures, neurotoxicity with burning in extremities, encephalopathy. *GI:* nausea, vomiting, diarrhea, stomatitis, GI lesions. *Respiratory:* interstitial pneumonitis, pneumothorax with high dose. *Hepatic:* cirrhosis, fibrosis (especially if on prolonged therapy); hepatotoxicity (most common with high-dose therapy). *GU:* severe nephropathy with hematuria and **renal failure**, elevated serum uric acid (most common with high-dose therapy). *Skin:* rash, pruritus, alopecia. *Hemic:* **leukemia**, thrombocytopenia, anemia (common). *Sensory:* photosensitivity. *Other:* fever, osteoporosis in children on long-term therapy

## Nursing Implications:

*Assess:* Establish baseline vital signs, weight, blood studies, hepatic function. Liver biopsy and renal studies are frequently done before therapy. TB test is recommended before psoriasis treatment; if positive, isoniazid is given with methotrexate and follow-up chest x-rays are done during therapy.

*Administer:* This drug has potentially severe toxic effects and should be given only under the supervision of a physician with training and experience in cancer chemotherapy. The drug's potential for toxic effects on health-care personnel as well as patients necessitates careful handling during preparation and administration. Generally, during preparation, latex gloves, a mask, and a solid front gown are worn, and a laminar flow hood is used. Gloves and gown may also be recommended for administration. Contaminated equipment, such as needles, syringes, vials, and unused medication, is disposed of properly. Cleanup of spills is carefully performed and accidental contact by patient or personnel receives prompt flushing and cleaning. *PO:* A 5 to 10-mg test dose is given 1 week before therapy for psoriasis. *IV:* Dilute vial with 2 to 25 ml of normal saline, sterile or bacteriostatic water (see package insert for recommendations for dilution). Hydrate patient well before high doses are given with alkaline solution, such as sodium bicarbonate, so that urine pH is 6.0 to 7.0. Continue increased hydration after dose. *IT:* Mix only with preservative-free solutions (preservative free Elliot's B, normal saline, 5% dextrose, lactated Ringer's). IT administration is done after a blood-free spinal tap with CSF equal to amount of injection removed first. Injected in 15 to 30 seconds. Care must be taken to avoid IT overdose. IT overdose is treated by allowing CSF to drain by a lumbar puncture. Systemic leukovorin calcium can be used to prevent or treat systemic toxicity.

*Monitor:* Watch patient for signs of infection with vital sign changes, fever, bleeding. Liver function tests and sometimes liver biopsy are done. Abnormal results necessitate decrease or stopping of dose. Monitor I & O and watch for signs of uricemia. Renal function tests should be done. WBC and platelet tests must be done at least weekly. Depression of bone marrow is an early sign of toxicity and necessitates stopping drug. GI tract should be checked for signs of lesions; mouth ulcers are the first sign of toxicity and must be promptly reported. *High-dose therapy:* After high-dose therapy, the serum drug level may be monitored for 48 to 72 hours; it should return below $10^{-7}$ to $10^{-8}$. High-dose therapy is followed by citrovorum factor to decrease toxicity for the hemic system; this therapy must be given promptly at the time ordered. Watch I & O. Replace all fluid loss and maintain good hydration with alkaline solutions. Copious urine output is essential. Check urine pH, BUN, creatinine, electrolytes, CBC platelets. Monitor for toxic effects of high-dose therapy such as pulmonary and central nervous system changes.

*Patient Teaching:* Avoid use of alcohol, which can increase hepatotoxicity. Avoid vitamin preparations unless prescribed by physician; vitamins with folic acid are not recommended. Perform good oral care. Report signs of side effects and toxicity such as mouth ulcers. Report symptoms of infection such as fever, sore throat, malaise. Avoid contact with persons with infections such as colds, influenza, chicken pox. Increase fluid intake. Use contraception for at least 12 weeks after therapy (men and women). Avoid exposure to ultraviolet light, which may worsen psoriasis. Prepare for possibility of alopecia.

**Drug Interactions:** Methotrexate is highly protein bound; displacement from protein-binding sites by other agents, such as aspirin, sulfonamides, phenytoin, can increase toxicity of methotrexate. Folic acid may increase action of the drug. Anticoagulant effects are increased with anticoagulant use. Suppresses immune response to immunizations. Live virus vaccines must not be given, nor oral polio vaccine to those in close contact with the patient on this drug due to the chance of infection with the virus; these vaccines are delayed at least 3 months after chemotherapy when the patient is in remission.

**Storage Requirements:** Store tablets in tightly covered containers at 15 to 30°C (59 to 86°F). Store injection vials at same temperature and protect from light.

---

## □ METHYLPHENIDATE (meth-ill-fen′i-date)

(Ritalin)

**Classification:** CNS stimulant

**Available Preparations:**
- 5, 10, 20-mg tablets
- 20-mg extended-release tablets

**Action and Use:** A derivative of piperidine that acts like amphetamine. Causes CNS and respiratory stimulation and has some sympathomimetic activity. May work by enhancing catecholamine effects in the reticular activating system, thereby affecting the cortex to improve attention span and task performance. It may also prevent flooding of sensory impulses into the cortex so that they enter in a more integrated manner. Used to treat children with attention-deficit disorder and adults with narcolepsy.

**Routes and Dosages:**
*PO:* For children 6 years or over: 5 mg before breakfast and lunch initially, increased in 5 to 10-mg increments weekly PRN or 0.25 mg/kg/day in 2 doses initially, increased by doubling weekly PRN; not to exceed 2 mg/kg/day or 60 mg/day.

**Absorption and Fate:** Well absorbed from GI tract. Distribution unknown but does cross into CNS. Metabolized drug excreted in urine. Duration of action: 3 to 6 hours after tablets and 8 hours after extended-release tablets. One-half of dose is present in urine by 6 hours.

**Contraindications and Precautions:** Pregnancy category C. Safe use in pregnancy and lactation is not established and, therefore, not recommended. Contraindicated in those with glaucoma, anxiety, agitation, motor tics, people with prior hypersensitivity to the drug, with a family history or Tourette's disease, and in children under 6 years. Cautious use in those with hypertension, seizures, EEG abnormalities, history of drug dependence

## Side Effects:

*CNS:* nervousness, insomnia, dizziness, drowsiness, psychosis. *CV:* hypertension, tachycardia, arrhythmia, palpitations, increased pulse. *GI:* anorexia, abdominal pain, weight loss particularly in children, gingival bleeding. *Skin:* hypersensitivity with rash, urticaria, dermatitis, bruising, hair loss. *Hemic:* erythema, thrombocytopenia, leukopenia, anemia, eosinophilia (rare). *Sensory:* blurred vision

## Nursing Implications:

*Assess:* Measure height and weight and plot on growth grid. Take baseline vital signs. Do CBC and platelet counts. Take history of previous drug therapy and reactions.

*Administer:* Schedule II drug under Federal Controlled Substances Act. *PO:* Tablets generally given before breakfast and lunch. Do not give late in afternoon or evening so sleep is not interrupted. Extended-release tablets are given once daily in early morning and should not be crushed or chewed.

*Monitor:* Patient is seen in office for regular visits when vital signs, height, weight, and CBC and platelet counts are done. Observe for signs of bleeding and bruising. Question parents and teachers about child's behavior and ability to concentrate and perform tasks. If drug is to be effective, behavior change occurs within 1 month.

*Patient Teaching:* Take drug as directed. Do not withdraw quickly; tapering is recommended under supervision of prescriber. Measure child's weight weekly and report weight loss. Report signs of bleeding, fever, sore throat, bruising. Report changes in child's ability to concentrate and general behavior. Drug-free holidays may be recommended occasionally to ascertain continued need for drug.

**Drug Interactions:** Use with pressor agents or MAO inhibitors can cause hypertensive crisis, therefore, concomitant use is generally avoided. Methylphenidate may decrease effects of guanethedine, bretylium. May decrease metabolism and thereby increase effects of coumarin preparations, phenobarbital, phenytoin, primidone, phenybutazine, imiprimine.

**Storage Requirements:** Store tightly covered in light-resistant containers at 15 to 30°C (59 to 86°F).

---

☐ **METHYLPREDNISOLONE ACETATE**    (meth-ill-pred-niss'oh-lone)

(depMedalone, Depoject, Depo-Medrol, Depopred-40, Duralone, Durameth, Enpak, Medrol, Medralone-40, Medrone-40, Mepred, Methylone, M-Prednisol, Pre-dep, Rep-Pred)

☐ **METHYLPREDNISOLONE (MEDROL)**

# ☐ METHYLPREDNISOLONE SODIUM SUCCINATE

(A-methaPred, Solu-Medrol, Solu-Medrone)

**Combination Products:** Methylprednisolone acetate with neomycin sulfate (Neo-Medrol Acetate)

**Classification:** corticosteroid, glucocorticoid

## Available Preparations:
- 2, 4, 8, 16, 24, 32-mg tablets
- 20, 40, 80 mg/ml (Acetate) for parenteral administration
- 40, 125, 500 mg, 1, 2 g (Sodium Succinate) for parenteral administration
- 40-mg rectal powder for suspension
- 0.25%, 1% topical ointment

**Action and Use:** Natural or synthetic, intermediate-acting glucocorticoid that has strong antiinflammatory, immunosuppressant, and metabolic actions. Used to treat diseases such as endocrine, collagen, dermatologic, allergy, and acute leukemia. Used with mineralocorticoids as replacement therapy in adrenocortical deficiencies. Topical form is a low potency and is nonfluorinated. Rectal form treats mild to moderate ulcerative colitis.

## Routes and Dosage:
*PO:*
- Adrenocortical Insufficiency: 0.117 to 1.66 mg/kg/day or 3.3 to 50 mg/$m^2$/day in 3 to 4 divided doses
- Antiinflammatory, Immunosuppressive: 0.4 to 1.67 mg/kg/day or 12.5 to 50 mg/$m^2$/day in 3 to 4 divided doses

*IM:* 0.03 to 0.2 mg/kg or 1 to 6.25 mg/$m^2$ 1 to 2 times per day
*IV:*
- Status Asthmaticus: Initial: 1 to 2 mg/kg/dose, then 1.6 mg/kg/day every 6 hours
- Shock: doses up to 30 mg/kg may be given.

Note: Dosage is determined by severity of condition and child's response. Intraarticular, intralesional and soft tissue dosages not established.
*Rectal:* 0.5 to 1 mg/kg or 15 to 30 mg/$m^2$ every 1 to 2 days for 2 or more weeks
*Topical:* apply as thin film, 1 to 2 times a day

**Absorption and Fate:** Absorption: PO, rapid, complete; IM sodium phosphate, rapid; IM acetate, slow but complete; topical, increased in inflamed or diseased skin or use of occlusive dressings; rectally, 20% and up to 50% if mucosa inflamed or damaged. Peak level: PO, 1 to 2 hours; IM acetate, 4 to 8 days. Duration: PO, 1.25 to 1.5 days; IM acetate, 1 to 4 weeks.

**Contraindications and Precautions:** Pregnancy category C and safety during lactation not established. Use caution in children; possible growth suppression. Contraindicated in hypersensitivity to drug or its components, sensitivity to corticosteroids, varicella, systemic fungal infections, nephrotic syndrome, acquired immune deficiency syndrome (AIDS), immunizations with live virus vaccines and oral polio virus vaccine, or contact with those who have had the vaccine. Use with caution in renal disease, hypertension, cardiac disease, congestive heart failure, diabetes, ulcerative colitis, gastrointestinal ulceration, hyperthyroidism, systemic lupus erythematosus, impaired hepatic function, osteoporosis, vaccinia, exanthema, Cushing's syndrome, seizures, myasthenia gravis, tuberculosis, ocular herpes simplex, hypoalbuminemia, emotional or psychotic tendencies.

**Side Effects:** Usually dependent on dosage and duration of treatment.
*CNS:* headaches, vertigo, euphoria, insomnia, **increased intracranial pressure** (papilledema), **psychotic behavior, seizures.** *CV:* edema, **hypertension, congestive heart failure.** *GI:* nausea, vomiting, change in appetite, gastrointestinal irritation, abdominal distention, pancreatitis, ulcerative esophagitis, peptic ulcer. *Skin:* impaired wound healing, thin fragile skin, petechia, ecchymosis, acne, facial erythema, increased sweating, may mask infections; Topical: burning, itching, irritation, dryness, folliculitis, hypertrichosis, hypopigmentation, allergic contact dermatitis, maceration of the skin, secondary infection, **skin atrophy, striae, miliaria.** *Hemic:* **thrombocytopenia.** *Endocrine:* **HPA-axis suppression,** menstrual irregularities, Cushing's states, **secondary adrenocortical, pituitary unresponsiveness.** *Musculoskeletal:* **suppression of bone growth, osteoporosis,** muscle weakness, **aseptic necrosis of femoral and humeral heads.** *Sensory:* Ophthalmic: **posterior subcapsular cataracts, increased intraocular pressure.** *Other:* sodium retention, potassium loss, **negative nitrogen balance, hypokalemia, hyperglycemia,** susceptibility to infections; Withdrawal symptoms: rebound inflammation, fatigue, weakness, fever, arthralgia, dizziness, lethargy, depression, fainting, orthostatic hypotension, dyspnea, anorexia, hypoglycemia, nausea and vomiting, shortness of breath, unusual weight loss

**Nursing Implications:**
*Assess:* Obtain baseline weight, height; before long-term therapy, obtain ECG, chest and spinal x-rays, glucose tolerance test, evaluation of HPA-axis function, and BP. Topical: observe, record appearance of involved area.
*Administer:* Best to calculate drug dosage in mg/m$^2$; reduces overdosage possibilities in very short or heavy children. *PO:* Take with food or milk to reduce GI irritation. Best to give daily dosage before 9 AM. It suppresses adrenal cortex activity less, which may reduce risk of HPA-axis suppression. Tablet can be crushed and mixed with small amount of food or fluid. *IM:* (Acetate) Depo-Medrol should not be diluted or mixed with other solutions.

Multidose use of vials may lead to contamination unless strict aseptic technique observed; preservative will prevent growth of most pathogenic organisms but not all. Do not use solution that is cloudy or contains a precipitate. Inject IM dosage deep into large muscle mass and do not use deltoid muscle. Burning and pain may occur with injection. Prevent leakage of drug into dermis and subcutaneous tissues because it may cause atrophy or abscesses. *IV:* Do not confuse Solu-Medrol with Solu-Cortef. Do not give acetate intravenously. Available as Mix-O-Vial so diluent is provided, but may be further diluted with 5% dextrose or normal saline. Give IV push dosage slowly over 3 to 5 minutes. Intermittent infusion maximum concentration is 60 mg/ml infused over 20 to 30 minutes. Compatible IV fluids $D_5W$, $D_5W/NS$, LR, amino acids 4.25%/D25%. Incompatible with aminophylline, calcium gluconate, cephalothin, insulin, nafcillin, tetracycline, and others; check with your pharmacist.
*Topical:* Cleanse with water before application or as physician prescribes. Apply thin coat, gently rubbing into area, avoiding eye area and mucous membranes. Do not cover with occlusive dressing unless directed by physician. If occlusive dressing is used, it should not remain in place for more than 16 hours; it increases incidence of side effects. Disposable diapers or plastic pants act as an occlusive dressing if covering medicated groin area.
*Monitor:* Monitor BP during infusion. Carefully assess of child's response to drug; necessary for dosage adjustments. Observe for side effects, especially hypocalcemia, signs of electrolyte imbalance, signs of adrenal insufficiency, symptoms of infections, or worsening of condition. Monitor BP and daily weights, report any sudden weight gain to the physician. With long-term usage, monitor serum electrolytes and height. Encourage well-balanced diet low in sodium, rich in potassium, calcium, vitamin K and D. Observe for ulcer development; if on long-term therapy, prophylactic antacids may be used. Encourage good hygiene and dental care (possible oral fungal infections). Tonometry (eye) examinations every 6 weeks. Diabetics may need increase in insulin due to steroid-induced hyperglycemia. Discontinuing of drug: dosage should be reduced gradually, especially after long-term usage so it does not cause acute life-threatening adrenal insufficiency. After discontinuation of short-term therapy (up to 5 days) with high dosage, adrenal recovery may occur within 1 week. After prolonged high-dose therapy, complete recovery of adrenal function may require up to 1 year. If infection occurs (topical, ophthalmic, otic), discontinue drug and inform physician. Itching can lead to scratching and introduction of infections. Younger children may need to be restrained especially during naps or at night; keep nails short and clean. Contact physician if itching persists.
*Patient Teaching:* Do not alter dosage or stop drug abruptly; it could cause very serious side effects, even death. Gradual tapering of dosage is necessary. Increasing amount of medication will not hasten healing process. Demonstrate how to apply topical medication, or dosing schedule for oral form. Monitor signs and symptoms of medication, symptoms of adrenal insufficiency or worsening of condition, and report to physician. Obtain daily weights; report any sudden weight gains to physician. Stress importance of close medical supervision and follow-up and regular ophthalmic examinations if on long-term therapy. Caution about receiving skin tests, vaccinations or other immunizations, or

coming in contact with persons receiving oral polio virus vaccine. Inform any health-care provider, including dentists, surgeons, or emergency care personal that child is on this medication. Child should carry a medical identification card. Observe for symptoms of infections. Do not use OTC medications without contacting health care provider. Topical: Do not use medication on areas other than those prescribed by physician.

**Drug Interactions:** This drug in combination with high dosage of acetaminophen may increase risk of hepatotoxicity. With analgesics and antiinflammatory drugs it may increase the risk of gastric ulceration. Amphotericin B and potassium-depleting diuretics increase risk of hypokalemia. Use with anabolic steroids may increase the risk of edema and acne. Drug in combination with anticoagulants may decrease anticoagulant effect. This drug used with anticonvulsants (Phenytoin) may lower seizure threshold. Use with vaccines, live virus, or other immunizations may potentiate replication of the vaccine virus, increasing chance for developing the viral disease.

**Laboratory Test Interferences:** May increase serum cholesterol, sodium and blood glucose. May decrease serum calcium, potassium, $T_4$, $^{131}I$ uptake, urine 17-hydroxysteroid and 17-ketosteroids. Tends to suppress skin tests; may give a false-negative result with nitroblue-tetrazolium for bacterial infection. Adrenal function assessed by ACTH stimulation or plasma cortisol may be decreased.

**Storage Requirements:** Store at 15 to 30°C (59 to 86°F). Discard parenteral form 48 hours after reconstitution.

---

□ **METOCLOPRAMIDE HYDROCHLORIDE**                    (met-oh-kloe'pra-mide)

(Clopra, Maxeran, Maxolon, Reglan)

**Classification:** cholinergic, antiemetic, dopamine receptor antagonist

**Available Preparations:**
- 5 mg/5ml oral solution
- 5, 10-mg tablets
- 5 mg/ml for parenteral administration

**Action and Use:** Increases upper gastric tract motility while lowering esophageal sphincter pressure. It also relaxes the pyloric sphincter and duodenal bulb as it increases peristalsis of duodenum and jejunum. Its cholinergic activity, however, does not stimulate gastric, biliary, or pancreatic secretions. Its dopamine-receptor antagonist properties gives it antiemetic and sedative capacities. Used in children for intubation of small intestine, management of gastric stasis and gastroesophageal reflux.

## Routes and Dosage:
*PO, IV:* Gastroesophageal Reflux:
- 1 to 6 year: 0.1 mg/kg/dose every 6 hours
- 6 to 14 years: 2.5 to 5 mg/dose every 6 hours
- adult: 10 mg/dose

**Absorption and Fate:** Rapidly absorbed form GI tract except with gastric stasis. Onset action: PO: 30 to 60 minutes; IM, 10 to 15 minutes; IV, 1 to 3 minutes. Duration of action: 1 to 2 hours. Half-life: 4 to 6 hours. 85% excreted unchanged in urine.

**Contraindications and Precautions:** Pregnancy category B. Excreted in breast milk, safety during lactation not established. Contraindicated in hypersensitivity to drug, sulfites, pheochromocytoma, seizure disorders, mechanical obstruction or perforation of GI tract. Use caution in GI hemorrhage, impaired renal or liver function, hypertension, congestive heart failure.

## Side Effects:
*CNS:* most frequent: restlessness, drowsiness, lassitude, fatigue; **extrapyramidal reactions** (dystonic reactions, usually high-dose antiemetic therapy for cancer treatment); insomnia, dizziness, headache. *CV:* transient hypertension. *GI:* constipation or diarrhea, dry mouth. *Skin:* maculopapular rash, urticaria, glossal or periorbital edema

## Nursing Implications:
*Assess:* Obtain baseline vital signs, P, BP, and respirations.
*Administer: PO:* For gastric reflux give 30 minutes before meal and at bedtime. *IV:* Give slow IV push undiluted (dosage under 10 mg) over 2 minutes. Rapid infusion causes restlessness, anxiety followed by drowsiness. Intermittent infusion dilute to 0.2 mg/ml and infuse over no less than 15 minutes. Compatible with $D_5W$, $D_5W/0.5\%NS$, NS, LR, Ringer's lactate. Protect intermittent infusions bags from light during infusion; use aluminum foil or dark plastic cover. Drug will decompose upon exposure to light. Consult pharmacist for drug incompatibilities. Discard open ampules.
*Monitor:* Observe for extrapyramidal reactions that can occur 24 to 48 hours after administration, more common in children. Symptoms include facial grimaces, rhythmic tongue, protrusions, involuntary limb movements, opisthonos, oculogyric crisis, laryngospasm. Treatment IM diphenhydramine: have emergency respiratory equipment available. Monitor vital signs.
*Patient Teaching:* Warn child or parent about side effects that may inhibit activity.

**Drug Interactions:** May potentiate depressive effects of opiates, analgesics, anticolinergics, sedatives, alcohol, barbiturates, or tranquilizers. This drug may effect GI transient time of some oral drugs especially drugs like digoxin (decrease absorption) and increase absorption of drugs from small intestine like acetaminophen, salicylates, diazepam, ethanol, levodopa, lithium, and tetracycline. Concurrent use with phenothiazines and butyrophenones increases incidence of extrapyramidal symptoms.

**Laboratory Test Interference:** Gonadorelin test altered by increasing serum prolactin levels.

**Storage Requirements:** Store at 15 to 30°C (59 to 86°F), in light-resistant container. Parenteral dilutions stable for 48 hours if protected from light.

---

## □ METRONIDAZOLE                              (me-troe-ni'da-zole)

(Apo-Metronidazole, Femazole, Flagyl, Flagyl IV, Flagyl IV RTU, Metro IV, Metryl IV, Neo-Tric, Novonidazole, PMS-Metronidazole, Protostat, Satric, Trikacide)

**Classification:** amebicide

### Available Preparations:
- 250, 500-mg tablets
- 250, 500-mg film-coated tablets
- 5 mg/ml for parenteral injection
- 500 mg or 100,000 U vaginal cream
- 500 mg or 100,000 U vaginal suppositories

**Action and Use:** Synthetic nitroimidazole derivative whose action is effective against trophozoites in intestinal lumen and wall and at extraintestinal sites. Also used as a trichomonacidal and bactericidal agent. Specific mechanism unknown but appears to work by binding and degrading DNA inside the organism. Used against *Entamoeba histolytica*, guinea worm, giardiasis, and trichomoniasis.

### Routes and Dosage:
*PO:*
- Amebiasis: 35 to 50 mg/kg/day in 3 divided doses for 5 to 10 days
- Guinea Worm: 25 mg/kg/day in 3 divided doses for 5 to 7 days
- Giardiasis: 15 mg/kg/day is 3 divided doses for 5 days
- Trichomoniasis: 15 mg/kg/day in 3 divided doses for 7 to 10 days

*PO, IV:* Bacteroides Meningitis: Loading dose: 15 mg/kg; then: neonates, under 7 days: 7.5 mg/kg/dose every 12 hour; neonates, over 7 days: 7.5 mg/kg/dose every 8 hours; children: 7.5 mg/kg/dose every 6 hours. (Maximum dosage 4 g/day)

**Absorption and Fate:** 80% absorbed from GI tract. Peak level: 1 to 2 hours. Half-life: 6 to 12 hours. 30 to 60% metabolized by liver and excreted in urine and feces.

**Contraindications and Precautions:** Pregnancy category B. Safe use during lactation not established. Manufacturer contraindicates use of IV or oral metronidazole in children except in amebiasis; however, oral form has been used for trichomoniasis, giardiasis, and guinea worm. Has been used experimentally in IV form in bacteroides meningitis. Contraindicated in hypersensitivity to drug or nitroimidiazole derivatives. Use caution in history of blood dyscrasias, hepatic impairments, patients on corticosteroids or predisposition to edema.

## Side Effects:
*CNS:* headache, dizziness, weakness, ataxia, confusion, irritability, depression, insomnia; **peripheral neuropathy**: numbness, tingling, paresthesia of extremity, **seizures** (rare). *CV:* **flattening of T wave** (rare). *GI:* nausea, anorexia, dry mouth, sharp unpleasant metallic taste, nausea, diarrhea, epigastric distress, constipation, antibiotic associated **pseudomembranous colitis** (rare). *GU:* dark or reddish brown urine, burning, dysuria, cystitis, polyuria, pelvic pressure. *Hemic:* **leukopenia** (rarely). *Other:* Hypersensitivity: urticaria, pruritus, erythematous rash, flushing, nasal congestion, fever, transient joint pains; Local: IV: thrombophlebitis

## Nursing Implications:
*Assess:* Obtain stool cultures according to agency policy (stool must be warm for detection of parasitic movement). Inspect and record appearance of stool. All family members need stool cultures. Obtain family history of home and sanitation conditions and presence of pets. Obtain baseline ophthalmic examination.

*Administer: PO:* Give with meals. Tablets may be crushed and mixed with food or fluid. IV: Solutions are diluted and ready to use. Flagyl IV is not and requires careful and special dilution process; because it is used so infrequently in children, consult your pharmacist. IV rate given over at least 1 hour. Do not mix with other solutions or drugs.

*Monitor:* Avoid extravasation and monitor for thrombophlebitis. Assess CNS and GI side effects. Stool cultures obtained weekly, then 1, 3, and 6 months after therapy stopped. Obtain stool cultures according to agency policy. Record number, frequency, and characteristics of stools. If not potty trained, keep tight fitting diapers or training pants on to prevent child from handling own fecal matter. Change diapers immediately after stools, dispose of properly and use good hand washing technique. Ophthalmic examinations should be done during therapy. Discontinue drug and report immediately to physician ophthalmic symptoms of blurred vision or eye pain, and skin rashes. Observe for overgrowth nonsusceptible organisms especially monilia.

*Patient Teaching:* Stress to all family members good hand washing techniques both before meals and after defecations. Use liquid soap; bar soap can harbor organisms for 18 hours. Discuss how disease transmitted and preventive measures and proper food preparation and handling. If child is in diapers, teach proper disposal of fecal matter. Observe for overgrowth of nonsusceptible organisms, ophthalmic side effects or skin symptoms, report to physician immediately. How to properly collect stool specimens. Importance of follow-up medical care.

**Laboratory Test Interferences:** Increased protein-bound serum iodine concentrations, decreased iodine-131 uptake, false-positive PKU. These may persist for 6 months.

**Storage Requirements:** Store at 15 to 30°C (59 to 86°F) in light-resistant container.

---

# ☐ MEZLOCILLIN SODIUM                                    (mez-loe-sill′in)

(Mezlin)

**Classification:** penicillin, extended spectrum

**Available Preparations:** 1, 2, 3, 4 g for parenteral administration

**Action and Use:** Mechanism similar to other penicillins that inhibit cell-wall synthesis in bacteria. Primarily used for *Klebsiella, Proteus vulgaris, Providencia rettgeri, Morganella morganii, P. mirabilis, Escherichia coli, Enterobacter, Serratia,* and *Pseudomonas aeruginosa* strains. Used in treatment of infections of GU tract, respiratory tract, intraabdominal, skin, soft tissue, and in septicemia and meningitis. Contains 1.75 to 1.85 mEq of sodium per gram of drug.

**Routes and Dosage:**
*IM, IV:*
- neonates, < 7 days: 75 mg/kg every 12 hours
- neonates, < 2000 g (over 8 days): 75 mg/kg every 8 hours
- neonates, > 2000 g (over 8 days): 75 mg/kg every 6 hours
- 1 month to 12 years: 50 to 75 mg/kg every 4 hours
- adult: 200 to 300 mg/kg/day in equally divided doses 4 to 6 hours. (Maximum not to exceed 24 g/day)

**Absorption and Fate:** Distributed in pleura, synovial, peritoneal, ascitic, wound, bile, bronchial secretions, tonsils, heart, gallbladder, adipose tissue, heart, bone, GU tissue, and meninges when inflamed. Peak level: neonates, IM or IV 30 minutes; children 2 to 17 years, IV 5 minutes after infusion. Half-life children, 0.83 to 0.97 hours; neonates, 2.4 to 4.47 hours. 16 to 42% bound to serum proteins; excreted in urine and small amount in bile.

**Contraindications and Precautions:** Pregnancy category B. Excreted in breast milk, use caution with lactation. Contraindicated if hypersensitivity to drug, penicillins, cephamycins, or cephalosporins. Use caution with sensitivity to multiple allergens, other drugs, renal impairment, bleeding tendencies or sodium restrictions.

## Side Effects:

*CNS:* headache, vertigo, lethargy, giddiness, neuromuscular hyperirritability, **seizures** (with high serum levels). *GI:* nausea, vomiting, abnormal taste, flatulence, loose stools, diarrhea (3%). *Hepatic:* transient elevation of SGOT, SGPT, LDH, alkaline phosphatase, bilirubin. *GU:* **acute interstitial nephritis:** rash, hematuria, cylindruria, eosinophilia, and renal failure. Transient increase in BUN and serum creatinine. *Hemic:* **anemi, eosinophilia, thrombocytopenia, leukopenia, neutropenia, abnormal prothrombin time and platelet aggregation** (with high doses). *Other:* Hypersensitivity: skin rashes, pruritus, urticaria, fever, serum sickness, **anaphylaxis** (increased incidence of hypersensitivity in cystic fibrosis patients); Local: IV: pain, vein irritation, erythema, phlebitis, thrombophlebitis, IM: pain, induration, erythema

## Nursing Implications:

*Assess:* Assess previous allergy to drug, penicillins, cephalosporins, other drugs, or history of allergies. Obtain cultures and sensitivity before treatment, but can start treatment before results. Obtain baseline data on renal, hepatic, hematological, potassium levels if on long-term therapy.

*Administer:* Powder and reconstituted solutions may darken upon storage but does not effect potency. Refrigerated, reconstituted solutions may have precipitate form; redissolve drug by raising solutions temperature to 37°C in warm water bath for 20 minutes then agitating vigorously. *IM:* Reconstitute each gram with 3 to 4 ml of sterile water or 0.5% lidocaine (without epinephrine) for injection and agitate vigorously to dissolve drug. Injection painful; minimize pain by injecting slowly over 12 to 15 seconds. IV: Reconstitute according to package inserts with sterile water, 0.9% normal saline, and 5% dextrose. Can give slow IV push over 3 to 5 minutes of dilution of 100 mg/ml. Preferred route intermittent infusion, minimum dilution of 80 mg/ml infused over 30 minutes. Compatible with $D_5W$, $D_5W/0.2\%$ NS, $D_5W/0.5\%NS$, $D_5W/NS$, NS, $D_{10}/W$, LR. Do not premix with aminoglycosides or other drugs; infuse separately. Incompatible with amphotericin B, chloramphenicol, lincomycin, oxytetracycline, polymyxin B, promethazine, tetracycline, and vitamins B with C. Using large vein with small bore needle may reduce local IV reactions.

*Monitor:* Check for hypersensitivity (especially in first 20 minutes of first dosage). Observe IV site for vein irritation and extravasation and change site every 72 hours. Monitor child for side effects. Closely observe for symptoms of bleeding; monitor platelet dysfunction and bleeding time especially on long term therapy. Monitor potassium and sodium levels, renal and hepatic function. Maintain flu levels for age group. Avoid prolonged use of drug because of overgrowth of nonsusceptible organisms. Duration of therapy usually 48 hours after symptoms subside or culture is negative. If given for **beta-hemolytic streptococcal infections**, 10-day course needed to prevent risk of acute rheumatic fever or glomerulonephritis.

## Drug Interactions:

Anticoagulants given with this drug may increase risk of bleeding. Erythromycin, tetracycline, and chloromycetin may decrease effects of mezlocillin. Probenecid increases serum concentrations and prolongs half-life of this drug.

**Laboratory Test Interferences:** Increased SGOT and SGPT.

**Storage Requirements:** Store powder at 15 to 30°C (59 to 86°F). Store reconstituted solutions for IM and IV according to package inserts.

---

# ☐ MICONAZOLE                              (mi-kon′a-zole)

(Micatin, Monistat)

**Classification:** antifungal

**Available Preparations:**
- 10 mg/ml for parenteral administration
- 2% lotion, cream, powder, aerosol, and aerosol powder for topical administration
- 2% cream for vaginal administration
- 100, 200 mg for vaginal suppositories

**Action and Use:** Inhibits the biosynthesis of ergosterol or other sterols, which alters the permeability of the cell. Intracellular constituents become necrotic. Parenteral form is used for fungal infections: candidiasis, coccidioido-mycosis, cryptococcosis, paracoccidioidomycosis, and chronic mucocutaneous candidiasis. Topical form used to treat tinea pedis, tinea cruris, tinea corporis, and cutaneous candidiasis.

**Routes and Dosage:**
*IV:* over 1 year: 20 to 40 mg/kg/day. (Maximum individual dose should not exceed 15 mg/kg/dose)
***Intrathecal (IT):*** 20 mg/dose every 1 to 2 days
***Topical:*** apply sparingly to affected area 2 times per day
***Vaginal:*** instill 1 applicatorful at bedtime for 7 days

**Absorption and Fate:** Distributed to body tissues and fluids, poor penetration in CSF, only achieved in significant levels by IT administration. 91 to 93% bound to serum proteins and metabolized by liver. Half-life phasic levels 0.4, 2.1, and 24.1 hours. Excreted primarily in feces with 10 to 14% in urine.

**Contraindications and Precautions:** Pregnancy category B. Safe use during lactation and in those under 1 year (parenteral) and 2 years (topical) not established. Contraindicated in hypersensitivity to this drug. Use caution with hepatic impairment.

**Side Effects:**
*CNS:* dizziness, drowsiness, headache; IT: arachnoiditis, transient saddle

numbness, **12th cranial nerve palsy, mild third ventricular hemorrhage**. *GI:* nausea, vomiting, anorexia. *GU:* topical: vaginal vulvovaginal burning, itching, irritation. *Skin:* IV: pruritus; topical: irritation burning, maceration. *Hemic:* transient decrease in hematocrit, normocytic or microcytic anemia, **thrombocytopenia**. *Other:* fever, chills, flushing, hyperlipidemia, serum triglycerides, hyponatremia; *Local:* phlebitis

## Nursing Implications:

*Assess:* Positively identify organism by culture or histological tests before starting drug. Obtain baseline hematocrit, hemoglobin, serum electrolytes, and lipids.

*Administer: IV:* If solution is dark in color, discard. Dilute further with normal saline or 5% dextrose to 1 mg/ml and infuse over 30 to 60 minutes. Compatible with $D_5W$, NS. Too rapid infusion may cause tachycardia or arrhythmias (cardiac arrest has occurred). To reduce vein irritation, use central venous catheter, or change infusion site every 2 to 3 days. Do not mix with other drugs. Child should be hospitalized for initial treatment and it is best to have physician present during first infusion.

*Topical:* Physician should specify how area should be cleaned before drug application. Use lotion for intertriginous areas. Apply cream sparingly rubbing into area. Do not use occlusive dressings. Avoid contact with eyes.

*Vaginal:* See Part I for insertion. Vegetable oil base of suppository may interact with latex of vaginal contraceptive diaphragms, so they should not be concurrently used. Vaginal cream does not have this base.

*Monitor: IV:* Monitor for cardiac arrhythmias during infusion and observe for signs of phlebitis. If nausea occurs, antiemetics may be given and avoid giving dosage near meal time. Observe for side effects. Pruritus may require diphenhydramine. Obtain periodic hematocrit, hemoglobin, serum electrolytes, and lipids. Therapy may be 6 to 12 weeks in duration or longer.

*Patient Teaching:* Teach proper application of topical forms of medication. If no improvement in 2 weeks, contact physician. Total therapy may take several months. With vaginal medication, the wearing of panty liner may prevent staining of undergarment. Do not apply other OTC over infected areas without contacting physician.

## Drug Interactions: Drug may interact with cyclosporine, phenytoin, and rifampin, altering metabolism of drugs. Used in combination with amphotericin B, antagonism may occur. Anticoagulant effect of coumarin drugs are enhanced with miconazole.

## Storage Requirements: Store at 15 to 30°C (59 to 86°F); protect from freezing. Reconstituted solutions stable 24 hours at room temperature.

---

## □ MIDAZOLAM                                    (mid′az-zoe-lam)

(Versed)

**Classification:** general anesthetic, anxiolytic

**Available Preparations:**
- 1, 5 mg/ml vials for parenteral use

**Action and Use:** This benzodiazepine has CNS depressant effects, acts to reduce anxiety, has muscle relaxant and amnesic effects. Interferes with an inhibitory neurotransmitter in the brain. Used for preoperative medication to provide sedation and amnesia in children over 2 years. Also useful before computerized tomography and for induction of anesthesia in children over 4 years. Used experimentally in oral form for children with night terrors. The drug has not been approved for use in children by the FDA, but is being used by clinicians for the above purposes.

**Routes and Dosages:** IM, IV
*IM:* Preoperative Medication: 0.08 to 0.2 mg/kg
Dose established by clinicians rather than manufacturers.

**Absorption and Fate:** Rapidly absorbed after IM administration and widely distributed to body tissues. Up to 97% bound to plasma proteins. Metabolized by the liver and excreted in the urine. For IM administration, onset of action is 5 to 15 minutes, with peak action in 20 to 60 minutes and duration generally about 2 hours. After IV administration, onset of action is 1 to 5 minutes and usual duration of action is 2 hours. The drug undergoes biphasic metabolism with initial half-life of 6 to 20 minutes and terminal half-life at 1 to 4 hours.

**Contraindications and Precautions:** Pregancy category D. Other benzodiazepines cross into breast milk, therefore, this drug is not recommended during lactation. Safety for children under 18 years not established. Contraindicated in those with hypersentivity to the drug and in acute narrow-angle glaucoma. Cautious use in pulmonary disease, renal dysfunction, and congestive failure.

**Side Effects:**
*CNS:* **excessive sedation**, headache, drowsiness, paradoxical agitation, tremors, and hyperactivity, euphoria, sleep disturbance, anxiety, restlessness, confusion, slurred speech. *CV:* **hypotension**, decreased heart rate, tachycardia and other cardiac changes. *GI:* nausea, vomiting, acidic taste, increased salivation, dry mouth, constipation. ***Respiratory:*** decreased respiratory rate, **apnea**. *Skin:* pain, erythema, induration at IV injection site, urticaria, rash, pruritus. *Sensory:* blurred vision, diplopia, nystagmus, blocked ears

**Nursing Implications:**
*Assess:* Establish baseline vital signs.
*Administer:* After administration bed rails are raised to safeguard patient.
*IM:* Compatible in same syringe with atropine, meperidine, morphine, scopolamine for up to 30 minutes. Compatible with fentanyl, hydoxyzine, prometha-

zine for 8 hours. *IV:* Compatible with 5% dextrose, saline, or Ringer's lactate solutions. Injected slowly over at least 2 minutes for sedation or 30 seconds for induction of anesthesia. The amount of drug to be injected can be added to 5% dextrose or saline to facilitate slow injection. IV use only with constant respiratory and cardiac monitoring; emergency equipment for respiratory support should be readily available during IV administration.

*Monitor:* Monitor blood pressure, watching for hypotension and respiratory rate especially during IV administration.

*Patient Teaching:* Avoid other CNS depressants.

**Drug Interactions:** Potentiation effects with other CNS depressants. Decreases need for some anesthetics during surgical procedure. Cimetidine or ranitidine may increase serum levels of midazolam.

**Storage Requirements:** Store in light-resistant containers at 15 to 30°C (59 to 86°F)

---

## □ MORPHINE  (mor'feen)

(Astromorph PF, MS Contin, MSIR, Roxanol, RMS)

**Combination Products:** Morphine and atropine sulfates

**Classification:** narcotic analgesic, opiate agonist

### Available Preparations:
- 10 mg/5ml, 20 mg/5 ml oral solution
- 20 mg/ml, 100 mg/5 ml oral concentrate solution
- 15, 30-mg tablets
- 10, 15, 30-mg soluble tablets
- 30-mg extended-release tablets
- 15 mg, 30 mg, 60-mg extended release, film coated tablets
- 0.5 mg/ml, 1 mg/ml, 2 mg/ml, 4 mg/ml, 5 mg/ml, 8 mg/ml, 10 mg/ml, 15 mg/ml vials for parenteral use; 1 mg/ml and 5 mg/ml injections for use with IV infusion device
- 5, 10, 20, 30-mg rectal suppositories

**Action and Use:** This is a phenathrene derivative of opium. It acts on the CNS by inducing neurotransmitters to produce analgesia, depresses cough by effect on cough center in medulla, and depresses respiration by effect on respiratory center in brainstem. This drug has strong analgesic effects and is used for relief of severe pain, and as a preoperative medication.

### Routes and Dosages:
*PO:* 0.3 mg/kg q4h
*SC, IM:* Pain: 0.1 to 0.2 mg/kg q4h PRN; not to exceed 15 mg/dose

*SC:* Severe Pain (i.e., cancer): maintenance: 0.025 to 1.79 mg/kg/hour (usually 0.06 mg/kg/hour)

*IV:* Severe Pain (i.e., cancer): 0.025 to 2.6 mg/kg/hour (usually 0.04 to 0.07 mg/kg/hour)

**Absorption and Fate:** Well absorbed from parenteral injection, less predictable from PO route; good from PR form. Widely distributed in the body; present in breast milk. Metabolized by the liver and excreted principally in urine. Peak action after PO is 60 minutes; after SC is 50 to 90 minutes; after IM is 30 to 60 minutes; after IV is 20 minutes. Analgesia present for up to 7 hours.

**Contraindications and Precautions:** Pregnancy category B. Contraindicated in prematures and other neonates, those with hypersensitivity to the drug, in patients with respiratory depression, comatose, elevated CSF pressure. Cautious use in infants and young children, those with asthma, hepatic or renal dysfunction, atrial flutter, tachycardia, colitis, hypothyroidism.

**Side Effects:**
*CNS:* **sedation**, dizziness, depression, **coma**, euphoria, restlessness, insomnia. *CV:* **circulatory depression** is potentially life threatening; orthostatic hypotension, palpitation, bradycardia, tachycardia (more common than with other opiates). *GI:* nausea, vomiting, constipation. ***Respiratory:*** **respiratory depression** (serious side effect). ***Hepatic:*** biliary spasm, increased serum amylase and lipase. *GU:* urinary retention, oliguria, stimulates release of vasopressin; impotence. *Skin:* rash, erythema, urticaria, pruritus, facial flushing indicate **hypersensitivity reaction**

**Nursing Implications:**
*Assess:* Assess type and degree of pain; use other pain control methods in addition to analygesic. Take baseline vital signs. Be certain respirations are within normal range.
*Administer:* Morphine is a Schedule II drug under the Federal Controlled Substances Act. 60 to 80 mg meperidine is approximately equivalent to 10 mg morphine sulfate in analgesic potency. Check time of last dose carefully before giving as well as currency of order. *PO:* Extended-release tablets should be swallowed whole. Dilute oral solution in at least 30 ml fluid. Read labels regarding strength carefully and use calibrated dropper dispensed with the solution. *IM, SC:* Incompatible with aminophylline, heparin, methicillin, nitrofurantoin, phenobarbital, sodium bicarbonate, and some other drugs. Consult pharmacist before placing in other solutions. *IV:* Given slowly with patient lying down. For IV push, dilute in at least 5 ml NS or bacteriostatic water and give over at least 5 minutes. For continuous infusion, dilute to 0.1 to 1 mg/ml in 5% dextrose and give by infusion device. Given for patient controlled analgesia by pump (PCA). ***Intrathecal, epidural use:*** **by specially trained personnel only**.
*Monitor:* Monitor vital signs every 15 to 30 minutes after administration. If hypotension occurs, or patients feel nausea or dizziness, have them lie down. After parenteral forms, patients are generally left in bed with side rails up.

Constantly evaluate respirations and level of consciousness during IV push administration. Evaluate pain in 30 minutes and record results. Observe for constipation.

*Patient Teaching:* Take drug only as directed and only for patient prescribed. Drug can alter mental alertness, therefore, avoid driving and adjust activities accordingly. Encourage adequate fluid intake, coughing, and deep breathing to avoid respiratory stasis. Prolonged use can be habit forming and the drug has been abused by health-care personnel. Instruct the correct use of the pump to patients using the drug for PCA.

**Drug Interactions:** Additive CNS effects with alcohol and other CNS depressants. Phenothiazines may antagonize action. Increased effects if given with dextroamphetamine, may increase effects of neuromuscular-blocking agents. May decrease effects of diuretics in congestive heart failure.

**Laboratory Test Interferences:** Increases serum amylase and lipase; delay drawing blood for these tests for 24 hours after the drug. False-positive urine glucose. Decreased serum and urine 17-ketosteroids and 17-hydroxysteroids.

**Storage Requirements:** Store in tightly covered, light-resistant containers at 15 to 30°C (59 to 86°F). Avoid freezing solutions.

---

# □ NAFCILLIN SODIUM

(naf-sill'in)

(Nafcil, Nallpen, Unipen)

**Classification:** antibiotic, penicillinase-resistant

## Available Preparations:
- 250 mg/5 ml oral solution
- 500-mg film-coated tablets
- 250-mg capsules
- 500mg, 1, 1.5, 2, 4 g for parenteral administration

**Action and Use:** Similar to penicillin in action but resistant to inactivation by penicillinase. Primarily use in penicillinase-producing *Staphylococcus aureus* and *S. epidermidis* infections. Each gram contains about 2.9 mEq sodium.

## Routes and Dosage:
*PO:*
- neonates: 30 to 40 mg/kg/day equally divided doses every 6 or 8 hours
- over 1 month: 50 to 100 mg/kg/day equally divided doses every 6 hours

*IM:* neonates:
- 20 mg/kg/day equally divided doses every 12 hours

- over 1 month: 50 mg/kg/day equally divided doses every 12 hours

However, some clinicians recommend the following dosages for neonates:

- < 7 days: 40 to 100 mg/kg/day equally divided doses every 12 hours
- 7 to 28 days: 60 to 200 mg/kg/day equally divided doses every 8 hours
- over 1 month: 50 to 200 mg/kg/day equally divided doses every 6 hours (severe infections every 4 to 6 hours).

*IV:* Manufacturer has not established dosage for neonates, however, some clinicians recommend the following dosages:

- < 7 days: 50 to 100 mg/kg every 12 hours
- 7 days to 1 month: 75 to 100 mg/kg every 8 hours
- over 1 month: 50 to 100 mg/kg/day equally divided doses every 6 hours (severe infections, 100–200 mg/kg/day every 4 to 6 hours)

**Absorption and Fate:** Absorption: poorly, erratically from GI site, rapidly from IM site. Distributed: synovial, pericardial, ascitic, pleural fluids, and into liver, bone, and bile. Peak level: PO, 30 to 120 minutes; IM, 30 to 120 minutes, IV at end of infusion. Half-life: 1 month to 14 years, 0.75 to 1.9 hours; neonates, 1.2 to 5.5 hours. 60% metabolized in liver; excreted by bile and small amount in urine.

**Contraindications and Precautions:** Pregnancy category B. Use caution during lactation. Manufacturer states safe use of IV form drug in neonates and infants not established. Contraindicated in hypersensitivity to drug, penicillins, cephalosporins, or cephamycins. Use caution with allergies, asthma, family history of allergies, renal or hepatic impairment.

**Side Effects:**

*GI:* nausea, vomiting and diarrhea. *GU:* **acute interstitial nephritis** (rare): rash, macroscopic or microscopic hematuria, azotemia, dysuria, oliguria, proteinuria. *Hepatic:* transient rise SGOT, SGPT, alkaline phosphatase. *Skin:* morbilliform, maculapapular, urticarial, or erythematous, rashes, pruritus (hypersensitivity). *Hemic:* **eosinophilia, anemia, neutropenia, thrombocytopenia, leukopenia, agranulocytosis, prolonged bleeding time** (rare). *Other:* Hypersensitivity: **serum sickness, anaphylaxis** (rare). *Local:* IM painful, sterile abscesses; IV phlebitis, thrombophlebitis, **extravasation causes severe chemical irritation that can result in full thickness skin loss and gangrene**

**Nursing Implications:**

*Assess:* Assess previous allergy to drug, penicillins, cephalosporins, other drugs, asthma, or family history of allergies. Obtain cultures and sensitivity before treatment, but can start treatment before results. Obtain baseline renal, hepatic, and hematologic data before therapy.

*Administer: PO:* Food interferes with drug absorption; give 1 hour before or 2 hours after meals. Refrigerate solution. Capsules may be taken apart and tablets crushed and mixed with small amount of food or fluid. Both forms buffered with calcium carbonate and can interact with other medications. *IM:* Reconstitute according to package inserts with either sterile or bacteriostatic water, 0.9% sodium chloride for injection. Injection painful. Do not use solutions with bacteriostatic water in neonates. *IV:* Reconstitute according to package insert with either sterile or bacteriostatic (do not use for neonates) water or 0.9% sodium chloride for injection. Can give slow IV push; dilute in 15 to 30 ml (2 to 40 mg/ml) and infuse over 5 to 10 minutes. Intermittent infusion: dilute to minimum 20 mg/ml infused in 30 to 60 minutes; maximum infusion time, 200 mg/minute. Compatible with $D_5W$, $D_5W/0.2\%NS$, $D_5W/0.5\%NS$, $D_5W/NS$, NS, LR, Normosol M or R, Ionosol I $D_5W$. Do not mix with any other drug; incompatible with aminoglycosides, succinylcholine, tetracyclines, and ascorbic acid and any additive changing solution pH below 5.0 or above 8.0. Give at least 1 hour before bacteriostatic antibiotics. Infuse drug only through patent tubing, **extravasation can cause severe skin damage**.

*Monitor:* IM site may develop sterile abscesses. Observe IV site for vein irritation and thrombophlebitis; change site every 24 to 48 hours. If pain occurs during infusion, stop IV flow and evaluate site. If extravasation occurs, local injury may be minimized by immediate infiltration of hyaluronidase at site. Monitor child for hypersensitivity (especially in first 20 minutes of first dosage), rash (onset and characteristics), and side effects. Watch for symptoms of superinfections or interstitial nephritis. Drug's sodium content may effect patient's sodium restrictions. Assess renal hepatic functions periodically during therapy. Hematological functions (differential leukocyte counts) should be done 1 to 3 times per week and observe for any symptoms of bleeding. Maintain fluid intake for age group. Therapy course varies and depends on severity and type of infection.

**Drug Interactions:** Erythromycin, tetracycline, chloramphenical may decrease the antibacterial effects of nafcillin. Anticoagulants given with this drug may increase risk of bleeding. Probenecid increases serum concentrations and prolongs half-life of this drug.

**Storage Requirements:** Store tablets and capsules at 15 to 30°C (59 to 86°F) protect tablets from light. Reconstituted, oral solution stable for 7 days if refrigerated; IM solutions stable at room temperature for 3 days and if refrigerated stable for 7 days. Consult package insert for stability of IV solutions.

---

# □ NALOXONE                               (nal-ox'one)

(Narcan)

**Classification:** narcotic antagonist

**Available Preparations:**
- 0.02, 0.4, 1 mg/ml vials for parenteral use

**Action and Use:** This thebaine derivative has little action except in the person who has received opiates. Although the exact mechanism of action is unknown, it is likely to compete with opiate receptors in the CNS. Used to treat overdose with narcotics and may be used in the neonate experiencing respiratory difficulty due to opiate treatment of the mother in labor and delivery. Uses not approved by the FDA include treatment of emetic effects of apomorphine, respiratory failure, shock, and opiate addiction.

## Routes and Dosages: SQ, IM, IV

**IV:** 0.005 to 0.01 mg at 2 to 3-minute intervals until effective; an IV infusion of 0.024 to 0.16 mg/kg/hour may be used alternatively; initially the infusion rate is generally 0.4 mg/hour. If IV is unavailable the drug is given IM or SC.
**IV:** Neonatal Depression: 0.01 mg/kg initially in umbilical vein at 2 to 3-minute intervals until effective. If umbilical vein unavailable the drug is given IM or SC.

## Absorption and Fate: Rapidly absorbed from parenteral routes and distributed into body tissues. Rapidly metabolized by the liver and excreted in the urine. Onset of action is 1 to 2 minutes after IV, 2 to 5 minutes after IM and SC. Peak action within 30 to 120 minutes. Duration of action about 45 minutes after IV route, longer after IM and SC. Half-life 3 hours in neonates, 60 to 90 minutes in others.

## Contraindications and Precautions: Pregnancy category B. Contraindicated in known hypersensitivity to the drug and for treatment of respiratory depression not caused by opiates. Cautious use in nursing mothers as it is unknown if it crosses to breast milk, in cardiovascular disease, neonates, or others dependent on opiates.

## Side Effects:

**CNS:** seizures (rare). **CV:** hypotension, hypertension, tachycardia; effects seen most often in those with CV disease or taking cardiac drugs. **GI:** nausea and vomiting (rare)

## Nursing Implications:

**Assess:** Take vital signs. Ascertain amount of opiate patient has received.
**Administer:** Resuscitative equipment and drugs should be readily available. High dose after surgery with opiate use is avoided as it causes nausea, vomiting, sweating, tachycardia. **IV:** Mix in 5% dextrose or normal saline to 4 μg/ml. Stable for 24 hours. Do not mix with solutions containing bisulfite, metabisulfite, or with alkaline solutions.
**Monitor:** Take vital signs frequently, particularly respirations. Even after successful treatment, vital signs must be taken frequently as naloxone has a short duration of action and the opiate action time may be longer, therefore, repeat doses of naloxone may be needed. Monitor postsurgical patients for bleeding as coagulation may be altered.

## Storage Requirements: Store in light-resistant containers at 15 to 30°C (59 to 86°F).

# ☐ NAPROXEN

(na-prox′en)

(Anaprox, Naprosyn)

**Classification:** nonsteroidal antiinflammatory, antirheumatic

## Available Preparations:
- 250, 375, 500-mg tablets
- 275, 550-mg film-coated tablets
- 125 mg/5 ml suspension

**Action and Use:** Interferes with action of prostaglandins, has an effect on the hypothalmus, and acts to block peripheral nerve transfer. Interferes with platelet aggregation, thereby prolonging bleeding time. Its analgesic effect is useful for mild to moderate pain such as postoperatively or during menstruation. Its antiinflammatory action makes it useful in rheumatoid arthritis; also used for osteoarthritis and ankylosing spondylitis.

## Routes and Dosages:
*PO:* Juvenile Rheumatoid Arthritis: 10 mg/kg/day in 2 doses

**Absorption and Fate:** Completely absorbed from GI tract with amount and speed of absorption decreased by food. Highly protein bound with distribution throughout the body. Crosses placenta and is present in breast milk. Metabolized by the liver and mainly excreted in the urine. Peak level reached in 2 to 4 hours for tablets and 1 to 2 hours for the salt preparations. Half-life: 13 hours.

**Contraindications and Precautions:** Pregnancy category B. Safe use during pregnancy has not been proven by study. Animal studies suggest the possibility of premature closure of the ductus arteriosus in the fetus and prolonged pregnancy due to uterine prostaglandin inhibition, therefore, use in the second half of pregnancy is not recommended. Present in breast milk, therefore, not recommended during lactation. Safety and efficacy in children under 2 years have not been demonstrated; its use when indicated for children 2 to 14 years should be supervised by a health-care provider. Film-coated tablets are not recommended for children. Contraindicated in those with allergy to this drug, aspirin, or other nonsteroidal antiinflammatories. Cautious use in GI disease such as ulcers, coagulation disorder, cardiac dysfunction, renal dysfunction, hypertension, hepatic dysfunction, asthma, congestive heart failure, mental depression, systemic lupus erythematosus.

## Side Effects:
*CNS:* dizziness, headache, fatigue, confusion, fever, mood changes and depression. *CV:* fluid retention and **congestive heart failure**, hypertension, palpitation, arrhythmias, anaphylaxis. *GI:* heartburn, nausea, vomiting, pain,

constipation, diarrhea, peptic ulcer, **GI bleeding**, dry mouth, gingivitis. **Respiratory:** bronchospasm, dyspnea, **anaphylaxis** (as allergic response). **Hepatic:** jaundice, hepatitis, altered liver enzymes. **GU:** polyuria, hematuria, proteinuria, oliguria. **Skin:** rash, urticaria, alopecia, Stevens-Johnson syndrome. **Hemic:** inhibited platelet action and **prolonged bleeding time**, neutropenia, agranulocytosis, aplastic anemia, **thrombocytopenia**, anemia. **Sensory:** blurred or disturbed vision, amblyopia, cataracts, tinnitus

## Nursing Implications:

**Assess:** History of prior allergy to this drug, aspirin, or other nonsteroidal antiinflammatories is taken. Patient with asthma is at higher risk for allergy. Visual disturbances and coagulation disorders need to be noted.

**Administer: PO:** Administration with food may help decrease GI discomfort, although this may also interfere with drug absorption. Tablet may be crushed and given in food if necessary, although a suspension form is available. The film-coated tablets cannot be accurately divided; it is recommended that children use the suspension or regular tablets instead. Both the film-coated tablets and suspension contain sodium that should be considered in the person with fluid and electrolyte or cardiac dysfunction.

**Monitor:** BUN, creatinine, SGOT, SGPT, serum potassium done in those with hepatic or renal dysfunction. Bleeding time monitored in those with coagulation disorder. If visual changes occur, an eye examination should be performed. Upper GI tests may be done if GI symptoms occur; stool for guaiac regularly performed. UA done periodically. Periodic physical assessments are useful as symptoms of illness may be masked.

**Patient Teaching:** Not intended for management of minor discomfort; usually used only in diseases such as juvenile rheumatoid arthritis in the pediatric population and its use is monitored by a health-care provider. For long-term use, the drug is taken with food to decrease GI discomfort. Take as directed; improvement may not be seen for about 2 weeks. Avoid alcohol and OTC drugs (such as acetaminophen) unless directed by prescriber. Drug can alter mental alertness; therefore, avoid driving and adjust activities accordingly. Report drug to other health-care providers such as dentists or surgeons. Report skin rash and flulike symptoms immediately as this may be an allergic reaction. Report visual changes and yellowing skin.

**Drug Interactions:** May displace other protein-bound drugs from binding sites. Increased risk of renal side effects with other drugs having similar effects such as acetaminophen and diuretics. Increased risk of GI side effects with other drugs having similar effects such as corticosteroids, potassium, aspirin. Potentiation of anticoagulant effects with drugs such as aspirin, heparin, and coumarin. Hypoglycemia with insulin. Decreased effect of antihypertensive medications such as hydralazine, furosemide, β blockers. Increased risk of hemic side effects with other drugs with same effect or with radiation. Increased serum lithium levels. Potential for decreased serum levels when given with aspirin; not recommended to be given with any other nonsteroidal antiinflammatory. Increased hyperkalemia with other drugs having the same effect such as potassium-sparing diuretics. Increased level and potentially toxic effects of methotrexate when given with this drug. Increased levels of aminoglycosides in prematures.

**Laboratory Test Interferences:** Prolongs bleeding time for about 1 day; no effect on prothrombin time or whole blood clotting time. Increased SGOT, SGPT, alkaline phosphatase, LDH, transaminase, BUN, creatinine, potassium, urine glucose, urine protein. False increase in 17-ketogenic steroids; does not influence 17-hydroxycorticosteroids; both of these tests, however, are delayed for 72 hours after last naproxen dose. Change urinary 5-hydroxyindoleacetic acid. Decreased blood glucose, plasma renin activity. Potential decreased urine output and uric acid.

**Storage Requirements:** Store at 15 to 30°C (59 to 86°F) in tightly closed, light-resistant containers. Do not freeze suspension.

---

## □ NIACIN

(Niac, Niacels, Niacinamide, Nicobid, Nicolar, Span Niacin)

**Classification:** nutritional supplement

**Available Preparations:**
*Niacin:*
- 50 mg/5 ml elixir
- 25, 50, 100, 250, 500-mg tablets
- 150, 250, 500, 750-mg extended-release tablets
- 125, 250, 300, 400, 500-mg capsules

*Niacinimide:*
- 50, 100, 500-mg tablets
- Available for IV infusion in combination vitamin/electrolyte solutions.

**Action and Use:** This water-soluble vitamin is a major cofactor for enzymes used in glycogenolysis, lipid metabolism, and tissue metabolism. Tryptophan is an amino acid that is converted to niacin in the body; niacin is also taken in directly and it is converted to the active substance niacinamide. 60 mg of dietary tryptophan converts to 1 mg niacin. Niacin may decrease synthesis of cholesterol, therefore, lowers serum cholesterol and triglyceride. It can cause peripheral vasodilation by direct effect on cutaneous vessels, although rarely used therapeutically for this effect. Deficiency results in pellagra with effects on the GI system, CNS, and skin. Used mainly in treatment of vitamin deficiency.

**Routes and Dosages:** PO, IM, IV
*PO:* Pellagra: 100 to 300 mg/day in divided doses
Nutritional supplement: 10 to 200 mg/day

**Absorption and Fate:** Readily and well absorbed from normal GI tract in stomach and small intestine. Widely distributed in body and present in breast milk. Metabolized in the liver and excreted in urine. Vasodilation effect occurs within 20 minutes of PO drug and lasts 20 to 60 minutes. Onset of action in lowering triglycerides occurs within several hours; in lowering cholesterol within several days. Peak levels in serum in 45 minutes. Half-life: 45 minutes. Therapeutic level for antilipemic action is 0.5 to 1.0 μg/ml.

**Contraindications and Precautions:** Pregnancy category C. Contraindicated in active hepatic disease, arterial bleeding, severe hypotension, active peptic ulcer, and prior hypersensitivity to the drug. Nicolar tablets contain tartrazine (yellow dye #5) and should not be given to those with tartrazine allergy. Cautious use in diabetics, glaucoma, hepatic dysfunction, stomach ulcer history, gallbladder dysfunction, allergy.

**Side Effects:**
*CNS:* dizziness, syncope, tingling skin. *CV:* hypotension, tachycardia. *GI:* heartburn, vomiting, stomach pain, increased GI motility, diarrhea. *Respiratory:* wheezing after IV form as **anaphylactic reaction**. *Hepatic:* jaundice, liver damage, abnormal liver function tests. *Skin:* tingling, itching, rash, redness, dryness, flushing. *Endocrine:* altered blood sugar in diabetics, hyperglycemia, glucosuria. *GU:* hyperuricemia. *Sensory:* blurred vision, amblyopia

**Nursing Implications:**
*Assess:* Obtain diet history. Baseline liver function studies and blood glucose are monitored. RDAs for niacin are:
- 0 to 6 months: 6 mg
- 6 to 12 months: 8 mg
- 1 to 3 years: 9 mg
- 4 to 6 years: 11 mg
- 7 to 10 years: 16 mg
- 11 to 18 years, male: 18 mg
- 11 to 14 years, female: 15 mg
- 15 to 18 years, female: 14 mg
- pregnancy: 15 mg
- lactation: 18 mg

*Administer:* Generally given PO unless patient can take nothing by mouth. Giving with meals will decrease GI distress. *IV:* Give slowly at less than 2 mg/minute. The parenteral niacinimide solution is incompatible with alkaline and strongly acidic solutions.

*Monitor:* Periodic liver function studies and blood glucose are performed particularly in those on long-term high-dose therapy. Side effects are relatively rare as excess amounts of this water-soluble vitamin are usually excreted. GI side effects and peripheral dilation are less of a problem if dosage is gradually increased to desired level. Record dietary intake. May occur with riboflavin deficiency so monitoring for it should occur.

***Patient Teaching:*** Take as directed. Limit alcohol intake. Get up slowly from supine position. Dietary teaching about sources of niacin should be done. These include organ meats, poultry, fish, beans, peas, peanuts, enriched cereals, wheat germ, milk, eggs.

**Drug Interactions:** Isoniazid can decrease niacin levels. Niacin potentiates antihypertensive effect of ganglionic blockers. Insulin requirements may be altered in diabetics.

**Laboratory Test Interferences:** False elevation of urinary catecholamines. False-positive urinary glucose by Benedict's reagent. Abnormal bilirubin, SGOT, SGPT, LDH, prothrombin time. Causes hypoalbuminemia.

**Storage Requirements:** Store tightly closed at 15 to 30°C (59 to 86°F). Protect solutions from freezing.

---

# □ NICLOSAMIDE                                    (ni-kloe′sa-mide)

(Niclocide)

**Classification:** anthelmintic

**Available Preparations:** 500 mg chewable tablet

**Action and Use:** Inhibits glucose uptake and mitochondrial oxidative phosphorylation in tapeworms. Effective against *Dipylidium caninum* (dog and cat tapeworm), *Diphyllobothrium latum* (fish tapeworm), *Hymenolepis diminuta* (rat tapeworm), *Hymenolepsis nana* (dwarf tapeworm), *Taenia saginata* (beef tapeworm), and *Taenia solium* (pork tapeworm). Not effective against *Cysticercus cellulosae*, the larval stage of pork tapeworm. When drug causes scolex to be dislodged from intestinal wall, the cestode may be partially or completely digested but this may also cause release of eggs into the host's intestine.

**Routes and Dosage:**
*PO:*
- Dwarf Tapeworm: over 2 years, 11 to 34 kg: 1 g as single dose, then 500 mg/day for 6 days; over 34 kg: 1.5 g as single dose, then 1 g/day for 6 days
- Other Tapeworms: over 2 years, 11 to 34 kg: 1 g as single dose; over 34 kg: 1.5 gm as single dose

**Absorption and Fate:** Very minimal absorption from GI tract. Metabolic fate of drug unknown. Excreted in feces.

**Contraindications and Precautions:** Pregnancy category B. Use with caution during lactation. Safe usage in children under 2 years has not been established. Contraindicated in hypersensitivity to drug.

## Side Effects:

*CNS:* headache, drowsiness, dizziness, weakness, irritability. *GI:* nausea, vomiting, abdominal pain, anorexia, diarrhea, pruritus ani, oral irritation, rectal bleeding bad taste in mouth, constipation. *Hepatic:* transient rise in SGOT. *Skin:* sweating, fever, rash, alopecia. *Other:* Rare: alopecia, rash, pruritus, flushing, hiccups cough, **hypotension**

## Nursing Implications:

*Assess:* Diagnosed through stool culture; follow your agency procedure for collection.

*Administer:* Tablet chewed or crushed and mixed with small amount of water to form a vanilla-flavored paste, do not swallow whole. Follow with fluids. Best to give with a small amount of food or light meal (breakfast). In treatment of dwarf tapeworm, it is necessary for all family members to be tested and treated.

*Monitor and Patient Teaching:* It is not necessary for purgation or dietary restrictions, but if child is constipated, a laxative may be necessary. Side effects are usually mild and drug is well tolerated in recommended doses. Presence of proglottids or eggs in stools for 7 days or longer indicates drug failure and repeat therapy is required. Child is considered cured if stool cultures are negative for ova and proglottids for 3 months. Prevention of reinfestation through good personal hygiene, hand washing, prevention of hand-to-mouth contamination, sanitary waste disposal, and proper cooking of pork, fish, and beef. If accidental ingestion of drug occurs, do not induce vomiting; fast-acting laxative or enema is used.

**Storage Requirements:** Store at 15 to 30°C (50 to 86°F) in tight container.

---

## □ NITROFURANTOIN,    (nye-troe-fyoor'an-toyn)
## NITROFURANTOIN
## SODIUM

(Apo-Nitrofurantoin, Furadantin, Furan, Furalan, Furantoin, Macrodantin, Nephronex, Nitrex, Novofuran, Sarodant)

**Classification:** antiinfective, urinary tract

## Available Preparations:
- 25 mg/ml oral (microcrystals) suspension
- 50, 100 mg (microcrystals) tablets
- 50, 100 mg (microcrystals) capsules
- 25, 50, 100 mg (macrocrystals) capsules

**Action and Use:** Antibacterial activity believed to be as result of interference with several bacterial enzyme systems. Used primarily in UTI or prophylaxis against UTI; active against *Escherichia coli*, Enterobacter, and a few strains of *Proteus*.

## Routes and Dosage:
*PO:* over 1 month: 5 to 7 mg/kg/day in equally divided doses every 6 hours
Prophylaxis: 1 to 2 mg/kg/day at hour of sleep or in 2 divided doses

**Absorption and Fate:** Appears most of drug absorbed in small intestine with absorption of microcrystal formulation fastest. Half-life: 20 minutes. 20 to 60% bound to plasma proteins. 30 to 50% excreted unchanged in urine.

**Contraindications and Precautions:** Pregnancy category B; but contraindicated near term, labor, and delivery. Safe use during lactation not established. Contraindicated in infants under 1 month, hypersensitivity to drug, anuria, oliguria, or creatinine clearance under 40 ml/minute. Use with caution with renal impairment, asthma, anemia, vitamin B deficiency, diabetes, electrolyte imbalances, G-6-PD deficiency, or debilitating disease conditions.

## Side Effects:
*CNS:* **peripheral neuropathy**, headache, vertigo, nystagmus, drowsiness. *GI:* anorexia, nausea, vomiting, abdominal pain and diarrhea (less common). *Resp:* **Hypersensitivity** (3 types) (1) **Acute:** chills, fever, cough, chest pain, **severe dyspnea**, pulmonary effusion (x-ray), may have erythematous maculopapular rash, urticaria. Can occur 8 hours to 3 weeks after therapy started; reversible if drug stopped. (2) **Subacute: tachypnea, dyspnea**, fever, cough, **interstitial pneumonitis lupus-like syndrome**. Occurs 1 month after initiation of therapy; recovery slower. (3) **Chronic:** malaise, **dyspnea on exertion**, cough, **altered pulmonary function**. After continuous therapy for 6 months or longer; permanent pulmonary damage may occur. *Hepatic:* **cholestatic jaundice, hepatic necrosis**. *GU:* dark yellow or brown color to urine, crystalluria. *Skin:* erythema multiforme, exfoliative dermatitis, **Stevens-Johnson syndrome**, photosensitivity, transient alopecia. *Hemic:* hemolytic anemia, **agranulocytosis**, leukopenia, eosinophilia, granulocytopenia, **thrombocytopenia, megaloblastic anemia**. *Other:* hypersensitivity: asthmatic attacks in those with history of asthma, **anaphylaxis**

## Nursing Implications:
*Assess:* Assess previous allergy to this drug. Assess renal function. Obtain cultures and sensitivity before treatment, but can start treatment before results. *Administer: PO:* May be given with food or milk. Macrocrystal size preferred because better tolerated, less nausea. Shake suspension well. Follow dosage with milk, fruit juice, or water. Capsules may be taken apart or tablets crushed for administration; however, contact with teeth may cause yellow staining. Contents can be mixed in small amount of food or fluid. Give with fluids and give oral hygiene after any crushed tablet or opened capsule. *Monitor:* Monitor child for hypersensitivity reactions: acute, subacute, and

chronic. Discontinue medication and inform physician. Watch for symptoms of superinfections, especially of urinary tract. Observe for symptoms of peripheral polyneuropathy; paresthesia, dysesthesia of lower extremities, muscle weakness, tingling; stop drug immediately. The severity of symptoms and recovery are not dose related and tend to occur in children with those illnesses listed in Contraindications and Precautions. Assess hepatic function with prolonged therapy. Maintain fluid intake for age group. Therapy course continued for 3 days after sterile urine culture.

***Patient Teaching:*** Take as scheduled and prescribed for full course of therapy. Inform child and parent of urine discoloration. Stop medication and call physician if tingling, numbness, or difficulty breathing occurs.

**Laboratory Test Interferences:** False-positive urine glucose with Clinitest and Benedict's test.

**Drug Interactions:** Probenecid and sulfinpyrazone combined with this drug decrease renal excretion of nitrofurantoin, thus prolonging serum levels and increasing its toxicity. Magnesium trisilicate antacids decrease absorption of this drug. Quinolone-derivative antiinfectives are antagonized by this drug.

**Storage Requirements:** Store at 15 to 30°C (59 to 86°F) in airtight, light-resistant containers. Drug decomposes on contact with any metal other than stainless steel.

---

# ☐ NITROPRUSSIDE SODIUM

(nye-troe-pruss'ide)

(Nipride, Nitropress)

**Classification:** vasodilator, antihypertensive

## Available Preparations:
- 50 mg/ml vials for parenteral use

**Action and Use:** This vasodilator relaxes smooth muscle in the vascular bed, thereby creating vasodilation and lowering blood pressure. No effect on uterine or duodenal smooth muscle or on myocardial contractility. Used in hypertensive crisis, left ventricular failure, and in surgery to decrease bleeding. Uses not approved at this time by the FDA include hypertension during surgery for pheochromocytoma, congestive heart failure, myocardial infarction, valvular regurgitation, ergot alkaloid overdose.

## Routes and Dosages:
***IV:*** 0.5 to 10 µg/kg/minute; average dose is 3 µg/kg/minute; not to exceed 10 µg/kg/minute

**Absorption and Fate:** Onset of action and peak action immediate; effect lasts only until 2 to 10 minutes after discontinuation of drug infusion. Rapidly metabolized by the liver and excreted mainly in urine. Half-life is a few minutes for the drug and 7 days for the metabolite thyocyanate; prolonged in renal dysfunction.

**Contraindications and Precautions:** Pregnancy category C. Safe use in pregnancy or lactation not established. Contraindicated in control of compensatory hypertension caused by congenital heart disease, during surgery in a patient with inadequate cerebral blood flow, and in emergency situations. Use with caution in hepatic or renal disease, hypothyroidism, hyponatremia, anemia, elevated intracranial pressure, pulmonary disease, and in those with decreased vitamin $B_{12}$.

**Side Effects:**
*CNS:* anxiety, apprehension, confusion, dizziness, muscle twitching, hyperreflexia, sweating. *CV:* **palpitation, lowered blood pressure, increase or decrease of pulse rate.** *GI:* nausea, vomiting, abdominal pain. *Other:* **Overdosage** manifested by weakness, fatigue, metabolic acidosis, tinnitus, blurred vision, confusion, loss of consciousness, nausea and vomiting, decreased reflexes, shortness of breath, shallow breathing, dilated pupils.

**Nursing Implications:**
*Assess:* Assess vital signs carefully. Assess for and correct hypovolemia and anemia.
*Administer:* 50 mg of drug is dissolved in 2 to 3 ml of solution and then added to 250 to 1000 ml or less of IV fluid for infusion. Dextrose in water is the only recommended infusion vehicle. Sterile water without preservative may be used to prepare solution. Solution will be slightly brownish colored. Increased discoloration, such as dark brown or blue, indicates need to discard solution. Wrap solution container in foil. Do not give in same solution with any other drugs. Use within 24 hours; if not wrapped from light, discard in 4 hours. Administer by infusion pump. Do not exceed 10 μg/kg/minute. Have 3% sodium nitrite solution and sodium thiosulfate solution readily available for treatment of potential thiocyanate poisoning (a breakdown product of the drug).
*Monitor:* Monitor vital signs, especially blood pressure, every few minutes. Keep systolic blood pressure above 60 mm Hg. Observe for side effects. If they occur, slow IV infusion rate. Monitor I & O. Monitor the blood level of thiocyanate if treatment is continued beyond 48 hours; not to exceed 100 μg/ ml. Serum cyanogen levels are done daily in patients with hepatic dysfunction. Monitor acid-base balance. Check IV infusion site often to identify infiltration. Replace with oral agents as soon as possible.

**Storage Requirements:** Store at 15 to 30°C (59 to 86°F). Protect reconstituted solution from heat and light. Cover vial of any unused solution with foil.

# ☐ NOREPINEPHRINE

(nor-ep-i-nef'rin)

(Levarterenol, Levophed)

**Classification:** catecholamine, α and β-adrenergic agent

## Available Preparations:
- 1 mg/ml ampule for parenteral use

**Action and Use:** A catecholamine similar to epinephrine and produced in the adrenal gland and sympathetic nervous system. Acts on α-adrenergic receptors producing peripheral vasoconstriction and on β-adrenergic receptors, increasing cardiac output. May cause hyperglycemia in high doses by inhibiting insulin release from the pancreas. Decreases blood flow to body parts other than the heart and brain; for example, decreases renal blood flow. Used in treatment of acute hypotensive states such as shock and myocardial infarction. Useful for temporary treatment of low blood pressure in cardiac arrest.

## Routes and Dosages:
*IV:*
- Hypotension: 2 μg/minute or 2 μg/m²/minute
- Cardiac Arrest: 0.1 μg/kg/minute; adjusted PRN to maintain adequate BP

**Absorption and Fate:** Rapid response after IV administration. Distributed in sympathetic nervous system tissue and does not cross blood-brain barrier. Metabolized in the liver and excreted in the urine. Effects last 1 to 2 minutes after administration.

**Contraindications and Precautions:** Pregnancy category D. May cause vasoconstriction in uterus and resultant fetal anoxia, therefore, should be avoided in pregnancy. Contraindicated in those with hypersensitivity to sulfites, patients with vascular thrombosis or hypoxia or hypercapnia, during general anesthesia with cyclopropane or halogentated hydrocarbons. Not to be given into leg veins of those with occlusive vascular disease or diabetes. Cautious use in those with hypertension or hyperthyroid.

## Side Effects:
*CNS:* headache, restlessness, anxiety, sweating, weakness, dizziness, tremor. *CV:* **tachycardia, elevated BP**, increased peripheral resistance, precordial pain, palpitation, reflex bradycardia, arrhythmias. ***Respiratory:*** **dyspnea**, apnea. *GU:* decreased renal perfusion and resultant decreased urinary output. *Skin:* tissue necrosis with extravasation. ***Other:*** **hypersensitivity** with photophobia, sweating, vomiting, seizures, angioedema, flushing, wheezing, hypertension.

## Nursing Implications:
*Assess:* Investigate patient history to rule out contraindications such as sulfite allergy. Persons with asthma are more likely to have such an allergy, therefore,

close observation of them would be needed. Hypovolemia should be corrected before or concurrent with norepinephrine use. Check vital signs, CVP or left ventricular filling pressure, EKG, intraarterial pressure, pulmonary arterial diastolic pressure, pulmonary capillary wedge pressure.

**Administer: IV:** 4 mg of norepinephrine is added to 1 L of 5% dextrose with or without normal saline (normal saline alone as solution should not be used; dextrose preserves the drug). Resultant solution contains 4 μg/ml and is stable for 24 hours at room temperature. If added to alkaline solutions, such as sodium bicarbonate, solution must be used immediately. Administered through plastic catheter deep into vein such as antecubital or femoral vein. Use a pump to regulate flow. Do not give with blood or plasma but administer in separate IV setup. A dose of 5 to 10 mg phentolamine is sometimes added to the liter of solution to minimize side effects in case of extravasation. Mixing with drugs other than phentolamine is not recommended. Have emergency drugs and equipment readily available. Propranolol may be used for arrhythmias and atropine for bradycardia. Drug is used for short-term treatment only and is slowly tapered before withdrawal.

**Monitor:** Check IV site frequently for signs of extravasation as the vasoconstriction effects of the drug can lead to tissue necrosis. Blanching along the vein is a common early indicator. If extravasation occurs, 5 to 10 mg phentolamine in 10 to 15 ml normal saline may be infiltrated into the affected area. Monitor BP during administration every 2 minutes until blood pressure reaches a level slightly below patient's normal reading; then take BP at least every 5 minutes while infusion continues. While infusion is tapered and after it is withdrawn, BP monitoring must continue. Monitor pulse, central venous pressure, intraarterial pressure, pulmonary arterial diastolic pressure, pulmonary capillary wedge pressure, EKG, urinary output. Watch for signs of peripheral vasoconstriction such as cold extremities.

**Drug Interactions:** Increased pressor effect and CNS stimulation with amphetamines and methylphenidate. Potential severe hypertension with MAO inhibitor. Increased risk of arrhythmia during general anesthesia with agents such as cyclopropane, enflurane, halothane, isoflurane, methoxyflurane. Atropine, tricyclic antidepressants, guanethidine, and some antihistamines may enhance the pressor effect. Furosemide or other diuretics and antihypertensives as well as lithium may decrease the pressor effect. Increased arrhythmias with digitalis and levodopa; EKG monitoring especially important and dosage lowering may be needed. Increased effects of both medications when given to patient on thyroid medication. Effects may be blocked in patient on propranolol.

**Storage Requirements:** Store in dark, tightly closed container to 15 to 30°C (59 to 86°F). Do not use solution if it is brown or a precipitate is present.

---

□ **NYSTATIN**                                                    (nye-stat'in)

(Mycostatin, Mykinal, Nadostine. Nilstat, Nyaderm, Nystex, O-V Statin)

**Combination Products:** Nystatin with triamcinolone acetonide (Mycolog-II, Myco-Triacet II, Mykacet, Mytrex F)

**Classification:** antifungal

**Available Preparations:**
- 100,000 U/ml oral suspension
- 500,000 U film-coated tablets
- 200,000 U oral lozenges
- 100,000 U/g powder, cream, ointment for topical application
- 100,000 U vaginal suppository

**Action and Use:** Binds to sterols in the fungal cell membrane and increases permeability with loss of cellular constituents and antifungal agent for candidiasis.

**Routes and Dosage:**
*PO:*
- premature, neonates: 100,000 U 4 times/day
- children: 400,000 to 600,000 U 4 times/day

*Topical:* Apply sufficient amount to affected areas once daily
*Vaginal:* 1 suppository at bedtime for 10 days

**Absorption and Fate:** Poorly absorbed from GI tract or intact skin and mucous membranes. Excreted primarily in feces as unchanged drug. Therapeutic level in vitro: 3 to 6.25 µg/ml.

**Contraindications and Precautions:** Pregnancy category C. Contraindicated in hypersensitivity to drug, for ophthalmic usage. Combination product contains corticosteroid and should be used with caution in children where systemic absorption is more likely to occur.

**Side Effects:**
*GI:* transient nausea, vomiting, diarrhea. *Skin:* rare topical irritation usually reaction to preservatives.

**Nursing Implications:**
*Assess:* Organism should be identified but therapy may be started before results. Observe mouth for characteristic white patches.
*Administer: PO:* After meals have child perform good oral hygiene; in those children too young to brush, clean mouth of food debris. Shake suspension well. Infants and young children who cannot follow directions, use swab to apply medication to mouth making sure to distribute drug to entire mouth area. Do not give fluids for 30 minutes after application. Children who can follow directions, have them swish fluid in mouth and hold in mouth for as long as possible before swallowing. Some suspensions contain as much as 50% sucrose, follow in 30 minutes with water or oral hygiene to remove sugar from

mouth. Lozenges should be given only if child can follow directions to allow tablet to dissolve in mouth for 30 minutes. Do not chew or crush lozenge. Vaginal tablet can be use for oral administration. ***Topical:*** Apply lotion and cream sparing to affected area with gloves or cotton swabs. Cream is preferred to ointment for intertriginous areas and powder is preferred over others if intertriginous area are moist. Powder should be applied so that child or health-care provider does not inhale particles. Freely dust powder on shoes and socks when treating feet. Do not use occlusive dressings in treatment of candidiasis because this creates environment that will foster growth of yeast. ***Vaginal:*** See Part I for instructions on suppository insertion. Applicator should be washed in hot soapy water after each usage.

***Monitor:*** Course of oral therapy usually 48 hours after symptoms have subsided or cultures returned to normal. All topical and vaginal preparations are continued for 2 weeks. Vaginal medication is given during menstruation. Relief of symptoms is usually evident in 48 to 72 hours. Discontinue medication and inform physician if skin irritation occurs.

***Patient Teaching:*** Therapy requires continuing medication as ordered by physician and not stopping medication when symptoms subside. Report any skin irritation immediately. Teach good hygiene techniques to prevent reinfection. Protect undergarments from vaginal drainage if using suppository. For oral infections, keep dental care items separate from other children and child should be supplied with new tooth brush or current one should be disinfected. Children should not share towels or clothes during treatment.

**Storage Requirements:** Store topical and oral suspension at 15 to 30°C (59 to 86°F) in tight containers. Refrigerate oral lozenge and vaginal tablet. All preparations should be protected from light. Nystatin has 1 to 4-year expiration date for time of manufacture.

---

# □ OXACILLIN SODIUM (ox-a-sill′in)

(Bactocill, Prostaphlin)

**Classification:** antibiotic, penicillinase-resistant

## Available Preparations:
- 250 mg/5 ml oral solution
- 250, 500-mg capsules
- 250, 500 mg, 1, 2, 4, 10 g for parenteral administration

**Action and Use:** Similar to penicillin in action but resistant to inactivation by penicillinase. Primarily use in penicillinase-producing *Staphylococcus aureus* and *S. epidermidis* infections. Each injectable gram contains about 2.8 to 3.1 mEq sodium and oral solution contains 0.8 mEq of sodium/5 ml.

## Routes and Dosage:
*PO:*
- over 1 month, under 40 kg: 50 mg/kg/day equally divided doses every 6 hours; (severe infections 100 mg/kg/day every 4–6 hours)
- over 40 kg: 500 mg every 4 to 6 hours

*IM, IV:* Manufacturer states limited data on safety in neonates; however, some clinicians recommend the following dosages:
- < 7 days, under 2000 g: 25 mg/kg every 12 hours; and over 2000 g: 25 mg/kg every 8 hours
- > 7 days, under 2000 g: 25–50 mg/kg every 8 hours; and over 2000 g: 25–50 mg/kg every 6 hours
- over 1 month, under 40 kg: 50 mg/kg/day every 6 hours: Severe infections: 100 to 200 mg/kg/day every 4 to 6 hours
- over 40 kg: 250-400 mg every 4 to 6 hours

**Absorption and Fate:** Absorption: rapidly but incompletely from GI site; rapidly from IM site. Distributed: synovial, pericardial, ascitic, pleural fluids, liver, bone, bile. Peak level: PO, 0.5 hours; IM, 0.5 hours; IV end of infusion. Half-life: 0.3 to 0.8 hours; neonates, 1.2 to 1.6 hours. 89 to 94% bound to serum proteins; excreted in urine.

**Contraindications and Precautions:** Pregnancy category B. Use caution during lactation. Manufacturer states safe use of drug in neonates not established. Contraindicated in hypersensitivity to drug, penicillins, cephalosporins, or cephamycins. Use caution with allergies, asthma, family history of allergies, renal or hepatic impairment.

## Side Effects:
*GI:* nausea, vomiting, diarrhea, glossitis, stomatitis, **pseudomembranous colitis**. *GU:* **acute interstitial nephritis** (rare): rash, macroscopic or microscopic hematuria, azotemia, dysuria, oliguria, proteinuria. *Hepatic:* transient rise SGOT, SGPT, alkaline phosphatase, **hepatic dysfunction** (with high dosage). *Skin:* morbilliform, maculopapular, urticarial, or erythematous, rashes, pruritus (hypersensitivity). *Hemic:* **eosinophilia, anemia, neutropenia, thrombocytopenia, leukopenia, agranulocytosis**. *Other:* Hypersensitivity: **serum sickness, anaphylaxis** (rare); Local: IM: painful, sterile abscesses; IV: phlebitis, thrombophlebitis.

## Nursing Implications:
*Assess:* Assess previous allergy to drug, penicillins, cephalosporins, other drugs, asthma, or family history of allergies. Obtain cultures and sensitivity before treatment, but can start treatment before results. Obtain baseline renal, hepatic, and hematologic data before therapy.
*Administer: PO:* Food interferes with drug absorption, give 1 hour before or 2 hours after meals. Solution refrigerated. Capsules may be taken apart and mixed with small amount of food or fluid. *IM:* Reconstitute according to package inserts with sterile water or 0.9% sodium chloride for injection. Shake vigorously to dissolve. Injection painful. *IV:* Reconstitute according to package

insert with sterile water or 0.9% sodium chloride for injection. Can give slow IV push; initial dilution of 100 mg/ml given over 10 minutes. Preferred route of intermittent infusion in dilution of 0.5 to 40 mg/ml infused no more than 100 mg/minute. Compatible with $D_5W$, $D_5W/LR$, NS, LR, amino acids 4.25%/ D 25%. Do not mix with any other drugs; incompatible with aminoglycosides, tetracyclines, levarterenol, metaraminol.

**Monitor:** IM site may develop sterile abscesses. Observe IV site for vein irritation and thrombophlebitis, change site every 48 hours. Monitor child for hypersensitivity (especially in first 20 minutes of first dosage), rash (onset and characteristics), and side effects. Watch for symptoms of superinfections or interstitial nephritis. Drug's sodium content may effect patient's sodium restrictions. Assess renal and hepatic functions periodically during therapy. Hematological functions (differential leukocyte counts) should be done 1 to 3 times per week and observe for any symptoms of bleeding. Maintain fluid intake for age group. Therapy course varies and depends on severity and type of infection.

**Drug Interactions:** Erythromycin, tetracycline, chloramphenical may decrease the antibacterial effects of oxacillin. Probenecid increases serum concentrations and prolongs half-life of this drug.

**Storage Requirements:** Store capsules at 15 to 30°C (59 to 86°F), protect tablets from light. Reconstituted oral solution stable for 3 days at room temperature and 7 days if refrigerated. Reconstituted parenteral forms stability varies, consult package insert for storage.

---

# □ OXANDROLONE                                    (ox-an'-droe-lone)

(Anavar)

## Classification: anabolic

## Available Preparations:
- 2.5 mg tablet

**Action and Use:** Related to methyltestostcrone and other androgenic hormones, but appears to have selective anabolic and few undesirable androgenic effects. Used in stimulate growth, to treat hereditary angioedema, and in treatment of congenital aplastic anemia.

## Routes and Dosage:
*PO:* 0.25 mg/kg/day in single dosage

**Absorption and Fate:** Half-life biphasic: 1st phase (distributive), 0.55 hours; 2nd phase (elimination), 9 hours. Excreted in urine and small amount in feces.

**Contraindications and Precautions:** Pregnancy category X. Safety during lactation not established. Contraindicated in premature infants, nephrosis, or the nephrotic phase of nephritis. Use with caution in prepubertal males and children because of premature epiphyseal closer, precocious sexual development in males and virilization in females. Use caution with patients taking insulin, ACTH, or corticosteroids.

## Side Effects:
*CV:* edema. *GI:* nausea, abdominal fullness, loss of appetite, vomiting. *Hepatic:* hepatotoxicity, **cholestatic jaundice** *GU:* phallic enlargement, clitoral enlargement (usually seen after 6 months of therapy). *Skin:* acne, especially in females and prepubertal males, hirsutism (usually seen after 6 months of therapy). *Endocrine:* hypercalcemia. *Musculoskeletal:* **Premature closure of epiphyseal**, especially in extended usage. *Metabolic:* increased serum cholesterol. *Other:* hypercalcemia; Females: hoarseness, deepening of voice, unusual hair growth or loss (may be nonreversible even with stopping drug), irregular menstruation; Prepubertal males: increased erections, unnatural hair growth, unexplained darkening of skin.

## Nursing Implications:
*Assess:* Wrist x-rays before treatment to establish level of bone growth. Accurate measurement of height to establish baseline before drug therapy.
*Administer: PO:* Give with food or milk if GI symptoms occur. Tablets can be crushed and mixed small amount of food or fluid.
*Monitor:* Frequent measurement of height preferably using same measuring device used to establish baseline. Because bone growth usually precedes linear growth, periodic x-rays of wrists (at least every 6 months) to assess drugs effects on growth. Observe for onset of secondary sexual characteristics and other side effects, e.g., hypercalcemia, hepatotoxicity, edema; inform physician immediately. Obtain periodic liver function tests to detect early signs of hepatotoxicity during chronic therapy. Monitor diabetic children closely for decreased blood sugar concentrations.
*Patient Teaching:* Drug does not enhance athletic abilities. Do not tamper with dosage thinking it will increase height. Take dose at same time of day. Monitor height according to physician recommendations. Be aware of any signs of secondary sexual characteristics, hypercalcemia and hepatotoxicity. Eat well balanced diet, high in iron to achieve maximum therapeutic effect.

## Drug Interactions:
With insulin, may decrease blood glucose and insulin requirements. Edematous patients on adrenal steroids or ACTH and this drug may have increased edema. Somatrem or somatropin may accelerate epiphyseal maturation.

## Laboratory Tests Interference:
Interferes with results of fasting blood sugar, glucose tolerance, thyroid tests, blood coagulation and it may increase creatine and creatinine excretion. May be effected for 2 to 3 weeks after therapy discontinued.

## Storage Requirements:
Store at 15 to 30°C (59 to 86°F) in light-resistant containers.

# ☐ PANCRELIPASE

(pan-kre-li'-pase)

(Cotazyme, Cotazyme-S, Ilozyme, Ku-Zyme HP, Pancrease, Viokase)

**Classification:** pancreatic enzyme

## Available Preparations:
- 16,800 U/7 g oral powder
- 8000, 11,000-U tablets
- 6000 U enteric-coated tablets
- 8000 U capsules
- 4000, 5000, 8000, 10,000, 12,000, 16,000-U enteric-coated capsules

**Action and Use:** Enzymes secreted by the pancreas that are essential for the digestion and absorption of fat, proteins, and carbohydrates. Help to restore to normal the abnormal biliary lipid composition, thereby preventing gallstone formation in patients with cystic fibrosis. The essential components are lipase (for digestion of fat), amylase (starch digesting enzymes), and trypsin and chymotrypsin (proteolytic enzymes for protein digestion). Used as replacement therapy for patients with pancreatic insufficiency, such as chronic pancreatitis, cystic fibrosis, ileal dysfunction.

## Routes and Dosage:
*PO:*
- 1 to 4 teaspoonsful of powder; 3 to 12 capsules or tablets, 1 to 3 enteric-coated capsules or tablets before each meal
- 1 to 2 teaspoonsful powder, 1 capsule or tablet before snack. (8000 U lipase usually given for each 17 g of dietary fat intake)
- Dosage has to be individualized; the therapeutic goal is to eliminate fecal excretion of fat and nitrogen
- Severe Cases: may have to increase dosage to hourly administration

**Contraindications and Precautions:** Pregnancy category C. Contraindicated in hypersensitivity to hog protein.

**Side Effects:** No effects in recommended dosage.
*GI:* mouth sores; high-dosage: nausea, cramping, diarrhea. *Other:* hyperuricosuria.

## Nursing Implications:
*Assess:* Note quantity and quality of stools, obtain weight.
*Administer: PO:* Drug given just before ingestion of food. Drug unpalatable in powder form. Avoid inhalation of powder; it should be mixed with small amounts of soft food or fluid. After drug is given, follow with food or at least 60 ml of fluid to remove drug from mouth. The proteolytic effects of enzymes will cause mouth sores. Plain tablet or capsule can be taken apart or crushed and mixed with food. May need concurrent administration of cimetidine and/or antacid to lower gastric pH (drug destroyed at pH under 4). Enteric-coated preparations are not to be chewed or crushed.

*Monitor:* Dosage adjustment is gauged reached by symptomatic improvement. Monitor quantity and quality of stools and weights.

*Patient Teaching:* Do not allow drug to dissolve in mouth. Medication must be taken with ingestion of all food. Parents and child must understand disease, dietary plan, and how drug works.

**Storage Requirements:** Store at 25°C (77°F) in tight dry containers.

---

## □ PANTOTHENIC ACID or CALCIUM PANTOTHENATE or DEXPANTHENOL

(Dexol, D-Pantothenyl, Panthoderm)

**Classification:** nutritional supplement

**Available Preparations:**
*Calcium pantothenate:* 30, 100, 109, 200, 218, 545-mg tablets
*Pantothenic Acid:*
- 50, 100, 200, 250, 500-mg tablets
- 1000-mg extended-release tablets

**Dexpanthenol:**
- 250 mg/ml vials for parenteral use
- 2% topical cream

**Action and Use:** This water-soluble B vitamin is a precursor of coenzyme A and is active in carbohydrate, protein, and fat metabolism. Active in forming healthy epithelium. Deficiency states are rare but may be manifested by fatigue, weakness, paresthesia, GI problems. Used in treatment of vitamin B deficiency, to stimulate peristalsis, and in treatment of skin itching, although the latter two uses are not approved by the FDA.

**Routes and Dosages:**
*PO:* 6 years and over: 37.5 mg each morning initially; increased by 18.75 increments weekly PRN; usual dose 55 to 75 mg/day; not to exceed 112.5 mg/day

**Absorption and Fate:** Readily absorbed as coenzyme A from intestine. Widely distributed in the body with large amounts in liver, kidney, heart, adrenals, and is present in breast milk. Not metabolized, with most excreted in urine and smaller amounts in stool. Normal serum pantothenic acid is 100 μg/ml or above.

**Contraindications and Precautions:** No problems in pregnancy documented. Safety in children not established. Contraindicated in paralytic ileus, hemophilia, previous hypersensitivity to the drug.

## Side Effects:
*GI:* cramping ***Hemic:*** prolonged bleeding time. ***Other:*** hypersensitivity response (rare): dyspnea, itching, rash, urticaria, hypotension, agitation

## Nursing Implications:
*Assess:* Serum pantothenate. Obtain diet history. History of low energy seen with deficiency. RDAs not available.
*Administer:* Because deficiencies are rare, usually given in combination with other B vitamins such as in malabsorption syndrome. Dexpanthenol incompatible with alkaline and strongly acidic solutions.
*Monitor:* Record dietary intake.
*Patient Teaching:* Take as directed. A normal diet supplies sufficient quantities. Pantothenic acid is present in all plant and animal foods with large amounts in salmon, liver, eggs, yeast.

**Drug Interactions:** May prolong muscle relaxation with succinylcholine; do not give within 1 hour of each other. Do not give within 12 hours of parasympathetics. Potentiates miotic effects of ophthalmic anticholinesterases.

**Laboratory Test Interferences:** Prolonged bleeding time.

**Storage Requirements:** Store tightly closed at 15 to 30%C (59 to 86°F). Protect solution from freezing.

---

## □ PEMOLINE                                              (pem'oh-leen)

(Cylert)

**Classification:** CNS stimulant

## Available Preparations:
- 18.75, 37.5, 75-mg tablets
- 37.5 mg chewable tablets

**Action and Use:** A derivative of oxazolidinone. Has similar action as amphetamine. CNS and respiratory stimulant and weak sympathomimetic. Mechanism of action unknown but may increase metabolism of dopamine in CNS. Increases activity and alertness. Used in children for treatment of attention-deficit disorder.

## Routes and Dosages:
*PO:* 6 years and over: 37.5 mg each morning initially; increased by 18.75 increments weekly PRN; usual dose 55 to 75 mg/day; not to exceed 112.5 mg/day

**Absorption and Fate:** Well absorbed from GI tract. Distribution unknown but does cross into CNS. About 90% bound to plasma proteins. Metabolized in the liver and excreted mainly in urine with small amounts in feces. Peak serum levels in 2 to 4 hours with duration of at least 8 hours. Therapeutic effects may not be evident for 2 to 3 weeks. Half-life is 2 to 12 hours.

**Contraindications and Precautions:** Pregnancy category B. Contraindicated in children under 6 years, in those with prior hypersensitivity to the drug, and patients with hepatic dysfunction. Cautious use with renal dysfunction.

**Side Effects:**
*CNS:* insomnia common during early therapy, which improves with continued therapy or dosage lowering; seizures, dizziness, headache, drowsiness, irritability, **depression**, dyskinetic movements, nervousness with large doses, Tourette's disorder. *CV:* **tachycardia** with overdose. *GI:* anorexia common during early therapy, which improves with continued therapy, weight loss, nausea, diarrhea. *Hepatic:* hepatitis, jaundice, elevated SGOT, SGPT, and alkaline phosphatase. *Skin:* rash (rare). *Hemic:* aplastic anemia (rare).

**Nursing Implications:**
*Assess:* Liver enzyme studies are done before therapy (SGOT, SGPT, alkaline phosphatase) and if elevated, drug is not used. Baseline height and weight are taken and recorded on growth grids. Neurological assessment to rule out motor tics in the child and Tourette's disorder in child and family is done; presence of these disorders is a contraindication to the drug.
*Administer:* This is a Schedule IV drug as classified by the Federal Controlled Substances Act. *PO:* Dose is given in early morning to prevent insomnia. Chewable tablet can be chewed or swallowed whole.
*Monitor:* Child's height and weight are monitored regularly and plotted on growth grid. If growth rate is slowing, drug is usually discontinued for several months. Liver function studies (SGOT, SGPT, alkaline phosphatase) are performed regularly and abnormalities reported as drug therapy will be discontinued in that case. Question family about common side effects such as anorexia, insomnia, behavior changes. Obtain periodic reports of school performance, attention span, and task completion from parents and teachers. Drug-free holidays are scheduled periodically to see if child is still benefiting from therapy. Drug can usually be discontinued by adolescence.
*Patient Teaching:* Parents should report behavior changes, school performance, appearance of jaundice, or other unexpected occurrences. Return for scheduled health-care visits so child's behavior, growth, and liver function can be monitored. Avoid driving and use of hazardous machinery. Insomnia and anorexia frequently decrease after continued therapy; meanwhile nutritious foods can be encouraged. The drug can produce dependence and has been abused, particularly by adults, therefore, encourage family only to use the drug for the child as prescribed.

**Drug Interactions:** Additive CNS stimulating effect with other CNS stimulants. Decreases seizure threshold so anticonvulsant dose may need altering.

**Laboratory Test Interferences:** Increase SGOT, SGPT, LDH.

**Storage Requirements:** Store in tightly closed containers at 15 to 30°C (59 to 86°F). Tablets expire 5 years after manufacture.

---

□ **PENICILLIN G BENZATHINE** (pen-i-sill'in)

(Bicillin, Bicillin L-A, Megacillin, Permapen)

**Combination Products:** 150,000 units penicillin G with 150,000 units penicillin G procaine /ml (Bicillin C-R); 300,000 units of penicillin G with 300,000 units penicillin G procaine /ml (Bicillin C-R); 450,000 units penicillin G with 150,000 units penicillin G /ml (Bicillin C-R)

**Classification:** antibiotic, natural penicillin

**Available Preparations:**
- 200,000-U tablet
- 300,000, 600,000 U for parenteral administration

**Action and Use:** Obtained from fermentation of *Penicillium chyrsogenum*; it acts by inhibiting cell-wall synthesis in bacteria. Frequently referred to as repository, depot, long-acting; slow absorption provides longest duration of any of the penicillins. Effective for infections caused by *Pneumococcus*, group A β-hemolytic streptococci, nonpenicillinase-producing staphylococci, meningococci, and gonococci. Used to treat infections of upper respiratory tract, skin, soft tissue, and prophylaxis for rheumatic fever, syphilis, and in follow-up therapy to parenteral penicillin G therapy.

**Routes and Dosage:**
*PO:*
- under 12 years: 25,000 to 90,000 U/kg/day equally divided doses every 6 to 8 hours
- over 12 years: 400,000 to 600,000 U/day every 4 to 6 hours

*IM:*
- neonates: 50,000 U/kg one dose
- children less than 27 kg: 300,000 to 600,000 U in one dose
- children over 27 kg: 900,000 U in one dose (some clinicians recommend 1.2 million units in one dose)
- adults: 1.2 million U in one dose

Rheumatic Fever Prophylaxis: 600,000 U every 2 weeks, or 1.2 million U every 4 weeks.

**Absorption and Fate:** Absorption: slowly, poorly from GI tract, IM very slowly. Peak level: PO, 6 hours; IM, 13 to 24 hours. Elimination is slow and therapeutic levels may range from 26 to 30 days after injection. Excreted by urine with rate dependent on renal maturity, dosage, and functional level of kidneys.

## Contraindications and Precautions: Pregnancy category B. Excreted in breast milk; use caution during lactation. Contraindicated in previous reactions to drug, penicillins, cephamycin, or cephalosporins; IV: avoid any peripheral nerves or blood vessels. Use caution with renal disease, asthma, allergies, family history of allergies, cystic fibrosis. Tablets contain FD&C yellow No. 5 dye, which may cause allergic reactions.

## Side Effects:

*CNS:* hallucinations confusion, lethargy, hyperreflexia, myoclonus, **seizures, coma, Hoigne's syndrome** (bizarre behavior, neurologic reactions following IM lasting 5 to 30 minutes) *GI:* nausea, vomiting, epigastric pain, diarrhea, **pseudomembranous colitis** (rare), stomatitis, glossitis, black tongue. *Skin:* contact dermatitis possible, infants can be sensitized in womb if mothers received drug. *Hemic:* **eosinophilia, hemolytic anemia, thrombocytopenia, leukopenia, thrombocytopenic purpura, agranulocytosis** (with high dosage). *Other:* Hypersensitivity: Type I: usually in 30 to 60 minutes: **anaphylaxis, bronchial asthma, angioedema**, urticaria, fever, **laryngospasm, hypotension**; Type II: hematologic reactions; Type III: serum sickness (1 to 7%), drug fever, **acute interstitial nephritis**, allergic vasculitis, Arthus phenomenon; Type IV: in 48 hours: urticarial erythematous morbilliform rashes, pruritus, **Stevens-Johnson syndrome**, exfoliative dermatitis: Local: pain with IM, induration if given subcutaneous, neurologic damage to nerves (nerve irritation, **dysfunction, paralysis**), sterile abscess, **embolic–toxic reactions**; following intravascular directly or near artery causing **thrombosis, neurovascular damage, gangrene, necrosis**, and **sloughing of tissue**

## Nursing Implications:

*Assess:* Assess previous allergy to drug, penicillins, cephalosporins, other drugs, asthma, or family history of allergies. Intradermal skin tests may detect previous drug sensitivity. Obtain cultures and sensitivity before treatment, but can start treatment before results. Obtain baseline renal, hepatic, and hematologic data before long-term therapy.

*Administer: PO:* Drug absorption hampered by food. Give 1 hour before or 2 hours after meals. Do not give with acidic fluids, drug is acid-labile. Tablet can be crushed and mixed with small amount of food or fluid. *IM:* Shake before withdrawal. Large doses may need to be divided and given in two different sites. Injection can cause major neurovascular damage if injected improperly. Use mid-lateral thigh under 2 years; but avoid overusage of this area in infants because it can cause quadriceps femoris fibrosis resulting in atrophy of muscle. If giving into gluteal area, avoid sciatic nerve. Injection may be painful; however, if child complains of severe pain or demonstrates symptoms of this, do not inject, choose alternate site.

*Monitor:* Observe IM sites for any symptoms of damage. Monitor for hypersensitivity reactions (allergy is unpredictable) that can occur 30 minutes to 10 days. Immediate reactions may be fatal; have emergency equipment and drugs available. If child has reaction, stop drug and notify physician immediately and monitor symptoms. Note reactions on chart and place in medical record, and inform parents. Observe for rash (onset and characteristics), side effects, and symptoms of superinfections. Assess renal, hepatic, and hematological functions with prolonged or high-dose therapy or with premature and neonates. Maintain hydration for age group. Therapy course varies with organism being treated and clinical response.

*Patient Teaching:* Take as prescribed for full course of therapy. Observe for side effects, especially hypersensitivity and report to physician. If allergic reaction occurs child should wear identification jewelry or carry ID card.

**Drug Interactions:** A synergistic effect may occur when combined with aminoglycosides. Erythromycin, tetracycline, and chloramphenicol decrease effects of penicillin. Salicylates and antiinflammatory agents (nonsteroidal) compete with this drug for protein binding sites and could increase penicillin half-life. It may cause breakthrough bleeding with oral contraceptives.

**Laboratory Test Interferences:** False-positive urine glucose with Clinitest and Benedict's test. Guthrie test for PKU unreliable in neonates. Use Glenn-Nelson method to determine 17-hydroxycorticosteroids in urine; others may result in false levels. False-positive direct Coombs' interferes with crossmatching procedures.

**Storage Requirements:** Store tablets at 15 to 30°C (59 to 86°F) in airtight containers. IM preparation store at 2 to 8°C.

---

## ☐ PENICILLIN G POTASSIUM

(pen-i-sill'in)

(Acrocillin, Benzylpenicillin, Burcillin-G, Cryspen, Deltapen, Falapen, Megacillin, Novopen-G, P-50, Pentids, Pfizerpen)

## ☐ PENICILLIN G SODIUM

(Crystapen)

**Classification:** antibiotic, natural penicillin

## Available Preparations:
- 200,000, 400,000 U/5 ml oral solution
- 200,000, 250,000, 400,000, 800,000-U tablets
- 1 million, 5 million, 10 million, 20 million units for parenteral administration
- 20,000, 30,000, 40,000 U/ml in 5% dextrose for parenteral administration

**Action and Use:** Obtained from fermentation of *Penicillium chyrsogenum*; acts by inhibiting cell-wall synthesis in bacteria. Frequently referred to as aqueous, crystalline penicillin; drug of choice for infections caused by *Pneumococcus*, group A β-hemolytic streptococci, nonpenicillinase-producing staphylococci, meningococci, and gonococci. Used to treat infections such as septicemias, pericarditis, endocarditis, pneumonia, and meningitis.

## Routes and Dosage:

*PO:*

- under 12 years: 25,000 to 90,000 U/kg/day equally divided doses every 6 to 8 hours
- over 12 years: 200,000 to 1.2 million U/day every 6 hours

### IM, IV:

- neonates < 7 days < 2000 kg: 50,000 to 150,000 U/kg/day equally divided doses every 12 hours; and > 2000 kg: same dosage every 8 hours.
- neonates < 7 days < 2000 kg: 75,000 to 200,000 U/kg/day equally divided doses every 8 hours; > 2000 kg: same dosage every 6 hours.
- 1 month to 12 years: 25,000 to 400,000 U/kg/day equally divided doses every 4 to 6 hours

**Absorption and Fate:** 15 to 30% absorbed from GI tract; IM rapidly absorbed. Widely distributed to body tissues and CSF absorption increased when meninges are inflamed. 45 to 68% bound to serum proteins. Peak levels: PO, 30 minutes; IM, 15 to 30 minutes; and IV, at end of infusion. Half-life: less than 6 days, 3.2 to 3.4 hours; 7 to 14 days, 0.9 to 2.2 hours; older children, 0.5 to 0.7 hours. Primarily excreted in urine, small amount in bile.

**Contraindications and Precautions:** Pregnancy category B. Excreted in breast milk; use caution during lactation. Contraindicated in previous reactions to this drug, penicillins, cephamycin, or cephalosporins. Use caution with renal disease, asthma, allergies, family history of allergies, cystic fibrosis. Pentids tablets and oral solution have FD&C yellow No. 5 dye, which may cause allergic reactions. Infants can be sensitized in womb if mothers received drug.

## Side Effects:

*CNS:* hallucinations, confusion, lethargy, hyperreflexia, myoclonus, **seizures, coma**. *GI:* nausea, vomiting, epigastric pain, diarrhea, **pseudomembranous colitis** (rare), stomatitis, glossitis, black tongue. *Hepatic:* transient rise SGOT, LDH with IM dose. *Skin:* contact dermatitis possible. *Hemic:* **eosinophilia, hemolytic anemia, thrombocytopenia, leukopenia, thrombocytopenic purpura, agranulocytosis**. *Other:* **hypokalemia, alkalosis, hypernatremia**; Hypersensitivity: Type I: usually in 30 to 60 minutes: **anaphylaxis, bronchial asthma, angioedema**, urticaria, fever, **laryngospasm, hypotension**; Type II: hematologic reactions; Type III: serum sickness (1 to 7%), drug fever, **acute interstitial nephritis**, allergic vasculitis, Arthus phenomenon; Type IV: in 48 hours: urticarial erythematous morbilliform rashes, pruritus, **Stevens-Johnson**

**syndrome**, exfoliative dermatitis; Jarisch-Herxheimer reaction with syphilis, Lyme disease: 2 to 12 hours after treatment: headache fever chills, sore throat, increased BP, arthralgia (subsides in 12 to 24 hours); Local: pain with IM, **neurologic damage to nerves** (nerve irritation, dysfunction, paralysis), sterile abscess; IV: phlebitis (rare)

## Nursing Implications:

*Assess:* Assess previous allergy to drug, penicillins, other drugs, cephalosporins, asthma, or family history of allergies. Intradermal skin tests may detect previous drug sensitivity. Obtain cultures and sensitivity before treatment, but can start treatment before results. Obtain baseline renal, hepatic, and hematologic data before long-term therapy.

*Administer: PO:* Drug absorption hampered by food. Give 1 hour before or 2 hours after meals. Do not give with acidic fluids, drug is acid-labile. Solution: refrigerate and measure with calibrated measuring device. Can crush tablet; mix in small amount of food or fluid. *IM, IV:* Reconstitute powder by lightly tapping vial to loosen powder. Hold vial horizontally and rotate while injecting stream of diluent against wall of vial. Shake vigorously to dissolve. *IM:* Reconstitute according to package inserts; can use 1% lidocaine (without epinephrine) as diluent. Injection may be painful. *IV:* Reconstitute, according to package insert, with sterile water, 0.9% sodium chloride, and 5% dextrose. Intermittent infused over 20 to 60 minutes diluted 1 to 5 million units in 50 to 100 ml. Continuous infusion over 24 hours dilute to less than 1 million U/ml. Compatible with $D_5W$, $D_5W/O.2\%$ NS, $D_5W/0.5\%$NS, $D_{10}W$, NS, LR. High-dose administration rate should be ordered by physician; should be given slowly to prevent electrolyte imbalance. Do not premix with strong acidic or basic drugs, inactivated by acids, alkalies, oxidizing agents, carbohydrate solutions with pH 8, or aminoglycosides. Check with pharmacist before adding any drugs, many incompatibilities.

tions with pH 8, or aminoglycosides. Check with pharmacist before adding any drugs, many incompatibilities.

*Monitor:* Observe IV site for vein irritation and extravasation. Monitor for hypersensitivity reactions (allergy is unpredictable) can occur 30 minutes to 10 days. Immediate reactions may be fatal; have emergency equipment and drugs available; more likely with high dosages given parentally. If child has reaction, stop drug and notify physician immediately and monitor symptoms. Note reactions on chart and place in medical record, and inform parents. Observe for side effects and symptoms of superinfections. Assess renal, hepatic, and hematological functions with prolonged or high-dose therapy or with premature and neonates. Electrolyte imbalance may occur if greater than 10 million units are given IV. Maintain hydration for age group. Therapy course varies with organism being treated and clinical response. If given for β-**hemolytic streptococcal infection**, 10-day course needed to prevent risk of acute rheumatic fever and glomerulonephritis.

*Patient Teaching:* Take as prescribed for full course of therapy. Observe for side effects, especially hypersensitivity and report to physician. If penicillin allergy occurs, child should wear identification jewelry or carry ID card. Store solution in refrigerator out of reach of children. Reconstituted solution should be discarded after 14 days if refrigerated. Do not share medication with others or family members.

**Drug Interactions:** A synergistic effect may occur when combined with aminoglycosides. Erythromycin, tetracycline, and chloramphenicol decrease effects of penicillin. Probenecid increases serum concentrations of penicillin. Salicylates and antiinflammatory agents (nonsteroidal) compete with this drug for protein-binding sites and could increase penicillin half-life. May cause breakthrough bleeding with oral contraceptives. Concomitant usage with potassium-sparing diuretics could cause hypokalemia.

**Laboratory Test Interferences:** False-positive urine glucose with Clinitest and Benedict's test. False increase in urine specific gravity high doses IV. Guthrie test for PKU unreliable in neonates. Use Glenn-Nelson method for determining urine 17-hydroxycorticosteroids; others may result in false levels. False-positive direct Coombs' interferes with cross-matching procedures.

**Storage Requirements:** Store tablets at 15 to 30°C (59 to 86°F); avoid excessive heat. Reconstituted solutions refrigerated stable for 14 days. Label suspension with date and time at reconstitution. Reconstituted parenteral form stable for 24 hours at room temperature or 7 days when refrigerated.

---

☐ **PENICILLIN G**                           (pen-i-sill'in)
   **PROCAINE**

(Ayercillin, Crysticillin A.S., Duracillin A.S. Wycillin)

**Combination Products:** 150,000 units penicillin G with 150,000 units penicillin G benzathine /ml (Bicillin C-R); 150,000 units penicillin G with 450,000 units of penicillin G benzathine /ml (Bicillin C-R)

**Classification:** antibiotic, natural penicillin

**Available Preparations:**
 ▪ 300,000, 500,000, 600,000 U for parenteral administration

**Action and Use:** Acts by inhibiting cell-wall synthesis in bacteria. Long-acting, relatively insoluble, slowly and absorbed from site. Effective for infections caused by *Pneumococcus*, group A β-hemolytic streptococci, nonpenicillinase-producing staphylococci, meningococci, and gonococci. Used to treat infections of upper respiratory tract, otitis media, skin, soft tissue, syphilis, gonorrhea, prophylaxis for rheumatic fever, and in follow-up therapy to parenteral penicillin G therapy.

## Routes and Dosage:
*IM:* Avoid usage in neonates due to sterile abscess or procaine toxicity
- infants over 1 month: 25,000 to 50,000 U/kg/day as single dose or 500,000 to 1 million U/m²/day (do not exceed adult dosage)
- over 12 years: 600,000 to 1.2 million U/day as single dose or twice daily

## Absorption and Fate:
IM very slowly absorbed. Peak level: 1 to 4 hour; slow release from IM site, drug levels detectable in 1 to 2 days. Renal excretion delayed in neonates, infants, renal impairment. Excreted usually within 36 hours.

## Contraindications and Precautions:
Pregnancy category B. Excreted in breast milk, use caution during lactation. Not recommended for usage with neonates. Contraindicated in previous reactions to drug, penicillins, cephamycin, cephalosporins, sensitivity to formaldehyde sulfoxylate (in Crysticillin) or procaine allergy, IV, and avoid injection into any peripheral nerves or blood vessels. Use caution in renal disease, asthma, allergies, family history of allergies, cystic fibrosis. Infants can be sensitized in womb if mothers received drug.

## Side Effects:
*CNS:* Hoigne's syndrome (bizarre behavior, neurologic reactions after IM injection, lasting 5 to 30 minutes). *Skin:* contact dermatitis possible. *Hemic:* **eosinophilia, hemolytic anemia, thrombocytopenia, leukopenia, thrombocytopenic purpura, agranulocytosis** *(with high dosage).* *Other:* Hypersensitivity: Type I: usually 30 to 60 minutes: **anaphylaxis, bronchial asthma, angioedema,** urticaria, fever, **laryngospasm,** hypotension; Type II: hematologic reactions; Type III: serum sickness (1 to 7%), drug fever, **acute interstitial nephritis,** allergic vasculitis, Arthus phenomenon; Type IV: in 48 hours: urticarial erythematous morbilliform rashes, pruritus, **Stevens-Johnson syndrome, exfoliative dermatitis;** Jarisch-Herxheimer reactions treatment of syphilis, Lyme disease; Local: less pain with IM except in doses above 600,000 U, induration if given subcutaneous; neurologic damage to nerves (nerve irritation, **dysfunction, paralysis**), sterile abscess, **embolic–toxic reactions:** following intravascular directly or near artery causing **thrombosis, neurovascular damage, gangrene, necrosis,** and **sloughing of tissue.**

## Nursing Implications:
*Assess:* Assess previous allergy to drug, penicillins, cephalosporins, other drugs, asthma, procaine, or family history of allergies. Intradermal skin tests may detect previous drug sensitivity. Obtain cultures and sensitivity before treatment, but can start treatment before results. Obtain baseline renal, hepatic, and hematologic data before long-term therapy.
*Administer: IM:* Shake before withdrawal. Large doses may need to be divided and given in two different sites. Injection causes major neurovascular damage if injected improperly. Use mid-lateral thigh under 2 years; but avoid overusage of this area in infants; causes quadriceps femoris fibrosis (atrophy of

muscle). Giving into gluteal area, avoid sciatic nerve. Injection may be painful; however, if child shows symptoms or complains of severe pain, do not inject but choose alternate site.

**Monitor:** Observe IM sites for any symptoms of damage; inform physician immediately. Monitor for hypersensitivity reactions (allergy is unpredictable); can occur in 30 minutes to 10 days. Immediate reactions may be fatal; have emergency equipment and drugs available. If child has reaction, stop drug and notify physician immediately and monitor symptoms. Note reactions on chart and place in medical record, and inform parents. Observe side effects and symptoms of superinfections. Assess renal, hepatic, and hematological functions with prolonged, high-dose therapy or with premature and neonates. Maintain hydration for age group. Therapy course varies with organism being treated and clinical response.

**Patient Teaching:** Report any symptoms of allergic response to physician. If allergic to penicillin child should wear identification jewelry or carry ID card.

**Drug Interactions:** A synergistic effect may occur when combined with aminoglycosides. Erythromycin, tetracycline, and chloramphenicol decrease effects of penicillin. Salicylates and antiinflammatory agents (nonsteroidal) compete with this drug for protein binding sites and could increase penicillin half-life. May cause breakthrough bleeding with oral contraceptives. Probenecid increases serum concentration of penicillin.

**Laboratory Test Interferences:** See penicillin G benzathine.

**Storage Requirements:** Store at 2 to 8°C (35 to 46°F).

---

## □ PENICILLIN V POTASSIUM
(pen-i-sill'in)

(Apo-Pen-VK, Beepen VK, Betapen-VK, Ledercillin VK, Nadopen-V, Novopen-VK, Penapar VK, Penicillin VK, Pen-V, Pen-Vee K, Robicillin VK, Uticillin VK, V-Cillin, VC-K, Veetids)

**Classification:** antibiotic, natural penicillin

**Available Preparations:**
- 125, 250 mg/5 ml oral solution
- 250, 500-mg tablets
- 125, 250, 500-mg film-coated tablets

**Action and Use:** Obtained from fermentation of *Penicillium chyrsogenum*; acts by inhibiting cell-wall synthesis in bacteria. Effective with mild to moder-

ately severe infections caused by *Pneumococcus*, group A β-hemolytic streptococci, nonpenicillinase-producing staphylococci, meningococci, and gonococci.
Used to treat infections such as otitis media, upper respiratory infections, Lyme
disease, and used for prophylaxis in endocarditis, pneumococcal infections, and
rheumatic fever.

## Routes and Dosage:

*PO:* under 12 years: 15 to 62.5 mg/kg/day equally divided doses every 6 to 8
hours; over 12 years: 250 to 500 mg every 6 hours

- Treatment of A β-hemolytic Streptococci: 125 to 250 mg every 6 to 8
  hours for 10 days
- Rheumatic Fever Prophylaxis: 125 to 250 mg twice a day
- Lyme Disease: under 9 years: 50 mg/kg daily in divided doses for 10 to
  12 days (do not give less than 1 g or more than 2 g daily)

**Absorption and Fate:** 60 to 73% absorbed from GI tract. Distributed to
body tissues especially kidneys, liver, skin, intestine. 78 to 89% bound to
serum proteins. Peak levels: 30 to 60 minutes. Half-life: 1 hour. 26 to 65%
excreted in urine; 32% excreted in feces.

**Contraindications and Precautions:** Pregnancy category B. Excreted
in breast milk; use caution during lactation. Contraindicated in previous reactions to drug, penicillins, cephamycin, or cephalosporins. Use caution in renal
disease, asthma, allergies, family history of allergies, cystic fibrosis, intestinal
hypermotility, nausea, vomiting. Veetids tablets and oral solution have FD&C
yellow No. 5 dye, which may cause allergic reactions. Penapar VK solution
contains aspartame that is metabolized to phenylalanine, affecting children with
PKU.

## Side Effects:

*GI:* nausea, vomiting, epigastric pain, diarrhea, **pseudomembranous colitis**
(rare), stomatitis, glossitis, black tongue. *Hemic:* **eosinophilia, hemolytic
anemia, thrombocytopenia, leukopenia, thrombocytopenic purpura, agranulocytosis.** *Other:* Hypersensitivity: Type I: usually 30 to 60 minutes: **anaphylaxis, bronchial asthma, angioedema,** urticaria, fever, **laryngospasm,**
hypotension; Type II: hematologic reactions; Type III: **scrum sickness** (1 to
7%), drug fever, **acute interstitial nephritis, allergic vasculitis, Arthus phenomenon**; Type IV: in 48 hours: urticarial erythematous morbilliform rashes,
pruritus, **Stevens-Johnson syndrome, exfoliative dermatitis**.

## Nursing Implications:

*Assess:* Assess previous allergy to drug, penicillins, cephalomporins, other
drugs, asthma, or family history of allergies. Intradermal skin tests may detect
previous drug sensitivity. Obtain cultures and sensitivity before treatment, but
can start treatment before results. Obtain baseline renal, hepatic, and hematologic data before long-term therapy.

*Administer: PO:* Drug absorption hampered by food. Give 1 hour before or

2 hours after meals. Can crush tablets; mix with small amount of food or fluid.
***Monitor:*** Monitor for hypersensitivity reactions (allergy is unpredictable) can occur in 30 minutes to 10 days. Immediate reactions may be fatal; have emergency equipment and drugs available. If child has reaction, stop drug and notify physician immediately and monitor symptoms. Chart reactions in medical record, and inform parents. Observe for side effects and symptoms of superinfections. Assess renal, hepatic, and hematological functions with prolonged or high-dose therapy or with premature and neonates. Maintain hydration for age group. Therapy course varies with organism treated and clinical response. If given for β-**hemolytic streptococcal infection**, 10-day course to prevent risk of acute rheumatic fever or glomerulonephritis.
***Patient Teaching:*** Take as prescribed for full course of therapy. Observe for side effects, especially hypersensitivity and report to physician. If allergic to penicillin, child should wear identification jewelry or carry ID card. Store solution in refrigerator out of reach of children (may be placed in opaque container toward back of shelf). Reconstituted solution should be discarded after 14 days if refrigerated.

**Drug Interactions:** A synergistic effect may occur when combined with aminoglycosides. Probenecid increases serum concentrations of penicillin. Salicylates and antiinflammatory agents (nonsteroidal) compete with this drug for protein-binding sites and could increase penicillin half-life. May cause breakthrough bleeding with oral contraceptives. Concomitant usage with potassium-sparing diuretics could cause hypokalemia.

**Laboratory Test Interferences:** See penicillin G benzathine.

**Storage Requirements:** Store tablets at 15 to 30°C (59 to 86°F), avoid excessive heat. Reconstituted solutions, refrigerated stable for 14 days. Label suspension with date and time at reconstitution.

---

## □ PENTAMIDINE ISETHIONATE     (pen-tam′i-deen)

(Lomidine, Nebu Pent, Pentam 300)

**Classification:** antiinfective, antiprotozoal

## Available Preparations:
- 300 mg for parenteral administration
- 300 mg for oral inhalation

**Action and Use:** Diamidine derivative antiprotozoal whose exact mechanism of action is unknown but appears to interfere with RNA and DNA, phospholipid, and protein synthesis in protozoa. Appears to vary its action in protozoa treated. Used in treatment of *Pneumocystis carinii* pneumonia in acquired immune deficiency syndrome (AIDS). Also used to treat visceral leishmaniasis caused by *Leishmania donovani* and African trypanosomiasis from the *Trypanosoma brucei gambiense* organism.

## Routes and Dosage:
*IM, IV:* *Pneumocystis carinii*: 4 mg/kg/dose every day for 12 to 14 days or 150 mg/m$^2$ once daily times 5 days, then 100 mg/m$^2$ once daily for 7 to 9 days (treatment for Pneumocystis pneumonia in AIDS may continue for 14–21 days); *Trypanosoma gambiense*: 4 mg/kg once daily for 10 days; *Leishmania donovani*: 2 to 4 mg/kg/dose every day for 15 days
Inhalation: prevention of Pneumocystic pneumonia dependent and type of nebulizer, delivery, and aerosol particle size. Follow your agency protocol. Respirgard II jet nebulizer has been used to deliver 300 mg once every 4 weeks.

## Absorption and Fate: 
Well adsorbed from IM site. IM peak level: 30 to 60 minutes. Distributed into body tissues and fluids, but does not appear to penetrate CNS. Primarily excreted in urine in biphasic manner; most of drug excrete in first 6 hours and in some patients small amounts were found for as long as 6 to 8 weeks.

## Contraindications and Precautions: 
Pregnancy category C and safe use during lactation not established. Use with caution in hypotension, hypoglycemia, hyperglycemia, hypertension, hypocalcemia, leukopenia, thrombocytopenia, anemia, hepatic and renal impairment, or diabetes mellitus.

## Side Effects:
*CNS:* dizziness, neuralgia, confusion, **hallucinations**. *CV:* **hypotension** (sudden and severe), **ventricular tachycardia**, ECG abnormalities, facial flushing. *GI:* anorexia, nausea, vomiting, metallic taste. *Hepatic:* increased SGOT, SGPT. *GU:* **nephrotoxicity**, increased serum creatinine and BUN, **acute renal failure**. *Skin:* generalized urticaria, maculopapular rash, pruritus, **toxic epidermal necrolysis**, **Stevens-Johnson syndrome**. *Hemic:* leukopenia, **thrombocytopenia** (severe), anemia (rare). *Endocrine:* **hypoglycemia**, **hyperglycemia**, hypocalcemia. *Other:* Local: IM: pain, erythema, tenderness, sterile abscess and induration in 10 to 20% patients; IV: phlebitis, facial flushing.

## Nursing Implications:
*Assess:* Obtain cultures to validate presence of organisms. Obtain baseline CBC, platelets, serum glucose, SGOT, SGPT, alkaline phosphatase, BUN, serum creatinine, urinalysis and vital signs, and ECG.
*Administer:* This drug may produce **severe hypotension** with single dose of either IM or IV; have emergency equipment available. *IM:* Reconstitute with 3 ml of sterile water, resulting dilution of 100 mg/ml. Injection painful. *IV:* Reconstitute with 3 to 5 ml of sterile water or 5% dextrose for injection. Then dosage should be further diluted in at least 50 ml of 5% dextrose and infused over a full 60 minutes. Do not infuse at faster rate because severe hypotension may result. If hypotension occurs, stop infusion and notify physician immediately; have emergency equipment available. Compatibility information not available. Do not mix with any solution or other drugs without consulting pharmacist. *Inhalation:* Experimental; follow agency protocol.

*Monitor:* This drug produces serious side effects; child must be carefully monitored and physician notified if they occur. Hypotension: Obtain BP every 15 minutes during IV therapy; IM take every 15 minutes for 1 hour; then every 30 minutes for 2 hours; then every 4 hours. Facial flushing may signal hypotension. Report immediately. Obtain ECG periodically. Hypoglycemia: (5 to 10% patients) usually occurs 5 to 7 days after therapy is initiated and can last for several days after drug is stopped (rarely it can occur for several months). Assess for symptoms of hypoglycemia or hyperglycemia. Obtain daily blood glucose. Have IV dextrose available. Nephrotoxicity: Assess for renal function by I & O, daily weights, and daily BUN and serum creatinine. Renal symptoms usually occur gradually about 2 weeks into therapy. Obtain periodic CBC, platelets, liver function tests, and serum calcium levels. Because this child is usually immune-suppressed, follow agency policy to prevent infections. Monitor respiratory function. Manufacturer has established hot line for emergency information on drug usage (312)34L-YPHO.

*Patient Teaching:* Immediately report any symptoms of hypoglycemia.

**Drug Interactions:** Do not use any other nephrotoxic drugs such as aminoglycosides, amphotericin B, capreomycin, colistin, cisplatin, methoxyflurane, polymyxin B, or vancomycin as renal effects may be additive.

**Storage Requirements:** Powder store at 2 to 8°C; protect from light. Reconstituted solutions stable for 48 hours at room temperature; protect from light. Manufacturer recommends unused portions be discarded.

---

# ☐ PENTOBARBITAL                                   (pen-toe-bar′bi-tal)

(Nembutal)

## Classification: barbiturate, sedative-hypnotic

## Available Preparations:
- 18.2 mg/5 ml elixir
- 50, 100-mg capsules
- powder
- 50 mg/ml vials for parenteral use
- 30, 60, 120, 200-mg rectal suppositories

**Action and Use:** This barbiturate acts at various CNS sites to cause sedation and drowsiness. This sedation may be preceded by euphoria or excitement. Respirations and GI tone are decreased. Used as a hypnotic for short-term treatment (under 2 weeks) of insomnia. May be used to treat status epilepticus and severe seizures. Used in conjunction with anesthesia or during short-term surgery. Although not approved by the FDA for that purpose, pentobarbital has been used to induce coma in increased intracranial pressure such as after head trauma, in Reye syndrome, and postdrowning.

**Routes and Dosages:** PO (pentobarbital or pentobarbital sodium), IM, IV, PR (pentobarbital sodium)
*PO:*
- Sedation: 2 to 6 mg/kg/day; not to exceed 100 mg/day
- Preoperative Medication: under 10 years: 5 mg/kg; 10 to 12 years: 100 mg

*IM:* Hypnosis: 2 to 6 mg/kg or 125 mg/m²; not to exceed 100 mg
*IV:* Initial Dose: 50 mg
*PR:*
- Hypnosis: 2 months to 1 year: 30 mg; 1 to 4 years: 30 to 60 mg; 5 to 12 years: 60 mg; 12 to 14 years: 60 to 120 mg
- Sedation: 2 to 6 mg/kg/day; not to exceed 100 mg/day

**Absorption and Fate:** Well absorbed from GI tract. 35 to 45% bound to plasma proteins. Metabolized by the liver and excreted in the urine. Onset of action: 15 to 60 minutes after PO or PR administration; peak action: 30 to 60 minutes; duration: 1 to 4 hours. Onset of action: 10 to 25 minutes after IM administration. Onset of action: 1 minute after IV administration; duration: 15 minutes. Therapeutic level to produce sedation is 1 to 5 µg/ml; levels above 10 µg/ml produce deep coma, levels above 30 µg/ml may be lethal.

**Contraindications and Precautions:** Pregnancy category D. Safety for children under 2 months not established. Contraindicated in those with bronchopneumonia, porphyria, barbiturate hypersensitivity. 100-mg nembutal sodium capsules contain tartrazine (yellow dye #5) and should not be used in those with tartrazine hypersensitivity. Must be discontinued if skin reaction occurs. Cautious use in cardiovascular disease and hypertension or hypotension (use oral routes only), in pain, depression, renal dysfunction, hepatic dysfunction.

**Side Effects:**
*CNS:* drowsiness, lethargy, headache, vertigo, mental depression, impaired motor skills. *CV:* vasodilation, **hypotension**. *GI:* nausea, vomiting, diarrhea, constipation. *Respiratory:* **respiratory depression, apnea, bronchospasm, laryngospasm**, especially with rapid IV injection. *Hepatic:* hepatitis, jaundice. *Skin:* thrombophlebitis at IV site; **hypersensitivity reaction** with rash, urticaria, dermatitis, systemic lupus erythematosus.

**Nursing Implications:**
*Assess:* Take baseline vital signs. Take history of allergy to barbiturates and respiratory disease.
*Administer:* Schedule II drug under Federal Controlled Substances Act. *PO:* Take on empty stomach. *IM:* Hypnotic doses given 30 to 60 minutes before bedtime. Do not use injection solutions that contain precipitate. Administer deep IM. *IV:* Do not use injection solutions that contain precipitate. Used only for anesthesia induction, severe seizures, or psychosis. Incompatible with many drugs, therefore, not recommended to be added to solution with other drugs. Usually given in 50 mg/ml concentration. Do not exceed 50 mg/minute for rate

of administration. IV push: 1–2 mg/kg given undiluted over 3–5 minutes. Emergency equipment and drugs must be readily available.

**Monitor:** Take vital signs frequently, every few seconds during IV administration, every few minutes after IM administration. CBC should be obtained periodically if used for more than brief therapy. Therapy with this drug usually does not exceed 2 weeks as treatment for insomnia; not generally effective for longer periods. Watch for sore throat, fever, bleeding, bruising that may indicate hemic effects and necessitate discontinuing drug. Observe for skin reactions as these can be fatal; drug must be discontinued; they may be preceded by fever, stomatitis, conjunctivitis, rhinitis.

**Patient Teaching:** Take as directed. Drug can alter mental alertness; therefore, avoid driving and adjust activities accordingly. Avoid alcohol and OTC drugs. Report fever, sore throat, bleeding, bruising, skin reaction immediately. Drug can be habit-forming and long-term use will require slow withdrawal.

**Drug Interactions:** Additive or potentiating effects with other CNS depressants. Possible decreased GI absorption of dicumarol. Increased metabolism and resultant decreases in levels of corticosteroids. Decreased absorption and levels of griseofulvin. Decreased half-life of doxycycline. Decreased effectiveness of birth control pills. Increased respiratory depressant effects with other drugs that have this side effect.

**Laboratory Test Interferences:** Elevated sulfobromophthalein if given within 24 hours before test.

**Storage Requirements:** Store oral and injectable preparations at 15 to 30°C (59 to 86°F). Store rectal suppositories at 2 to 8°C (35 to 46°F).

---

## □ PERMETHRIN                                    (per-meth′rin)

(Nix)

**Classification:** pediculocide

**Available Preparations:**
   1% lotion

**Action and Use:** Synthetic pyrethroid used to kill *Pediculus capitis* (head louse). Drug adsorbed through arthropods chitinous exoskeleton where it acts on membrane of nerve cell disrupting the sodium channel current delaying repolarization and causing paralysis.

**Routes and Dosage:**
**Topical:** Head Louse: Apply 25 to 50 ml of solution to hair and scalp; Rinse after minutes, dry with clean towel. (see **Administer** for how to apply)

**Absorption and Fate:** Less than 2% absorbed. Duration of action: 14 days.

**Contraindications and Precautions:** Pregnancy category B. Safety during lactation not established. Dosage not established in those under 2 years. Contraindicated in hypersensitivity to drug or its components, allergy to chrysanthemums, acutely inflamed or raw scalp.

## Side Effects:
*Skin:* pruritus, erythema, burning, numbness, stinging, or tingling, rash.

## Nursing Implications:
*Assess:* Carefully inspect and note extent and amount of infestation. Pediculosis confirmed by finding lice or eggs (nits).

*Administer: Topical:* Head louse: Shake well before usage. Do not treat child's hair in bath tub or shower because of risk of getting lotion in eyes and mucous membranes. Shampoo, rinse, and dry hair with regular shampoo. Apply about 25 to 50 ml of lotion to dry hair making sure entire scalp and hair covered (wet). Take care not to get lotion in eyes or other mucous membranes. If lotion gets into eyes, flush with copious amounts of water. Leave on for 10 minutes. Rinse hair well (cup or glass prevents lotion from getting into eyes or ears); a rinsing solution of 1/2 water and 1/2 white vinegar may aid in nit removal. It is not necessary, but fine-toothed comb can be used to comb hair to remove nits. Pay particular attention to nape of neck and area behind ears. This is a single treatment drug; however, may be repeated in 7 days if lice are seen. With all infestations, fresh bedding should be placed on bed; then all bedding, personal clothes, and towels that child used should be washed in hot water and dried on hot dryer setting. Combs and hair-care items can be boiled or washed in solution of drug. Items that cannot be washed should be dry cleaned (stuffed animals etc.), placed in dryer for 20 minutes on hot setting, or sealed in airtight plastic bags for 2 weeks. Vacuum carpets and upholstered furniture. Floors should be damp mopped. All family members should be examined and treated if infected.

*Monitor:* If child is hospitalized during this infestation, take proper isolation precautions used by agency. Assess skin for healing and notify physician if condition does not improve or worsens. Check child in 1 week for symptoms of disease. Notify schools, nursery school, and day-care centers.

*Patient Teaching:* Parent and child should understand that this is a contagious condition and why it has to be treated. Head lice is a result of contact with someone with disease and not indicative of poor hygiene. Explain how to apply and prevent reinfestations or spreading of pediculosis. Thick applications will not hasten healing and may cause irritation. School, day-care centers, or child's preschool should be informed of infestation to prevent spread to other children.

**Storage Requirements:** Store at 15 to 30°C (59 to 86°F) in light-resistant containers.

---

## □ PHENOBARBITAL (fee-noe-bar'bi-tal)

(Barbita, Luminal, Solfoton)

**Combination Products:** Dilantin with phenobarbital kapseals

**Classification:** anticonvulsant, barbiturate, sedative, hypnotic

## Available Preparations:
- powder
- 15 mg/5 ml elixir
- 8, 15, 16, 30, 32, 60, 65, 100-mg tablets
- 16-mg capsules
- 30 mg/ml, 60 mg/ml, 65 mg/ml, 130 mg/ml vials for parenteral use
- 120-mg powder for parenteral use

Also available in capsules with 100 mg of phenytoin and 16 or 32 mg of phenobarbital

**Action and Use:** Causes CNS depression. Raises threshold for electrical stimulation of motor cortex and reduces transmission of impulses in nerve cells. Has sedative and hypnotic actions. Used for all types of seizures except absence (petit mal), for example, in tonic-clonic (grand mal), partial seizures, febrile seizures, and status epilepticus. Also used for preoperative sedation.

**Routes and Dosage:** PO, SQ, IM, IV
*PO:*
- Seizures: 3 to 5 mg/kg/day or 125 mg/day
- Febrile Seizures: 3 to 4 mg/kg/day for prophylaxis
- Sedation: 6 mg/kg/day or 180 mg/m²/day in 3 doses
- Preoperative Sedation: 1 to 3 mg/kg preop

*IM:* Preoperative Sedation: 16 to 100 mg 60 to 90 minutes before surgery
*IV:* Status Epilepticus: 15–20 mg/kg over 10–15 minutes.

**Absorption and Fate:** Absorbed slowly from GI tract and quickly from rectal or parenteral administration. About 20 to 45% bound to plasma proteins. Metabolized by the liver and excreted in urine. Onset of action after IV administration is 5 minutes and peak action is in 30 minutes. Peak serum levels after PO administration occur in 8 to 12 hours and peak CNS levels occur in 10 to 15 hours. Duration of action after parenteral forms is 4 to 6 hours. PO half-life of 2 to 6 days is quite long, thereafter, 3 to 4 weeks of oral drug is needed to reach steady-state blood levels of the drug. Parenteral half-life is 110 hours. Therapeutic levels are 10 to 20 µg/ml, with levels above 50 µg/ml life threatening.

**Contraindications and Precautions:** Pregnancy category D. Can cause fetal damage when administered to pregnant women, especially in first trimester. Anticonvulsants, however, should not be discontinued if the women's risk of seizure is high; benefits and risks must be studied. Bisulfate preparation contraindicated in those hypersensitive to sulfites. Contraindicated in those hypersensitive to barbiturates. Cautious use in hepatic, renal, cardiac, respiratory disease, and during lactation.

## Side Effects:

**CNS:** drowsiness, ataxia, irritability, headache; these symptoms may decrease as therapy continues. Can cause paradoxical excitement, hyperactivity, sleep disturbance, impaired memory, and school difficulties. **GI:** nausea, vomiting. **Hepatic:** jaundice, hepatitis. **GU:** renal damage. **Skin:** rash, dermatitis. **Hemic:** lowered RBC levels, bone marrow suppression (rare). **Metabolic:** hypocalcemia.

## Nursing Implications:

**Assess:** Baseline CBC, liver function tests; UA should be performed. History of child's performance in school is obtained.

**Administer:** Schedule IV drug under Federal Controlled Substances Act. Phenobarbital is the oral form and phenobarbital sodium is the parenteral preparation. When the drug is to be discontinued or another anticonvulsant is to be substituted, dosages are slowly tapered rather than being withdrawn suddenly. **PO:** Tablet may be crushed and mixed with a small amount of food. **IM:** Inject deep into muscle. Avoid SC injection that may lead to tissue necrosis and intraarterial injection that can cause pain and arterial spasm. **IV:** Solution can be added to most IV solutions such as saline, 5% dextrose, lactated Ringer's. Reconstituted solution must be administered within 30 minutes or discarded. Do not use parenteral solution if a precipitate is visible. Generally phenobarbital should not be given with other drugs in the same IV as it has many drug incompatibilities. Administer slowly over 3–5 minutes at a rate not to exceed 2 mg/kg/minute or 30 mg/minute. IV route is usually used only in emergency treatment of seizures.

**Monitor:** Observe state of consciousness especially during and after parenteral administration. **IV:** observe for respiratory depression and hypotension. Take vital signs. CBC, liver function tests, renal function tests are performed regularly. The child on long-term therapy should be observed for behavior in the classroom and ability to perform cognitively. Be alert for signs of hypocalcemia; vitamin D supplements may be given to prevent this side effect. Observe the IV site carefully during IV administration. Discontinue the injection if pain, color changes in skin near IV site, or lack of therapeutic action occur. If extravasation occurs, 0.5% procaine hydrochloride can be injected into the site and moist heat applied.

**Patient Teaching:** Return for scheduled visits with health-care provider. Do not discontinue drug, increase dosage, or change forms without consultation with prescriber. Do not take other drugs or alcohol. Report increasing dizziness, lethargy, ataxia, changes in school performance and achievements.

## Drug Interactions:
May increase or decrease phenytoin serum levels. Decreases amount of the anticoagulant dicumarol from GI tract. Decreases levels of corticosteroids, tricyclic antidepressants, griseofulvin, doxycycline, and digitoxin in the serum. Additive CNS depressant effects with alcohol and other CNS depressants.

## Laboratory Test Interferences:
Increases serum phosphatase.

**Food Interactions:** Can decrease the body's vitamin D and folate levels.

**Storage Requirements:** Store at 15 to 30°C (59 to 86°F). Discard parenteral solutions if a precipitate is visible.

---

## □ PHENTOLAMINE

(Regitine)

**Classification:** alpha-adrenergic blocking agent, antihypertensive

### Available Preparations:
- 5-mg vial for parenteral use (available with 25 mg of mannitol)

**Action and Use:** Blocks α-adrenergic receptors, thereby decreasing peripheral resistance and causing peripheral vasodilation. Increases cardiac output, stimulates gastric secretion, and counteracts hypertension caused by epinephrine and norepinephrine. Used to diagnose pheochromocytoma and to treat hypertension before and during surgery for pheochromocytoma. May be useful to prevent tissue necrosis after intravenous administration or extravasation of norepinephrine.

### Routes and Dosages:
*IM:*
- Diagnosis of Pheochromocytoma: 3 mg
- Hypertension: 1 mg or 0.1 mg/kg or 3 mg/m$^2$ 1 to 2 hours before surgery for pheochromocytoma

*IV:*
- Diagnosis of Pheochromocytoma: 1 mg or 0.1 mg/kg or 3 mg/m$^2$
- Hypertension: 1 mg or 0.1 mg/kg or 3 mg/m$^2$ 1 to 2 hours before surgery for pheochromocytoma; same dose may be repeated during surgery PRN

*Infiltration:* 5 to 10 mg is added to 10 ml normal saline and infiltrated into norepinephrine IV extravasation site.

**Absorption and Fate:** Pharmacokinetics mostly unknown. Peak action in 2 minutes, with duration of 15 to 20 minutes. Half-life following IV administration is 19 minutes. Drug appears to be eliminated mainly in urine.

**Contraindications and Precautions:** Pregnancy category C. Unknown if the drug appears in breast milk. Contraindicated in those with hypersensitivity to the drug, after myocardial infarction, coronary insufficiency, angina. Cautious use in gastritis and peptic ulcer.

### Side Effects:
*CNS:* weakness, dizziness, flushing. *CV:* **hypotension**, orthostatic hypoten-

sion, **tachycardia, arrhythmias**, angina, **myocardial infarction**. *GI:* nausea, vomiting, abdominal pain, diarrhea, exacerbation of peptic ulcer. *Other:* nasal stuffiness.

## Nursing Implications:
*Assess:* Establish baseline vital signs. With patient in supine position and at rest, obtain stabilized blood pressure by taking readings every 10 minutes for at least 30 minutes.

*Administer:* Equipment for constant BP monitoring should be available. Emergency resuscitative equipment and personnel should be available. *IM or IV:* Reconstitute with 1 ml sterile water; solution will contain 5 mg/ml. Stable 48 hours at room temperature; do not store or refrigerate reconstituted solution. For diagnosis of pheochromocytoma, the IV injection is given rapidly. *Monitor:* Take blood pressure every 30 seconds for 3 minutes after IV, then every 1 minute for 7 minutes, then at least every 5 minutes for 30 to 45 minutes. When given IV for diagnosis of pheochromocytoma, blood pressure peak decrease is at 2 minutes and returns to normal in 15 to 30 minutes. Take blood pressure at least every 5 minutes for 30 to 45 minutes after IM administration. Peak action on blood pressure is expected in 20 minutes with normal reading returning in 30 to 45 minutes. A decrease of at least 35 mm Hg in systolic pressure and 25 mm Hg in diastolic pressure is a positive response in the test for pheochromocytoma.

*Patient Teaching:* Have patient lie supine and relax in a quiet darkened room to establish baseline blood pressure. Remain lying down until medication effects have worn off and someone is present to assist with dangling and ambulation.

**Drug Interactons:** May decrease effects of dopamine, ephedrine, epinephrine, methoxamine, phenylephrine. Increased orthostatic hypotension and bradycardia with guanethidine.

**Storage Requirements:** Store at 15 to 30°C (59 to 86°F). Do not store or refrigerate reconstituted solution.

---

## □ PHENYLEPHRINE                                              (fen-ill-ef′rin)

(Al-Dilate, AK-Nefrin, Ak-Vernacon, Alconefrin, Allerest Nasal, Coricidin Nasal Mist, Cyclomydril, doktors, Duration Mild, I-Liqui-Tears Plus, I-Phrine, I-White, Isopto Frin, Murocoll-2, Mydfrin, Neo-Synephrine, Nostril, Ocu-Phrin, Optised, Prefrin, Relief, Rhinall, Sinarest Nasal, Sinex, Sinophen Intranasal, Vacon, Vasosulf)

**Combination Products:** Duo-Medihaler (with isoproterenol)

**Classification:** decongestant, mydriatic, sympathomimetic

## Available Preparations:
- 10 mg/ml vial for parenteral use
- 0.12, 0.125, 1, 10 % ophthalmic solutions
- 0.125, 0.16, 0.2, 0.25, 0.5, 1 % nasal drops
- 0.2, 0.25, 0.5, 1 % nasal spray
- 0.5 % nasal jelly

Also available in 240 μg metered spray with isoproterenol 160 μg

**Action and Use:** This sympathomimetic acts on α-adrenergic receptors, causing vasoconstriction, increased peripheral resistance, increased blood pressure, and possibly reflex bradycardia. It does not stimulate β-adrenergic receptors. It leads to vasoconstriction in the respiratory system, and dilates the pupil of the eye. Phenylephrine is used parenterally to cause vasoconstriction and restore blood pressure during shock. It is sometimes added to local anesthetic solutions to cause vasoconstriction at the site and slow absorption of the anesthetic. It produces mydriasis without cyclopegia during ophthalmic examinations. Oral inhalation causes constriction in bronchioles and relieves congestion. Nasal preparations are applied topically to reduce congestion during upper respiratory infections.

**Routes and Dosages:** SC, IM, IV, ophthalmic, nasal, inhalation
**SQ, IM:**
- Hypotension: 0.1 mg/kg or 3 mg/m²; repeat in 1 to 2 hours PRN
- Hypotension During Spinal Anesthesia: 0.044 to 0.088 mg/kg
- Addition to Local Anesthetic: 0.05 mg/ml (1:20,000); add 1 ml phenylephrine to 20 ml anesthetic

**Ophthalmic:** Mydriasis: 1 drop of 2.5% solution, repeat in 1 hour PRN
**Nasal:**
- birth to 2 years: 2 to 3 drops of 0.125% solution in each nostril q3–4h PRN
- 2 to 6 years: 2 to 3 drops of 0.125 or 0.16% solution in each nostril q4h PRN
- 6 to 12 years: 2 to 3 drops of 0.25% solution in each nostril q3–4h PRN or 1 to 2 sprays of 0.25% spray in each nostril q3–4h

**Inhalation:** 1 inhalation; repeat in 2 to 5 minutes PRN; up to 4 to 6 times/day; not to exceed 2 inhalations at a time or 6 doses/day

**Absorption and Fate:** Immediate effect after IV with duration of 15 to 20 minutes. After IM, peak effect in 10 to 15 minutes and duration of ½ to 2 hours. After SC, effects occur in 10 to 15 minutes with duration of 3 hours. Effects seen in 15 to 20 minutes after inhalation with a duration of 2 to 4 hours. Effects after nasal administration last for 1/2 to 4 hours. With ophthalmic administration, peak effect occurs in 15 to 60 minutes with 2.5% solution and effects last 3 hours. With 10% ophthalmic solution, peak occurs in 10 to 90 minutes and effects last 3 to 7 hours. The drug is metabolized in the liver and intestines and excretion is not known.

**Contraindications and Precautions:** Pregnancy category C. Administration in late pregnancy could cause fetal anoxia and bradycardia. Unknown distribution into breast milk. The 10% ophthalmic solution is contraindicated in children under 1 year; generally 2.5% ophthalmic solution is used for all children. Contraindicated in severe hypertension, coronary disease, ventricular tachycardia, peripheral or mesenteric vascular thrombosis, and in those hypersensitive to the drug. Ophthalmic forms should not be used in those with narrow-angle glaucoma. Use in local anesthetics applied to fingers, toes, ears, nose; genitalia is contraindicated. The parenteral solution contains metabisulfite and should not be used in those with sulfite allergy. Cautious use in hyperthyroidism, diabetes, arteriosclerotic changes, cardiac disease, children with low body weight.

## Side Effects:
*CNS:* restlessness, nervousness, anxiety, tremor, headache, **seizures**. *CV:* **hypertension, palpitation**, chest pain, reduced blood flow, **severe bradycardia, decreased cardiac output**. *GI:* vomiting. *Respiratory:* increased pulmonary arterial pressure; rebound congestion after local applications. *Skin:* pallor, blanching, necrosis after extravasation. *Sensory:* stinging, tearing, blurred vision, local allergy after eye instillation, photosensitivity.

## Nursing Implications:
*Assess:* Establish baseline vital signs. Be certain patient treated wih parenteral forms is adequately hydrated as hypovolemia increases side effects.
*Administer:* Have phentolamine available to treat IV overdose and levodopa for ophthalmic overdose. *IV:* Use antecubital fossa rather than ankle or hand due to danger of extravasation. For direct IV injection, dilute 1 ml of drug with 9 ml sterile water. For IV infusion, dilute further with 5% dextrose or saline. Solution stable for 48 hours. Incompatible with iron, oxidizing agents, metals. When infusion is stopped it should be tapered gradually. *Ophthalmic:* Use 2.5% solution for children. 10% solution must not be given to children under 1 year. *Nasal:* Use smallest strength that produces desired effect.
*Monitor:* Blood pressure, central venous pressure, and EKG are monitored during IV doses. I & O measures are important. Observe for desired and side effects of medication, depending on route of administration. Systemic absorption from topical applications can occur.
*Patient Teaching:* Use only in amounts prescribed. Do not increase doses of nasal and inhalation routes. Teach correct administration of doses.

## Drug Interactions:
Increased pressor effects with guanethidine, tricyclic antidepressants, atropine. Cardiac arrhythmias may occur with digitalis, anesthetics, mercurial diuretics. MAO inhibitors may lead to severe hypertension. Alpha-adrenergic agents block pressor response. The inhaler is not to be used with epinephrine or other sympathomimetics due to potential tachycardia and arrhythmia.

## Storage Requirements:
Store at 15 to 30°C (59 to 86°F). Protect from light and freezing. Solution that is discolored brown or has a precipitate should not be used.

---

## □ PHENYTOIN
(fen'i-toy-in)

(Dilantin, Diphenylan)

**Combination Products:** Dilantin with phenobarbital kapseals

**Classification:** anticonvulsant, antiarrhythmic (Class IB)

### Available Preparations:
- 30 mg/5 ml, 125 mg/5 ml suspension
- 50-mg chewable tablets
- 30, 100-mg capsules, extended, and prompt action
- 50 mg/ml vials for parenteral use

Also available in capsules with 100 mg of phenytoin and 16 or 32 mg of phenobarbital

**Action and Use:** Controls seizure propagation by modifying the activities of ions such as sodium, potassium, and calcium and prevents seizure discharge from seizure foci. Acts as an antiarrhythmic similar to lidocaine or quinidine; decreases contraction force, improves atrioventricular conduction, and prolongs the refractory period. Used for control of tonic-clonic (grand mal) and partial seizures with complex symptomatology (psychomotor), as well as seizures caused by factors other than epilepsy. May be used in status epilepticus, particularly in combination with diazepam. Although not approved by the FDA for these purposes, it has been used in certain types of tachycardia and in arrhythmias, especially those caused by digitalis overdose.

**Routes and Dosages:** PO, IM (rare), IV
*PO:* Seizures: 5 mg/kg or 250 mg/m$^2$/day in 2 to 3 doses initially; adjusted as needed; not to exceed 300 mg/day; usual maintenance dose is 4 to 8 mg/kg/day or 200 mg/day. Loading dose may be used to reach therapeutic serum levels more quickly. Dose is 500 to 600 mg in several doses over 24 hours, followed by the lower maintenance dose.
*IM:* only used temporarily in patient unable to take PO form. Reduce usual oral dose by one-half and give IM. Upon return to PO form dose by that route is reduce by one-half for 1 week due to possibility of slow release of the drug from IM storage locations.
*IV:* Status Epilepticus: 250 mg/m$^2$ or 10 to 15 mg/kg, not to exceed 20 mg/kg/day

**Absorption and Fate:** Well absorbed from GI tract; unpredictable IM absorption. Highly (95%) protein bound. Metabolized mainly in the liver and excreted in the urine. Peak levels after capsule administration is 1.5 to 3 hours; after extended-release capsules, 4 to 12 hours. The half-life for neonates under 1 month is 60 hours; for children older than 1 month about 22 hours. Therapeutic serum level is 7.5 to 20 μg/ml.

**Contraindications and Precautions:** Pregnancy category D. Not to be given during pregnancy unless clearly needed because of risk of fetal hydantoin syndrome. Not given during lactation. Contraindicated in those with previous hypersensitivity to the drug, sinus bradycardia, heart block. Use is discontinued if a rash or lymphadenopathy occurs during therpay. Preparation containing sodium bisulfite is not given to those with sulfite allergy. Use with caution in respiratory depression, congestive failure, especially IV form.

## Side Effects:

*CNS:* **confusion, drowsiness** during early therapy, dizziness, headache; nystagmus, diplopia, and ataxia are early signs of intoxication. *CV:* **cardiovascular arrest** and **hypotension** with IV use. *GI:* nausea, vomiting, anorexia, decreased taste, weight loss. *Skin:* pain and necrosis at injection site; rash or **severe dermatitis** with fever; lupus erythematosus, Stevens-Johnson syndrome; hirsutism particularly in females. *Hemic:* **thrombocytopenia, leukopenia**, granulocytopenia, pancytopenia, anemia. *Endocrine:* hyperglycemia. *Other:* lymphadenopathy, hypertrichosis, osteomalacia, gingival hyperplasia especially in children.

## Nursing Implications:

*Assess:* Baseline CBC, liver function tests, and UA are done. Take vital signs especially before IV administration. Ask about rash or lymphadenopathy with previous phenytoin therapy. A previous exfoliative, purpuric, or bullous rash is contraindication to future phenytoin therapy.

*Administer:* The chewable tablets and suspension are phenytoin and other preparations (capsules and parenteral solution) are phenytoin sodium. 100 mg of phenytoin sodium is equivalent to about 92 mg of phenytoin, a factor that may require dosage regulation if this form of drug is changed. Bioavailability of all products differs depending on manufacturer so therapeutic levels must be monitored during change of products. Have patient bring usual product to the hospital for administration there when hospitalized. Vitamin D supplements may be ordered. *PO:* Shake suspension well. Chew chewable tablets to aid in dissolution. Regular tablets can be crushed and capsule opened and given in small amounts food or fluid. The PO form should be given with food or fluid to prevent gastric irritation. *IM:* IM route is used only if patient cannot take oral form. If long-term, oral preparations should be given through a gastric tube. IM bioavailability is variable, therefore, serum levels and side effects must be monitored carefully. *IV:* Solution should be clear. Can use solution with slight yellow color but not if precipitate is present. Give at rate of 0.5 to 1.5 mg/kg/minute. Incompatible with many other drugs in same IV solution, therefore, generally given alone. Inject normal saline to flush line after IV administration. If given in IV solution, normal saline is used, a 0.22-$\mu$m filter is in place, and the solution is given immediately after preparation. Have emergency drugs and equipment readily available.

*Monitor:* CBC, liver function studies, UA are done monthly. Serum levels of drug are monitored. Side effects are observed for, particularly rash or lymphadenopathy that may necessitate drug withdrawal. Observe for and record seizures, neuropathy, mental changes. Watch for gingival hyperplasia, a common occurrence in children. *IV:* observe for irritation and necroses which can occur even without infiltration.

***Patient Teaching:*** Family should report seizure activity. Teach emergency care for seizure occurrence. Teach to avoid alcohol and other CNS depressants, including OTC drugs. Return for scheduled appointments as serum levels may indicate need for dosage adjustment. Do not change forms or companies of drug used without discussion with prescriber and close monitoring for effects. Child should wear medical alert band stating seizure disorder and use of phenytoin. Drug can alter mental alertness; therefore, avoid driving cars and adjust activities accordingly. Gingival hyperplasia may be prevented somewhat by good oral hygiene (daily brushing, flossing, gum massage). Oral care must be started in the infant as soon as teeth erupt. If excessive, hyperplasia may be removed surgicaly although it can grow back. Report progress of the child in the classroom, as well as presence of disruptive behavior.

**Drug Interactions:** A number of drugs may decrease serum phenytoin levels; these include CNS depressants, antacids, barbiturates, folic acid, rifampin. Valproic acid may increase or decrease phenytoin levels. Increased sedation if given with primidone. Phenytoin can decrease serum digitoxin levels. Disulfiram can increase phenytoin levels.

**Food Interactions:** May interfere with vitamin D metabolism, therefore, a supplement may be ordered and diet should be high in vitamin D (dairy products, fish). May interfere with folic acid metabolism, therefore, observation of folate deficiency (neuropathy, mental changes) should occur.

**Laboratory Test Interferences:** Decreases protein bound iodine, thyroxine levels, 17-hydroxycorticosteroids, 17-ketosteroids. Increases $T_3$ uptake, serum alkaline phosphatase, glucose, BSP.

**Storage Requirements:** Store at 15 to 30°C (59 to 86°F) in tightly closed containers. Avoid freezing of oral and parenteral solutions.

□ **PIPERAZINE ADIPATE**

(Entacyl)

□ **PIPERAZINE CITRATE**                                        (pi'per-a-zeen)

(Antepar, Bryrel, Pin-Tega Tabs, Pipril, Ta-Verm, Veriga, Vermazine, Vermirex)

**Classification:** anthelmintic

## Available Preparations:

- 500 mg/5 ml oral solution
- 250, 500-mg tablet

**Action and Use:** Mechanism unknown; believed to paralyze the musculature of parasite resulting in removal of the organism by intestinal peristalsis of the host. Most effective against roundworm (*Ascaris lumbricoides*) and pinworm (*Enterobius vermicularis*).

## Routes and Dosage:
*PO:*

- Pinworms: 65 mg/kg/day once per day or 1 g/m$^2$/day, for 7 days; may repeat in 1 week. (Maximum dose of 2.5 mg/day)
- Roundworms: 75 mg/kg/day once per day or 2 g/m$^2$/day, for 2 days. (Maximum dose 3.5 g/day)

**Absorption and Fate:** Well absorbed from GI tract. Excreted unchanged in urine.

**Contraindications and Precautions:** Pregnancy category C. Contraindicated in hypersensitivity to drug or its salts, seizure disorders and with impaired renal or hepatic function. Use with caution in anemia, severe malnutrition, and prolonged usage in children.

## Side Effects:

*CNS:* headache, dizziness, ataxia, tremors, choreiform movements, muscular weakness, hyporeflexia, paresthesia, nystagmus, sense of detachment, **memory defect, convulsions, EEG changes**. *GI:* nausea, vomiting, diarrhea, abdominal pain. *Hemic:* **hemolytic anemia.** *Sensory:* blurred vision, **paralytic strabismus**, cataracts. *Other:* Hypersensitivity: urticaria, erythema multiform purpura, fever, productive cough, arthralgia, lacrimation, bronchospasm.

## Nursing Implications:

*Assess:* Obtain pinworm test during night or when child is sleeping, then worms migrate to perianal area to deposit their eggs. Commercial test kit available or can use scotch tape with sticky side to outside of tongue blade. Obtain test by carefully exposing buttocks and pressing tape to anal area. Wash hands well after test. Round worm diagnosed through stool samples; follow your agency procedure for collection.

*Administer:* Tablet can be crushed and mixed with small amount of food to administer. Can be given with food to reduce GI upset. Shake suspension well.

*Monitor and Patient Teaching:* Pinworms: A highly contagious female can deposit 17,000 eggs a night; ova mature within 3 to 8 hours. Ova also spread by hand-to-mouth contact and through inhalation. All members of family should be treated. All bed linen, towels, undergarments, and personal clothes should be washed. Carpets should be vacuumed, floors damp mopped, toilets disinfected daily. Infected child should sleep alone with tight-fitting underwear or diapers. Cut nails and keep clean. Change linens, bedclothes, and underwear daily. This disease does not indicate family has unclean home. However, good hand washing is important to prevent spread of disease. Round-worm: Common where human wastes are used as fertilizer. Occasionally worm may migrate to mouth, nose, or rectum. Good hand washing and washing raw vegetables and fruits. If CNS side effects occur withhold drug and notify physician. Caution parents not to give more frequently than prescribed because of neurotoxicity. With all infestations teach parent how to obtain stool culture.

**Drug Interactions:** Usage of chlorpromazine and this drug may cause seizures. Pyrantel pamoate and this drug, possible pharmacological antagonism.

**Laboratory Test Interferences:** May cause increase serum uric acid.

**Storage Requirements:** Store at 15 to 30°C (50 to 86°F) in tight container.

---

## □ PNEUMOCOCCAL POLYSACCHARIDE VACCINE

(noo-moe-cock'al)

(Pneumovax)

**Classification:** immunization

**Available Preparations:** single and 5-dose vials for parenteral use

**Action and Use:** Stimulates body production of antibodies against disease caused by *Streptococcus pneumoniae* (pneumococcus). The 23-valent vaccine is used for children over 2 years who have chronic illness.

**Routes and Dosages:**
*IM, SC:* over 2 years: 0.5 ml one time dose

**Absorption and Fate:** Adequate immune response is achieved in most recipients 2 to 3 weeks after administration.

**Contraindications and Precautions:** Contraindicated in pregnancy. Use with caution in lactation. Not used for those under 2 years. Contraindicated in those with hypersensitivity to vaccine components, such as thimerosal, a mercury derivative used as preservative, and phenol. Booster doses are generally contraindicated. (Some patients with Hodgkin's disease may have inadequate response and require a booster dose 3 to 4 months after chemotherapy and radiation are completed.) Delay administration in those with active infection. The vaccine is not recommended for HIV-infected children who are asymptomatic, but is recommended for symptomatic children.

## Side Effects:
*Skin:* erythema and pain at injection site. ***Musculoskeletal:*** myalgia. *Other:* fever, **anaphylaxis (rare)**.

## Nursing Implications:
*Assess:* Identify target groups for immunization. It is recommended for children over 2 years with chronic illness associated with risk of pneumococcal disease. These include asplenia, sickle cell disease, nephrotic syndrome, immunosuppressive states, symptomatic HIV-infected children, and children with cerebral spinal fluid leaks.
*Administer:* The vaccine is to be given only once. Do not confuse with influenza vaccine that is given annually. Epinephrine 1:1000 and resuscitative equipment should be readily available in case of anaphylaxis. The vaccine does not replace the need for penicillin prophylaxis for pneumococcal exposure, as antibody response is not immediate. *IM:* Give into deltoid of older children or lateral thigh of young child. Avoid intravenous or intradermal administration.
*Monitor:* Observe child for 20 minutes after immunization for signs of anaphylaxis.
*Patient Teaching:* A mild analgesic, such as acetaminophen, may relieve side effects.

**Drug Interactions:** Immunosuppressive therapy may decrease response to the vaccine, therefore, vaccine should be deferred until 10 to 14 days after therapy is completed.

**Storage Requirements:** Refrigerate at 2 to 8°C (35 to 46°F) in the refrigerator rather than on door where temperature variations are greater.

---

## ☐ POLIO-INACTIVATED VACCINE

(poe'lee-oh)

(IPV)

**Classification:** immunization

**Available Preparations:** 1-ml ampule and 10-ml vial for parenteral use

**Action and Use:** A suspension of the three types of polio virus that stimulates body production of polio antibody against all types of polio. Used for initial series in previously unimmunized adults and in children for whom OPV live virus vaccine is contraindicated, such as when a child or family member is immunosuppressed, or when a child is HIV-infected, whether symptomatic or asymptomatic.

### Routes and Dosages:
*SC:* four 1.0-ml doses; the first three at 1 to 2-month intervals; the fourth, 6 to 12 months after the third.

### Absorption and Fate: Four doses produce immunity in 95% of recipients.

### Contraindications and Precautions: The vaccine is contraindicated in pregnancy, and in those with known hypersensitivity to neomycin and streptomycin. Delay immunization in those with active infection.

### Side Effects:
*Skin:* erythema, tenderness, rash. *Other:* fever, **hypersensitivity reaction** to trace amounts of neomycin and streptomycin used in vaccine preparation

### Nursing Implications:
*Assess:* Take history of allergy to neomycin or streptomycin. Check records of young children for adequacy of immunization.
*Administer:* If series is interrupted, there is no need to restart; begin with next scheduled dose. Epinephrine 1:1000 and resuscitative equipment should be readily available in case of anaphylaxis. The National Childhood Vaccine Injury Act requires recording of patient's name, address, route and site of administration, lot number and manufacturer of vaccine, date of immunization, as well as the name, address, and title of the person who administers the vaccine.
*Monitor:* Observe for 20 minutes after immunization for anaphylaxis. Severe reactions, such as anaphylaxis, are reported to the United States Department of Health and Human Services (see Appendix J).
*Patient Teaching:* Teach parents when child is to return for next immunization in the series and to bring immunization records with them.

### Storage Requirements: Refrigerate at 2 to 8°C (35 to 46°F) in body of refrigerator rather than on door where temperature variations may be greater. Avoid freezing. Discard solution with cloudiness or color change.

---

### ☐ POLIO-TRIVALENT ORAL POLIO VACCINE                      (poe'lee-oh)

(OPV, Orimune)

### Classification: immunization

### Available Preparations:
- single-dose plastic dispensers
- multiple-dose glass bottles with dropper

**Action and Use:** A suspension of live attenuated polio virus that stimulates body production of polio antibodies against all three types of polio. Used for initial series and booster in childhood against all three types of polio.

**Routes and Dosages:**
*PO:* 0.5 ml or 2 drops, or entire content of single-dose dispenser at 2, 4, 15 to 18 months, and 4 to 6 years (a total of 4 doses). For those children not immunized in infancy, 2 doses are given 6 to 8 weeks apart, and a third dose is given 6 to 12 months later. If the third dose is given after 4 years of age, the fourth dose is not needed.

**Absorption and Fate:** After PO ingestion, live polio virus multiplies and is present in the gastrointestinal tract for 4 to 6 weeks. Excreted during that time in the feces. Immune response is present 7 to 10 days after administration. Immunity occurs in 95% of recipients after 3 doses.

**Contraindications and Precautions:** Not to be given to pregnant women. Contraindicated in children who are HIV-infected, whether symptomatic or asymptomatic, who are receiving steroids or other immunosuppressants, who have an immune deficiency disease, or who have a family member with an immune deficiency disease, and in adults who have never received oral polio before. Polio immunization with OPV is not recommended for those over 18 years living in the United States. (Inactivated polio vaccine) (IPV) may be used for most of these cases. Children who have received immune serum globulin in the last 90 days and those with a current febrile or acute illness should have immunizatin delayed.

**Side Effects:**
*CNS:* rare incidence of contraction of **polio disease** by the patient (1 in 8.7 million) or a family member (1 in 5 million) occurs; the latter is infected by contact with the live virus in the feces where it is excreted.

**Nursing Implications:**
*Assess:* A physical examination is done to rule out active infection. Review of records and history should rule out immunosuppression in the patient and close family members. If parents have not been immunized against polio, they should be informed of the slight risk (1 in 5 million) of polio disease in contacts of persons vaccinated. They may choose to become immunized with IPV before the infant's immunization with OPV to avoid this risk. Check records of young children for adequacy of immunization. If one or more doses were given at an earlier time, start with the next scheduled dose and complete the series. It is not necessary or advisable to start the series again.
*Administer:* The National Childhood Vaccine Injury Act requires recording of the patient's name, address, route and site of administration, lot number and manufacturer of vaccine, date of immunization, as well as the name, address, and title of the person who administers the vaccine.

The third dose may be given at 15 to 18 months at the same visit as the measles–mumps–rubella vaccine or the DTP. Doses of OPV should be given at least 6 weeks apart to ensure adequate immune response. *PO:* Solution can be thawed by gently rotating container in hand or allowing to sit at room temperature for a few moments. See storage requirements for important information. Doses are generally administered by dropping the liquid directly into the child's mouth.

*Monitor:* Severe reaction of contraction of polio is reported to the United States Department of Health and Human Services (see Appendix J).

*Patient Teaching:* Teach parents to wash hands thoroughly after diaper change or when assisting child during toileting for at least 4 weeks after immunization. Careful cleaning or disposal of diapers is recommended. Teach child to wash hands after bowel movements if old enough to attend to own toileting. Teach parents when child is to return for next polio immunization and have them bring immunization records with them. Breast feeding does not interfere with the efficacy of the vaccine administered to the breast-fed infant.

**Drug Interactions:** Disseminated disease is a potential in the patient who is on immunosuppressants, therefore, the vaccine should not be given in these cases.

**Storage Requirements:** Keep frozen (-10°C or 14°F). May refreeze unopened vials if temperature did not exceed 8°C (46°F) during the thaw period. Each vial can go through no more than 10 thaw–freeze cycles. Unopened thawed containers may be kept no more than 30 days at 2 to 8°C (35 to 46°F) in refrigerator. Opened vials may be kept at the same refrigeration for no more than 7 days. A clear marking system must be devised so that a vaccine that is potentially ineffective can be discarded.

---

□ **POLYMYXIN SULFATE**                    (pol-i-mix'in)

(Aerosporin)

**Combination Products:** Ophthalmic: Polymyxin B used with drugs such as gramicidin, neomycin sulfate hydrocortisone, bacitracin and oxytetracycline hydrochloride; Otic: Polymyxin B, hydrocortisone and neomycin sulfate (Cortisporin, Octicair, Otocort); Topical: Polymyxin B, bacitracin and neomycin sulfate

**Classification:** antiinfective, polymyxin

**Available Preparations:** 500,000 units for parenteral administration

**Action and Use:** Obtained from cultures of *Bacillus polymyxa*. Damages the cytoplasmic membrane of bacteria by cationic detergent action causing leakage of the essential intracellular metabolites. Treats many strains of gm− bacteria except *Proteus* and *Neisseria*. Used primarily to treat organisms resisant to other antibiotics due to toxicity of drug. Drug of choice for urinary tract infections, septicemia and meningitis caused by *Ps. aeruginosa.* Intrathecal (IT) administration is only route for treatment of meningeal infections with this drug. Combination products are used to treat susceptible organisms of eye and external ear.

## Routes and Dosage:
*IM:*
- infants to 2 years: up to 40,000 U/kg/day
- over 2 years: 25,000 to 30,000 U/kg/day in equally divided doses every 4 to 6 hours

*IV:*
- infants to 2 years: up to 40,000 U/kg/day
- over 2 years: 15,000 to 25,000 U/kg/day in equally divided doses every 12 hours. (Maximum IV dose is 25,000 U/kg/day)

Dosage and frequency decreased in patients with renal impairment
*IT:*
- under 2 years: 20,000 U/day for 3 to 4 days, then 25,000 U every other day for 2 weeks or until spinal cultures negative
- over 2 years: 50,000 U/day for 3 to 4 days, then 50,000 U once every other day for 2 weeks or until spinal cultures are negative

**Absorption and Fate:** Peak levels: IM, 2 hours; IV, within 10 minutes of infusion. Distributed to body tissues except CSF. Not highly bound to plasma proteins and half-life is 4.3 to 6 hours. 60% drug excreted unchanged in urine.

**Contraindications and Precautions:** Pregnancy category B. IM not recommended in infants and children, unless absolutely necessary, due severe pain at injection site. Contraindicated in hypersensitivity to this drug or renal failure. Use caution in neonates, infants, or in impaired renal function. Parenteral and intrathecal drug should be administered only to hospitalized children.

**Side Effects:** More likely seen with high dosages or impaired renal function.
*CNS:* facial flushing, circumoral or peripheral paresthesia, numbness, muscle weakness, slurred speech, dizziness, vertigo, ataxia, blurred vision, irritability, **confusion, coma, seizures, neuromuscular blockade with apnea** *GU:* **nephrotoxicity**: albuminuria, cylindruria, azotemia, hematuria, increased blood−drug level without increasing dose. *Skin:* pruritus, urticaria, rash. *Other:* Hypersensitivity: fever, eosinophilia, **anaphylaxis**; Local: IM: severe pain; IV: thrombophlebitis; IT: meningeal irritation, fever, headache, stiff neck, increased leukocytes and protein in CSF.

## Nursing Implications:
*Assess:* Assess previous allergy to this drug. Obtain cultures and sensitivity

before treatment, but can start treatment before results. Obtain baseline renal function data and serum electrolytes.

***Administer: IM:*** Reconstitute with 2 ml of sterile water, 0.9% sodium chlorine, or 1% procaine hydrochloride for injection. Injection extremely painful. ***IV:*** 500,000 U dissolved in 300 to 500 ml of 5% dextrose (dilution of 1667 to 1000 U/ml), infused over 1 to 2 hours. Compatible with $D_5W$, NS, and diphenhydramine and hydrocortisone sodium succinate. Avoid premixing with other drugs or solutions. ***IT:*** Reconstitute with 10 ml of 0.9% sodium chloride in sterile syringe. Do not use procaine hydrochloride for reconstitution. Administer according to hospital policy for intrathecal administration.

***Monitor:*** IM injection causes severe pain that radiates along peripheral nerves for 40 to 60 minutes after injection. Ice pack may ease some discomfort. Observe IV site for extravasation and thrombophlebitis; use large vein with small-bore needle. Monitor for nephrotoxicity and neurotoxicity (symptoms usually occur in first 4 days of therapy). Assess renal function by I & O, weights, surum drug levels, and BUN and serum creatinine. Neurotoxicity can be difficult to detect in infants and young children because of their inability to verbalize. Watch for symptoms of superinfections. Maintain fluid intake for age group. IT: assess for meningeal irritation.

**Drug Interactions:** Avoid giving with other neurotoxic drugs such as aminoglycosides, amphotericin B, capreomycin, methoxyflurane, polymyxin B sulfate, vancomycin, anticholinesterases, antineoplastics, quinidine, and quinine. Curariform muscle relaxants, such as (ether, tubocurarine, succinylcholine, gallamine, decamethoniuma, and sodium citrate, may enhance neuromuscular reactions of polymyxin B. Cephalothin and this drug may cause increased nephrotoxic effect.

**Storage Requirements:** Store sterile powder at 15 to 30°C and protected from light. Aqueous solutions with pH of 5 to 7.5 can remain stable for 6 months at 2 to 8°C; (35–46°F) however, after diluted stable for only 72 hours if refrigerated.

---

□ **POTASSIUM, POTASSIUM ACETATE, POTASSIUM CHLORIDE**
(poe-tass'ee-um)

(Cena-K, Kaochlor, Kaon-CL, Kato, Kay Ciel, K-Dur, Klor-10%, Klor-Con, Klotrix, K-Lyte, K-Tab, Micro-K, Potachlor, Potage, Potasalan, Potassine, Rum-K, Slow-K, Ten-K)

# ☐ POTASSIUM GLUCONATE

(Bayon, Kaon, Kao-Nor, Kaylixir, K-G Elixir)

**Combination Products:** Kolyum, Tri-K

**Classification:** electrolyte

## Available Preparations:
***Potassium acetate:***   2, 4 mEq ampules for parenteral use
***Potassium chloride:***
- 4, 13.4 mEq enteric-coated tablets
- 6.7, 8, 10, 20 mEq extended-release tablets
- 8, 10 mEq capsules
- 5, 6.7, 10, 13.3 mEq/5 ml oral solution
- 1.5, 2, 2.4, 3, 3.2 mEq/ml parenteral solution

Also available in combination with saline, dextrose, lactated Ringer's, potassium bicarbonate, potassium gluconate, and potassium citrate
***Potassium gluconate:***
- 2, 5 mEq tablets
- 6.7 mEq/5 ml elixir

Also available in combination with potassium chloride, potassium citrate, and ammonium chloride.

**Action and Use:** The main intracellular cation responsible for isotonicity, nerve impulse, skeletal and cardiac muscle contraction, carbohydrate metabolism, transferring glucose to glycogen, protein synthesis, and acid-base balance. Used to treat hypokalemia caused by conditions such as vomiting, nasogastric suction, and diuretic use.

## Routes and Dosages:
*PO:*
- Potassium Chloride: 15 to 40 mEq (1 to 3 g potassium chloride)/m²/day or 1 to 3 mEq (75 to 225 mg potassium chloride)/kg/day in divided doses
- Potassium Gluconate and its combination products: 20 to 40 mEq/m²/day or 2 to 3 mEq/kg/day in divided doses
- Potassium Acetate, Potassium Bicarbonate, Potassium Citrate Combination: 15 to 30 mEq/m² or 2 to 3 mEq/kg/day in divided doses

*IV:* Potassium Acetate: up to 40 mEq/m²/day or 3 mEq/kg/day (not to exceed 3 mEq/kg/day)

**Absorption and Fate:** Well absorbed from small intestine. Present in body fluids. Excreted by kidneys. Normal serum levels are 3.5 to 5.0 mEq/L or up to 6 to 7.7 mEq/L in neonates.

**Contraindications and Precautions:** Pregnancy category C. Contraindicated in severe renal dysfunction, hyperkalemia, acute dehydration; capsule and tablet forms not used with delayed GI emptying. Cautious use in metabolic acidosis, heart block, trauma, such as burns, myotonia congenita, renal dysfunction, diarrhea.

**Side Effects:**
*CNS:* confusion, tiredness, weakness; all signs of hyperkalemia. *CV:* bradycardia, hypotensin with hyperkalemia. *GI:* nausea, vomiting, diarrhea, GI distress and ulceration.

**Nursing Implications:**
*Assess:* Serum pH and electrolytes especially if potassium and magnesium are taken.
*Administer: PO:* Give after meals with generous amount of water. *IV:* Given slowly, diluted in IV fluid. Infusion rate not to exceed 0.02 mEq/kg/minute or 0.5 to 1 mEq/kg/hour.
*Monitor:* Monitor serum pH and electrolytes, particularly potassium and magnesium. Renal function is assessed by tests such as creatinine. Assess I & O. EKGs are done with careful monitoring in those on digitalis. *IV:* Monitor EKG and serum potassium.
*Patient Teaching:* Return for scheduled health-care visits. Take as directed with ample fluid. Teaching about potassium-rich foods is needed; these include oranges, banana, tomato, broccoli, legumes, meats, raisins, potatoes, peanut butter, whole grains, and milk.

**Drug Interactions:** Corticosteroids can decrease drug's action. Use with other drugs causing GI upset, such as nonsteroidal antiinflammatories, can increase that side effect. Increased GI upset with heparin. Hyperkalemia with potassium-sparing diuretics, blood transfusion, captopril. Decreased vitamin $B_{12}$ absorption with extended-release forms.

**Food Interactions:** Foods with high potassium content can increase risk of hyperkalemia. Other products, such as salt substitutes and some OTC medications, also contain significant amounts of potassium.

**Storage Requirements:** Store in tightly covered, light-resistant containers at 15 to 30°C (59 to 86°F). Protect solutions from freezing.

---

□ **PRAZIQUANTEL**                              (pray-zi-kwon'tel)

(Biltricide)

**Classification:** anthelmintic

**Available Preparations:**   600-mg film-coated tablet

**Action and Use:** Exact mechanism of activity unknown but appears to cause an increase in permeability of worms' cell membrane, resulting in an increase of calcium ion uptake. This causes contraction and paralysis of worms' musculature leading to dislodgment of suckers; the worms are then passed into the liver where phagocytosis from the host occurs. Drug effective against schistosomes (blood flukes), trematodes (liver, lung, intestinal flukes), and cestodes (tapeworm). Active against cysticerosis (larval stage) of cestodes.

## Routes and Dosage:
*PO:* over 4 years:
- Schistosoma: 60 mg/kg given in 3 equally divided doses over 4 to 6 hours in 1 day; or 40 mg/kg/dose as single dose
- Trematodes: 75 mg/kg given 3 equally divided doses over 4 to 6 hours in 1 day (dosage may vary with different species)
- Cestodiasis: 25 mg/kg/dose as single dose
- Cysticercosis: 50 mg/kg/day in divided doses 3 times a day for 14 days

**Absorption and Fate:** 80% drug absorbed from GI tract. Peak levels: 1 to 3 hours. Half-life: 0.8 to 1.5 hours; of metabolites: 4 to 5 hours. Excreted mainly in urine.

**Contraindications and Precautions:** Pregnancy category B. Safe usage not established in those under 4 years. Contraindicated in hypersensitivity to drug, during lactation, and for 72 hours after ingestion of last dose of drug, intraocular cysticercosis.

## Side Effects:
*CNS:* malaise, headache, dizziness (occurs in 90%); drowsiness, giddiness; **CSF reaction: neurologic signs and symptoms, seizures, intracranial hypertension**. *GI:* occasional abdominal pain, nausea (90%); vomiting, anorexia, diarrhea; crampy abdominal pain, fever, bloody stools usually 1 hour after taking drug. *Hepatic:* transient rise in SGOT, SGPT; no evidence of adverse hepatic effects. *Other:* maculopapular rash, pruritus, urticaria, fever, myalgia or arthralgia, hypotension and palpitation.

## Nursing Implications:
*Assess:* Parasites are diagnosed through stool samples; follow your agency procedure for collection. Lung fluke infestation may be confirmed through sputum tests. Obtain dietary histories, e.g., ingestion of raw fish, crabmeat, crayfish, watercress, improperly cooked pork or beef, or if human sewage is used to fertilize vegetables and fruits. Some of these infestations are rare in the United States, therefore, information on travel to other countries is necessary.
*Administer:* Tablet is not to be chewed due to bitter taste. Tablet is easily divided due to scoring (divides into 4 segments). Tablet should not be crushed, but mixing segment with jelly may enable small child to swallow drug. Praziquantel is very soluble in water, resulting in a bitter-tasting solution that may

cause vomiting and gagging; do not mix in juice. Follow tablet with fluid so tablet is rinsed from mouth. Administer with food.

**Monitor and Patient Teaching:** Side effects occur more frequently in those with heavy infestations. In treatment of cysticercosis: because of adverse CNS symptoms, corticosteroids may be used concurrently in those with cerebral cysticercosis infestations. It is usually not necessary for purgation or dietary restrictions, but if child is constipated a laxative may be necessary. A mild purgative and saline purge may be given in conjunction with treatment for *T. solium* infestations. Child is considered cured if stool cultures are negative for ova and proglottids for 3 months. Reinfestations prevented through good personal hygiene, hand washing, prevention of hand to mouth contamination, sanitary waste disposal, not eating watercress, swimming in infested water, and proper cooking of pork, crabmeat, crayfish, fish, and beef. Teach parent how to obtain stool culture.

**Drug Interaction:** May cause synergistic effect when used with oxamniquine.

**Storage Requirements:** Store at 15 to 30°C (50 to 86°F) in tight container.

---

□ **PREDNISOLONE** (pred-niss'oh-lone)

(Cortalone, Delta-Cortef, Inflamase, Novoprednisolone, Prelone Predoxine)

□ **PREDNISOLONE ACETATE**

(Articulose, Deltastab, Econopred, Key-Pred, Predate, Pred Mild, Savacort)

□ **PREDNISOLONE SODIUM PHOSPHATE**

(Ak-Pred, Codelsol, Hydeltrasol, Key-Pred-SP, Metreton, Predate-S, PSP-IV)

□ **PREDNISOLONE TEBUTATE**

(Hydeltr-TBA, Metalone TBA, Nor-Pred TBA, Predate-TAB, Predcor-TBA, Prednisol TBA)

**Combination Products:** Prednisolone acetate with atropine sulfate (Mydrapred); prednisolone acetate with sulfacetamide sodium (Blephamide, Liquifilm, Sulfacort, and others); prednisolone acetate with neomycin sulfate, polymyxin B sulfate (Poly-Pred); prednisolone sodium phosphate with sulfacetamide sodium (Optimyd, Vasocidin)

**Classification:** corticosteroid, glucocorticoid

## Available Preparations:
- 5 mg/5 ml, 15 mg/5 ml oral solution
- 5-mg tablet
- 20, 25, 50 mg/ml for parenteral administration
- 0.125%, 1% ophthalmic solution
- 0.12%, 0.125%, 1% ophthalmic suspension
- 0.5% otic solution

**Action and Use:** Natural or synthetic, intermediate-acting glucocorticoid that has strong antiinflammatory, immunosuppressant, and metabolic actions. Used to treat diseases such as endocrine, collagen, dermatologic, allergy, and acute leukemia. Used with mineralocorticoids as replacement therapy in adrenocortical deficiencies.

## Routes and Dosage:
*PO:* 0.14 to 2 mg/kg/ day or 4 to 60 mg/m$^2$/day in 4 divided doses.
*IM:* Acetate: 0.04 to 0.25 mg/kg or 1.5 to 7.5 mg/m$^2$ 1 to 2 times per day
*IM, IV:* Sodium Phosphate: 0.04 to 0.25 mg/kg or 1.5 to 7.5 mg/m$^2$ 1 to 2 times per day
Note: Dosage determined by severity of condition and child's response. When used in combination with long-acting glucocorticoids, an alternate-day dose therapy is given, especially with those receiving doses larger than required for replacement therapy; to decrease risk of growth suppression.
*Ophthalmic:* 1 to 2 drops of suspension or solution into conjunctival sac every hour during day and every 2 hours at night or 1 to 2 drops every 3 to 12 hours.
*Otic:* 3 to 4 drops of solution into ear canal 2 to 3 times a day.

**Absorption and Fate:** Absorption: PO, rapid, complete; IM sodium phosphate, rapid; IM acetate, slow but complete. Peak effect: PO, 1 to 2 hours. Duration: PO, 1.25 to 1.5 days; IM acetate, up to 4 weeks. Metabolized by liver and excreted primarily by kidney.

**Contraindications and Precautions:** Pregnancy category C and safety during lactation not established. Intraarticular, intrabursal, intradermal, or intralesional dosages not established for children. Use caution in children, possible growth suppression; not recommended for long-term usage. Contraindicated in hypersensitivity to drug or its components, sensitivity to corticosteroids, varicella, systemic fungal infections, nephrotic syndrome, acquired immune deficiency syndrome (AIDS), immunizations with live virus vaccines, and oral polio virus vaccine or contact with those who have had the vaccine. Use with caution in renal disease, hypertension, congestive heart failure, cardiac disease, diabetes, ulcerative colitis, gastrointestinal ulceration, hyperthyroidism, systemic lupus erythematosus, impaired hepatic function, osteoporosis, vaccinia, exanthema, Cushing's syndrome, seizures, myasthenia gravis, tuberculosis, ocular herpes simplex, hypoalbuminemia, emotional or psychotic tendencies.

**Side Effects:** Usually dependent on dosage and duration of treatment.
***CNS:*** headaches, vertigo, euphoria, insomnia, **increased intracranial pressure** (papilledema), **psychotic behavior, seizures**. ***CV:*** edema, **hypertension, congestive heart failure**. ***GI:*** nausea, vomiting, change in appetite, gastrointestinal irritation, abdominal distention, pancreatitis, ulcerative esophagitis, peptic ulcer. ***Skin:*** impaired wound healing, thin fragile skin, petechia, ecchymosis, acne, facial erythema, increased sweating, may mask infections. ***Hemic:*** **thrombocytopenia**. ***Endocrine:*** **HPA-axis suppression**, menstrual irregularities, Cushing's states, **secondary adrenocortical, pituitary unresponsiveness**. ***Musculoskeletal:*** **suppression of bone growth, osteoporosis**, muscle weakness, **aseptic necrosis of femoral and humeral heads**. ***Sensory:*** Ophthalmic: **posterior subcapsular cataracts, increased intraocular pressure**. ***Other:*** sodium retention, potassium loss, **negative nitrogen balance, hypokalemia, hyperglycemia**, susceptibility to infections; Withdrawal symptoms: rebound inflammation, fatigue, weakness, fever, arthralgia, dizziness, lethargy, depression, fainting, orthostatic hypotension, dyspnea, anorexia, hypoglycemia, nausea and vomiting, shortness of breath, unusual weight loss.

## Nursing Implications:

***Assess:*** Obtain baseline weight and height; before long-term therapy, obtain ECG, chest and spinal x-rays, glucose tolerance test, evaluation of HPA-axis function, and BP before therapy. Ophthalmic: do not use if eye is infected. Otic: do not use if external ear is infected.
***Administer:*** Best to calculate drug dosage on mg/m²; reduces overdosage possibilities in very short or heavy children. ***PO:*** Take with food or milk to reduce GI irritation. Best to give daily dosage before 9 AM; it suppress adrenal cortex activity less, which may reduce risk of HPA-axis suppression. Tablet can be crushed and mixed with small amount of food or fluid. ***IM:*** Shake well (acetate) before withdrawal. Do not use deltoid muscle. Prevent leakage of drug into dermis and subcutaneous tissues because it may cause atrophy or abscess.
***IV:*** Sodium phosphate is form of drug used for IV and is commercially diluted. Can further dilute with 5% dextrose or NS. Rarely given IV in children; consult pharmacist for dilutions, rates of infusion, and compatibilities.
***Ophthalmic:*** See Part I for instillation. Shake suspension. Remove contact lenses before usage and consult physician when child may begin wearing them again. ***Otic:*** See Part I for instillation.
***Monitor:*** Monitor BP during infusion. Carefully assess child's response to drug; necessary for dosage adjustments. Observe for side effects, especially hypocalcemia, signs of electrolyte imbalance, signs of adrenal insufficiency, symptoms of infections, or worsening of condition. Monitor BP and daily weights, report any sudden weight gain to the physician. With long-term usage, monitor serum electrolytes and height. Encourage well-balanced diet low in sodium, rich in potassium, calcium, vitamins K and D. Observe for ulcer development; if on long-term therapy, prophylactic antacids may be used. Encourage good hygiene and dental care (possible oral fungal infections). Tonometry (eye) examinations every 6 weeks. Diabetics may need increase in insulin due to steroid-induced hyperglycemia. To discontinue, drug dosage should be reduced gradually, especially after long-term usage so it does not cause acute

life-threatening adrenal insufficiency. After discontinuation of short-term therapy (up to 5 days) with high dosage, adrenal recovery may occur within 1 week. After prolonged high-dose therapy, complete recovery of adrenal function may require up to 1 year. If infection occurs (ophthalmic, otic), discontinue drug and inform physician.

**Patient Teaching:** Do not alter dosage or stop drug abruptly, it could cause very serious side effects, even death. Gradual tapering of dosage is necessary. Increasing amount of medication will not hasten healing process. Demonstrate how to instill ophthalmic or otic forms, or dosing schedule for oral form. Monitor signs and symptoms of medication, symptoms of adrenal insufficiency, or worsening of condition; report to physician. Obtain daily weights; report to physician any sudden weight gains. Stress importance of close medical supervision and follow-up. Regular ophthalmic examinations if on long-term therapy. Caution about receiving skin tests, vaccinations, or other immunizations, or coming in contact with persons receiving oral polio virus vaccine. Inform any health-care provider, including dentists, surgeons, or emergency care personnel that child is on this medication. Child should carry a medical identification card. Observe for symptoms of infections. Do not use OTC medications without contacting health-care provider.

**Drug Interactions:** This drug in combination with high dosage of acetaminophen may increase risk of hepatotoxicity. With analgesics and antiinflammatory drugs, increased risk of gastric ulceration. Amphotericin B and potassium-depleting diuretics increase risk of hypokalemia. Use with anabolic steroids may increase the risk of edema and acne. Drug in combination with anticoagulants may decrease anticoagulant effect. This drug used with anticonvulsants (phenytoin) may lower seizure threshold. Use with vaccines, live virus, or other immunizations may potentiate replication of the vaccine virus, increasing chance for developing the viral disease.

**Laboratory Test Interferences:** May increase serum cholesterol, sodium and blood glucose. May decrease serum calcium, potassium, $T_4$, $^{131}I$ uptake, urine 17-hydroxysteroid and 17-ketosteroids. Tends to suppress skin tests; may give a false-negative result with nitroblue-tetrazolium for bacterial infection. Adrenal function assessed by ACTH stimulation or plasma cortisol may be decreased.

**Storage Requirements:** Store at 15 to 30°C (59 to 86°F). Protect from light and freezing.

# □ PREDNISONE (pred′ni-sone)

(Apo-Prednisone, Colisone, Cortan, Deltasone, Liquid Pred, Meticorten, Novoprednisone, Orasone, Panasol, Prednicen-M, SK-Prednisone, Sterapred, Winpred)

**Classification:** corticosteroid, glucocorticoid

## Available Preparations:
- 5 mg/5 ml oral syrup and solution
- 1, 2.5, 5, 10, 20, 25, 50-mg tablets
- 5-mg film-coated tablets

**Action and Use:** Natural or synthetic, intermediate-acting glucocorticoid that has strong antiinflammatory, immunosuppressant, and metabolic actions. Treats diseases such as collagen, dermatologic, allergy, acute leukemia, and respiratory distress syndrome.

## Routes and Dosage:
*PO:*
- 0.14 to 2 mg/kg/day or 40 to 60 mg/m$^2$/day in equally divided doses 4 times a day
- Nephrosis: 2 mg/kg/day 3 to 4 times per day until urine is protein free for 5 days or for 28-day course. (Maximum of 80 mg/day). For persistent proteinuria may increase to 4 mg/kg/dose every other day for additional 28 days. Maintenance: 2 mg/kg/dose every other day for 28 days and to discontinue taper over 4 to 6 weeks
- Asthma: Acute: 0.5 to 1 mg/kg/day for 3 to 5 days. (Maximum of 20 to 40 mg/day) Severe: 5 to 10 mg/day or 10 to 30 mg every other day, taper to aerosol corticosteroids

Note: Dosage determined by severity of condition and child's response.

**Absorption and Fate:** Absorbed rapidly and almost completely orally. Peak level: 1 to 2 hours. Half-life: 3.4 to 3.8 hours. Duration: 1.25 to 1.5 days. Metabolized by liver and excreted primarily by kidney.

**Contraindications and Precautions:** Pregnancy category C. Safety during lactation not established. Use caution in children; possible growth suppression. Contraindicated in hypersensitivity to drug or its components, sensitivity to corticosteroids, varicella, systemic fungal infections, acquired immune deficiency syndrome (AIDS), immunizations with live virus vaccines and oral polio virus vaccine, or contact with those who have had the vaccine. Use with caution in renal disease, hypertension, congestive heart failure, thromboembolic disorders, diabetes, metastatic cancer, ulcerative colitis, gastrointestinal ulceration, impaired hepatic function, systemic lupus erythematosus, osteoporosis, vaccinia, exanthema, Cushing's syndrome, seizures, myasthenia gravis, tuberculosis, ocular herpes simplex, hypoalbuminemia, emotional or psychotic tendencies.

**Side Effects:** Usually dependent on dosage and duration of treatment. *CNS:* euphoria, insomnia, pseudotumor cerebri, **psychotic behavior**. *CV:* edema, **hypertension, congestive heart failure**. *GI:* nausea, vomiting, increased appetite, gastrointestinal irritation, pancreatitis, peptic ulcer. *Skin:* impaired wound healing, thin fragile skin, petechia, ecchymosis, acne, facial erythema, increased sweating, may mask infections. *Hemic:* **thrombo-**

cytopenia. *Endocrine:* HPA-axis suppression, menstrual irregularities, Cushing's states, **secondary adrenocortical, pituitary unresponsiveness**. *Musculoskeletal:* **suppression of bone growth, osteoporosis**, muscle weakness. *Sensory:* Ophthalmic: **posterior subcapsular cataracts, increased intraocular pressure**. *Other:* **negative nitrogen balance**, sodium retention, **hypokalemia, hyperglycemia**, susceptibility to infections; Withdrawal symptoms: rebound inflammation, fatigue, weakness, arthralgia, fever, dizziness, lethargy, depression, fainting, orthostatic hypotension, dyspnea, anorexia, hypoglycemia, nausea and vomiting, shortness of breath, unusual weight loss.

## Nursing Implications:
*Assess:* Obtain baseline weight and height; before long-term therapy, obtain ECG, chest and spinal x-rays, glucose tolerance test, evaluation of HPA-axis function, and BP before therapy.

*Administer:* Dosage based on child's response to drug and severity of condition rather than strictly based on weight or body surface. *PO:* Take with food or milk to reduce GI irritation. Tablets can be crushed and mixed with small amount of food of fluid. Tablets are very bitter. If child is able to swallow capsules, they can be placed in a gelatin capsule and taken. Follow with fluids to cleanse child's palate. Best to give daily dosage before 9 AM. It suppress adrenal cortex activity less, which may reduce risk of HPA-axis suppression. Alternate-day therapy recommended to reduce growth retarding effects.

*Monitor:* Carefully assess child's response to drug; necessary for dosage adjustments. Observe for side effects, especially hypocalcemia, signs of adrenal insufficiency, symptoms of infections, or worsening of condition. Monitor BP and daily weights, report any sudden weight gain to the physician. With long-term usage, monitor serum electrolytes and height. Encourage well-balanced diet low in sodium and encourage good hygiene and dental care (possible oral fungal infections). Tonometry (eye) examinations every 6 weeks. Discontinuing of drug, dosage should be reduced gradually, especially after long-term usage so it does not cause acute life-threatening adrenal insufficiency. After discontinuation of short-term therapy (up to 5 days) with high dosage, adrenal recovery may occur within 1 week. After prolonged high-dose therapy, complete recovery of adrenal function may require up to 1 year.

*Patient Teaching:* Do not alter dosage or stop drug abruptly, it could cause very serious side effects, even death. Gradual tapering of dosage is necessary. Increasing amount of medication will not hasten healing process. Dosing schedule should be discussed and written down to increase compliance. Monitor signs and symptoms of medication, symptoms of adrenal insufficiency or worsening of condition, and report to physician. Obtain daily weights; report any sudden weight gain to physician. Stress importance of close medical supervision and follow-up. Regular ophthalmic examinations if on long-term therapy. Caution about receiving skin tests, vaccinations, or other immunizations, or coming in contact with persons receiving oral polio virus vaccine. Inform any health-care provider, including dentists, surgeons, or emergency care personal that child is on this medication. Child should carry a medical identification card. Observe for symptoms of infections. Do not use OTC medications without contacting health-care provider.

**Drug Interactions:** This drug in combination with high dosage of ace-taminophen may increase risk of hepatotoxicity. When used with asparaginase, may increase hyperglycemia. With analgesics and antiinflammatory drugs, it may increase the risk of gastric ulceration. Amphotericin B and potassium-depleting diuretics increase risk of hypokalemia. Use with anabolic steroids may increase the risk of edema and acne. Drug in combination with anticoagulants may decrease anticoagulant effect. This drug used with anticonvulsants (phenytoin) may lower seizure threshold. Use with vaccines, live virus, or other immunizations may potentiate replication of the vaccine virus, increasing chance of developing the viral disease.

**Laboratory Test Interferences:** May increase serum cholesterol, sodium and blood glucose. May decrease serum calcium, potassium, $T_4$ [131]I uptake, urine 17-hydroxysteroid and 17-ketosteroids. Tends to suppress skin tests; may give a false-negative result with nitroblue-tetrazolium for bacterial infection. Adrenal function assessed by ACTH stimulation or plasma cortisol may be decreased.

**Storage Requirements:** Store at 15 to 30°C (59 to 86°F). Protect from light and freezing.

---

## ☐ PRIMIDONE                                    (pri'mi-done)

(Mysoline)

**Classification:** anticonvulsant

### Available Preparations:
- 250 mg/5 ml suspension
- 50, 250-mg tablets

**Action and Use:** Related to the barbiturate-derived anticonvulsants such as phenobarbital. Metabolized into phenobarbital and other substances in the body. Used in partial seizures, particularly those with complex symptomatology (psychomotor seizures) as well as akinetic and tonic-clonic (grand mal) seizures.

### Routes and Dosages:
*PO:*
- under 8 years: 50 mg at h.s. for 3 days; 50 mg BID for the next 3 days; 100 mg BID for the next 3 days, and then maintenance dose of 125 to 250 mg TID or 10 to 25 mg/kg/day or 1.25 g/m²/day given in 3 doses/day
- 8 years and older: 100 to 125 mg at h.s. for 3 days; 100 to 125 mg BID for the next 3 days, 100 to 125 mg TID for the next 3 days, and then maintenance dose of 250 mg TID; may be increased slowly, not to exceed 2 g/day given in 3 doses.

**Absorption and Fate:** Well absorbed from GI tract. Metabolized by the liver into phenobarbital and other substances and excreted in the urine. Peak level is in 4 hours. Half-life of the drug is reported to range from 10 to 20 hours; however, the metabolites may have a longer half-life of 24 to 48 hours. Therapeutic level is 5 to 12 μg/ml.

**Contraindications and Precautions:** Pregnancy category D. Safe use in pregnancy and lactation is not established, therefore, its use is avoided if possible. The infant of a lactating mother on the drug is observed so that breast-feeding can be discontinued if infant's sedation is observed. Contraindicated in those with previous hypersensitivity to barbiturates and those with porphyria. Use with caution in children with attention-deficit disorder, respiratory, renal, hepatic disese.

**Side Effects:**
*CNS:* **drowsiness**, dizziness, headache; paradoxical excitement particularly in children with attention-deficit disorder; nystagmus and **ataxia** signal drug toxicity. *GI:* nausea, vomiting, anorexia. *Skin:* rash, alopecia. *Hemic:* **leukopenia, eosinophilia, megaloblastic anemia.**

**Nursing Implications:**
*Assess:* Obtain history of previous drug allergy.
*Administer:* Tablet can be crushed and administered with a small amount of food or fluid. Give with food if GI discomfort occurs. Do not withdraw drug quickly; doses should be tapered even when changing to a different anticonvulsant. Folic acid supplements can be given to treat the side effect of megaloblastic anemia.
*Monitor:* CBC, SMA-12, and serum levels are done at least every 6 months. Record seizure activity. Gather information about the child's behavior, activity level, and school performance.
*Patient Teaching:* Drug can alter mental alertness; therefore, avoid driving and adjust activities accordingly. Avoid alcohol and other CNS depressants. Report changes in behavior, school performance, and seizure activity. Wear an identification bracelet stating child has seizures and is on medication. Avoid OTC medications. Return for scheduled appointments with prescriber. Inform health-care provider of seizure activity before child receives DPT immunization.

**Drug Interactions:** Increased phenobarbital level if given with that drug. Isoniazid and phenytoin can increase primidone's levels. May decrease effects of adrenocorticosteroids, anticoagulants, antidepressants, carbamazepine, dacarbazine, quinidine, and others. Increases excretion of ascorbic acid. Increased metabolism of theophylline. Decreases absorption of vitamin $B_{12}$ and decreases level of vitamin D.

**Laboratory Test Interferences:** False-positive phentolamine test. Can decrease serum bilirubin.

**Storage Requirements:** Store in tightly closed containers at 15 to 30°C (59 to 86°F). Avoid freezing. Expiration date is 5 years from manufacturing date.

---

## ☐ PROCAINAMIDE (proe-kane-a′mide)

(Procan, Promine, Pronestyl, Rhythmin)

**Classification:** antiarrhythmic (class IA)

### Available Preparations:
- 250, 500, 750 mg, 1-g extended-release tablets
- 250, 375, 500-mg film-coated tablets
- 250, 375, 500-mg capsules
- 100, 500 mg/ml vials for parenteral use

**Action and Use:** Similar to quinidine in action. Depresses myocardial activity by suppressing excitability and automaticity, delaying conduction, and prolonging refractory period. Little effect on cardiac output. May not alter or may increase pulse rate slightly. Causes vasodilation, decreases peripheral resistance, and may decrease blood pressure. Used to treat arrhythmias such as atrial fibrillation, premature ventricular contractions, ventricular tachycardia, and paroxysmal atrial tachycardia. Useful to maintain normal sinus rhythm with digitalis toxicity and surgery.

### Routes and Dosages:
*PO:* 40 to 60 mg/kg/day or 1.5 g/m²/day in 4 to 6 doses; not to exceed 4 g/day
*IM:* 20 to 30 mg/kg/day in 4 doses; not to exceed 4 g/day
*IV:* 2 to 5 mg/kg, not to exceed 100 mg; dose repeated at 10 to 30-minute intervals, not to exceed 30 mg/kg/24 hours.
Or an IV dose of 3 to 6 mg/kg over 5 minutes and maintenance IV of 0.02 to 0.08 mg/kg/minute may be used.
Dosages established by clinicians not the manufacturer.

**Absorption and Fate:** Absorbed well from GI tract, although this can be affected by intestinal pH, presence of food, and other factors. Widely distributed in body tissues. Only 15 to 20% bound to plasma proteins. Peak action at the end of IV infusion, 15 to 60 minutes after IM, and 60 to 90 minutes after PO administration. Duration of activity 3 hours and 8 hours for extended-release form. Half-life: 2.5 to 4.5 hours and prolonged in renal dysfunction. Widely distributed in body tissues. Eliminated in both unchanged and metabolized forms in the urine. Therapeutic level is 4 to 8 µg/ml and should be measured 24 hours after initial dose.

**Contraindications and Precautions:** Pregnancy category C. Excreted in breast milk, therefore, should be avoided during lactation. Safety in children has not been established. Contraindicated in those hypersensitive to the drug, in those with AV block, atypical ventricular tachycardia. Pornestyl Filmlok tablets contain tartrazine (yellow dye #5) and should be avoided in those with allergy to that dye. Injectable form may contain sulfites and should not be used in those with sulfite allergy. Cautious use in hypotension, hepatic failure, electrolyte imbalance, asthma, severe digitalis toxicity, congestive heart failure, lupus erythematosus, ventricular tachycardia in coronary occlusion, bundle branch block.

## Side Effects:

**CNS:** dizziness, depression, **confusion, drowsiness.** **CV:** **severe hypotension, myocardial depression, conduction block, arrhythmia, tachycardia** with high serum level. **GI:** nausea, vomiting, diarrhea, bitter taste. **Skin:** lupus-like syndrome in those on chronic therapy; skin rash (rare), itching. **Hemic:** **agranulocytosis, thrombocytopenia.**

## Nursing Implications:

**Assess:** Baseline vital signs, EKG, CBC

**Administer: PO:** Extended-release tablets not generally used in children. Check apical and radial pulses before giving dose. Give 1 hour before or 2 hours after meal with glass of water. May be given with food if GI distress occurs. Tablet (except extended-release) may be crushed if necessary. **IV:** Dilute in 5% dextrose and administer no faster than 25 to 50 mg/minute or over a period of 15 minutes. Diluted solution is stable 24 hours at room temperature or 7 days if refrigerated. May be incompatible with many drugs. Solution may turn slightly yellow but should not be used if darker than light amber. Keep patient supine to avoid orthostatic hypotension.

**Monitor:** Monitor heart rate and BP during infusion. If irregular pulse, flushing of face, loss of consciousness, arrest occur, stop infusion and notify physician. If EKG indicates 50% widening of QRS, prolonged PR interval, or if blood pressure drops 15 mm Hg or more, infusion is stopped and physician notified. Measure I & O and electrolyte status. Monitor temperature frequently; fever may necessitate stopping drug. Take plasma procainamide levels 24 hours after dose with desired range of 4 to 8 $\mu$g/ml. Above 8 $\mu$g/ml can indicate toxicity. Monitor periodically patients on long-term therapy for CBC, agranulocytosis, bleeding, lupus-like syndrome, CV changes, respiratory difficulty, LE cell preparation, antinuclear antibody (ANA) titer, procainamide, and N-acetylprocainamide (NAPA) levels.

**Patient Teaching:** Take drugs at same times each day, on empty stomach if possible. Avoid driving or adjust hazardous activities accordingly if dizziness occurs. Make position changes slowly. Instruct patient or family in pulse taking before each dose. Keep record of pulses for prescriber. If sore mouth, fever, difficulty breathing, or fatigue occur, notify prescriber. Perform good oral hygiene. Take and record daily weight; report increasing weight and signs of edema. Instuct other physicians and dentists if on this medication and wear medic alert identification. Store tightly closed and away from light and moisture (not in bathroom).

**Drug Interactions:** Additive effects with other antiarrhythmics. Increased atropine-like side effects with antihistamines, antidyskinetics, antimuscarinics like atropine. Increased leukopenia and thrombocytopenia with bone marrow depressants. Increased hypotension with bretylium and cholinergics. Increased effects of neuromuscular blocking agents requires careful monitoring after surgery. Cimetidine may inhibit clearance of the drug and its metabolites, leading to procainamide toxicity.

**Laboratory Test Interferences:** Increased alkaline phosphatase, bilirubin, lactic dehydrogenase, SGOT, SGPT. Invalidates bentiromide test, edrophonium test. Can cause positive Coombs' test. Alters ANA titer, leukocyte count, and causes EKG changes such as widening of QRS and prolonging of PR and QT.

**Storage Requirements:** Store tablets between 15 and 30°C (59 and 86°F) in tightly closed containers away from moisture. Injection solution may be stored at 15 to 30°C (59 to 86°F). Refrigeration is acceptable and may deter yellowish coloring. Protect solution from light and avoid freezing.

---

## ☐ PROCARBAZINE                          (proe-kar'ba-zeen)

(Matulane)

**Classification:** antineoplastic, hydrazine derivative

**Available Preparations:**   50-mg capsules

**Action and Use:** Appears to have several actions that block inclusion of necessary substances into DNA and RNA. Damages DNA, inhibits protein synthesis, and inhibits mitosis. Cell-cycle specific for C phase of cell division. Acts as monoamine oxidase inhibitor. Used in treatment of late stage Hodgkin's disease and non-Hodgkin's lymphoma. Used experimentally in some solid tumors, such as brain tumors, although not approved by the FDA for this purpose.

### Routes and Dosages:
*PO:* 50 mg/m$^2$/day for 1 week; then 100 mg/m$^2$/day; maintenance dose: 50 mg/m$^2$/day
- Brain Tumors: 75 mg/m$^2$ (1 dose) q 4–6 wk
- Hodgkin's Disease: 100 mg/m$^2$/day for 14 days (MOPP therapy protocol)

**Absorption and Fate:** Well absorbed from GI tract. Distributed in body tissues especially in liver, kidneys, intestines, skin, and CNS. Metabolized by the liver and excreted mainly in urine. Peak level is 1 hour and half-life, 10 minutes.

**Contraindications and Precautions:** Pregnancy category D. Not to be used in pregnant or lactating women unless benefits outweigh risks. Contraindicated in those hypersensitive to the drug, in myelosuppression evidence by bone marrow aspiration, and in those with chicken pox or herpes zoster infection. Not to be given concurrently with sympathomimetics, local anesthetics, tricyclic antidepressants, foods with high tyramine content, or alcohol. Cautious use in hepatic or renal disease and infection.

### Side Effects:
*CNS:* paresthesia, headache, depression, dizziness, anxiety, drowsiness. Tremors, seizures, and coma are more common in children. Drug should be stopped if paresthesia, neuropathy, or confusion occur, although these are infrequent. *GI:* severe nausea and vomiting, diarrhea, constipation, abdominal pain, stomatitis, dry mouth; drug dosage may be altered if stomatitis or diarrhea occur. *Respiratory:* cough, pneumonitis. *GU:* potential suppression of spermatogenesis and testicle atrophy, urinary tract infections. *Skin:* rash, dermatitis. *Hemic:* marked **bone marrow suppression** with **leukopenia**, anemia, and **thrombocytopenia;** increased bleeding tendency. *Other:* gynecomastia in prepubertal and beginning puberty males, vision and speech disturbance.

### Nursing Implications:
*Assess:* CBC and bone marrow studies are done before instituting therapy. Hepatic and renal studies should be performed. Question history of prior radiation therapy or chemotherapy since this drug is generally held until at least 1 month after other therapy.
*Administer:* This drug has potentially severe toxic effects and should be given only under the supervision of a physician with training and experience in cancer chemotherapy. The drug's potential for toxic effects on health-care personnel as well as patients necessitates careful handling during preparation and administration. *PO:* Given once daily orally.
*Monitor:* Blood studies are done frequently including WBC, hemoglobin, hematocrit, differential, reticulocyte count, platelet count. Bone marrow study may be done 2 to 8 weeks after therapy begins. Dosage is altered if WBC count is 4000/mm³ or less and platelets are 100,000/mm³ or less, or bleeding occurs. Renal and hepatic studies including BUN, UA, serum transaminase, alkaline phosphatase, SGPT, SGOT, bilirubin, creatinine, LDH, uric acid are performed weekly. One month should pass after other chemotherapy or radiation before beginning procarbazine, unless the protocol for drug therapy varies such as with MOPP or ABVD when procarbazine is started 2 weeks after other drugs. Measure vital signs and I & O.
*Patient Teaching:* Avoid persons with infections such as colds, influenza, chicken pox. Report signs of infection such as fever, sore throat, malaise.

Report signs of bleeding such as bruising and hematuria. Avoid alcohol and cigarettes, and tyramine-containing foods such as cheese, bananas, yogurt, sour cream, chicken liver, pickled herring, meat tenderizer, canned figs, raisins, avocados, soy sauce, tea, coffee, wine, even for 2 weeks after last dose. The drug causes drowsiness in some, therefore, caution against driving or operating hazardous machinery if this occurs. Avoid OTC medications such as nose drops and cough medicines. Avoid sun exposure. Encourage nutritious diet and small feedings to minimize nausea. Increase fluid intake. Return for scheduled follow-up and laboratory work.

**Drug Interactions:** Increases depressant effects of alcohol and CNS depressants such as barbiturates, hypotensives, phenothiazines. With narcotic analgesics, can cause severe hypertension, excitation, hyperpyrexia, vascular collapse. Can lead to hypertensive crisis, hyperpyrexia, convulsions if given with tricyclic antidepressants, MAO inhibitors, tyramine-containing foods. If given with antihypertensives, hypotension can occur. May increase hypoglycemic effects of insulin and oral hypoglycemics. Suppresses immune response to immunizations. Live virus vaccines must not be given, nor oral polio vaccine to those in close contact with the patient on this drug due to the chance of infection with a virus; these vaccines are delayed at least 3 months after chemotherapy when the patient is in remission.

**Food Interactions:** Can lead to hypertensive crisis if given with tyramine-containing foods. The MAO inhibitor effects continue for 2 weeks after the last dose of the drug is given, therefore, food–drug interactions can occur during that time. See foods to avoid in Patient Teaching section.

**Storage Requirements:** Store in tightly covered and light-resistant containers. Keep at 15 to 30°C (59 to 86°F).

---

## □ PROMETHAZINE (proe-meth'a-zeen)

(Anergan 25, Pentazine, Phenazine, Phencen, Phenergan, Phenoject, Prorex, V-Gan)

**Combination Products:** Mepergan, Phenergan-D, Phenergan VC syrup, Promethazine HC1 VC Plain syrup, Prothazine

**Classification:** phenothiazine, antihistamine, antiemetic

## Available Preparations:
- 6.25 mg/5 ml, 25 mg/5 ml oral solution
- 12.5, 25, 50-mg tablets

- 25 mg/ml, 50 mg/ml ampules for parenteral use
- 12.5, 25, 50-mg rectal suppositories

Also available in capsules with meperidine, solution with phenylephrine, tablets with pseudoephedrine, and injection solution with meperidine.

**Action and Use:** This phenothiazine derivative is a sedative, acts as an antihistamine, antiemetic, anticholinergic, and has local anesthetic effects. Used as a preoperative medication for sedative and antiemetic effects, and in postoperative care in combination with analgesics. Used to manage motion sickness and allergy. Has been used experimentally in Rh-sensitized women after the 16th week of pregnancy to lessen effects of hemolytic disease of the newborn.

**Routes and Dosages:**
*PO:* Antihistamine: 0.125 mg/kg/dose q6h during day and 0.5 mg/kg at h.s. PRN
*IM:* Preoperative Medication: 12.5 to 25 mg or 0.5 to 1.1 mg/kg
*IM, PR:* Nausea and Vomiting: 0.25 to 0.5 mg/kg or 7.5 to 15 mg/m$^2$ 4 to 6 times/day

**Absorption and Fate:** Well absorbed from GI tract and parenteral injection. Distributed widely in body tissues and over 90% bound to plasma proteins. Metabolized in the liver and excreted by urine and feces. Onset of action: 3 to 5 minutes for IV route, 20 minutes for other routes; duration of action: 2 to 8 hours.

**Contraindications and Precautions:** Pregnancy category C. Contraindicated in neonates, acutely ill or dehydrated children, vomiting of unknown origin, Reye syndrome, hepatic disease, hypersensitivity to phenothiazines, narrow-angle glaucoma, bone marrow depression, coma. Preparations with sulfites are contraindicated in those with sulfite hypersensitivity. Cautious use in children with sleep apnea, those with family history of sudden infant death syndrome (SIDS), respiratory dysfunction, asthma, peptic ulcer.

**Side Effects:**
*CNS:* **dizziness, confusion,** fatigue, incoordination, insomnia, nervousness, seizures, akathisia, dystonia especially in acutely ill or dehydrated children.
*CV:* **tachycardia, bradycardia.** *GI:* anorexia, nausea, vomiting, constipation, dry mouth. *Respiratory:* **increased sleep apnea,** asthma, nasal stuffiness. *Hepatic:* jaundice. *Skin:* urticaria, dermatitis. *Hemic:* **leukopenia,** agranulocytosis, thrombocytopenic purpura. *Sensory:* photosensitivity, blurred vision.

**Nursing Implications:**
*Assess:* Establish baseline vital signs. Physical assessment to rule out acute illness and dehydration.
*Administer: PO:* Give with food or fluid to decrease gastric upset. Tablet may be crushed and mixed with food or fluid. *IM:* Inject slowly and deeply

into muscle mass. Massage site well. Patient should be supine during and after injection in case of hypotension. Raise side rails on bed after administration.
***Monitor:*** Frequent vital sign checks. Monitor toxic effects of antineoplastic drugs whose toxicity is manifested by nausea and vomiting, as these effects may be masked by the drug.
***Patient Teaching:*** Avoid driving and hazardous activities, i.e., children are not advised to ride bicycle. Good oral hygiene and nutritious food can decrease some side effects.

**Drug Interactions:** Additive or potentiation effects with other CNS depressants. This drug could potentially reverse the effect of epinephrine and lower blood pressure; norepinephrine or phenylephrine should be used instead.

**Laboratory Test Interferences:** False-positive pregnancy tests. May decrease response of intradermal allergy tests within 4 days of promethazine. Can interfere with ABO blood grouping.

**Storage Requirements:** Store in tightly covered, light-resistant containers with oral and parenteral preparations at 15 to 30°C (59 to 86°F); avoid freezing. Rectal suppositories should be kept refrigerated at 2 to 8°C (35 to 46°F). Expiration date is 2 to 5 years after manufacture.

---

# ☐ PROPANTHELINE BROMIDE                    (proe-pan'the-leen)

(Banlin, Norpanth, Noropropanthil, Pro-Banthine, Propanthel, Robantaline)

**Classification:** anticholinergic

**Available Preparations:**   7.5, 15 mg tablets

**Action and Use:** Drug with anticholinergic properties that reduces gastrointestinal motility and contraction of smooth muscles of the bladder, and decreases gastric, salivary, and pancreatin secretions. Used as an antispasmodic agent in bladder and ureteral control, as well as for a variety of gastrointestinal disorders (e.g., gastritis or hypermotility of the GI tract).

**Routes and Dosage:**
***PO:*** 1.5 mg/kg/day in 4 divided doses or 2.5 mg/kg every hour.

**Absorption and Fate:** Incompletely absorbed from PO route. Peak plasma level about 2 hours. Metabolized in upper small intestine and liver. Duration of action about 6 hours. Metabolites and a small amount of unchanged drug excreted in urine.

**Contraindications and Precautions:** Pregnancy category C and safety during lactation not established. Safety and efficacy has not been established in children. Contraindicated in hypersensitivity to drug, obstruction of bladder or GI tract, paralytic ileus, intestinal atony, unstable cardiac conditions in acute hemorrhage, toxic megacolon, and narrow-angle glaucoma. Use caution with autonomic neuropathy, hepatic or renal impairment, ulcerative colitis, hyperthyroidism, coronary heart disease, congestive heart failure, hypertension, cardiac arrhythmias, spastic paralysis, brain damage, hiatal hernia, or biliary tract disease.

## Side Effects:
*CNS:* dizziness, light-headedness, drowsiness, weakness, headache, insomnia, confusion, hyperexcitability. *CV:* palpitations, tachycardia. *GI:* dry mouth, constipation, nausea, vomiting, **paralytic ileus**, loss of taste. *GU:* urinary hesitancy, retention. *Skin:* urticaria, pruritus, decreased sweating. *Sensory:* EENT blurred vision, mydriasis, **increased intraocular pressure**. *Other:* fever, allergic reaction, **anaphylaxis**.

## Nursing Implications:
*Assess:* Obtain baseline vital signs.
*Administer: PO:* Give 30 minutes before meals and at bedtime. Tablet can be crushed, mixed with amounts of food or fluids. Drug is bitter tasting, therefore, follow with fluids to relieve bad taste.
*Monitor:* Use with caution in hot and humid climates because of potential of heat stroke caused by drug. Monitor vital signs and side effects. Early CNS symptoms may indicate overdosage. Sugarless gum or hard candy may relieve dry mouth symptoms.
*Patient Teaching:* Drug can cause blurred vision; adjust activities accordingly.

**Drug Interactions:** Do not give at same time of other drugs, it tends to delay absorption of these drugs. May increase digoxin levels when given with slow dissolving tablets of digoxin. Do not give with corticosteroids, causes increased intraocular pressure.

**Storage Requirements:** Store at 15 to 30°C (59 to 86°F); drug expires 2 years from date of manufacture.

---

## □ PROPARACAINE HYDROCHLORIDE
(proe-par'a-caine)

(Ak-Taine, Alcaine, Kainair, Ocu-Caine, Ophthaine, Ophthetic)

**Combination products:** proparacaine hydrochloride 0.5% with fluorescein sodium 0.25% (fluoracaine)

**Classification:** anesthetic, ophthalmic (local)

**Available Preparations:** 0.5% drops for ophthalmic administration

**Action and Use:** Short-acting, local anesthesia that inhibits initiation and transmission of nerve impulses in the neuronal membrane. Used to anesthetize the eye for tonometry or gonioscopy, for the removal of foreign bodies, sutures, or for diagnostic conjunctival scraping.

**Routes and Dosage:**
*Ophthalmic:* Instill 1 drop of a 0.5% solution 30 seconds before diagnostic test, procedure, or suture removal; may repeat every 5 to 10 minutes for 5 to 7 doses

**Absorption and Fate:** Absorbed rapidly after instillation. Onset of action: 13 to 20 seconds; duration: 15 minutes or longer; increases with repeated doses.

**Contraindications and Precautions:** Pregnancy category C. Contraindicated in hypersensitivity to this drug. Use with caution in ocular inflammation or infection, cardiac disease, or hyperthyroidism.

**Side Effects:**
*Skin:* rash, drying and cracking if drug contacts skin, especially the fingertips. *Sensory:* stinging, burning, conjunctival redness (may last several hours after application); immediate hypersensitivity reaction (rare): diffuse epithelial keratitis, **sloughing of necrotic epithelium, corneal filaments, iritis.** *Other:* (rare) systemic toxicity, blurred vision, dizziness, muscle twitching, convulsions, CNS stimulation or depression, increased sweating, weakness and irregular heartbeat.

**Nursing Implications:**
*Administer: Ophthalmic:* Do not use if solution is amber in color. Read medication label carefully. Ophthaine bottle is similar to hemoccult container. For instillation, see Part I. Wash hands after instillation to prevent localized skin reactions to drug.
*Monitor:* Observe for symptoms of hypersensitivity. Protect the child's eye from injury as the cornea is anesthetized and blink reflex is temporarily absent. Delay in corneal epithelial healing can occur with prolonged usage.
*Patient Teaching:* Instruct child not to rub eye because a corneal abrasion could occur. The blink reflex is temporarily eliminated.

**Laboratory Test Interferences:** This drug may inhibit the growth of certain organisms altering cultures taken for eye infections. Prevent by using new, previously unopened bottle before culture.

**Storage Requirements:** Store unopened containers at 15 to 30°C (59 to 86°F) in light-resistant containers; protect from freezing. Refrigerate open containers to prevent solution from amber discoloration.

# ☐ PROPOXYPHENE                              (pro-pox'i-feen)

(Darvon, Doraphen, Doxaphene, Profene, ProPox, Propoxycon)

**Combination Products**: Bexophene, Darvon Compound, Dolene, Genagesic, Wygesic. Also available in combination with aspirin, caffeine, acetaminophen.

**Classification**: narcotic agonist analgesic

## Available Preparations:
- 50 mg/5 ml oral suspension
- 100-mg film-coated tablets
- 32, 65-mg capsules

**Action and Use**: A synthetic narcotic related to methadone. It acts on the CNS by inducing neurotransmitters to produce analgesia. It has little antitussive action, unlike related drugs. Its metabolite has a local anesthetic effect. Used in treatment of mild to moderate pain; often used in combination with other analgesics such as aspirin and acetaminophen.

## Routes and Dosages:
*PO:* over 12 years: 65 mg q4h PRN

**Absorption and Fate**: Well absorbed and distributed to body tissues, including brain. Highly protein bound. Metabolized in the liver and eliminated in the urine. Onset of action is in 15 to 60 minutes; duration: 4 to 6 hours. Peak action is in 120 minutes and half-life is 6 to 12 hours for propoxyphene and 30 to 36 hours for the metabolite norpropoxyphene.

**Contraindications and Precautions**: Pregnancy category C; D for prolonged use. Not accepted for use in children; children over 12 years are sometimes given dose similar to adult dose. Contraindicated in those with hypersensitivity to the drug, those with respiratory depression, comatose, elevated CSF pressure. Cautious use in those with asthma, hepatic or renal dysfunction, seizures, atrial flutter, tachycardia, colitis, hypothyroidism.

## Side Effects:
*CNS:* **sedation**, dizziness, depression, **coma**, euphoria, restlessness, insomnia. *CV:* **circulatory depression**, **orthostatic hypotension**, palpitation, bradycardia, tachycardia. *GI:* anorexia, nausea, vomiting, constipation. ***Respiratory:*** **respiratory depression.** ***Hepatic:*** biliary spasm, increased serum amylase and lipase. *GU:* urinary retention, oliguria, stimulates release of vasopressin, impotence. *Skin:* rash, erythema, urticaria, pruritus, facial flushing indicates hypersensitivity reaction.

## Nursing Implications:
*Assess:* Assess type and degree of pain; use other pain control methods in addition to analgesic. Take baseline vital signs.

*Administer:* A schedule IV drug under the Federal Controlled Substances Act. Check time of last dose carefully before giving, as well as currency of order.

*Monitor:* Monitor vital signs every 30 to 60 minutes after administration. If hypotension occurs, or patients feel nausea or dizziness, have them lie down. Evaluate pain in 30 to 60 minutes and record results. Observe for constipation.

*Patient Teaching:* Take drug only as directed and only for patient prescribed. Drug can alter mental alertness, therefore avoid driving and adjust activities accordingly. Encourage adequate fluid intake, coughing, and deep breathing. Prolonged use can be habit forming.

**Drug Interactions:** Additive CNS effects with alcohol and other CNS depressants. Phenothiazines may antagonize action. Increased effects if given with dextroamphetamine. May increase effects of neuromuscular blocking agents. May decrease effects of diuretics in congestive heart failure.

**Laboratory Test Interferences:** Increases serum amylase and lipase; delay drawing blood for these tests for 24 hours after the drug. False-positive urine glucose. Decreased serum and urine 17-ketosteroids and 17-hydroxysteroids. Increased SGOT, SGPT, LDH, bilirubin, akaline phosphatase. Delayed gastric emptying. Increased CSF pressure.

**Storage Requirements:** Store tightly closed at 15 to 30°C (59 to 86°F).

---

□ **PROPRANOLOL**                                    (proe-pran'oh-lole)

(Inderal, Inderal LA, Ipran)

**Combination Products:** Inderide LA, Interide 40/25, 80/25

**Classification:** antihypertensive, β-adrenergic blocker, antiarrythmic (class II), antianginal

**Available Preparations:**
- 10, 20, 40, 60, 80, 90-mg tablets
- 60, 80, 120, 160-mg extended-release tablets
- 1 mg/ml ampule for parenteral use

Also available in extended-release capsules and tablets in combination with hydrochlorothiazide.

**Action and Use:** A $\beta_1$ and $\beta_2$-adrenergic blocking agent. Reduces sympathetic output in the myocardium, thereby prolonging AV nodal induction, reducing heart rate, depressing automaticity. Decreases myocardial oxygen consumption, enhances oxygen delivery to tissues, and enhances platelet aggregation. Used for treatment of cardiac arrhythmias, including those caused by digitalis toxicity, for hypertension, prevention of migraine headaches, management of angina, control of symptoms of pheochromocytoma, short-term treatment of thyrotoxicosis, and in essential tremors. Nonapproved uses include management of paroxysmal cyanosis of tetralogy of Fallot, anxiety states, other tremors.

## Routes and Dosages: PO, IV
*PO:*

- Hypertension: 0.5 to 1 mg/kg/day initially in 2 doses; increases as needed, generally to 1 to 5 mg/kg/day in 2 to 4 doses
- Maintenance: 2 to 4 mg/kg/day in 2 or more doses; not to exceed 16 mg/kg/day
- Tachyarrhythmias in Neonates with Thyrotoxicosis: 2 mg/kg/day; not approved by FDA

*IV:* 10 to 20 μg/kg/ over 10 minutes; not approved by FDA

## Absorption and Fate: Well absorbed from GI tract but with variable concentrations in plasma of different people. Highly bound to plasma proteins. Metabolized by liver and distributed widely in body tissues. Metabolites excreted mainly in urine. Appears in plasma 30 minutes after PO dose with peak level reached in 60 to 90 minutes. Peak level reached 1 minute after IV administration. Half-life in 3.5 to 6 hours after PO; 10 minutes initially after IV with 2.3 hours in terminal phase. Therapeutic level is 50 to 100 mg/ml.

## Contraindications and Precautions: Pregnancy category C. Safe use in children has not been established. Small amounts are present in breast milk, therefore, if a woman breastfeeds a baby while on the drug, the baby should be monitored for bradycardia. Contraindicated with sinus bradycardia, some types of heart block, severe congestive heart failure, history of bronchospasm or asthma, cardiogenic shock, malignant hypertension, Raynaud's syndrome. Cautious use with diabetes, renal or hepatic impairment, compensated congestive heart failure, sinus node dysfunction, thyrotoxicosis (may mask hyperthyroidism). Children with Down's syndrome may have increased bioavailability, therefore, a cautious approach and careful dose management is wise. When a patient on the drug has surgery there is a possibility of hypotension or bradycardia that is not responsive to usual measures.

## Side Effects:
*CNS:* dizziness, irritability, sleepiness, weakness, confusion. *CV:* **bradycardia, hypotension**, palpitations, **arrythmia**, syncope, shock, angina, **heart failure, heart block**, peripheral arterial insufficiency; sudden withdrawal may exacerbate angina or contribute to **myocardial infarction. GI:** nausea, vomiting, diarrhea, cramping. ***Respiratory:* dyspnea, bronchospasm. *Hepatic:*** elevated BUN. *Skin:* skin and nail changes. ***Endocrine:*** may mask symptoms of hypoglycemia; causes hyperglycemia by blocking insulin release from pancreas. ***Sensory:*** disturbed vision or hearing with chronic use; effect reversed with drug withdrawal. ***Other:* Allergic response**

## Nursing Implications:

***Assess:*** Take baseline blood pressure and pulse before giving dose.

***Administer: PO:*** Take apical pulse before giving drug; report significant variations before giving drug. Give either with or between meals, following the same pattern so absorption remains the same. Drug should be discontinued 48 hours before surgery; discontinued by gradual tapering over 1 to 2 weeks. ***IV:*** Give over 10 minutes while monitoring CVP, EKG, BP, pulse. Compatible with normal saline.

***Monitor:*** Monitor CVP, EKG, BP during IV infusion. The drug promotes sodium retention, therefore, weight and BP monitoring are needed. Pulse, I & O, and observations for symptoms of heart failure are performed. Monitor patients with renal or hepatic dysfunction carefully for side effects or toxic effects. Diabetics require close monitoring due to effect of drug on blocking insulin release and masking hypoglycemia.

***Patient Teaching:*** Take before meals if possible. If taken with meals to decrease GI irritation, take consistently with meals to promote uniform absorption. (When given with meals, the total amount will be absorbed over a longer period of time.) Check pulse as directed; notify physician before giving if under indicated amount. Sodium restriction may be recommended. Avoid prolonged exposure of extremities to cold temperature. Do not take OTC medications unless instructed by physician.

**Drug Interactions:** Additive cardiac depressant effects with other antiarrhythmics and digitalis. Increased cardiac depressant effect with IV phenytoin, digitalis. Hypoglycemia can occur if insulin is given. Barbiturates enhance metabolism of propranolol. Increased hypotensive effect when given with phenothiazines, diuretics, or other antihypertensives. Decreased hypotensive effect when given with nonsteroidal antiinflammtories, estrogen. Cimetidine can reduce clearance and cause increased β-adrenergic blockade. Antagonizes effects of sympathomimetics; marked with isoproterenol; epinephrine is used cautiously with propranolol due to resultant bradycardia. Atropine may decrease bradycardic effect. Increased risk of bradycardia and hypotension with anesthetics. Hypertension may occur if given with MAO inhibitor that is then discontinued; these drugs should not be given together. Decreased reflex tachycardia and decreased blood pressure may occur if given with nitroglycerin; increased serum concentration of both drugs occurs if given with phenothiazines. Inhibits effects of xanthines. May decrease theophylline clearance.

**Laboratory Test Interferences:** Increased BUN in those with heart disease. Increased creatinine, aminotransferase, alkaline phosphatase, lactic dehydrogenase. False elevation of urinary catecholamine. Increased antinuclear antibody titers. Increased lipoproteins, potassium, triglyceride, uric acid, LDH.

**Storage Requirements:** Store at 15 to 30°C (59 to 86°F) in tightly closed, light-resistant containers.

# ☐ **PROTAMINE** (proe'ta-meen)

(Protamine)

**Classification:** heparin antidote

## Available Preparations:
- 50, 250-mg vials for parenteral use
- 10 mg/ml vial for IV use

**Action and Use:** A protein prepared from fish sperm or testes that combines with heparin to form a stable salt. Protamine is a weak anticoagulant but is not used for this purpose; the combination of heparin–protamine does not act as an anticoagulant. Protamine is used in treatment of heparin overdose.

## Routes and Dosages:
**IV:** Dosage determined by coagulation studies, dose of heparin, type of heparin, and time since heparin injection. Generally 1 mg protamine is given for every 90 units of beef-derived heparin, or 100 units of pork-derived heparin calcium, or 115 units of pork-derived heparin sodium. In consideration of time dose of protamine is:
- 1 to 1.5 mg for 100 units of heparin in last few minutes
- 0.5 to 0.75 mg for 100 units of heparin 30 to 60 minutes before
- 0.25 to 0.375 mg for 100 units of heparin 2 hours or more before;

Or, following IV infusion of heparin, 25 to 50 mg protamine may be given.

After SC injection of heparin, 25 to 50 mg protamine may be used as a loading dose with continuous IV infusion to follow with remainder of dose over 8 to 16 hours.

Dose of protamine not to exceed 50 mg in 10 minutes.

**Absorption and Fate:** Onset of action: 30 seconds to 1 minute, neutralization of heparin within 5 minutes, and duration of action 2 hours.

**Contraindications and Precautions:** Pregnancy category C. Unknown if drug is present in breast milk, therefore, lactation is not recommended during its use. Safety in children has not been established, although it is used in this age group. Contraindicated in those hypersensitive to the drug. Cautious use in those who most commonly demonstrate hypersensitivity (those with fish allergy, previous protamine or protamine-containing insulin injection, and men who are infertile or who have had a vasectomy).

## Side Effects:
**CV:** hypotension, bradycardia, flushing. **GI:** nausea, vomiting. **Respiratory:** pulmonary hypertension, dyspnea. **Hemic:** heparin rebound with bleeding 8 to 9 hours and up to 18 hours after protamine dose. **Other:** hypersensitivity with angioedema, urticaria, anaphylaxis; feeling of warmth, back pain, weakness

## Nursing Implications:

*Assess:* Blood coagulation studies such as ACT, APTT, TT are performed. Previous hypersensitivity to the drug, as well as history of prevous protamine or protamine-containing insulin, fish allergy, or men with vasectomies or infertility. Baseline vital signs especially blood pressure are taken. Patient blood volume should be adequate; hydration may be needed.

*Administer:* Be prepared to treat shock. *IV:* Add 5 ml of bacteriostatic water with benzyl alcohol or sterile water to 50-mg vial and shake or use prepared injection solution; both solutions will contain 10 mg/ml. Do not use bacteriostatic water with benzyl alcohol preservative for injection into newborns. Administer drug by slow IV injection over 1 to 3 minutes. Dose not to exceed 50 mg in 10 minutes. Incompatible with antiinfectives such as penicillins and cephalosporins; use in IV with other additives discouraged. Solution reconstituted with sterile water should be used immediately. If reconstituted with bacteriostatic water with benzyl alcohol solution is stable at room temperature for 72 hours.

*Monitor:* Coagulation studies are done 5 to 15 minutes after drug is given and repeated in 2 to 8 hours (ACT, APTT, TT). Monitor blood pressure every 15 minutes for 2 to 3 hours.

## Storage Requirements: Store powder at 15 to 30°C (59 to 86°F). Store injection solution at 2 to 8°C (35 to 46°F). Avoid freezing.

---

## □ PYRIDOXINE

(Beesix, Hexa-Betalin, Pyroxine, Rodex, TexSix T.R., Vitamin B-6)

## Classification: nutritional supplement

## Available Preparations:
- 10, 25, 50, 100, 200, 250, 500-mg tablets
- 500-mg extended-release tablets
- 25, 50, 100, 500-mg capsules
- 100, 150-mg extended-release capsules
- 100 mg/ml vials for parenteral use

## Action and Use: This water-soluble B vitamin is used as a coenzyme in protein, fat, and carbohydrate metabolism. It assists in converting tryptophan to niacin and helps to synthesize heme and some regulatory compounds in the CNS. Deficiency is manifested by CNS changes such as seizures, especially in children; by skin changes and irritation, and by sideroblastic anemia. Used in treatment of dietary deficiency and in familial pyridoxine deficiency. The latter may be manifested as seizures in infancy. Used in treatment of isoniazid, hydralazine, and cycloserine toxicity when it decreases incidence of seizures. Unapproved uses include treatment of acne and other skin conditions, nausea

and vomiting of pregnancy, psychosis and depression, asthma, absence seizures, and other numerous conditions.

## Routes and Dosages: PO, IM, SQ, IV
*PO:*
- Nutritional Supplement: 2 to 10 mg/day for 3 weeks, then 2 to 5 mg/day
- Pyridoxine Deficiency Syndrome: infants: 2 to 10 mg/day; children: 30 to 50 mg/day

*IM, IV:* Seizures in Pyridoxine-Deficient Infant: 10 to 100 mg

## Absorption and Fate: Well absorbed from GI tract. Stored in liver, muscle, and brain. Crosses placenta and present in high amounts in fetus. Present in breast milk. Although pyridoxine in not bound to plasma proteins, its metabolite pyridoxal phosphate is highly bound. Metabolized in the liver and excreted in urine. Half-life is 15 to 20 days and usual serum level is 30 to 80 ng/ml.

## Contraindications and Precautions: Pregnancy category C. Large doses in pregnancy may lead to pyridoxine deficiency and resultant seizures in newborns. Contraindicated in its IV form during heart disease and not given to those with prior hypersensitivity to the vitamin.

## Side Effects:
*CNS:* headache, somnolence, paresthesia, sensory neuropathy with numbness and clumsiness; symptoms seen with chronic overdose. *GI:* nausea. *Skin:* burning at injection site. *Other:* rare hypersensitivity

## Nursing Implications:
*Assess:* Obtain diet history.
RDAs for pyridoxine are:
- 0 to 6 months: 0.3 mg
- 6 to 12 months: 0.6 mg
- 1 to 3 years: 0.9 mg
- 4 to 6 years: 1.3 mg
- 7 to 10 years: 1.6 mg
- 11 to 14 years: 1.8 mg
- 15 to 18 years: 2.0 mg
- pregnancy: 2.6 mg
- lactation: 2.5 mg

*Administer:* Drug is usually given PO. IM and IV forms used in newborn seizure treatment.
*Monitor:* Monitor seizure activity if used as treatment for newborn seizures. Seizure usually is interrupted within 2 to 3 minutes after drug is given. Be alert for neurological side effects in thsoe on chronic overdose. There is no proven benefit for megatherapy.
*Patient Teaching:* Nutritional counseling may be needed. Dietary sources for

pyridoxine include meats, whole grains, corn, banana, potato, green leafy vegetables, green beans. Discourage use of megadoses.

**Drug Interactions:** Chloramphenicol, hydralazine, immunosuppressants, isoniazid, and oral contraceptives are among the drugs that can increase pyridoxine requirements. Decreases effect of levodopa in parkinsonism.

**Laboratory Test Interferences:** False-positive urobilinogen with Ehrlich's test. Increased SGOT and decreased folic acid.

**Storage Requirements:** Store at 15 to 30°C (59 to 86°F) in tightly closed containers. Protect solution from freezing and excessive heat.

---

□ **PYRIMETHAMINE**                                (peer-i-meth′a-meen)

(Daraprim)

**Combination Products:** 25 mg Pyrimethamine with 500 mg sulfadoxine (Fansidar)

**Classification:** antimalarial

**Available Preparations:** 25 mg tablets

**Action and Use:** Folic acid antagonist whose action blocks conversion of dihydrofolic acid to functional form of tetrahydrofolic acid. Because folate is depleted, the protozoa is unable to synthesize nucleic acid. This drug interferes with action in synthesis just prior to point of sulfonamides; use with sulfonamides causes a synergistic effect. Principally active against asexual erythrocytic forms of malarial plasmodia; arrests sporogony in mosquitoes but does not destroy gametocytes. Used for treatment and prophylaxis of malaria; in combination with sulfonamides in treatment of resistant form of *Plasmodium falciparum* and this combination treatment is also used for toxoplasmosis.

**Routes and Dosage:** *PO:*
- Suppression or chemoprophylaxis malaria: over 10 years: 0.5 mg/kg/week (maximum dose, 25 mg/week); 4 to 10 years: 12.5 mg/week; under 4 years: 6.25 mg/week
- Suppression or chemoprophylaxis of *P. falciparum* malaria: 0.25 mg/kg once per week with dapsone 2 mg/kg once per week
- Treatment of Chloroquine-resistant *P. falciparum* malaria (in combination with quinine sulfate and sulfadoxine): less than 10 kg: 6.25 mg/day for 3 days; 10 to 20 kg: 12.5 mg/day for 3 days; 20 to 40 kg/day: 12.5 mg/day for 3 days; adults: 25 mg/day for 3 days
- Toxoplasmosis (with trisulfapyrimidine or sulfadiazine): Initial, 1 mg/kg/day in 2 equally divided dose for 2 to 4 days, then 0.5 mg/kg/day once

or in 2 equally divided doses for 4 weeks; or clinicians recommend 2 mg/kg/day for 3 days then 1 mg/kg/day for 4 weeks
■ Pyrimethamine and Sulfadoxine suppression or chemoprophylaxis of malaria: 2 to 11 months: ⅛ tablet every week; 1 to 3 years: ¼ tablet every week; 4 to 8 years: ½ tablet every week; 9 to 14 years: ¾ tablets every week; over 14 years: 1 tablet every week

**Absorption and Fate:** Well absorbed from GI tract. Peak level in 2 hours. Distributed mainly to spleen liver, kidneys, lungs; 80% bound to plasma proteins. Half-life 54 to 148 hours. Excreted primarily in urine.

**Contraindications and Precautions:** Pregnancy category C. Use with caution during lactation. Pyrimethamine and sulfadoxine is contraindicated in nursing mothers and in those under 2 years. Contraindicated in hypersensitivity to drug, megaloblastic anemia caused by folate deficiency, chloroguanide-resistant malaria. Use with caution in seizure disorders, G-6-PD deficiency. Pyrimethamine and sulfadoxine, use caution with impaired renal and hepatic function, severe allergies, or bronchial asthma.

**Side Effects:**
**CNS:** malaise, fatigue, irritability; high dosage: ataxia, tremors, **seizures**, **respiratory failure**. **GI:** anorexia, nausea, vomiting, atrophic glossitis or gastritis. **Hemic:** **agranulocytosis**, **aplastic anemia**, **megaloblastic anemia**, leukopenia, **thrombocytopenia**, **pancytopenia**. **Other:** Hypersensitivity: (pyrimethamine and sulfadoxine): serum sickness, urticaria, pruritus, photosensitivity, exfoliative dermatitis, **erythema multiforme**, **Stevens-Johnson syndrome**, **toxic epidermal necrolysis**.

**Nursing Implications:**
**Assess:** History of travel or exposure. Obtain blood studies to identify organism.
**Administer:** PO: For prophylaxis give drug on same day of each week. Centers for Disease Control (CDC) recommends that treatment should start 1 to 2 weeks before travel to endemic area and continue for 6 weeks after leaving area. Take with meals to decrease gastric distress. Tablet or capsule can be crushed or capsule taken apart and mixed with small amount of food or fluid. A suspension can be made from crushed tablets by your pharmacist, shake well before usage. If sucrose solution is used as vehicle for tablets, store at room temperature and discard in 5 to 7 days.
**Monitor:** Observe for side effects and monitor closely. Side effects from pyrimethamine and sulfadoxine have been fatal, causing severe hypersensitivity reactions and hepatic effects; therefore, it is recommended that this drug only be used when risk of chloroquine-resistant *P. falciparum* is substantial. Obtain CBC, platelet counts twice weekly during therapy. Leucovorin may be given if folic acid-deficiency occurs. Periodic blood samples should be obtained to check on progress of disease. Dosage for toxoplasmosis is near toxic levels.
**Patient Teaching:** Importance of taking drug only as directed and not missing doses. Observe for any signs and symptoms of side effects and contact

physician immediately if they occur. Take precautions for mosquito control while in infested areas. Fatalities have occurred with accidental ingestion.

**Drug Interactions:** Use with *p*-aminobenzoic acid (PABA) interferes with action of this drug.

**Storage Requirements:** Store at 15 to 30°C (59 to 86°F) in tight, light-resistant containers. Drug darkens on exposure to light.

---

## □ QUINACRINE HYDROCHLORIDE

(kwin′a-kreen)

(Atabrine)

**Classification:** anthelmintic

**Available Preparations:** 100 mg tablet

**Action and Use:** Mechanism of action is unknown against *Giardia lamblia*. Action against cestodes appears to occur by causing scolex to be dislodged from intestine. Used for *Dipylidium caninum* (dog and cat tapeworm), *Diphyllobothrium latum* (fish tapeworm), *Hymenolepis diminuta* (rat tapeworm), *Hymenolepsis nana* (dwarf tapeworm), *Taenia saginata* (beef tapeworm), and *Taenia solium* (pork tapeworm) infestations. Also used to treat malaria caused by *Plasmodium malariae*, *P. vivax*, and *P. faiciparum*.

**Routes and Dosage:** *PO:*
- Giardiasis: 2 mg/kg 3 times per day for 5 to 7 days. (Maximum dosage 300 mg/day)
- Cestodiasis: 15 mg/kg/day in 2 divided doses 1 hour apart
- Malaria (acute attack): 1 to 4 years: 100 mg 3 times on day one, then 100 mg daily for 6 days; 4 to 8 years: 200 mg 3 times on day one, then 100 mg twice daily for 6 days; over 8 years: 200 mg every 6 hours for 5 doses, then 100 mg 3 times/6 days
- Suppression of Malaria: under 8 years: 50 mg/day
- over 8 years: 100 mg/day (therapy usually continues for 1 to 3 months)

**Absorption and Fate:** Readily absorbed from GI tract. Peak plasma level in 8 hours. Widely distributed to body tissues. Metabolic fate unknown. Excreted primarily in urine.

**Contraindications and Precautions:** Pregnancy category C. Use with caution in those under 1 year. Contraindicated in hypersensitivity to drug, psoriasis, porphyria, and those receiving primaquine. Use with caution in severe cardiac, renal, or hepatic disease, history of psychosis, alcoholism deficiency.

## Side Effects:

*CNS:* severe headache, drowsiness, dizziness, weakness, transient toxic psychosis of 2 to 4 weeks; long-term therapy: nightmares, restlessness, **confusion**, irritability, aggressive behavior, **seizures**. *GI:* nausea, vomiting, abdominal pain, anorexia, diarrhea. *Hepatic:* hepatitis. *Skin:* pleomorphic skin eruptions, blue and black skin and nail pigmentation, contact dermatitis, **exfoliative dermatitis**. *Hemic:* **blood dyscrasias**, **aplastic anemias**. *Sensory:* Long-term therapy: visual halos, blurred visions, focusing difficulty. *Other:* rare: alopecia, rash, pruritus, flushing, hiccups, cough, hypotension, increased liver function tests.

## Nursing Implications:

*Assess:* Intestinal disease: Diagnosed through stool culture; follow your agency procedure for collection. Malaria diagnosed through blood smears. Obtain baseline CBC and ophthalmologic examinations if on long-term therapy.

*Administer:* Tablet can be crushed and mixed with small amount of food or fluid. Tablet extremely bitter. If child is unable to tolerate taste of tablet and is able to swallow capsule, contents of tablet can be placed in gelatin capsule. Have child suck on ice or flavored ice treat before taking drug. Follow with fluids of child's choice to remove taste from mouth. Giving sodium bicarbonate with each dose will reduce nausea and vomiting. If given for cestodes, a bland, nonfat, liquid or semisolid diet is recommended for 24 to 48 hours before medication dosage. A saline enema is usually given the night before medication dosage.

*Monitor and Patient Teaching:* Inform family that the drug may cause yellow pigmentation to skin, blue-black discoloration to nails, ears, or nose, and acid urine will turn yellow. This dissipates in 2 weeks after last drug dosage. For long-term therapy, periodic CBC and ophthalmologic examinations should be obtained. Inform physician if sensory symptoms or CNS signs occur. Do not ingest alcohol while on this drug. Cestodiasis: 2 hours after last dose of drug, follow with saline enema. Do not discard stool without inspection for scolex, which will be stained yellow from quinacrine. Do not put toilet paper in with fecal matter. Passage of worm usually occurs in 4 to 12 hours. If scolex is not found, and stool is ova-free in 3 to 6 months of therapy, considered cured. Reinfestations prevented through good personal hygiene, hand washing, prevention of hand to mouth contamination, sanitary waste disposal, and proper cooking of pork, fish, and beef. Giardiasis: Three negative stool specimens on alternate days usually indicated cure of disease. Infestation is usually caused by fecal-contaminated water. Prevention aided by proper food and water hygiene. Malaria: Therapy is usually for 1 to 3 months.

## Drug Interactions:

Alcohol and this drug may produce disulfiram-like reaction. Primaquine toxicity increased when used with this drug.

## Laboratory Test Interferences:

May increase urine and serum cortisol levels. Mattingly method for 11-hydroxycorticosteroid concentrations may be elevated.

**Storage Requirements:** Store at 15 to 30°C (50 to 86°F) in tight container.

---

☐ **QUINIDINE**                                               (kwin'i-deen)
**GLUCONATE**

(Duraquin, Quinate, Quinaglute Dura-tabs, Quinalan)

☐ **QUINIDINE**
**POLYGALACTURONATE**

(Cardioquin)

☐ **QUINIDINE SULFATE**

(Apo-Quinidine, Cin-Quin, Novoquinidin, Quindex Extentabs, Quinora)

**Classification:** antiarrhythmic (class IA)

**Available Preparations:**
- 100, 200, 300-mg sulfate tablets
- 275-mg polygalacturonate tablets
- 30-mg extended-release sulfate tablets
- 324, 330-mg extended-release gluconate tablets
- 80 mg/ml gluconate vial for parenteral use
- 200 mg/ml sulfate vial for parenteral use

**Action and Use:** Acts as a cardiac depressant, prolonging conduction intervals and refractory period, reduces excitability and automaticity. Likely inhibits potassium movement across cell membranes. Reduces vagal tone. May produce peripheral vasodilation. Used in treatment of cardiac arrhythmias such as atrial fibrillation, atrial flutter, premature systoles, paroxysmal supraventricular and ventricular tachycardia.

**Routes and Dosages:**
*PO:* Quinidine Polygalacturonate: 30 mg/kg/day or 900 mg/m$^2$/day in 5 doses
*IM, IV:* Quinidine Gluconate: 30 mg/kg/day or 900 mg/m$^2$/day in 5 doses
Doses are established by clinicians rather than manufacturers. Doses of other forms of quinidine have not been established for children. The preparations of sulfate, gluconate, and polygalacturonate are *not* equivalent. Approximately 200 mg of sulfate, 267 mg of gluconate, and 275 mg of polygalacturonate are equivalent.

**Absorption and Fate:** PO form well absorbed. Widely distributed in body tissues and 70 to 80% is protein bound. Metabolized by the liver and excreted in urine. Rate of excretion increases with a urinary pH of 6 or less; decreases in alkaline urine. Peak level at end of IV infusion, at 1 hour after IM, and 1 to 1.5 hours after PO sulfate form and 3 to 4 hours after PO gluconate form. Duration of action: 6 to 8 hours after regular tablets or capsules and 12 hours after extended-release tablets. Half-life averages 6 hours but may range from 3 to 16 hours with great individual variation. Therapeutic level: 3 to 6 µg/ml with levels taken 24 hours after therapy begins; 8 µg/ml is toxic level.

## Contraindications and Precautions: Pregnancy category C for sulfate and gluconate, X for polygalacturonate. Drug present in breast milk, therefore, not recommended during lactation. Safety in children has not been established. Contraindicated in hypersensitivity to the drug, those with complete AV block, digitalis toxicity with AV conduction problems, intraventricular conduction defects. Cautious use in heart block, asthma, electrolyte imbalance especially hypokalemia, congestive heart failure, hypotension, digitalis toxicity, infection and fever, renal dysfunction, hepatic dysfunction, hyperthyroidism, psoriasis.

## Side Effects:
*CNS:* headache, fever, tremors, hearing disturbance, seizures, dizziness, fainting, confusion. *CV:* **severe hypotension**, paradoxical tachycardia, **heart block**, arrhythmia, congestive heart failure, widened QRS. *GI:* nausea, vomiting, diarrhea, cramping, bitter taste. *Hepatic:* hepatitis, jaundice, elevated SGOT, alkaline phosphatase. *Skin:* rash, urticaria, pruritus, psoriasis. *Sensory:* disturbed vision, ringing of ears, loss of hearing. *Hemic:* thrombocytopenia, anemia, leukopenia, bleeding. *Endocrine:* decreased blood glucose. *Other:* systemic lupus erythematosus-like syndrome, hypersensitivity with sensory disturbance, hemic changes, skin reactions, **anaphylaxis**

## Nursing Implications:
*Assess:* Quinidine gluconate, polygalacturonate, and sulfate are administered PO; the gluconate preparation is also given IM and IV. Check order carefully as doses of each preparation are not equivalent. Do not confuse this drug with quinine sulfate. Obtain baseline vital signs, EKG, CBC.

*Administer: PO:* Give between meals unless GI upset occurs; then administer with small amount of food. *IM:* Painful and erratic absorption. *IV:* Dilute in 5% dextrose and administer slowly over 5 to 10 minutes while monitoring blood pressure and EKG. Give while supine. Solution stable 24 hours at room temperature. Incompatible with several drugs, should be given alone.

*Monitor:* Monitor BP and EKG constantly during infusion. Report QRS widening of 25%; 50% widening indicates toxicity and dose should be stopped. If on continued therapy, monitor CBC, hepatic function tests, renal function tests, I & O, daily weight, serum potassium, serum quinidine. Be alert for signs of hypersensitivity such as sensory changes, hemic changes, and anaphylaxis. A test dose may be given before therapy begins.

*Patient Teaching:* Take at same time each day. Take weight daily and report increases as well as edema. Avoid caffeine, smoking, excess citrus juices, OTC medications. Wear medic alert identification. Be alert for and report signs of bleeding. Encourage good oral hygiene.

**Drug Interactions:** Additive cardiac depressant effects with other antiarrhythmics. Increased digitalis levels with digoxin. Additive hypoprothrombinemia with coumarin. Increased atropine-like effects with antimuscarinics. Potentiation of hypotension with antihypertensives. Cimetidine prolongs clearance and increases quinidine levels. Increased effects of neuromuscular blocking agents require close monitoring after surgery. Increased quinidine effects with potassium. Anticonvulsants increase rate of metabolism.

**Food Interactions:** Urinary alkalizers increase toxic effects of quinidine; examples include antacids, large amounts of vegetables, milk or citrus juice, carbonic anhydrase inhibitors.

**Storage Requirements:** Store tightly covered between 15 and 30°C (59 and 86°F). Protect from light and freezing. Do not use discolored injection solution.

---

## □ QUININE SULFATE                                    (kwye'nine)

(Legatrin, Novoquine, Quin-260, Quinamm, Quinine, Quinite, Quintrol, Q-Vel, Strema)

**Combination Products:** Quinine sulfate with vitamin E (M-KYA, Q-vel)

**Classification:** antimalarial

**Available Preparations:**
- 260, 325-mg tablets
- 130, 200, 300, 325-mg capsules

**Action and Use:** Exact mechanism of action unknown but appears to interfere with parasite's ability to bind and alter plasmodial DNA. Also exerts a curare-like effect on musculature and reduces the tetanic stimulation response of skeletal muscles. Used to treat chloroquine-resistant malaria from *Plasmodium falciparum*. Over 12 years, used to treat nocturnal recumbency leg cramps.

**Routes and Dosage:**

*PO:*
- Uncomplicated Chloroquine-Resistant *P. falciparum* Malaria: 25 mg/kg/day in equally divided doses 3 times a day for 3 days. (Maximum 650 mg/dose)
- Nocturnal Recumbency Leg Cramps: over 12 years: 200–300 mg at hs

**Absorption and Fate:** Almost completely absorbed from GI tract. Peak level: 1 to 3 hours. Widely distributed to body tissues; 70% bound to plasma proteins. Half-life: 11 to 12 hours. Excreted in urine (increased when urine acidic) and feces.

**Contraindications and Precautions**: Pregnancy category X. Use with caution during lactation. Contraindicated in hypersensitivity to drug, G-6-PD deficiency, tinnitus, optic neuritis, history of black water fever. Use with caution in those with atrial fibrillation.

**Side Effects:**
*CNS:* **cinchonism syndrome:** tinnitus, headache, nausea, slight visual disturbances; (severe) deafness, confusion, apprehension, restlessness, vertigo. *CV:* **ventricular tachycardia,** anginal symptoms. *GI:* nausea, vomiting, epigastric pain. *Hemic:* **thrombocytopenic purpura,** hypoprothrombinemia, **agranulocytosis** (rare). *Endocrine:* hypoglycemia. *Sensory:* blurred vision, scotomata, photophobia, diplopia, constricted visual fields, night blindness, **optic atrophy** (rare). *Other:* Hypersensitivity: flushing, intense, generalized pruritus, fever, urticarial or papular rash, facial edema, hemoglobinuria, **asthma** (rare)

**Nursing Implications:**
*Assess:* History of travel or exposure. Obtain blood studies to identify organism.
*Administer:* PO: Take with meals to decrease gastric distress. Tablet should be swallowed whole, it has an extremely bitter taste and is irritating to gastric mucosa. If tablet or capsule is to be given to young child, crush or take capsule apart; mix with small amount of food or fluid. Give child ice to suck on or frozen-flavored ice treat before medication. Follow with fluid of choice and oral hygiene to rid mouth of unpleasant taste. Parenteral form of quinine sulfate is available from U.S. Centers for Disease Control. Consult your pharmacist for information on administration.
*Monitor:* Observe for cinchonism syndrome and monitor closely. Plasma levels of drug should not reach above 10 μg/ml or severe symptoms of cinchonism may occur. Blood studies for organisms may need to be done every 8 hours to chart progress of disease.
*Patient Teaching:* Observe for any symptoms of cinchonism and report to health care provider.

**Drug Interactions:** Causes increased plasma level of digoxin and digitoxin when taken with this drug. Antacids containing aluminum may decrease absorption of this drug. Cimetidine increases half-life of quinine. This drug when used with neuromuscular blocking agents may cause respiratory depression. Quinine increases the hypoprothrombinemic effect of warfarin and other anticoagulants. Sodium bicarbonate, acetazolamide, and other drugs that increase urinary pH are given with this drug; it can cause quinine toxicity.

**Laboratory Test Interference:** Interferes with 17-hydroxycorticosteroids (Reddy-Jenkins-Thorn) and 17-ketogenic steroids (Zimmerman method) resulting in false-positive tests

**Storage Requirements:** Store at 15 to 30°C (59 to 86°F) in tight, light-resistant containers. Drug darkens on exposure to light.

## ☐ RABIES VACCINE, HUMAN DIPLOID CELL

(rae'bees)

(HDCV, Imovax, Rabies vaccine, RVA, WYVAC)

**Classification:** immunization

**Available Preparations:** 2.5 IU single-dose vials

**Action and Use:** Induces antibody formation to rabies virus. Used for treatment of persons exposed to rabies disease.

**Routes and Dosages:** IM, ID (for preexposure prophylaxis only)
**IM:** Postexposure Prophylaxis: six 1.0-ml doses (2.5 IU) with the first dose as soon as possible after exposure, additional doses on days 3, 7, 14, 28, and 40 *or* five 1.0-ml doses of RVA on days 0, 3, 7, 14 and 28
**ID or IM (HDCV):** Preexposure Prophylaxis: 3 doses with the second on day 7 and the third on day 21 or 28

**Absorption and Fate:** Three doses create adequate immune response in 99% of those vaccinated. Rabies antibody is present 7 to 10 days after the first injection. Therapeutic level is 1.5 titer by rapid fluorescent-focus inhibition test or serum antibody of 0.5 IU/ml.

**Contraindications and Precautions:** May be used in pregnancy if needed because of the potential severe outcome of rabies disease. Unknown if fetal harm can be caused by the vaccine but no documented abnormalities have occurred. Safe use of the intradermal vaccine in children is not established but no specific hazards are expected. Cautious use with history of hypersensitivity to the vaccine or neomycin. In such a case, antihistamines can be used concurrently; observation of patient and availability of epinephrine should be ensured. Side effects other than anaphylaxis are not reason to withhold future doses.

### Side Effects:
**CNS:** headache, neurological effects (rare) such as Guillain-Barré syndrome, transient neuroparalysis. **GI:** nausea, abdominal pain. **Skin:** pain, erythema, swelling, itching at injection site. **Musculoskeletal:** muscle aches. **Other:** fever, chills, immune complexlike reaction (rare) after booster dose, rare **anaphylaxis.**

### Nursing Implications:
**Assess:** Before rabies treatment is begun, the prescriber considers the need for prophylaxis. The prevalence of rabies in the area, the type of animal involved, type of attack, and extent of exposure are considered. Carnivorous wild animals such as skunks, raccoons, foxes, coyotes, and bobcats, are most commonly infected. An unprovoked attack is more likely to indicate a rabid animal. Contamination of an open wound with animal saliva is the usual means

of rabies transmission. Question previous reaction to the vaccine or neomycin. **Administer:** An animal bite should be washed immediately with soap and water. Epinephrine 1:1000 and resuscitative equipment should be available in case of anaphylaxis. **IM:** Reconstitute single dose vial of 2.5 IU of Imovax with 1 ml of sterile water for injection, shake gently, and administer entire contents of vial (approximately 1 ml) immediately. Inject into deltoid muscle or upper outer quadrant of gluteal muscle. Lateral thigh is to be used in infants and small children. Aspirate and discard if blood is withdrawn; the injection will need to be prepared again and administered in a different site. When the first dose of HDCV is given, one dose of Rabies Immune Globulin, Human (RIG) or antirabies serum equine (ARS) is also administered in previously nonimmunized persons. RIG is preferred as it rarely causes adverse reactions and ARS causes serum sickness in over 40% of recipients. **ID:** Imovax is the only preparation used intradermally. It is used only for preexposure prophylaxis for those at high risk of contact with rabid animals. Reconstitute with provided diluent, gently shake, and administer entire solution (approximately 0.1 ml) immediately. Give into lateral aspect of upper arm over deltoid area. If not given intradermally, another intradermal injection should be repeated at a different site.

**Monitor:** Observe for 20 minutes after immunization for signs of anaphylaxis or other unfavorable reaction.

**Patient Teaching:** Instruct patient when to return for next dose.

**Drug Interactions:** Immunosuppressive drugs can lessen immune response. They should be avoided or, if used concurrently, antibody serum titers for rabies should be measured to ensure adequate response. RIG may partially suppress response to rabies vaccine. Chloroquine may decrease antibody response.

**Storage Requirements:** The powders are refrigerated at 2 to 8°C (35 to 46°F) in body of the refrigerator rather than on the door where temperature variations may be greater. Avoid freezing. Using reconstituted vaccine immediately.

---

# □ RANITIDINE HYDROCHLORIDE

(ra-nye'te-deen)

(Zantac)

**Classification:** antihistamine, $H_2$-receptor antagonist

## Available Preparations:
- 75 mg/5 ml oral solution
- 150, 300-mg tablet
- 25 mg/ml for parenteral administration
- 0.5 mg/ml in 0.45% sodium chloride for parenteral administration

**Action and Use:** Inhibits histamine action at the $H_2$-histamine receptor sites of parietal cells, prohibiting basal and nocturnal secretion of gastric acid. It also suppresses the gastric acid secretion caused by food, insulin, bentazole, amino acids, and pentogastrin. Used for treatment of active GI hemorrhage or peptic ulcer disease, hypersecretory syndrome, and gastroesophageal reflux.

**Routes and Dosage:**
*PO:* 2 to 4 mg/kg/day in equally divided doses every 12 hours
*IM, IV:* 1 to 2 mg/kg/day in equally divided doses every 6 to 8 hours
Adult: 50 mg every 6–8 hours (maximum daily dosage 400 mg)

**Absorption and Fate:** Rapidly absorbed from gastric tract. Peak level: PO: 2 to 3 hours; IM: 15 minutes. Half-life: 1.8 to 2 hours. Metabolized in liver; primarily excreted in urine. Duration of action: basal, 4 hours, nocturnal, 12 hours.

**Contraindications and Precautions:** Pregnancy category B; excreted in breast milk and not recommended during lactation. Safe use in those under 12 years not established due to lack of controlled studies, thus risk versus benefit must be evaluated. Contraindicated in hypersensitivity to this drug. Use caution with hepatic or renal function impairment.

**Side Effects:**
*CNS:* headache (3%), dizziness, malaise, insomnia. *CV:* bradycardia, tachycardia, PVCs (rare). *GI:* nausea, constipation, abdominal discomfort (mild and transient). *Hepatic:* increase in SGOT, SGPT, alkaline phosphatase, LDH, total bilirubin, jaundice. *GU:* transient elevation serum creatinine. *Skin:* maculopapular rash, urticaria, pruritus. *Hemic:* leukopenia, granulocytopenia, agranulocytosis, thrombocytopenia. *Other:* **Hypersensitivity:** bronchospasm, fever, eosinophilia, rash; Local: burning and pruritus at IV site.

**Nursing Implications:**
*Assess:* Important to have ruled out malignant GI neoplasm before therapy is started.
*Administer: PO:* Unaffected by food, usually given with or after meals. Tablet may be crushed, mixed with small amounts food and fluid. Physician should specify dosing schedule; if given once a day, take at bedtime for best results. *IM:* Do not use if discolored or has precipitate. Injection may cause burning. *IV:* For those over 12 years: each 50 mg of drug must be diluted with at least 20 ml of 0.9% sodium chloride, 5% dextrose, or other compatible IV solutions; infuse slowly over at least 5 minutes. Rapid administration may cause bradycardia, tachycardia, or PVCs. Preferred route, intermittent infusion with dilution of 50 mg/50 to 100 ml infused over 15 to 20 minutes. Compatible with $D_5W$, $D_{10}W$, NS, LR, 5% sodium bicarbonate. Data on incompatibility not available; consult your pharmacist. Limited usage in those under 12 years.
*Monitor:* Assess for side effects; notify physician if they occur. Monitor blood counts, renal and hepatic function during therapy. Assess medication's effectiveness by assessing symptoms of entity being treated. Oral therapy for peptic ulcer continues for 4 weeks.

***Patient Teaching:*** Drug dosage must be followed and given at time ordered. Notify physician if side effects occur; importance of close medical follow-up while on this medication. Parents and child need to understand diet, drug therapy, and disease entity for effective treatment of ulcers. Do not take any OTC drugs without consulting physician or pharmacist.

**Drug Interactions:** Antacids decrease action of this drug; give 1 hour before or 1 hour after ranitidine. Propantheline bromide decreases absorption and increases peak serum concentration of this drug. Check with pharmacist before adding any drugs to child's therapy. Smoking decreases drug's effectiveness.

**Laboratory Test Interference:** False-positive for urine proteins using Multistix. May inhibit cutaneous histamine response of skin allergens causing false-positive results.

**Storage Requirements:** Store at 15 to 30°C (59 to 86°F) in light-resistant containers. Store parenteral form below 25°C. Diluted parenteral form stable for 48 hours at room temperature.

---

## □ RIBAVIRIN
rye-ba-vye′rin)

(Tribavirin, Vilona, Viramid, Virazole)

**Classification:** antiviral, respiratory

**Available Preparations:** 6 g/100 ml sterile solution for nebulization

**Action and Use:** Action not completely known but appears to interfere with RNA and DNA synthesis, inhibiting viral replication. It seems to deplete intracellular nucleotide pools. Active against many RNA and DNA viruses, but it is primarily used in hospitalized infants and children against severe lower respiratory infections caused by respiratory syncytial virus (RSV).

**Routes and Dosage:**
***Inhalation:*** 190 μg/L in mist by Viratek small-particle aerosol generator (SPAG-2) administered per oxygen hood, face mask, or oxygen tent at rate of 12.5-L mist per minute over 12 to 18 hours for minimum of 3 to a maximum of 7 days

**Absorption and Fate:** Systemically absorbed from respiratory tract, which is effected by tidal volume and respiratory rate. Highest plasma concentrations are achieved by aerosol generator with endotracheal tube. Distributed in highest concentrations to respiratory secretions and erythrocytes. Half-life: 9.5 hours. 30 to 55% excreted in urine and 15% in feces in 72 hours.

**Contraindications and Precautions:** Pregnancy category X. Contraindicated in hypersensitivity to drug, with pregnancy or lactation, and in women or girls who may become pregnant; manufacturer recommends not using in infants requiring assisted ventilation. Use with caution in chronic obstructive lung disease or asthma.

## Side Effects:

*CV:* hypotension, **cardiac arrest**. *Resp:* worsening of respiratory function, **dyspnea**, **bacterial pneumonia**, **pneumothorax**, ventilator dependence. *Skin:* rash. *Hemic:* reticulocytosis, **anemia**. *Sensory:* erythema of eyelids, conjunctivitis

## Nursing Implications:

*Assess:* Virus heat labile and susceptible to destruction through freezing or thawing; thus, specimen collection critical and agency collection policy should be closely followed. Treatment may start before culture but it should not continue beyond 24 hours without confirmation.

*Administer:* Drug most effective if used in first 3 days of onset of disease. Not to be used with mild or moderate infections. Some agencies currently recommend that women or men who are planning pregnancy (within 90 days), or women who are pregnant or lactating, not work with children receiving this drug. Family or visitors should be questioned about pregnancy before allowing visitation. Drug is teratogenic in almost all animal studies performed thus far, but there is no pertinent human data yet. Some employees working with this drug have experienced headaches, burning nasal passages and eyes, and crystallized soft contact lenses. Some agencies place child in negative airflow room and use strict isolation techniques. They wear protective goggles, respirator masks (1 per person, changing every 8 to 12 hours), gowns, gloves, and hat to protect against these symptoms. Visitors are required to use same isolation gear. Follow your agency policies for your protection and respiratory isolation in caring for these patients. Before usage of SPAG-2 be familiar with operation of device; this is the only aerosol generating device that should be used. Add 50 to 100 ml of sterile water (*without additive*) to reconstitute 6-g vial. If solution has any particulate matter or discoloration, discard. Place entire solution in the Erlenmeyer flask reservoir of SPAG-2, then further dilute to final volume of 300 ml. This provides solution containing 20 mg/ml. Then attach to hood, face mask, or oxygen tent. **Do not administer any other areosol medications**. Some clinicians have used drug with ventilators but the precipitate of drug may cause increased positive-end expiratory pressures and positive inspiratory pressure. "Rain out" term used for accumulation of fluid in tubing, which  may also occur. If using ventilator apparatus, must be checked for adequate ventilation and gas exchange at least every 2 hours.

*Monitor:* When fluid in reservoir becomes low or in 24 hours discard and replace with fresh solution. This drug treatment must be given with replacement fluid therapy and supportive respiratory care. Assess respiratory function carefully and if any sudden deterioration, discontinue drug and immediately inform physician. Children need emotional support due to isolation techniques and respiratory difficulty, all which may frighten them.

*Patient Teaching:* An informational pamphlet is available from ICN Pharmaceuticals Inc (drug manufacturer) explaining RSV virus and reasons for therapy.

**Drug Interactions:** Potentials for drug interactions have not been fully evaluated. It appears that zidovudine antiviral activity against HIV may be antagonized by this drug. Some evidence that usage with other antiviral agents may enhance this drugs activity.

**Laboratory Test Interference:** Has not been evaluated.

**Storage Requirements:** Store at 15 to 25°C (59 to 78°F). Reconstituted solution stable for 24 hours at 20 to 30°C (68 to 86°F).

---

## □ RIBOFLAVIN

(Vitamin B-2)

**Classification:** nutritional supplement

**Available Preparations:**
- 5, 10, 25, 50, 100-mg tablets
- 10, 25, 50, 100-mg capsules

**Action and Use:** This water-soluble B vitamin is used in metabolism and oxidation–reduction processes. It is a coenzyme in protein metabolism, therefore, when protein requirements increase, so also does riboflavin need. Necessary for erythrocyte integrity and in pyridoxine metabolism. Deficiency results in angular stomatitis, glossitis, normochromic anemia, skin changes, cheilosis, corneal vascularization, which causes eye symptoms such as strain, itching, burning, and light sensitivity. Used in treating deficiency states such as in malabsorption syndrome and in states of increased protein requirements.

**Routes and Dosages:**
*PO:*
- Nutritional Supplement: 600 μg/1000 calories in diet
- Deficiency: over 12 years: 3 to 10 mg/day for several days

**Absorption and Fate:** Well absorbed from GI tract, particularly by active transport in duodenum. Increased absorption when given with food. Distributed throughout body with greater amounts in liver, spleen, kidneys, heart. 60% bound to plasma proteins. Metabolized in GI tract and liver and probably excreted mainly in urine. Half-life of 1 hour or more. Conversion to coenzyme occurs in cytoplasm of most tissues

**Contraindications and Precautions:** Pregnancy category A.

## Side Effects:
*GU:* yellow urine with large doses

## Nursing Implications:
*Assess:* Obtain diet history. CBC performed. Urinary ribloflavin and erythrocyte riboflavin may be done to determine deficiency. Urinary riboflavin under 27 μg/g creatinine, or urinary riboflavin of less than 50 μg/day, or erythrocyte riboflavin of under 10μg/dl erythocytes are abnormal. The RDAs for riboflavin are:

- 0 to 6 months: 0.4 mg
- 6 to 12 months: 0.6 mg
- 1 to 3 years: 0.8 mg
- 4 to 6 years: 1.0 mg
- 7 to 10 years: 1.4 mg
- 11 to 14 years, males: 1.6 mg
- 15 to 18 years, males: 1.7 mg
- 11 to 18 years, females: 1.3 mg
- pregnancy: 1.5 mg
- lactation: 1.7 mg

*Administer:* May be given with food.

*Monitor:* If given for deficiency the anemia and ocular symptoms improve within a few days, therefore, monitoring should occur and dosage be decreased. CBC done regularly. Newborns under phototherapy need close monitoring as riboflavin's sensitivity to light can cause decomposition of the vitamin during phototherapy for hyperbilirubinemia.

*Patient Teaching:* Discourage megadoses. Dietary teaching is indicated. Teens are especially vulnerable to deficiency in times of increased growth and stress; teaching is required. Sources of riboflavin include milk, eggs, organ meat, enriched grains, mushrooms, and green leafy vegetables.

## Drug Interactions: The phenothiazines and tricyclic antidepressants may increase the requirement for riboflavin.

## Laboratory Test Interferences: In high doses can cause false elevation of urinary catecholamines and urobilinogen with Ehrlich's test.

## Storage Requirements: Store in tightly closed, light-resistant container at 15 to 30°C (59 to 86°F).

---

## □ RIFAMPIN                                        (rif'am-pin)

(Rifadin, Rimactane, Rofact)

## Combination Products: 300 mg rifampin with 150 mg isoniazid (Rifamate)

**Classification:** antibiotic, antitubercular

**Available Preparations:** 150, 300-mg capsules

**Action and Use:** Derived from *Streptomyces mediterranei*, inhibits DNA-dependent RNA polymerase synthesis in susceptible bacteria undergoing cell division. Effective against *Mycobacterium tuberculosis* in treatment of tuberculosis, *Neisseria meningitidis* elimination of carrier state, certain gram-positive cocci and gram-negative bacilli. May be used prophylactically in those exposed to *Haemophilus influenzae* type B. Treats leprosy in combination with Dapsone or other antiinfective.

## Routes and Dosage:
*PO:*
- Antituberculosis: over 5 years: 10 to 20 mg/kg/day (maximum dosage 600 mg/day). Some clinicians recommend: under 5 years: 10–20 mg/kg/day (maximum dose for those under 1 week is 10 mg/kg/day). Refampin in combination with isoniazide: limit dosage to 15 mg/kg/day and isoniazide to 10 mg/kg/day
- Meningococcus carriers or meningitis prophylaxis: 3 months to 1 year: 5 mg/kg twice daily for 2 days; over 1 to 12 years: 10 mg/kg twice daily for 2 days (maximum dosage 600 mg/day); over 12 years: 10–20 mg/kg/day for 4 days
- *Haemophilus Influenzae* Type B Prophylaxis: up to 1 month: 10 mg/kg/day for 4 days; over 1 month: 20 mg/kg/day for 4 days. (Maximum dosage 600 mg/day)

**Absorption and Fate:** Well absorbed from GI tract. Peak levels: 2 hours. Well distributed to body tissues and fluids including CSF. Half-life: 2 to 5 hours. Metabolized by liver; drug and its metabolites excreted by bile and a small amount by urine. Therapeutic level: 0.1 to 0.5 μg/ml.

**Contraindications and Precautions:** Pregnancy category C. Drug excreted in breast milk. Contraindicated in hypersensitivity to drug or rifamycins. Use caution hepatic function impairment and alcoholism.

## Side Effects:
*CNS:* headache, fatigue, drowsiness, ataxia, dizziness, confusion, generalized numbness. *GI:* heartburn, epigastric distress, nausea, vomiting, anorexia, diarrhea, flatulence, sore mouth and tongue. *Hepatic:* transient rise in SGPT, SGOT, alkaline phosphatase, bilirubin, **jaundice and hepatitis** (rare). *GU:* hematuria, hemoglobinuria, increased BUN and serum uric acid, **renal insufficiency, acute renal failure** (rare). *Hemic:* thrombocytopenia, leukopenia, purpura, hemolytic anemia. *Musculoskeletal:* muscle weakness, joint and extremity pain. *Other:* reddish orange color to urine, feces, saliva, sweat, tears; Hypersensitivity: flulike syndrome with fever, headache, chills, dizziness, dyspnea; pruritus, rash, urticaria, sore mouth, sore tongue, exudative conjunctivitis.

## Nursing Implications:

*Assess:* Obtain diagnostic cultures. Obtain baseline liver function studies SGPT, SGOT, alkaline phosphatase, bilirubin. Renal and hematopoietic status studies may also be obtained.

*Administer: PO:* Give 1 hour before meals or 2 hours after for maximum absorption; however, if GI irritation occurs may take with food. Capsule can be taken apart and mixed with food; the drug is unstable in solution so best not to mix with fluids. Pharmacist can make a suspension of capsules that is stable for 4 weeks. This drug is usually given concurrently with at least one other antitubercular medication for tuberculous treatment and therapy length varies from 6 to 9 months.

*Monitor:* Assess for symptoms of jaundice and other side effects. Periodic hepatic, renal, and hematopoietic examinations should be obtained.

*Patient Teaching:* Inform parent and child of harmless discoloration of body fluids; however, soft contact lenses will be permanently stained. Report any symptoms of side effects immediately, especially hepatic symptoms. Medication must be taken as prescribed and do not stop therapy; it could result in hepatorenal reaction when drug is resumed. Its important to have close medical follow-up.

**Drug Interactions:** Alcohol causes increased risk for hepatotoxicity. Aminosalicylic acid may impair GI absorption of rifampin. Concurrent administration of ketoconazole and this drug cause decreased serum levels of ketaconazole. This drug causes liver enzymes to inactivate these barbiturates, corticosteroids, digitalis derivatives, quinidine, dapsone, cyclosporine, chloramphenicol, oral anticoagulants, estrogens and oral contraceptives. Clofazimine decreases the absorption of rifampin.

**Laboratory Test Interference:** Interferes with serum folate and vitamin $B_{12}$. Interferes with contrast media for gallbladder tests.

**Storage Requirements:** Store at 15 to 30°C (59 to 86°F); protect from light, air, and excessive heat.

---

## ☐ SILVER SULFADIAZINE
(sul-fa-dye′a-zeen)

(Silvadene, Thermazene)

**Classification:** antiinfective, sulfonamide derivative

**Available Preparations:** 1% cream for topical administration

**Action and Use:** Acts on cell membrane and cell wall and does not appear to react like other sulfonamides by inhibiting the biosynthesis of folic acid. Used topically for treatment of second and third degree burns to prevent infection.

## Routes and Dosage:

*Topical:* Apply 16 mm ($^1/_{16}$ inch) thickness to entire debrided burn area 1 to 2 times a day

## Absorption and Fate:

When applied to second degree burns, sulfadiazine appears to be systemically absorbed. This is after the compound reacts with sodium chloride and proteins releasing sulfadiazine.

## Contraindications and Precautions:

Pregnancy category C and D near term. Contraindicated if nursing, premature, neonates, and infants under 2 months; allergy to drug or any its components, sulfonamides, methyparaben, or asthmatic. Use caution in renal or hepatic impairment.

## Side Effects:

*Skin:* pain and burning after application, rashes, pruritus. *Hemic:* reversible leukopenia (after first 4 days). *Other:* If applied to extensive burn area may have adverse reaction similar to other sulfonamides.

## Nursing Implications:

*Assess:* Accurate assessment and recording of appearance of wound site. Obtain baseline information (especially if large area involved), vital signs, weight, hematologic and renal function.

*Administer: Topical:* Cream is white in color; it reacts with heavy metals causing darkening, if this occurs discard cream. Apply aseptically with sterile gloves to wound in $^1/_{16}$-mm thickness. Wound should be cleaned according to orders but can use bath, shower, or whirlpool (preferred) before application. Maintain room temperature when dressing changed. Keep wound covered with medication at all times. Treated area usually left open but if dressing used, only thin layer is necessary.

*Monitor:* Accurate observation and recording of wound progression. Assess for symptoms of superinfections and septicemia. Observe for side effects of medication and hypersensitivity reactions. If this occurs, contact physician. If large burn area, use flow charts to monitor vital signs, weight, I & O, sulfonamides side effects, and laboratory information. Use of therapeutic play can help child handle dressing changes. May need analgesic before dressing change and drug application. Duration of therapy is until wound healed or site ready for grafting.

*Patient Teaching:* If parents caring for child at home, teach how to apply and not to use more medication then prescribed. To observe for symptoms of infections and importance of close medical follow-up.

## Storage Requirements:

Store at 15 to 30°C in light-resistant containers, avoiding excessive heat.

---

## □ SODIUM BICARBONATE

(soe'dee-um bey-car'bun-ate)

(Baking soda, Bell-Ans, citrocarbonate, Neut, Soda Mint)

**Classification:** anticid, alkalizer

## Available Preparations:
- 300, 325, 520, 600, 625, 650-mg tablets
- Powder
- Powder for solution
- 4, 4.2, 5, 7.5, 8.4% ampules and vials for parenteral use
- 4, 4.2% solution for nebulization

**Action and Use:** This alkalinizing agent dissociates into sodium and bicarbonate in the body, thus providing bicarbonate ions for replacement in disease states. Increases blood and urinary pH, buffers hydrogen ions, and neutralizes gastric acid as it increases gastric pH. Used to correct metabolic acidosis in conditions such as cardiac arrest and severe diarrhea, prevent uric acid crystallization of urine, and as a gastric antacid. Topical powders may be used to relieve minor skin discomfort.

## Routes and Dosages:
*PO:*
- Antacid: 6 to 12 years: 1.9 to 3.9 g in water (effervescent tablets); 6 to 12 years: 520 mg (tablets)
- Urinary Alkalization: 1 to 10 mEq/kg/day or 12 to 120 mg/kg/day

*IV:*
- Cardiac Arrest: 1 mEq/kg initially, then 0.5 mEq/kg q10 min
- Metabolic Acidosis: 2 to 5 mEq/kg over 4 to 8 hours; not to exceed 8 mEq/kg/day in children under 2 years

**Absorption and Fate:** Dissociates rapidly into sodium and bicarbonate ions. Immediate peak level after IV infusion. Duration of action is short, especially in those with normal kidney function. Duration of antacid effect is 20 to 60 minutes with a longer effect when given after meals.

**Contraindications and Precautions:** Pregnancy category C. Safe in low doses in pregnancy, although high doses can contribute to systemic alkalosis, increased serum sodium, and resultant edema and weight gain. Caution must be used in children particularly under 2 years and IV infusion must be slow (see Administration Section). Antacids not generally recommended in children under 6 years. Contraindicated in metabolic or respiratory alkalosis, hypocalcemia, excess chloride use. Cautious use in congestive heart failure, sodium retention, renal dysfunction, patients on corticosteroids, hypertension. Cautious use of antacids and continued diagnosis in patients with syumptoms of possible appendicitis or GI bleeding.

## Side Effects:
*CNS:* confusion, **seizures** in those with ketoacidosis, weakness, headache. *CV:* irregular pulse. *GI:* distention, flatulence with PO form, cramps. *Skin:* necrosis with extravasation. Other: metabolic alkalosis, hypercalcemia, tetany, hyperirritability, sodium and water retention, weight gain, edema, **hypokale-**

mia; in children under 2 years, rapid IV injection can lead to elevated sodium levels, decreased CSF pressure, and **intracranial hemorrhage.**

## Nursing Implications:

*Assess:* Measure urinary pH, vital signs for IV forms.

*Administer: PO:* Do not give with milk or other calcium as milk–alkali syndrome may result (anorexia, nausea, vomiting, headache, hypercalcemia, metabolic alkalosis, confusion, urinary dysfunction). *IV:* Dilute with sterile water, saline, or 5% dextrose. The 7.5% solution is stable in syringe for 100 days if refrigerated or 45 days at room temperature. Assure adequate ventilation during administration. Incompatible with many drugs, therefore, not recommended for mixing; avoid giving with calcium. Given slowly IV to infants and children. Rate of 10 ml/minute in children under 2 years may cause excessive sodium levels, decreased CSF, intracranial hemorrhage. Dose not to exceed 8 mEq/day with slow IV infusion of 4.2% solution or 1:1 dilution of 7.5% or 8.4% solution with 5% dextrose. Sodium bicarbonate is given early in resuscitation as metabolic acidosis occurs soon as a result of insufficient oxygen at the cellular level. Cardiac arrhythmias are more likely in metabolic acidosis.

*Monitor:* Monitor arterial blood pH, serum bicarbonate levels, renal function, urinary pH, $PO_2$, $PCO_2$. Monitor IV site carefully as extravasation can lead to necrosis. If on chronic oral form, do periodic weight check, observe for edema.

*Patient Teaching:* Discourage patients from using OTC for gastric distress; antacids with less side effects are available. Take antacids with water, not milk or calcium. Maximum antacid use is 2 weeks without physician instructions. Do not use in children under 6 years unless directed by a physician. Be aware of OTC products that contain sodium such as Alka-Seltzer, Bi-So-Dol, and Bromo-Seltzer; read labels. Topical: soak, use 1/2 cup of baking powder in tub of warm water. For paste, use 3 parts baking soda to 1 part water. Be cautious that children do not drink the prepared solution or paste.

## Drug Interactions:

Antacid may alter rate of absorption of any other drug. For example, may decrease absorption of digoxin and iron and increase rate of naproxen absorption. In general other drugs must be spaced at least 1 hour apart in time from sodium bicarbonate. Absorption of some aspirin preparations increases with sodium bicarbonate; aspirin excretion is enhanced, therefore, dosage may need to be increased. Increased excretion of aspirin and decreased excretion of amphetamines and quinidine due to increased urinary pH. In general will decrease excretion of basic drugs and increase excretion of acidic drugs.

## Laboratory Test Inferences:

PO form alters gastric acid secretion test; withhold on day of test. Increases blood and urinary pH. Reduced serum potassium. Increased blood lactate. False-positive urinary protein by some methods. Elevated urinary urobilinogen.

## Storage Requirements:

Store in tightly closed containers at 15 to 30°C (59 to 86°F). Do not use solution if a precipitate is present. Note expiration date.

---

# □ SOMATREM

(soe'ma-trem)

(Protropin)

**Classification:** pituitary hormone, growth

**Available Preparations:** 5 mg (10 units) per vial for parenteral administration

**Action and Use:** Synthetic recombinant DNA product structurally identical to pituitary hormone with the addition of another amino acid. It stimulates growth by increasing number and size of organ and muscle cells, as well as linear cartilaginous skeletal growth. Used to treat growth failure in those with pituitary growth hormone failure, e.g., pituitary dwarfism or growth failure from cranial irradiation.

## Routes and Dosage:
*IM:* 0.05 to 0.1 international unit (IU)/kg every other day or 3 times per week. (Minimum of 48 hours between dosage)

**Absorption and Fate:** About 90% metabolized by liver. Half-life: 20 to 30 minutes with longer lasting effects. Excreted in urine.

**Contraindications and Precautions:** Pregnancy category C. Contraindicated in epiphyseal closure, intracranial lesions, or sensitivity to benzyl alcohol, or those with sensitivity to somatropin. Use with caution in diabetics, untreated hypothyroidism, or previous intracranial lesion.

## Side Effects:
*CV:* hypertension, atherosclerosis (high-dosage therapy). *Endocrine:* **hypothyroidism, hyperglycemia.** *Musculoskeletal:* acromegalic features of hand, face and feet, organ enlargement (with high-dosage therapy). *Other:* **antibodies to this drug** (30 to 40% in 3 to 6 months); Local: pain and swelling at site of injection.

## Nursing Implications:
*Assess:* Obtain baseline thyroid function tests, blood and urine glucose, and bone age determination (wrist x-rays). Growth hormone work up to establish diagnosis to rule out multiple pituitary hormone deficiency. If previous intracranial lesion, establish presence of current tumor activity.
*Administer: IM:* Reconstitute vial with bacteriostatic water included. Inject into vial by aiming so fluid will hit against side of vial. Gently roll vial between palms; **do not shake contents.** Do not use if solution has particulate matter or is cloudy. Avoid injecting into subcutaneous tissue, it may increase antibody development. Injection painful. Discard unused portion.
*Monitor:* Assessment of growth levels at periodic intervals either every 6 or

12 months. Assess urine and blood glucose levels and thyroid levels. Although antibodies form, they rarely interfere with drug therapy. Therapy continued as long as child responds to drug or until mature adult height or epiphyses close. *Patient Teaching:* Parents and child should be counseled so that they understand drug's action and develop realistic ideas about goals of treatment. Monitor for symptoms of glucose intolerance and hyperglycemia. Importance of close medical follow-up. If child develops limp, or complains of hip or knee pain, he should be evaluated by physician immediately for slipped capital femoral epiphyses, which can occur in children with endocrine disorders.

**Drug Interactions:** Thyroid hormones, estrogens, androgens, and anabolic steroids may increase epiphyseal growth closure. ACTH and corticotropin in large dosages with this drug may inhibit growth response to somatrem.

**Laboratory Test Interference:** $T_4$, radioactive iodine uptake, and thyroxine binding capacity can be slightly lower. Glucose tolerance decreased with high dosage.

**Storage Requirements:** Store at 2 to 8°C (36 to 46°F), protect from freezing.

---

## □ SPIRONOLACTONE                    (speer-on-oh-lak'tone)

(Aldactone)

**Combination Products:** Aldactazide

**Classification:** diuretic

**Available Preparations:**
- 25, 50, 100-mg tablets
- 25, 50-mg tablets with hydrochlorothiazide

**Action and Use:** Competitively antagonizes the effect of aldosterone in distal renal tubules, causing sodium and chloride excretion without creating additional potassium loss. Possible antiandrogenic effect. Used as a diuretic, particularly in combination with others to reduce potassium loss. Used for primary hyperaldosteronism, women with polycystic ovary syndrome.

**Routes and Dosages:**
*PO:*
- Hypertension and Edema: 3.3 mg/kg/day in 1 to 4 doses or 60 mg/m²/day in 2 to 4 doses; give 5 days and adjust upward PRN
- Aldosteronism: 125 to 375 mg/m²/day in divided doses

**Absorption and Fate:** Well absorbed from GI tract with 90% bioavailable. 90% bound to plasma proteins. Metabolized by the liver and excreted in urine and bile. Peak level of the drug is 1 to 2 hours and of metabolites is 2 to 4 hours. Maximum diuretic effect occurs 3 days after drug therapy begins and continues for 2 to 3 days after drug withdrawal. Half-life is 13 to 24 hours when given 1 to 2 times/day or 9 to 16 hours when given QID.

**Contraindications and Precautions:** Pregnancy category D. Contraindicated in anuria, renal failure, hyperkalemia, or if BUN or creatinine are two times normal levels. Cautious use with BUN of 40 mg/dl or more or in hepatic or renal dysfunction, diabetes, hyponatremia, metabolic or respiratory acidosis.

**Side Effects:**
*CNS:* lethargy, confusion, fatigue, dizziness, headache. *CV:* **arrhythmia** (resulting from hyperkalemia). *GI:* nausea, vomiting, anorexia, abdominal cramps, diarrhea, dry mouth, thirst. *Hepatic:* elevated BUN. *GU:* menstrual abnormalities, breast enlargement. *Metabolic:* **hyperkalemia** if renal failure develops or if on potassium supplements, **metabolic acidosis**, hyponatremia (especially with cirrhosis patients). *Skin:* rash, urticaria, sweating.

**Nursing Implications:**
*Assess:* Obtain baseline CBC, BUN, creatinine, EKG, serum electrolytes, weight, and vital signs, especially blood pressure.
*Administer:* Tablets may be crushed and given in suspension of cherry syrup. Suspension is refrigerated and discarded 1 month after compounding. Give with food to enhance absorption and decrease GI upset. Given 5 days and dosage adjusted; if not effective in 5 days, patient is switched to another diuretic.
*Monitor:* Continue to monitor serum potassium and sodium, vital signs especially blood pressure, I & O, and daily weight. Watch for signs of hyperkalemia (paresthesias, confusion, weakness, cardiac irregularities). If giving combination product with hydrochlorothiazide, hypokalemia may occur. BUN, creatinine, EKG are monitored periodically. If given to diabetic, monitor blood glucose carefully as hyperglycemia may result.
*Patient Teaching:* Avoid excess intake of potassium such as potassium supplements and sodium-free salt unless also taking a potassium-depleting diuretic. Teach the signs of hyperkalemia (paresthesia, confusion, weakness) and teach to report. Report sore throat, fever, malaise, bleeding, or bruising.

**Drug Interactions:** Increased blood glucose in those on insulin. Hyperkalemia may result if potassium supplement is given; note that whole blood also contains potassium. Increased hyperkalemia may occur with captopril, therefore, drug should be used with caution. May reduce excretion of digoxin; may inhibit inotropic effect of digitalis. Diuretic effect may decrease if salicylates are also given. Increased potassium excretion may occur with corticosteroids. Acidosis may occur if given with ammonium chloride. Nonsteroidal antiinflammatories, estrogen, sympathomimetics can decrease the antihypertensive effect. Increased diuresis with other diuretics. Decreased blood pressure with other antihypertensives. Lithium will have reduced renal clearance and is not recommended for use with potassium-sparing diuretics. Do not use with other potassium-sparing drugs.

**Laboratory Test Interferences:** Interferes with fluorescent measurement of quinidine and lactic dehydrogenase. May elevate BUN, creatinine, plasma renin activity, magnesium, potassium, uric acid. Falsely elevates plasma digitalis level. May increase blood glucose in diabetics. Increases urinary calcium and decreases serum sodium. Causes inaccurate plasma and urinary 17-hydroxycorticosteroids.

**Storage Requirements:** Store at 15 to 30°C. Protect from light. Solution is kept at 2 to 8°C (35 to 46°F).

---

## ☐ SULFAMETHOXAZOLE                    (sul-fa-meth-ox′a-zole)

(Gamazole, Gantanol, Urobak)

**Combination Products:** 500 mg sulfamethoxazole and 100 mg phenazopyridine HCl (Azo Gantanol, Azo-Sulfamethoxazole)

**Classification:** antibiotic, sulfonamide

### Available Preparations:
- 500 mg/5 ml oral suspension
- 500 mg, 1-g tablets

**Action and Use:** Prevents incorporation of $p$-aminobenzoic acid (PABA) into dihydrofolate, inhibiting the biosynthesis of folic acid, which is necessary for susceptible pathogen growth.

### Routes and Dosage:
*PO:* over 2 months: loading dosage: 50 to 60 mg/kg/ times 1 dose; then maintenance: 25 to 30 mg/kg/ twice daily. (Maximum dosage 75 mg/kg/day) Some clinicians recommend. initial dosage: 1.2 g/m²; then 0.6 g/m² twice daily.

**Absorption and Fate:** Not well absorbed from GI tract. Peak level: 3 to 4 hours. Distributed into body tissues and fluids. 50 to 70% bound to plasma proteins. Excreted primarily in urine.

**Contraindications and Precautions:** Pregnancy category B, near term D. Contraindicated during lactation, first 2 months life (may cause kernicterus in infants), combination form in children under 12 years, hypersensitivity to this drug, sulfonamides. Use with caution in impaired renal or hepatic function, bronchial asthma, allergies, G-6-PD deficiency, or blood dyscrasias.

### Side Effects:
*CNS:* headache, lethargy, nervousness, ataxia, mental depression, **seizures,**

hallucinations. *GI:* nausea, vomiting, diarrhea, GI pain, stomatitis, **pseudo-membranous enterocolitis**, pancreatitis. *Hepatic:* jaundice. *GU:* crystalluria, increased BUN and serum creatinine, renal colic, **oliguria**, hematuria, proteinuria, rarely **interstitial nephritis**. *Skin:* erythematous, maculopapular, morbilliform rashes, urticaria. *Hemic:* **granulocytopenia, agranulocytosis, aplastic anemia, leukopenia, neutropenia, thrombocytopenia, hemolytic anemia**. *Other:* Hypersensitivity: **epidermal necrolysis, Stevens-Johnson syndrome, exfoliative dermatitis, allergic myocarditis**, arthralgia, pruritus, fever, **serum sickness**, photosensitive, **anaphylaxis**.

## Nursing Implications:

*Assess:* Assess if previous allergy to drug combination or sulfonamides. Obtain cultures and sensitivity before treatment, but can start treatment before results. Obtain baseline CBC, UA, renal function tests, especially if on therapy longer than 2 weeks.

*Administer: PO:* Shake suspension well. Tablet may be crushed, mixed with a small amount of food or fluid. Give on empty stomach 1 hour before meals or 2 hours after meals; however, if nausea occurs, can give with a small amount of food. Follow dosage with as much fluids as child will take to prevent crystalluria.

*Monitor:* Observe for sore throat, fever, skin rash, and sore mouth; signs of blood dyscrasias. Observe for side effects. Assess CBC and renal function during therapy. Report hematological symptoms immediately; stop medication. Maintain daily hydration level for child's age and maintain alkaline urine to prevent crystalluria (may need to give sodium bicarbonate if this occurs).

*Patient Teaching:* Take as prescribed for full course of therapy. Observe for side effects and importance of maintaining hydration levels. Protect child from sun. Store suspension at room temperature.

## Drug Interactions:
Used in combination with coumarin may prolong prothrombin time. Can displace methotrexate and salicylates from protein-binding sites when used concurrently. Local anesthetics that are derivatives of *p*-aminobenzoic acid (procaine, tetracaine) may antagonize antibacterial activity of this drug.

## Storage Requirements:
Store at 15 to 30°C (59 to 86°F); light-resistant containers.

---

## □ SULFASALAZINE                                    (sul-fa-sal′a-zeen)

(Azulfidine, Azulfidine En-Tabs, Salazopyrin, SAS-500)

## Classification: antibiotic, sulfonamide

## Available Preparations:
- 250 mg/5 ml oral suspension
- 500-mg tablets
- 500-mg enteric-coated tablets

**Action and Use:** Exact mechanism of action against ulcerative colitis and Crohn's disease is unknown but it appears to deliver the antibacterial action of sulfapyridine and antiinflammatory action of 5-aminosalicylic acid to the colon. It also appears to reduce *Clostridium* and *Escherichia coli* in the stool, interferes with the synthesis of prostaglandins, and alters the absorption of electrolytes and fluids in the colon.

## Routes and Dosage:
*PO:* Over 2 years: Initial Dosage: 40 to 60 mg/kg/day in 3 to 6 equally divided doses; Maintenance: 30 mg/kg/day in 4 equally divided doses

**Absorption and Fate:** 85 to 90% passes into colon; sulfapyridine rapidly absorbed, where 5-aminosalicylic acid minimally absorbed. Sulfapyridine peak level in 1.5 to 6 hours. Half-life: 5.7 to 10.4 hours. Excreted in urine; unchanged or as metabolites of drugs.

**Contraindications and Precautions:** Pregnancy category B, near term D. Contraindicated during lactation, first 2 years of life, hypersensitivity to this drug, sulfonamides, and intestinal or urinary tract obstructions. Use caution in impaired renal or hepatic function, bronchial asthma, porphyria, allergies, G-6-PD deficiency, or blood dyscrasias.

## Side Effects:
*CNS:* headache, lethargy. *GI:* nausea, vomiting, diarrhea, GI distress. *GU:* crystalluria, hematuria, orange-yellow color to alkaline urine. *Skin:* orange-yellow color to skin, photosensitive. *Other:* Hypersensitivity: urticaria, rash, serumlike sickness **Stevens-Johnson syndrome** (rare), fever, serum sickness.

## Nursing Implications:
*Assess:* Assess if previous allergy to drug combination or sulfonamides. Obtain cultures and sensitivity before treatment, but can start treatment before results. Obtain baseline CBC and UA, especially if on long-term therapy.
*Administer: PO:* Shake suspension well. Regular tablet may be crushed and given with a small amount of food. Do not crush enteric-coated tablet. Give on empty stomach 1 hour before meals or 2 hours after meals and dosing intervals should not exceed 8 hours. Follow dosage with as much fluids as child will take to prevent crystalluria.
*Monitor:* If GI upset occurs can give after meals; spread dosage more evenly spaced; may need to start with lower dosage or use enteric-coated tablets. Some patients may pass enteric-coated tablets into stools without disintegrating; stop enteric-coated tablets and contact physician. Observe for hypersensitivity and side effects. This drug may inhibit folic acid absorption, resulting in possible deficiency. Assess CBC and UA function during therapy. Maintain daily hydration level for child's age to prevent crystalluria.
*Patient Teaching:* Take as prescribed for full course of therapy. Importance of continual medical supervision. Observe for side effects and importance of maintaining hydration levels. If taking enteric-coated tablet, observe stools for passage of tablets. Protect child from sun. Store suspension at room temperature.

**Drug Interactions:** Used with other antibiotics may alter intestinal flora and metabolism of sulfasalazine. Sulfasalazine chelates iron, inhibiting the drug's absorption. Used in combination with coumarin may prolong prothrombin time. Can displace methotrexate and phenytoin from protein-binding sites when used concomitantly.

**Storage Requirements:** Store at 15 to 30°C (59 to 86°F) in light-resistant containers.

---

## □ SULFISOXAZOLE                              (sul-fi-sox'a-zole)

(Barazole, Gantrisin, G-Sox, J-Sul, Lipo Gantrisin, Rosoxol, Novosoxazole, Sosol, Soxa, Soxomide, Sulfagan, Urisoxin, Urizole, Velmatrol)

**Combination Products:** Sulfisoxazole and erythromycin ethylsuccinate (Pediazole)

**Classification:** antibiotic, sulfonamide

### Available Preparations:
- 500 mg/5 ml oral solution
- 500 mg/5 ml oral suspension
- 500-mg tablets
- 500-mg film-coated tablets
- 400 mg/ml for parenteral administration
- 4% ophthalmic ointment and solution

**Action and Use:** Prevents incorporation of *p*-aminobenzoic acid (PABA) into dihydrofolate, inhibiting the biosynthesis of folic acid that is necessary for susceptible pathogens' growth. Active against both gram-positive and gram-negative bacteria such as *Staphylococcus*, *Streptococcus*, *Escherichia coli*, *Proteus*, and *Haemophilus influenzae* (especially ampicillin-resistant strains in otitis media).

### Routes and Dosage:
*PO:* over 2 months: Loading dosage: 75 mg/kg or 2 g/m$^2$ times 1 dose; Maintenance: 150 mg/kg/day or 4 g/m$^2$/day in equally divided doses every 4 to 6 hours. (Maximum dosage 6 g/day)
*IV:* Loading dosage: 50 mg/kg times 1 dose; Maintenance: 100 mg/kg/day every 6 hours
*Ophthalmic:*
- Drops: instill 1 to 2 drops of 4% solution into conjunctival sac every 8 hours
- Ointment: instill 1-cm strip into conjunctival sac every 8 hours

**Absorption and Fate:** Well absorbed from GI tract. Peak level: PO, 2 to 4 hours; IV, 30 minutes after infusion. Distributed into extracellular spaces. Half-life ranges from 4.6 to 7.8 hours. 95% excreted in urine in 24 hours.

**Contraindications and Precautions:** Pregnancy category B, near term D. Contraindicated during lactation, first 2 months life (may cause kernicterus in infants), hypersensitivity to this drug, sulfonamides, porphyria or intestinal and urinary obstruction. Use with caution in impaired renal or hepatic function, bronchial asthma, allergies, blood dyscrasias, or G-6-PD deficiency.

## Side Effects:
*CNS:* headache, lethargy, nervousness, ataxia, mental depression, **seizures**, hallucinations. *GI:* nausea, vomiting, diarrhea, GI pain, stomatitis, **pseudomembranous enterocolitis**, pancreatitis. *Hepatic:* jaundice. *GU:* crystalluria, increased BUN and serum creatinine, renal colic, **oliguria**, hematuria, proteinuria, **interstitial nephritis** (rare). *Skin:* erythematous, maculopapular, morbilliform rashes, urticaria. *Hemic:* **granulocytopenia, agranulocytosis, aplastic anemia, leukopenia, neutropenia, thrombocytopenia, hemolytic anemia.** *Sensory:* Ophthalmic: itching, redness, burning, blurred vision. *Other:* Hypersensitivity: **epidermal necrolysis, Stevens-Johnson syndrome, exfoliative dermatitis, allergic myocarditis**, arthralgia, pruritus, fever, **serum sickness**, photosensitive, **anaphylaxis**.

## Nursing Implications:
*Assess:* Assess if previous allergy to drug combination or sulfonamides. Obtain cultures and sensitivity before treatment, but can start treatment before results. Obtain baseline CBC, UA, renal function tests, especially if therapy longer than 2 weeks. Ophthalmic: note and record appearance of eye.
*Administer: PO:* Shake suspension well. Tablet may be crushed, mixed and given with a small amount of food. Give on empty stomach 1 hour before meals or 2 hours after meals; however, if nausea occurs can give with a small amount of food. Follow dosage with as much fluids as child will take to prevent crystalluria. *IV:* Intermittent infusion: dilute with sterile water to maximum 50 mg/ml concentration and infuse over 20 to 30 minutes. Compatible with D$_5$W, NS, D$_{10}$W, LR, and dextrose–saline combinations. Some drugs compatible, check with pharmacist, but as general rule do not mix with other drugs. *Ophthalmic:* See Part I for instillation in children. Inform child that medication may sting and that ointment will blur vision for several minutes after instillation.
*Monitor:* Observe IV site for extravasation. Assess outcome of ophthalmic preparation. Observe for sore throat, fever, skin rash, and sore mouth; signs of blood dyscrasias. Observe for hypersensitivity and side effects. Assess CBC and renal function during therapy. Report hematological symptoms immediately; stop medication. Maintain daily hydration level for child's age and maintain alkaline urine to prevent crystalluria (may need to give sodium bicarbonate if this occurs).
*Patient Teaching:* Teach parent how to instill medication. Take as prescribed for full course of therapy. Observe for side effects and maintain hydration levels. Protect child from sun. Store suspension at room temperature. Consult physician before taking OTC medications.

**Drug Interactions:** Used in combination with coumarin may prolong prothrombin time. Can displace methotrexate, phenytoin, and salicylates from protein-binding sites when used concurrently. Local anesthetics that are derivatives of *p*-aminobenzoic acid (procaine, tetracaine) may antagonize antibacterial activity of this drug.

**Storage Requirements:** Store at 15 to 30°C (59 to 86°F) in light-resistant containers and avoid freezing.

---

## ☐ TERBUTALINE SULFATE

(ter-byoo'te-leen)

(Brethaire, Brethine, Bricanyl)

**Classification:** adrenergic, bronchodilator

### Available Preparations:
- 2.5, 5-mg tablets
- 200 μg/metered spray oral inhalation
- 1 mg/ml for parenteral administration

**Action and Use:** A synthetic sympathomimetic amine that stimulates β-adrenergic receptors causing relaxation of smooth musculature of bronchial tree and peripheral vasculature. Used as a bronchial dilator in treatment of symptoms of asthma, bronchial, and emphysema. Also used to stop uterine contractions in premature labor.

### Routes and Dosage:
*PO:* over 12 years: 0.05 mg/kg/dose 3 times per day. (Maximum dosage 7.5 mg/day)
*SC:*
- under 12 years: 0.005 to 0.010 mg/kg/dose (maximum dosage 0.25 mg/dose every 15 to 20 minutes 2 times per day)
- over 12 years: 3.5–5 μg/kg (maximum dosage 0.5 mg in 4 hours); dosage established by clinicians

*Inhalation:* Nebulization: 2 inhalations (400 μg) every 4 to 6 hours for continuous treatment

**Absorption and Fate:** Onset of action: PO, 1 to 2 hours; SC, 15 minutes; inhalation 5, to 30 minutes. Peak effect: PO, 2 to 3 hours; SC, 30 to 60 minutes; inhalation, 5 to 60 minutes. Duration of action: PO, 4 to 8 hours; SC, 1.5 to 4 hours. Metabolized in liver and 60% excreted unchanged in urine.

**Contraindications and Precautions:** Pregnancy category B. Use caution during lactation. Not recommended by manufacture for usage in those under 12 years. Contraindicated in hypersensitivity to drug or any of its ingredients, MAO inhibitors, sensitivity to other sympathomimetic drugs. Use caution in asthma, diabetes mellitus, hypertension, hyperthyroidism, history of seizures, cardiac disease.

## Side Effects:

**CNS:** nervousness, tremors, lethargy, dizziness, headache, sweating. **CV:** palpitations, **tachycardia**, **dysrhythmia**, **altered ECG readings** (rare). **GI:** nausea, vomiting. **Sensory:** dry nose, mouth, and throat; tinnitus.

## Nursing Implications:

**Assess:** Assess respiratory status and obtain baseline pulse.

**Administer: PO:** Tablets can be crushed and mixed with small amounts of food or fluid. Do not crush extended-release tablets. If GI irritation occurs give with food. **SC:** Do not use if solution is discolored. Give SC in lateral deltoid area. Carefully check dosage—making an error in decimal point could be fatal; double check with RN. Monitor pulse; more likely to experience cardiac symptoms with this route. If no significant clinical improvement in 15 to 30 minutes after initial dosage, may repeat. If condition does not improve in 15 to 30 minutes after second dosage, do not repeat. Contact physician, other measures may be needed. **Inhalations:** Assemble according to package insert. Shake container well and administer as described in Part I. If second inhalation is prescribed manufacture recommends that 1 minute elapses between doses.

**Monitor:** Monitor response to medication. Maintain hydration for age group. Monitor pulse in response to SC injection.

**Patient Teaching:** Proper usage and care of inhaler should be taught and it is beneficial to have child demonstrate inhaler usage. Inhaler should not be used more frequently than prescribed; if symptoms worsen contact physician. If paradoxical bronchospasms occur, discontinue immediately. Do not use any inhalers other than those ordered by physician. Tolerance can develop with long-term therapy.

**Drug Interactions:** MAO inhibitors used with this drug can cause hypertensive crisis, do not use this drug within 11 days of MAO inhibitor. Avoid usage with other sympathomimetic amines because of additive effects. Effects of β-adrenergic blocking agents antagonize bronchodilation effects of this drug.

**Storage Requirements:** Store at 15 to 30°C (59 to 86°F) in light-resistant containers. Do not store aerosol at temperatures above 30°C and avoid placing near heat or in direct sunlight.

---

## □ TERFENADINE                                    (ter-fin'a-deen)

(Seldane)

**Classification:** antihistamine

**Available Preparations:** 60 mg tablets

**Action and Use:** Butyrophenone derivative that competes with histamine for $H_1$-receptor sites of effector cells. By blocking the histamine it decreases the allergic reactions. Does not cross blood-brain barrier, therefore, does not appear to have incidence of CNS symptoms of other antihistamines. Used to relieve seasonal nasal rhinitis and pruritus.

**Routes and Dosage:**
*PO:*
- 3 to 6 years: 15 mg 2 times per day
- 7 to 12 years: 30 mg 2 times per day
- over 12 years: 60 mg 2 times per day

**Absorption and Fate:** Absorbed well from GI tract. Peak level: 1 to 2 hours. Biphasic half-life: 3.5 hours, 16 to 23 hours. Duration of action: 12 hours. Excreted primarily in feces.

**Contraindications and Precautions:** Pregnancy category C. Use during lactation not recommended. Safe use in those under 12 years not established, but has been used without toxicity in limited number of 3 to 12-year olds. Contraindicated if hypersensitive to drug. Use caution with lower respiratory disease or asthma.

**Side Effects:**
*CNS:* drowsiness (less pronounced), dizziness, headaches, nervousness, insomnia, tremors, confusion (rare). *GI:* abdominal distress, nausea, vomiting, diarrhea, dry mouth (less 5%). *Hepatic:* mild increase SGOT, SGPT. *Resp:* increased thick secretions, **wheezing**, **chest tightness**. *GU:* urinary retention or frequency. *Skin:* rash, urticaria.

**Nursing Implications:**
*Administer: PO:* May give with food or milk to reduce GI distress. Can crush tablet and mix with small amount of food or fluid.
*Patient Teaching:* Take only as directed and only under physician's supervision in those under 12 years. Observe for side effects and maintain hydration. Assess relief of symptoms. If CNS symptoms occur, may require adjustment of behavior, e.g., skate boarding, bike riding, and other activities requiring mental alertness. Chewing sugarless gum or sucking on sugarless candy may relieve dry mouth.

**Laboratory Test Interferences:** May suppress reactions to skin testing, discontinue drug 4 days before testing.

**Storage Requirements:** Store at 15 to 30°C (59 to 86°F), in tight, light-resistant containers.

# ☐ TERPIN HYDRATE
(ter'pin)

**Combination Products:** Terpin hydrate with codeine; terpin hydrate with dextromethorphan hydrobromide (Terphan); terpin hydrate with codeine sulfate (Prunicodeine)

**Classification:** antitussive; expectorant

## Available Preparations:
- 85 mg/5 ml oral elixir
- elixir and solution are available in combination products

**Action and Use:** Appears to act by directly stimulating secretory glands of respiratory tract to increase respiratory tract fluid. Efficiency of this drug as an expectorant is not established. Used as vehicle for antitussive of codeine and dextromethorphan. Alcohol content 42.5%.

## Routes and Dosage:
*PO:* Dosage for children under 1 year must be individualized by physician
- 1 to 4 years: 20 to 25 mg 3 to 4 times per day
- 5 to 9 years: 40 to 45 mg 3 to 4 times per day
- 10 to 12 years: 85 mg 3 to 4 times per day
- over 12 years: 170 mg 3 to 4 times per day or 200 mg every 4 hours. (Maximum dosage 1.2 g/day)

**Contraindications and Precautions:** Pregnancy category C. Due to high alcohol content it should not be used for self-medication in those under 12 years. Contraindicated in hypersensitivity to drug, peptic ulcer, diabetes mellitus.

## Side Effects:
*GI:* nausea, vomiting

## Nursing Implications:
*Assess:* cough: type, characteristics, and frequency.
*Administer: PO:* Taking with food may decrease epigastric distress. Combination products containing codeine classified as Schedule V drug.
*Monitor:* Drug should not be used when coughing is necessary to remove sputum from lungs as immediately postoperatively or for infrequent coughs. Monitor response to medication. Maintain hydration for age group.
*Patient Teaching:* Take drug only as prescribed. Children under 12 years should be given this drug *only* under physician's care due to very high alcohol content. Carefully measurement to avoid overdosage. A cough that lasts longer than 1 week should be evaluated by a physician. Humidifiers: avoiding inhalation of irritants such as smoke, cleaners, dust, and others may aid in cough depression. Do not consume alcohol while on this drug.

**Storage Requirements:** Store at 15 to 30°C (59 to 86°F) in tight container.

---

□ **TETRACAINE**                                                    (tet′ra-caine)
**HYDROCHLORIDE**

(Anacel, Pontocaine)

**Classification:** anesthetic, ophthalmic (local)

**Available Preparations:** 0.5% drops and ointment for ophthalmic administration

**Action and Use:** Local, short-acting anesthesia that inhibits the initiation and transmission of nerve impulses in the neuronal membrane. Used to anesthetize eye for tonometry, gonioscopy, the removal of foreign bodies or sutures. A topical preparation of tetracaine, adrenalin, and cocaine (TAC) is sometimes used in children.

**Routes and Dosage:**
*Ophthalmic:*
- Drops: Instill 1 to 2 drops of a 0.5% solution just before procedure
- Ointment: Pediatric dosage is not established

**Absorption and Fate:** Absorbed rapidly after instillation. Onset of action: about 15 seconds; duration: 10 to 20 minutes (average 15 minutes or longer).

**Contraindications and Precautions:** Pregnancy category C. Contraindicated if intolerant of ester-type local anesthetics (benzocaine, procaine, etc), PABA, or parabens. Use with caution in ocular inflammation, infection, or plasma cholinesterase deficiency.

**Side Effects:**
*Skin:* rash, drying and cracking if drug contacts skin, especially fingertips. *Sensory:* stinging, burning, conjunctival redness (may occur in 30 seconds after application); immediate hypersensitivity reaction (rare): diffuse epithelial keratitis, sloughing of necrotic epithelium, corneal filaments, iritis. *Other:* (rare) systemic toxicity, blurred vision, dizziness, muscle twitching, convulsions, CNS stimulation or depression, increased sweating, weakness, and irregular heatbeat.

**Nursing Implications:**
*Administer: Ophthalmic:* Do not use solution if cloudy or contains crystals. For instillation, see Part I.

*Monitor:* Observe for symptoms of hypersensitivity. Protect child's eye from injury as the cornea is anesthetized and the blink reflex is temporarily absent. Delay in corneal epithelial healing can occur with prolonged usage.

*Patient Teaching:* Instruct child not to rub eye after instillation because he could cause a corneal abrasion. Blink reflex is temporarily eliminated.

**Drug Interactions:** Cholinesterase inhibitors may inhibit metabolism of tetracaine, increasing the anesthetic effect and risks of toxicity. Drug interferes with the antibacterial activity of sulfonamides. Wait 30 minutes after tetracaine dosage before instilling sulfonamide in the eye.

**Laboratory Test Interferences:** This drug may inhibit the growth of certain organisms, altering cultures taken for eye infections. Prevent by using new, previously unopened bottle before culture.

**Storage Requirements:** Store at 15 to 30°C (59 to 86°F) in tightly closed containers. Protect from light and freezing.

---

## □ TETRACYCLINE HYDROCHLORIDE                    (tet-ra-sye'kleen)

(Achromycin, Achromycin V, Amer-Tet, Bicycline, Brodspec, Cefracycline, Centet-250, Cycline, Cyclopar, Maso-Cycline, Medicycline, Neo-Tetrine, Novotetra, Panmycin, Sarocycline, Scotrex, Sumycin, Tetracyn, Tetra-C, Tetraclor, Tetra-Co, Tetracyn, Tetralan, Tetram, Tetramax, Tetralean, Trexin, Tetracap, Topicycline)

**Combination Products:** Tetracycline hydrochloride with amphotericin B (Mysteclin-F); tetracycline hydrochloride with procaine hydrochloride

**Classification:** antiinfective, tetracycline

**Available Preparations:**
- 125 mg/5 ml oral suspension
- 250, 500-mg film-coated tablets
- 100, 250, 500-mg capsules
- 250, 500 mg for parenteral administration
- 1% suspension and ointment ophthalmic application
- 0.22% suspension, 3% ointment for topical application

**Action and Use:** Inhibits protein synthesis by blocking binding of 30S ribosomal subunit of susceptible organism. Active against variety of gram-positive organisms (staphylococci, streptococci, pneumococci, *Clostridia*); gram-negative organisms (meningococci, gonococci, *Haemophilus influenzae*,

*Escherichia coli, Enterobacter, Klebsiella*). High percentage (10 to 40%) of gram-negative organisms are resistant to drug.

**Routes and Dosage:** Not recommended in children under 8 years
*PO:* over 8 years: 25 to 50 mg/kg/day equally divided doses every 6 hours or 0.6 to 1.2 g/m²/day
*IM:* Over 8 years: 15 to 25 mg/kg/day in 2 to 3 divided doses. (Maximum single daily injection is 250 mg)
*IV:* over 8 years: 12 mg/kg/day in 2 divided doses but may be increased to 10 to 20 mg/kg/day depending on severity of infection
*Ophthalmic:*
- Prophylaxis Neonatal Gonococcal Ophthalmic: instill 0.5 to 2 cm strip ointment or 1 to 2 drops suspension into conjunctival sac within 1 hour after delivery
- Ocular Infections: Instill 0.5 to 2 cm strip ointment or 1 to 2 drops suspension into conjunctival sac 2 to 4 times per day
*Topical:*
- Solution: Safe use of Topicycline under 11 years not established. Acne: applied to cleansed skin morning and evening
- Ointment: Apply sparingly to cleansed infected area 2 to 3 times/day

**Absorption and Fate:** Absorption: 75 to 80% drug from GI tract; IM poorly and erratically; topical preparations virtually none, unless used in excess. Drug distributed to most body tissues and fluids; concentrated in bone, liver, spleen, tumors, teeth. Peak level: 2 to 4 hours. Half-life: 6 to 12 hours, reduced in renal impairment. Excreted primarily unchanged by urine and feces.

**Contraindications and Precautions:** Pregnancy category D; not recommended during last half of pregnancy or lactation. American Academy of Pediatrics recommends this drug only be used under unusual circumstances in children under 9 years of age. Causes skeletal retardation in infants and neonates and permanent staining (yellow gray to brown) of deciduous and permanent teeth. Contraindicated in hypersensitivities to drug, sulfite allergies. Use caution in renal or hepatic function impairment, diabetes insipidus.

**Side Effects:**
*CNS:* dizziness, vertigo, ataxia, drowsiness, fatigue, increased **intracranial pressure** and bulging fontanels in infants. *CV:* pericarditis. *GI:* nausea, vomiting, diarrhea, loose stools, flatulence, anorexia, epigastric distress, stomatitis, glossitis, dysphagia, black hairy tongue, esophageal ulceration, oral candidiasis, **pseudomembranous colitis**, **staphyloccocal enterocolitis**. *Hepatic:* **hepatotoxicity** (IV dosages over 2 g). *GU:* vaginal candidiasis, increased BUN. *Skin:* photosensitivity, maculopapular, erythematous rashes, urticaria, onycholysis, discoloration of nails; Topical: local burning, stinging, treated areas will fluoresce under ultraviolet light; Ophthalmic: lacrimation, burning, foreign body sensation. *Hemic:* leukocytosis, neutropenia, eosinophilia. *Other:* Local: IM pain and induration, IV thrombophlebitis; skeletal retardation and tooth staining in young children.

## Nursing Implications:

*Assess:* Obtain baseline renal, hepatic, and hematological data if long-term therapy anticipated. Obtain cultures before therapy.

*Administer:* Check for outdated drug, can cause nephrotoxicity. *PO:* Give on empty stomach 1 hour before or 2 hours after meals; food or dairy products decrease adsorption by 50% or more. Shake suspension well. Regular tablets can be crushed and capsules taken apart, mixed with small amount of food or fluid. Give with as much water as child will take after tablets and capsules to prevent esophageal irritation. If child has reflux, do not give dosage just before bedtime to prevent esophageal irritation. *IM:* Rarely used because of erratic absorption and pain upon injection. *IV:* Parenteral preparations for IM and IV not interchangeable, make sure have correct form (IM contains **procaine HCl**). Discard any solutions that are dark or cloudy. Reconstitute 250 mg with 5 ml sterile water for injection. Do not give IV push. Dilute with at least 100 to 1000 ml of compatible IV solution. Minimum dilution is 10 mg/ml infused over 40 to 60 minutes. Do not exceed rate of 100 mg in 5 minutes. Compatible with $D_5W$, $D_5W/NS$, $D_{10}W$, NS, LR, and others. Drug unstable in acid solutions, has many incompatibilities, avoid mixing with other drugs. *Ophthalmic:* See Part I for instillation of drops or ointments. After given for prophylaxis ophthalmia neonatorum, do not flush medication from eye, excess may be wiped away. Use new tube or single unit for each neonate. *Topical:* Apply sparingly as thin film to cleansed skin.

*Monitor:* IV can cause thrombophlebitis; start oral therapy as soon as possible to replace IV administration. Assess hepatic, renal, and hematologic function periodically. Assess for side effects and report immediately to physician. Superinfections may occur. Maintain fluid intake for age group.

*Patient Teaching:* Teach proper administration, instillation and application of prescribed preparations. Maintain good oral hygiene, and inspect mouth daily for signs of superinfections. Importance of following dosage schedule and taking for entire duration even if symptoms dissipate. Inform physician of any side effects. Avoid exposure to sun or sunlamps. Do not take outdated medication. Do not take OTC medications without contacting physician.

**Drug Interactions:** Tetracycline readily chelates with divalent or trivalent cations, thus drugs containing aluminum, calcium, magnesium, iron, zinc (e.g., antacids, iron preparations, mineral supplements, laxatives) should not be given concurrently but 3 hours after or 2 hours before. May potentiate effects of oral anticoagulants. Corticosteroids may mask signs of superinfections. Antidiarrheal agents with kaolin, pectin, or bismuth subsalicylate impair absorption of oral form of this drug. Methoxyflurane anesthesia used with tetracycline may produce fatal nephrotoxicity.

**Laboratory Test Interference:** False-positive urinary catecholamines may result. False-negative urine glucose with Clinistix and TesTape. IV tetracycline containing ascorbic acid can cause false-positive urine glucose with Benedict's and Clinitest.

**Storage Requirements:** Store at 15 to 30°C in tight containers. Preparations darken on exposure to sunlight and moist air. Reconstituted parenteral forms stable for 24 hours at room temperature.

---

## □ THEOPHYLLINE
(thee-off'i-lin)

(Accurbron, Aerolate, Aquaphyllin, Asmalix, Bronkodyl, Duraphyl, Elixicon, Elixomin, Elixophyllin, Lanophyllin, Liquophylline, Lixolin, Lodrane, PMS Theophylline, Pulmophylline, Quibron-T, Respbid, Slo-Bid, Slo-Phyllin, Somophyllin, Somophyllin-12, Sustaire, Theobron SR, Theo-Dur Sprinkle, Theo-Dur, Theo-24, Theolair, Theolixir, Theon, Theophyl, Theospan, Uniphyl)

## □ THEOPHYLLINE SODIUM GLYCINATE

(Acet-Am, Synophylate)

**Combination Products:** Available in combination with antitussives, expectorants, sedatives, and sympathomimetics

**Classification:** spasmolytic, xanthine bronchodilator

**Available Preparations:**
- 110 mg/5 ml oral elixir
- 27 mg/5 ml, 50 mg/5 ml oral solution
- 100, 125, 200, 250, 300-mg tablets
- 100, 200, 250, 300, 400, 450, 500-mg extended-release tablets
- 100-mg chewable tablet
- 100, 200, 250-mg oral capsules
- 50, 60, 65, 75, 100, 125, 130, 200, 250, 260, 300-mg extended-release oral capsules
- 0.4, 0.8, 1.6, 2, 3.2, 4 mg/ml all in 5% dextrose for parenteral administration

**Action and Use:** Methyl xanthine derivative that is an enzyme inhibitor of phosphodiesterase, which results in increased concentrations of cyclic AMP, causing relaxation of bronchial smooth muscles. It may have an effect on adenosine receptors, intracellular calcium, and protaglandin antagonism. Used for the symptomatic relief of bronchial asthma, reversible bronchospasm of chronic bronchitis and emphysema. Also used in treatment of Cheyne-Stokes respiration, apnea, and bradycardia in prematures and bronchospasms associated with cystic fibrosis. Theophylline sodium glycinate contains 49% anhydrous theophylline. Liquid preparations vary in content of sugar and alcohol with different brands. Some preparations are sugar-free and alcohol-free.

## Routes and Dosage:
*PO:*

Bronchospasm: Loading Dosage: 0.8 mg/kg/dose to obtain each 2 mg/L desired increase in serum theophylline level

Maintenance:

- birth: to 2 months: 3 to 6 mg/kg/day in equally divided doses every 8 hours
- 2 to 6 months: 6 to 15 mg/kg/day in equally divided doses every 6 hours
- 6 to 12 months: 15 to 22 mg/kg/day in equally divided doses every 6 hours
- 1 to 9 years: 20 to 22 mg/kg/day in equally divided doses every 6 hours. (Maximum dosage 24 mg/kg/day)
- 9 to 12 years: 16 to 20 mg/kg/day in equally divided doses every 6 hours. (Maximum dosage 20 mg/kg/day)
- 12 to 16 years: 16 to 18 mg/kg/day in equally divided doses every 6 hours. (Maximum dosage 18 mg/kg/day)
- over 16 years (adult): 13 mg/kg/day in equally divided doses every 6 hours. (Maximum dosage 13 mg/kg/day or 900 mg/day)

The same dosage is used in extended-release preparations but drug is given every 8 to 12 hours

*PO, IV:* (Dosage not well established and must be individualized.)

Neonatal Apnea: Loading Dosage: 1 **mg/kg for each 2 µg/ml increase in serum theophylline level desired**

Maintenance:

- prematures at birth (gestational age up to postnatal age of 40 weeks): 1 mg/kg every 12 hours
- term neonates at birth or 40 weeks postconception (up to 4 weeks postnatal): 1 to 2 mg/kg every 8 hours
- 4 to 8 weeks postnatal: 1 to 3 ml/kg every 6 hours

*IV:*

Bronchospasm: Loading Dosage: 4.7 mg/kg for 1 dose only

Maintenance:

- 6 months to 9 years: 1.2 mg/kg/hour for 12 hours, then 1 mg/kg/hr
- 9 to 16 years: 1 mg/kg/hour for 12 hours, then 0.8 mg/kg
- over 16 years (nonsmoker): 0.7 mg/kg/hour for 12 hours, then 0.5 mg/kg/hr

**Dosage is individualized and should be based on serum concentrations**.

**Absorption and Fate:** Peak level: PO, liquid 1 hour, plain tablets 2 hours, chewable tablets 1 to 1.5 hours, enteric-coated tablets 5 hours, extended-release tablets or capsules 4 to 7 hours; IV within 30 to 60 minutes. Mean half-life: neonates and prematures 24+ hours; over 6 months 3.7 + 1.1 hours. Half-life decreased by fever or smoking. Half-life increased by alcoholism, decreased hepatic or renal function, congestive heart failure, or some antibiotics. Therapeutic level: neonatal apnea, 5 to 15 μg/ml, bronchodilator 10 to 20 μg/ml. Excreted in urine.

**Contraindications and Precautions:** Pregnancy category C. Distributed in breast milk and can cause irritability in nursing infants. Dosage in those younger than 1 year must be individualized and used with caution. Contraindicated in hypersensitivity to drug or xanthines (caffeine), preexisting cardiac arrhythmias. Use caution in children, peptic ulcer, hyperthyroidism, diabetes mellitus, renal or hepatic disease, hypertension, cor pulmonale, compromised cardiac or circulatory function.

**Side Effects:**
**CNS:** headaches, restlessness, dizziness, irritability, insomnia, muscle twitching, **seizures**. **CV:** palpitations, **sinus tachycardia**, extrasystoles, flushing, **marked hypotension, circulatory failure, cardiac arrest**. **GI:** nausea, vomiting (due in part to CNS stimulation), bitter aftertaste, epigastric pain, anorexia, diarrhea. **Resp:** tachypnea. **Skin:** urticaria, exfoliative dermatitis. **Other:** hyperglycemia, inappropriate ADH; Local: redness, pain at IV site.

**Nursing Implications:**
**Assess:** Assess respiratory status and vital signs. Obtain weight; dosage based on lean body mass, drug not distributed to fatty tissues. If child on any form of theophylline, ask when last dose was given and it may be necessary to obtain drug level before starting this drug.
**Administer: PO:** Food delays the absorption of this drug, but when GI irritation occurs it can be taken with food. Follow drug with at least full glass of water. Lowering dosage may be necessary if GI irritation occurs. Dosage individualized. Oral dosage can also be given by nasogastric tube. Plain tablets can be crushed and mixed with small amounts of food or fluids. Extended-release tablets should not be crushed or chewed. Chewable form is to be chewed, not swallowed whole. **IV:** (Aminophylline is the preferred form of parenteral theophylline.) Crystallization may occur if drug solution falls below 8.0 pH, do not use if crystals visualized. Make sure you have IV form before usage and verify theophylline content. Drug is commercially diluted with dextrose; do not add any drugs or fluids to this injection; dosages are titrated to specific levels. If added as piggyback to other IV fluids, stop other fluid flow during infusion and do not administer through blood. **Administering faster than 25 mg/minute may result in circulatory failure or excessive serum concentrations of drug**. Administration rate is usually over 25 to 30 minutes. Continuous infusion delivered at rate of 0.9 to 1.5 mg/kg/hour. Do not use continuous infusions for neonates. Incompatible with acid solutions, alkali labile drugs (penicillin G, isoproterenol, thiamine), vitamin B complex, vitamin B with C, insulin, phenytoin, methylprednisolone and many others. Check with pharmacist prior to mixing with any drug.

*Monitor:* Carefully monitor respiratory status. Theophylline preparations have low therapeutic index; thus, optimum serum levels between 10 and 20 μg/ml should be maintained. Peak level of 6 to 10 μg/ml for neonatal apnea. Toxic symptoms are more likely to occur when serum drug level is over 20 μg/ml. Drug levels need to be monitored frequently. If theophylline levels rise above 20 μg/ml, notify physician at once. With drug serum level above this dosage adjustment is necessary. With intermittent infusions, monitor drug serum levels within 4 to 6 hours of last IV dosage. Assess vital signs and I & O during IV infusion. Monitor IV site for pain and inflammation. Change IV tubing every 24 hours.

*Patient Teaching:* Report any CNS, cardiac, or GI side effects to physician. Monitor respiratory response. Maintain hydration for weight. Do not use any OTC drug that may contain ephedrine, which can cause excessive CNS symptoms. Take drug as directed and take at same time of day every day to maintain blood levels of drug. Drug is meant for control of asthma under physician's supervision. It is important that child and parent understand asthma and its pharmacological treatment.

**Drug Interactions:** Phenytoin and barbiturates decrease this drug's blood levels. This drug decreases therapeutic effectiveness of lithium and furosemide. Beta-adrenergic blockers (especially propranolol and nadolol) may induce bronchospasms when used with this drug. Erythromycin, cimetidine, troleandomycin decrease the hepatic clearance of this drug. This drug may enhance the toxic potential of cardiac glycosides. Adrenergics may increase CNS stimulation. Lithium decreases effectiveness of theophylline and phenobarbital may increase the metabolism of this drug.

**Food Interactions:** Charcoal-broiled foods may delay theophylline clearance and half-life by 50%, because of high polycyclic content.

**Laboratory Test Interference:** Produces false-positive serum uric acids with Bittner or colorimetric method.

**Storage Requirements:** Store at 15 to 30°C (59 to 86°F), protect from freezing. Exposure of some liquid preparations to refrigeration may cause crystallization to occur but they will redissolve upon reaching room temperature.

---

# □ THIAMINE

(Betalin S, Bewon, Biamine, Vitamin B-1)

**Classification:** nutritional supplement

**Available Preparations:**
- ■ 5, 10, 25, 50, 100, 250, 500-mg tablets

- 2.25 mg/5 ml elixir
- 100, 200 mg/ml vials for parenteral use

**Action and Use:** This water-soluble B vitamin combines with ATP and the resultant coenzyme is active in carbohydrate metabolism. Crucial as coenzyme in normal function of brain, nerves, muscles, and heart. Deficiency is manifested by beriberi and Wernicke's encephalopathy, but may present with a wide range of symptoms due to the effect on carbohydrate, protein, and fat metabolism. Used in treatment of deficiency syndrome and as a supplement in those with conditions such as hyperthyroidism and malabsorption. Thiamine deficiency rarely occurs alone.

**Routes and Dosages:**
*PO:*
- Nutritional Supplement: infant: 0.3 to 0.5 mg/day
                               child: 0.5 to 1.0 mg/day
- Deficiency: 10 to 50 mg/day in divided doses
- Beriberi: infant: 10 mg/day

*IM, IV(slow):* Severe Deficiency in Critical Illness: 10 to 25 mg

**Absorption and Fate:** Well absorbed from GI tract principally in duodenum. Absorption slowed but not decreased with meals; amount decreased with alcohol ingestion. Normal absorption dependent on active transport. Distributed throughout body tissues and present in breast milk. Metabolized in liver and excreted in urine.

**Contraindications and Precautions:** Pregnancy category X. Contraindicated in prior hypersensitivity to thiamine.

**Side Effects:**
*Skin:* urticaria, pruritus. *Other:* wheezing, weakness, cyanosis, **hypotension** and other symptoms of **anaphylaxis** with IV administration.

**Nursing Implications:**
*Assess:* Obtain diet history; be alert for intake of raw fish that can decrease thiamine absorption. Prior history of hypersensitivity to thiamine injection is ascertained. A test dose may be administered by intradermal skin test before parenteral injection.
RDAs of thiamine are:
- 0 to 6 months: 0.3 mg
- 6 to 12 months: 0.5 mg
- 1 to 3 years: 0.7 mg
- 4 to 6 years: 0.9 mg
- 7 to 10 years: 1.2 mg
- 11 to 18 years, males: 1.4 mg
- 11 to 18 years, females: 1.1 mg
- pregnancy: 1.4 mg

■ lactation: 1.5 mg

**Administer:** **IV:** Given slowly. Incompatible with carbonates, citrates, barbiturates; unstable in sodium bisulfite solution, therefore, should be used immediately if added to these solutions.

**Monitor:** A common deficiency state that can occur within 10 days of dietary deficiency includes depression, decreased concentration, disinterest; monitor those at risk. Monitor the symptoms of deficiency closely as improvement in neuritis, heart failure, and other symptoms shown within hours of IV administration. Cardiovascular and GI complications will completely improve with treatment; neurological symptoms will improve but some residual may remain with prolonged or severe deficiency. Can cause lactic acidosis so pH should be monitored.

**Patient Teaching:** Megadoses are not recommended. Dietary teaching is appropriate. Dietary sources of thiamine include legumes, potatoes, yeast, enriched cereals, whole grains, meats, nuts. Increased need for calories increases need for thiamine.

**Drug Interactions:** May increase effects of neuromuscular blocking agents.

**Laboratory Test Interferences:** False-positive uric acid and urobilinogen with Ehrlich's test. Large doses may interfere with serum theophylline measurement.

**Storage Requirements:** Store tightly closed in light-resistant containers at 15 to 30°C (59 to 86°F). Protect injectable solution and elixir from freezing.

---

## □ THIOGUANINE OR TG OR 6-TG OR 6-THIOGUANINE

(thye-oh-gwah'neen)

**Classification:** antineoplastic, antimetabolite

**Available Preparations:** 40-mg tablets

**Action and Use:** This antimetabolite is converted intracellularly to ribonucleotides that block synthesis of purine and thus interferes with DNA manufacture. Acts in S phase of cell division. Used to treat acute and chronic myelogenous leukemia, lymphocytic leukemia, and chronic myelogenous leukemia.

**Routes and Dosages:** PO
**PO:** 2 mg/kg/day; increase with caution to 3 mg/kg/day if no remission in 4 weeks; alternatively 75 to 100 mg/m²/day

Combination Therapy: 75 to 200 mg/m²/day in 1 to 2 doses until remission is achieved, then 2 mg/kg/day as maintenance therapy; alternatively 30 to 60 mg/m²/day for 14 days.

**Absorption and Fate:** Variable absorption from GI tract. Incorporated into bone marrow cells; not present in therapeutic levels in CNS. Rapidly metabolized in the liver and excreted in the urine. Peak level in 8 hours. Half-life biphasic with 25 minutes initially and 6 hours in the terminal stage.

**Contraindications and Precautions:** Pregnancy category X. Avoid use in pregnancy and lactation. Potential for fetal effects when father takes the drug should be considered. Not to be used if prior therapy with the drug was ineffective, or in infections such as chicken pox or herpes zoster. Use with caution in infections and decrease dosage when used in the patient with renal or hepatic disease.

## Side Effects:

*GI:* nausea, vomiting, anorexia; **stomatitis** and **diarrhea** may be symptoms of toxicity. *Hepatic:* jaundice, elevated serum hepatic enzymes. *GU:* hyperuricemia. *Skin:* rash (uncommon). *Hemic:* **leukopenia** after 2 to 4 weeks, thrombocytopenia, anemia; **myelosuppression** (major toxic effect).

## Nursing Implications:

*Assess:* Establish baseline CBC, vital signs, hepatic function.
*Administer:* This drug has potentially severe toxic effects and should be given only under the supervision of a physician with training and experience in cancer chemotherapy. The drug's potential for toxic effects on health-care personnel, as well as patients, necessitates careful handling during preparation and administration. Increase fluid intake to avoid hyperuricemia. *PO:* Tablets only are available. An oral suspension may be prepared from them by the pharmacist.
*Monitor:* Watch patient for signs of infection such as fever, sore throat. Observe for bruising. Observe oral membranes and stools for signs of GI toxic effects. CBC is done at least weekly. Rapidly falling leukocytes necessitate alteration of therapy. Protect patient from sources of infection; instituting reverse isolation if needed. Liver function studies, such as BUN, serum transaminase, alkaline phosphatase, bilirubin, are done at least weekly; abnormalities or jaundice necessitate stopping drug. Creatinine, LDH, and uric acid levels may also be done.
*Patient Teaching:* The patient must report signs of GI toxicity (stomatitis and diarrhea) and hepatotoxicity (jaundice) immediately. Observe for signs of infection such as fever, sore throat, bruising, malaise. Avoid persons with infection such as colds, chicken pox, influenza. Return for follow-up care as scheduled.

**Drug Interactions:** Although similar to 6-mercaptopurine, this drug does not need to be reduced in dosage when allopurinol is given concurrently. Depresses immune response to immunization. Live virus vaccines must not be given, nor oral polio vaccine to those in close contact with the patient on this drug due to the chance of infection with a virus; these vaccines are delayed until at least 3 months after chemotherapy when the patient is in remission.

**Storage Requirements:** Store in tightly closed containers between 15 and 30°C (59 and 86°F).

---

## □ THIABENDAZOLE

(thye-a-ben'da-zole)

(Mintezol)

**Classification:** anthelmintic

**Available Preparations:**
- 500 mg/5 ml oral suspension
- 500-mg chewable tablet

**Action and Use:** Mechanism is known; has been shown to interfere with enyzmatic activity of the parasite. Active against visceral and cutaneous creeping eruption (larva migrans), hookworm (ancylostome), roundworm (*Ascaris lumbricoides*), pinworm (*Enterobius vermicularis*), whipworm (*Trichuris trichiura*), and threadworm (*Strongyloides stercoralis*).

**Routes and Dosage:**
*PO:* under 70 kg: 25 mg/kg or 650 mg/m$^2$
over 70 kg: 1.5 g. (Maximum dosage 3 g/day)
- Strongyloidiasis: above dosage 2 times per day for 2 days
- Cutaneous Larva Migrans: above dosage 2 times per day for 2 to 5 days
- Visceral Larva Migrans: above dosage 2 times per day for 7 days
- Trichinosis: above dosage daily 2 times per day for 2 to 4 days
- Ascariasis, Hookworm, Trichuriasis: above dosage daily twice a day for 2 days

**Absorption and Fate:** Rapidly and well absorbed from GI tract. Peak level 1 hour. Metabolized in liver. Excreted in urine (90%) and feces (5%) as unchanged drug and metabolites.

**Contraindications and Precautions:** Pregnancy category C. Use with caution during lactation. Use with children under 13.6 kg only if benefits outweigh risks. Contraindicated in hypersensitivity to drug. Use with caution in hepatic or renal dysfunction, severe malnutrition, anemia, or when vomiting might be dangerous to child.

**Side Effects:**
*CNS:* dizziness, headache, drowsiness, weariness, giddiness, tinnitus, irritability, seizures. *CV:* hypotension, bradycardia. *GI:* anorexia, nausea, vomiting,

diarrhea, epigastric distress. *Hepatic:* increase SGOT, jaundice, **parenchymal liver damage**. *GU:* malodorous urine, crystalluria, hematuria, enuresis. *Skin:* rash, pruritus, erythema multiforme. *Hemic:* leukopenia. *Sensory:* abnormal sensation in eyes, blurred vision, drying of mucous membranes of mouth, nose, eye. *Other:* flushing, **hyperglycemia, lymphadenopathy**.

## Nursing Implications:

*Assess:* Obtain pinworm test during night or when child sleeping; then worms migrate to perianal area to deposit their eggs. Commercial test kit available or can use scotch tape with sticky side to outside of tongue blade. Obtain test by carefully separating buttocks and pressing tape to anal area. Wash hands well after test. Other parasites are diagnosed through stool samples; follow your agency procedure for collection. Sputum samples may be checked for strongyloidiasis.

*Administer:* Tablet chewed or can be crushed and mixed with small amount of food to administer, but do not swallow tablet whole. Check for loose teeth before giving chewable tablet. Suspension, shake well and measure with calibrated measuring device. Give after meal. Laxatives, special diets, or enemas are not required.

*Monitor and Patient Teaching:* Side effects usually mild occurring 3 to 4 hours after taking drug and lasting up to 2 to 8 hours. Drug can alter mental alertness and CNS; adjust activities accordingly. Pinworms: Highly contagious, female can deposit 17,000 eggs a night, then dies; ova mature within 3 to 8 hours. All members of family should be treated. All bed linen, towels, undergarments, and personal clothes should be washed. Carpets should be vacuumed, floors damp mopped, toilets disinfected daily. Infected child should sleep alone with tight-fitting underwear or diapers. Cut nails and keep clean. Change linens, bedclothes, and underwear daily. This disease does not indicate family has unclean home; however, good hand washing is important to prevent spread of disease. Hookworm: Avoid going barefoot. Pica may contribute to this disease. Proper disposal of human sewage. Roundworm: Common where human wastes are used as fertilizer. Occasionally worm may migrate to mouth, nose, or rectum. Whipworm: Infestation from contaminated ground. Good hand washing and washing raw vegetables and fruits. Cutaneous Larva Migrans: Because child is infested from infected dog or cat, animals, especially puppies, should be treated for worms early in life. With all infestations, teach parent how to obtain stool culture.

**Drug Interactions:** This drug may compete with other drugs metabolized in liver, therefore, those drugs should be used with caution.

**Storage Requirements:** Store at 15 to 30°C (50 to 86°F) in tight container.

---

☐ **THIORIDAZINE**                    (thye-or-rid′a-zeen)

(Mellaril)

**Classification:** antipsychotic, phenothiazine

## Available Preparations:
- 25, 100 mg/5 ml suspension
- 30, 100 mg/ml concentrated solution
- 10, 15, 25, 50, 100, 150, 200-mg tablets
- 10, 15, 25, 50, 100, 150, 200-mg film-coated tablets

**Action and Use:** This piperidine derivative of phenothiazine is similar in action to chlorpromazine. It blocks dopamine receptors in the CNS and inhibits the chemoreceptor trigger zone in the medulla. Has strong anticholinergic and sedative effects and weak extrapyramidal and antiemetic effects. Used as an antipsychotic agent, particularly in combative, aggressive children with attention-deficit disorder.

## Routes and Dosages:
*PO:* 2 to 12 years: 0.5 to 3 mg/kg/day or 10 mg BID or TID; initial dose may be 25 mg BID or TID if child is hospitalized and in severe psychosis. Dosage is gradually increased until desired behavior is seen; maximum dose is 3 mg/kg/day.

**Absorption and Fate:** Well absorbed from GI tract. Widely distributed in the body and crosses the blood-brain barrier; present in high concentrations in brain. Highly bound to plasma proteins. Extensively metabolized by the liver and excreted principally in urine. Takes about 5 days to achieve full therapeutic effect. Multiphasic metabolic pattern with early half-life 4 to 10 hours and late half-life 26 to 36 hours.

**Contraindications and Precautions:** Pregnancy category C. Contraindicated in children under 2 years, in those with prior hypersensitivity to phenothiazines, often manifested as jaundice; those with CNS depression, comatose, subcortical damage, bone marrow suppression, and tablets containing yellow dye #5 are not to be given to those with yellow dye #5 (tartrazine) hypersensitivity. Cautious use in cardiovascular disease, seizure disorders, hepatic or renal disease, glaucoma, children with acute illness or dehydration, hypocalcemia, previous reaction to insulin, and in those taking drugs, such as antineoplastics, with which nausea and vomiting may signal toxic effects.

## Side Effects:
*CNS:* Dystonic reactions especially in children with acute illness or dehydration, manifested by neck spasm, torticollis, rigid back, opisthotonos, tics, TMJ dysfunction, tongue spasm, difficult swallowing, sweating, fever; effects in 24 to 48 hours of dose and relief obtained with anticholinergics. Motor restlessness especially in children with acute illness or dehydration, manifested by foot tapping, excess movement, insomnia; effects generally in 2 to 3 days after therapy begins. Other CNS effects include tardive dyskinesia, neuroleptic malignant syndrome, drowsiness, restlessness, insomnia, depression, weakness, headache, **seizures**, hyperthermia, hypothermia. *CV:* hypotension, tachycardia, syncope, **EKG changes;** effects usually end in 30 to 120 minutes. *GI:* ano-

rexia, constipation, dry mouth, diarrhea, paralytic ileus. ***Respiratory:*** **laryngospasm**, bronchospasm, anaphylaxis (rare). ***Hepatic:*** **cholestatic jaundice** after 2 to 4 weeks of therapy; effect seen in some newborns whose mothers received phenothiazines in pregnancy; elevated bilirubin, alkaline phosphatase, transaminases. ***Skin:*** pruritus, photosensitivity, urticaria, dermatitis, hyperpigmentation; contact dermatitis upon skin contact with solutions. ***Hemic:*** **agranulocytosis, leukopenia, eosinophilia, thrombocytopenia, aplastic anemia**; all rare but potentially fatal. ***Endocrine:*** glycosuria, gynecomastia. ***Sensory:*** ocular changes.

## Nursing Implications:

***Assess:*** CBC, liver function studies are done before therapy. Establish baseline vital signs. Physical assessment to rule out acute illness and dehydration. ***Administer:*** Avoid contact of solutions with skin. ***PO:*** Give with food or fluid to decrease gastric upset. Tablet may be crushed and added to small amount of food. Concentrate is mixed just before giving in juice, milk, water, or carbonated drink.

***Monitor:*** Vital sign checks especially during initial therapy. CBC periodically during long-term therapy. Weekly urine bilirubin during first month and serum bilirubin, alkaline phosphatase, transaminase regularly. Take temperature. Monitor urine glucose. Periodic eye examinations if on long-term therapy. Monitor hearing if patient also is on ototoxic drugs; monitor toxic effects of antineoplastic drugs if patient on concurrent therapy with drugs whose toxicity is manifested by nausea and vomiting, as above effects may be masked by phenothiazines.

***Patient Teaching:*** Take drug as directed. Drug can alter mental alertness; therefore, avoid driving and adjust activities accordingly. Report continued insomnia or other side effects as they usually decrease with time. Good oral hygiene and nutritious food can decrease some side effects. Urine may turn red in color.

## Drug Interactions: Additive effects with other CNS depressants. It can decrease phenytoin metabolism, has additive hypotensive effects with β blockers, additive effects with tricyclic antidepressants. Phenothiazines reverse effects of epinephrine and lower blood pressure; these two drug should not be given together; effect not seen with norepinephrine or phenylephrine. Phenobarbital increases excretin of the drug. Acute encephalopathy possible when given with lithium.

## Laboratory Test Interferences: False-positive urobilinogen, amylase, uroporphrins, porphobilinogens, 5-hydroxyindolacetic acid, phenylketonuria, pregnancy tests. May elevate serum bilirubin, alkaline phosphatase, transaminase, PBI, other liver function tests.

## Storage Requirements: Store in tightly covered, light-resistant containers at 15 to 30°C (59 to 86°F). Avoid freezing.

# □ **THIOTHIXENE**                    (thye-oh-thix′een)

(Navane)

**Classification:** antipsychotic

## Available Preparations:
- 5 mg/ml oral concentrate solution
- 1, 2, 5, 10, 20-mg capsules
- 2 mg/ml vials for parenteral use
- 10 mg with mannitol for parenteral use

**Action and Use:** Similar in action to phenothiazines. Blocks dopamine receptors in the CNS; acts at the subcortical level; has cholinergic and adrenergic blocking effects on autonomic nervous system. Has sedative, hypotensive, weak anticholinergic, and perhaps antiemetic effects. Used in treatment of psychotic disorders.

## Routes and Dosages:
*PO:* over 12 years: 2 mg TID initially; increased to a maximum of 60 mg/day in 2 to 3 divided doses
*IM:* over 12 years: 4 mg BID to QID; increased to a maximum of 30 mg/day in 2 to 3 divided doses

**Absorption and Fate:** Well absorbed from GI tract and IM injection. Widely distributed in body. Metabolized in the liver and excreted principally in the liver. Onset of action 1 to 6 hours after IM, days to weeks after PO. Remains in the body several weeks after administration. Distribution half-life is 3.5 hours; elimination half-life 34 hours.

**Contraindications and Precautions:** Pregnancy category C. Similar drugs can cause hyperreflexia in infants when mother has taken them during pregnancy. Not approved for use in children under 12 years. Contraindicated in coma, CNS depression, CV collapse, blood dyscrasia, prior hypersensitivity. Cautious use in CV disease, seizure disorder, glaucoma, patients with akathisia, restlessness.

## Side Effects:
*CNS:* Dystonic reactions especially in children with acute illness or dehydration, manifested by neck spasm, torticollis, rigid back, opisthotonos, tics, TMJ dysfunction, tongue spasm, difficult swallowing, sweating, fever; effects in 24 to 48 hours of dose and relief obtained with anticholinergics. Motor restlessness especially in children with acute illness or dehydration, manifested by foot tapping, excess movement, insomnia; effects generally in 2 to 3 days after therapy begins. Drowsiness is common but may improve with continued therapy. Other CNS effects include tardive dyskinesia, neuroleptic malignant syndrome, restlessness, insomnia, depression, weakness, headache, **seizures**, hy-

perthermia, hypothermia. *CV:* hypotension, tachycardia, syncope, **EKG changes**; effects often improve with continued therapy. *GI:* anorexia, constipation, dry mouth, diarrhea, paralytic ileus. *Respiratory:* **laryngospasm, bronchospasm, anaphylaxis** (rare). *Hepatic:* **cholestatic jaundice** after 2 to 4 weeks of therapy; elevated bilirubin, alkaline phosphatase, transaminases. *Skin:* pruritus, photosensitivity, urticaria, dermatitis, hyperpigmentation; contact dermatitis upon skin contact with solutions. *Hemic:* **agranulocytosis, leukopenia, eosinophilia, thrombocytopenia, aplastic anemia**; all rare but potentially fatal. *Endocrine:* glycosuria, gynecomastia, amenorrhea, lactation. *Sensory:* ocular changes.

## Nursing Implications:

*Assess:* CBC, liver function studies are done before therapy. Establish baseline vital signs. Physical assessment to rule out acute illness and dehydration.
*Administer:* Avoid contact of solutions with skin. *PO:* Capsules may be opened and mixed with a small amount of food. Oral concentrate solution should be diluted in a cup of fluid such as water, juice, or carbonated drink.
*IM:* Reconstitute with sterile water for injection. Solution will be stable for 48 hours at room temperature. Give into upper outer quadrant of buttock. Have patient remain supine for at least 30 minutes after administration in case of hypotension.
*Monitor:* Vital sign checks especially during initial therapy. CBC periodically during long-term therapy. Monitor I & O. Weekly urine bilirubin during first month and serum bilirubin, alkaline phosphatase, transaminase regularly. Take temperature. Monitor urine glucose. Periodic eye examinations if on long-term therapy. Monitor hearing if patient also is on ototoxic drugs; monitor toxic effects of antineoplastic drugs if patient on concurrent therapy with drugs whose toxicity is manifested by nausea and vomiting as above effects may be masked by phenothiazines.
*Patient Teaching:* Take drug as directed and return for follow-up care. Avoid driving and operating hazardous machinery. Do not take OTC drugs or alcohol. Use sunscreen if exposed to sunlight.

**Drug Interactions:** Additive effects with other CNS depressants, anticholinergics, antihypertensives.

**Storage Requirements:** Store at 15 to 30°C (59 to 86°F) in tightly closed, light-resistant containers.

---

## ☐ TICARCILLIN DISODIUM

(tye-kar-sill'in)

(Ticaripen, Ticar)

**Classification:** penicillin, extended spectrum

**Available Preparations:** 1, 3, 6, 20, 30 g for parenteral administration

**Action and Use:** Mechanism similar to other penicillins that inhibit cell-wall synthesis in bacteria. Can be inactivated by penicillinase-producing staphylococci, and is primarily used for *Proteus vulgaris, Providencia rettgeri, Morganella morganii, P. Mirabilis, Escherichia coli, Enterobacter*, and *Pseudomonas aeruginosa* strains; may be useful in *Bacteroides* infection with large doses. Used in treatment of infections of GU tract, respiratory tract, intraabdominal, skin, soft tissue, and in septicemia and meningitis. Contains 5.2 to 6.5 mEq of sodium per gram of drug.

### Routes and Dosage:
*IM, IV:* over 1 month, less than 40 kg (uncomplicated UTI): 50 to 100 mg/kg in equally divided doses every 6 or 8 hours
*IV:* Neonates less than 2000 g
   ■ under 7 days: 150 mg/kg/day in equally divided doses every 12 hours
   ■ over 7 days: 225 mg/kg/day in equally divided doses every 8 hours
Neonates over 2000 g
   ■ under 7 days: 225 mg/kg/day in equally divided doses every 8 hours
   ■ over 7 days: 300 mg/kg/day in equally divided doses every 8 hours
   ■ over 1 month: 200 to 300 mg/kg/day equally divided doses every 4 to 6 hours
Note: Dosages based on normal renal function.

**Absorption and Fate:** Distributed in pleura, synovial, peritoneal, sputum, lymph, interstitial, kidneys, bile, and meninges when inflamed. Peak level: neonates IM, 1 hour; older children, 30 to 75 minutes. Peak level IV at the end infusion or within 30 minutes. Half-life: 1.3 to 5.6 hours in neonates, 0.9 hours in children. 45 to 65% bound to plasma proteins. Excreted in urine and feces. Peak serum concentrations 125–150 μg/ml with serum through concentrations 25–50 μg/ml.

**Contraindications and Precautions:** Pregnancy category B. Excreted in breast milk, use caution with lactation. Contraindicated if hypersensitivity to this drug, penicillins, or cephalosporins. Use with caution in sensitivity to multiple allergens, other drugs, renal impairment, bleeding tendencies, or sodium restrictions.

### Side Effects:
*CNS:* neuromuscular irritability, **seizures** (with high serum levels). *GI:* nausea, vomiting, abnormal taste, flatulence, loose stools, diarrhea. *Hepatic:* elevation of SGOT, SGPT, LDH, alkaline phosphatase, bilirubin, **reversible hepatitis** (rare). *GU:* **acute interstitial nephritis** (rare). *Hemic:* **anemia, eosinophilia, thrombocytopenia, leukopenia, neutropenia, abnormal prothrombin time and clotting time** (with high doses). *Other:* Hypersensitivity: skin rashes, pruritus, urticaria, drug fever, **anaphylaxis**; hypernatremia, hypokalemia; Local: IV: pain, vein irritation, phlebitis; IM pain, induration.

### Nursing Implications:
*Assess:* Assess previous allergy drug, penicillins, cephalosporins, other

drugs, or history of allergies. Obtain cultures and sensitivity before treatment, but can start treatment before results. Obtain baseline data on renal, hepatic, hematological, potassium levels if on long-term therapy.

***Administer: IM:*** Reconstitute each gram with 2 ml with sterile water, 0.9% sodium chloride, or 0.5% lidocaine (without epinephrine) for injection. Do not exceed 2 g in any one site. Injection painful, may minimize pain by giving slowly (over 12 to 15 seconds). Do not use bacteriostatic preparations containing benzyl alcohol with neonates. ***IV:*** Reconstitute according to package inserts with sterile or bacteriostatic water. Can give IV push dilution to less than 200 mg/ml and infuse over 10 minutes. Intermittent infusion preferred: dilute to 10 to 50 mg/ml infused over 30 to 120 minutes. Compatible with $D_5W$, $D_5W/0.2\%$ NS, $D_5W/0.5\%NS$, NS, LR. Do not premix with aminoglycosides; avoid mixing with other drugs; infuse separately. Use of large vein with small-bore needle may reduce local IV reactions.

***Monitor:*** Check for hypersensitivity (especially in first 20 minutes of first dosage). Observe IV site for vein irritation and extravasation and change site every 72 hours. Monitor child for hypersensitivity and side effects. Closely observe for symptoms of bleeding; monitor platelet dysfunction and bleeding time especially on long-term therapy. Monitor potassium and sodium levels, renal and hepatic function. Maintain fluid levels for age group. Avoid prolonged use of drug because of overgrowth of nonsusceptible organisms.

**Drug Interactions:** Anticoagulants given with this drug may increase risk of bleeding. Erythromycin, tetracycline, and chloromycetin may decrease effects of ticarcillin. Probenecid increases serum levels of ticarcillin.

**Laboratory Test Interferences:** Increased SGOT and SGPT. Bleeding time and hemoglobin may be increased; hematocrit decreased.

**Storage Requirements:** Store powder at 15 to 30°C (59 to 86°F). Store reconstituted solutions according to package insert.

---

# ☐ TOBRAMYCIN SULFATE
(toe-bra-mye′sin)

(Nebcin, Tobrex, Alcon)

**Classification:** aminoglycoside

## Available Preparations:
- 10 mg, 20 mg, 40 mg, 1 ml for parenteral administration
- 0.3% drops and ointment for ophthalmic administration

**Action and Use:** Obtained from cultures of *Streptomyces tenebrarius*, inhibits protein synthesis by binding irreversibly to bacterial ribosomes. Active against both gram-positive and gram-negative bacteria, such as *Staphylococcus, Enterobacter, Citrobacter, Escherichia coli, Proteus, Klebsiella, Serratia, Providencia,* and *Pseudomonas.* Treats infections of bone, skin, urinary tract, gastrointestinal tract, and neonatal and bacterial septicemias. Ophthalmic preparations treat topical infections of external eye and adnexa (ointment preferred).

## Routes and Dosage:
*IM, IV:*
- prematures, < 34 weeks, < 1.25 kg: 3 mg/kg every 24 hours
- prematures, < 34 weeks, > 1.2 kg: 2.5 mg/kg every 18 hours
- prematures, > 34 weeks: 2.5 mg/kg every 12 hours
- neonates to 1 year: 2.5 mg/kg every 8 hours. (Do not exceed 4 mg/kg/day)
- over 1 year: 2.5 to 3 mg/kg/day in divided doses every 8 hours

Note: Dosages based on normal renal function. Impaired renal function dosage based on creatinine clearances. Treatment duration should be limited to 7 to 10 days.

*Ophthalmic:* Drops: instill 1 to 2 drops into conjunctival sac every 4 hours; severe infection 2 drops every hour, initially
Ointment: instill 1-cm strip ointment into conjunctival sac every 8 to 12 hours; severe infection every 3 to 4 hours

## Absorption and Fate:
IM rapidly adsorbed. Distributed mainly to extracellular fluids; CSF concentrations slightly increased when meninges inflamed. Ocular absorption increased if cornea abraded; drug cleared from eye surface in 15 to 30 minutes. Peak level: IM, 25 to 45 minutes; IV, 25 to 45 minutes after infusion. Half-life: newborns, less than 1500 g, over 8 hours; 1500 to 2500 g, 6 to 8 hours; more than 2500 g, 4 hours; older infants and children, 2 hours. Therapeutic level: 4 to 12 µg/ml. Excreted unchanged into urine.

## Contraindications and Precautions:
Pregnancy category D; safety during lactation not established. Use caution in premature infants and neonates due to renal immaturity. Contraindicated in hypersensitivity to drug or other aminoglycosides and in renal failure. Use caution in renal function impairment or eighth cranial nerve impairment.

## Side Effects:
*CNS:* confusion, **neurotoxicity**: numbness, tingling, muscle twitching, seizures; **neuromuscular blockade**: muscle weakness, respiratory depression, lethargy, headache. *GI:* nausea, vomiting, loss of appetite. *Hepatic:* increased bilirubin, SGOT, SGPT, hepatomegaly, **hepatic necrosis**. *GU:* **nephrotoxicity**: blood or casts in urine, proteinuria, increased BUN and serum creatinine, decreased urine creatinine clearance and specific gravity, **renal failure**. *Skin:* rash, burning, edema. *Hemic:* eosinophilia, anemia, leukopenia, agranulocytosis, thrombocytopenia. *Sensory:* ophthalmic: burning, stinging, blurred vision, photosensitivity; **ototoxicity**: eighth cranial nerve damage: permanent hearing loss, vertigo, loss of balance, tinnitus; **cochlear damage**: high frequency hearing loss detected only at first by audiometric testing.

## Nursing Implications:

***Assess:*** Obtain cultures and sensitivity before treatment, but can start treatment before results. Obtain baseline weights, BUN, creatinine levels, audiogram and vestibular function tests before therapy. Assess and record appearance of eye irritation.

***Administer: IM:*** Occasional report of pain at injection site. ***IV:*** Do not give IV push. Dilute in 25 to 100 ml of 5% dextrose or 0.9% sodium chloride (amount of solution depending on child's fluid requirements), drug maximum concentration 1 mg/ml. Infuse over 20 to 60 minutes. Do not infuse in less than 20 minutes, causes peak serum levels to exceed 12 μg/ml. Compatible with $D_5W$, $D_5W/NS$, $D_{10}W$, NS, Normosol, Dextran-40 10%/$D_5W$, check with pharmacists for others. Do not premix with other medications and infuse separately. After infusion flush line with NS or 5% dextrose. ***Ophthalmic:*** Carefully clean exudate from eye. Instill as described in Part I. After instillation of drops, apply light pressure on lacrimal sac for 1 to 2 minutes after instillation to minimize systemic absorption. If ointment, tell child vision will be blurred for several minutes.

***Monitor:*** Observe for signs of respiratory depression during IV infusion. Peak blood levels drawn 1 hour after IM dosage; 30 to 60 minutes after infusion ends. Desirable peak concentrations are 4 to 10 μg/ml and maximum trough concentrations (drawn just before next dose) should be 2 μg/ml. Measurements above these levels are associated with increased incidence of toxicity. Maintain daily hydration levels for age. If no response in 3 to 5 days, therapy should be discontinued. Usually continue ophthalmic preparations for 48 hours after infection controlled. Use a ticking watch to daily monitor child's ability to hear. Observe for symptoms of deafness and vestibular dysfunction (nausea, vomiting, and vertigo). Renal function assessed by I & O, daily weights, urine specific gravity, urinalysis, creatinine levels, and BUN. Report any side effects immediately to physician. Observe for superinfections. If therapy continues for more than 10 days, daily renal function tests and weekly audiograms should be obtained.

***Patient Teaching:*** Teach parents to observe for symptoms of hearing, vestibular, renal function loss, and overgrowth of infections. Teach parents proper eye instillation techniques. If no improvement in 3 to 5 days, notify physician. Observe for superinfections. When using drug for ocular infection, do not share towels, wash cloths, pillow cases, make-up, or this medication with other family members. Do not wear contact lenses while using eye medication.

**Drug Interactions:** Tobramycin used in combination with other aminoglycosides, amphotericin B, bacitracin (parenteral), capreomycin, cephalosporins, colistin, cisplatin, ethacrynic acid, furosemide, mannitol, methoxyflurane, polymyxins, or vancomycin causes increased chance of ototoxicity, neurotoxicity, or nephrotoxicity. Masked symptoms of ototoxicity can occur when used with dimenhydrinate. Neuromuscular blockade may occur with halogenated hydrocarbon inhalation anesthetic, citrate-anticoagulated blood transfusion, and neuromuscular blocking agents combined with tobramycin. Parenteral penicillins, such as carbenicillin and ticarcillin, inactivate this drug.

**Storage Requirements:** Store at 15 to 30°C (59 to 86°F). After reconstitution, stable if refrigerated for 96 hours, at room temperature stable for 24 hours.

---

## □ TOLAZOLINE (toe-laz'a-leen)

(Priscoline)

**Classification:** pulmonary antihypertensive, vasodilator

**Available Preparations:** 25 mg/ml for parenteral administration

**Action and Use:** A derivative of imidazoline that is structurally related to phentolamine. has a histamine type reaction on peripheral vascular smooth muscle causing relaxation and vasodilation. Has weak and incomplete α-adrenergic blocking action. Increases peripheral blood flow, heart rate, cardiac output, blood pressure, secretions of gastrointestinal tract and respiratory system. Used in treatment of persistent pulmonary hypertension in newborns. The drug has been used for other purposes such as treatment of spastic peripheral vascular problems, but is not approved for such uses by the FDA.

### Routes and Dosages:
*IV:* 1 to 2 mg/kg by scalp vein over 5 to 10 minutes initially; then maintenance infusion of 1 to 2 mg/kg/hour; tapered when arterial blood gas results are stable

**Absorption and Fate:** Rapid absorption with heavy distribution to the liver and kidneys. Excreted mainly as unchanged drug in urine. Onset of action in 30 minutes with peak effect in 30 to 60 minutes. Half-life in newborns ranges from 1.5 to 41 hours, with 3 to 10 hours usual range; half-life is inversely related to urine output.

**Contraindications and Precautions:** Pregnancy category C. Distribution in breast milk unknown. Contraindicated in those with hypersensitivity to the drug, with hypotension, in coronary artery disease, and after cerebrovascular accident. Cautious use in mitral stenosis, acidosis, gastritis, peptic ulcer.

### Side Effects:
*CNS:* tingling, paresthesia, sweating, headache, dizziness. *CV:* **systemic hypotension**, postural hypotension, **tachycardia**, **arrhythmias**, angina, **myocardial infarction**, **marked hypertension**. *GI:* nausea, vomiting, activation of ulcers, GI hemorrhage, diarrhea. *Respiratory:* pulmonary hemorrhage. *GU:* oliguria, hematuria. *Hemic:* agranulocytosis, thrombocytopenia, pancytopenia. *Other:* goose bumps from pilomotor action.

## Nursing Implications:

***Assess:*** Take baseline vital signs, CBC, blood gases, blood pH, electrolytes, EKG.

***Administer:*** Given only when facilities and personnel are available for constant monitoring (in NICU). Drug therapy may be preceded with antacids to prevent GI side effects. ***IV:*** Compatible with most IV solutions. Avoid diluents with benzyl alcohol in preparing solutions for newborns. Initial dose given over 10 minutes by scalp vein. Maintenance dose should be given by infusion device. Dose is reduced in those with oliguria. Dose generally tapered and stopped by at least 36 to 48 hours.

***Monitor:*** Continual monitoring of pulse, blood pressure, EKG are done. Frequent blood gases, electrolytes, CBC, blood pH, and hematest of gastric aspirate needed. Monitor urine output. Be prepared to provide cardiovascular and respiratory support. Overdose is manifested by flushing, goose bumps, hypotension, shock. Head should be placed downward, and IV infusion and ephedrine are given.

**Drug Interactions:** With alcohol, causes acetaldehyde accumulation and disulfiram-like reaction. Initial decreased, then increased blood pressure with epinephrine or norepinephrine. May decrease effects of dopamine, ephedrine, and phenylephrine.

**Laboratory Test Interferences:** Decreased potassium or chloride in serum.

**Storage Requirements:** Store at 15 to 30°C (59 to 86°F) and protect from light.

---

## ☐ TRIAMCINOLONE                    (trye-am-sin'oh-lone)

(Aristocort, Kenacort, Ledercort)

## ☐ TRIAMCINOLONE ACETONIDE

(Acetospan, Adcortyl, Azmacort, Cenocort A-40, Cinonide, Kenaject, Kenalog, Kenalone, Tramacort, Triacet, Triaderm, Triam-A, Tri-Kort, Trianide, Triamonide-40, Trilog, Trymex)

## ☐ TRIAMCINOLONE DIACETATE

(Amcort, Aristocort Forte, Aristocort Intralesional, Articulose-L.A., Cenocort Forte, Cinalone, Cino-40, Tracilon, Triam-Forte, Triamolone, Trilone, Tristoject)

# ☐ TRIAMCINOLONE HEXACETONDIDE

(Aristospan, Lederspan)

**Combination Products:** Triamcinolone acetonide with nystatin (Myco II, Myco-Aricin, Mycolog, Myco-Triacet, and others)

**Classification:** corticosteroid, glucocorticoid

## Available Preparations:
- 2 mg/5 ml, 4 mg/5 ml oral syrups
- 1, 2, 4, 8-mg tablets
- 3, 10, 40-mg/ml (acetonide) for parenteral administration
- 25, 40 mg/ml (diacetate) for parental administration
- 5, 20 mg/ml (hexacetonide)
- 100 metered spray for oral inhalation
- 0.025%, 0.1% topical lotion
- 0.025%, 0.1%, 0.5% topical cream and ointments
- 0.2 mg per 2-second spray topical aerosol
- 0.1% topical paste

## Action and Use:
Natural or synthetic, intermediate-acting glucocorticoid with strong antiinflammatory, immunosuppressant, and metabolic actions; essentially devoid of mineralocorticoid activity. Treats diseases such as collagen, dermatologic, allergy, acute leukemia, and others. It is used with mineralocorticoids in treatment of adrenocortical insufficiency. Topical preparations fluorinated. Oral inhalation form controls symptoms of chronic bronchial asthma.

## Routes and Dosage:
**PO:** 0.117 to 1.66 mg/kg/day or 3.3 to 50 mg/m$^2$/day in 4 divided doses
Note: With acute leukemia may require initial doses 2 mg/kg/day
**IM:** 6 to 12 years: 0.03 to 0.2 mg or 1 to 6.25 mg/m$^2$ every 1 to 7 days (acetonide); over 12 years: 40 to 80 mg every 4 weeks as needed (acetonide); over 6 years: 40 mg repeated at 4 week intervals (diacetate)
Intralesional: 1 mg/ injection site at weekly intervals
Note: Dosage determined by severity of condition and child's response.
**Oral Inhalation:** 6 to 15 years: 1 to 2 inhalations (0.1 to 0.2 mg or 100 to 200 g) 3 to 4 times a day. (Maximum dosage 1.2 mg/day, 12 inhalations)
**Topical:**
- Lotions: apply 0.025% sparingly, 1 to 2 times a day; 0.1% daily
- Creams and Ointments: apply 0.025% thin film, twice a day; 0.1 to 0.5% daily
- Aerosol: apply 0.015% once or twice a day

## Absorption and Fate:
Well absorbed from all sites; topical absorption increased in inflamed or diseased skin, with usage of occlusive dressings. Peak

level: PO, 1 to 2 hours; IM (acetonide), 24 to 48 hours. Half-life: 2 to 5 hours. Duration: PO, 2.25 days; IM acetonide, 1 to 6 weeks; IM diacetate, 4 days to 4 weeks. Metabolized in liver and excreted primarily in urine.

**Contraindications and Precautions:** Pregnancy category C. Safety during lactation not established. Dosages not established; IM under 6 years, intraarticular, intrabursal, or tendon-sheath (hexacetonide) dosages in children. Use caution in children and adolescents; possible growth suppression. Contraindicated in hypersensitivity to drug or its components, sensitivity to corticosteroids, varicella, systemic fungal infections, acquired immune deficiency syndrome (AIDS), immunizations with live virus vaccines and oral polio virus vaccine or contact with those who have had the vaccine. Use with caution in renal disease, hypertension, congestive heart failure, cardiac disease, diabetes, ulcerative colitis, gastrointestinal ulceration, hyperthyroidism, impaired hepatic function, systemic lupus erythematosus, osteoporosis, vaccinia, exanthema, Cushing's syndrome, seizures, myasthenia gravis, tuberculosis, ocular herpes simplex, hypoalbuminemia, emotional or psychotic tendencies.

**Side Effects:** Usually dependent on dosage and duration of treatment.
*CNS:* headaches, vertigo, euphoria, insomnia, **increased intracranial pressure** (papilledema), **psychotic behavior, seizures.** *CV:* edema, sodium retention, potassium loss, **hypertension, congestive heart failure.** *GI:* nausea, vomiting, change in appetite, gastrointestinal irritation, abdominal distention, pancreatitis, ulcerative esophagitis, peptic ulcer. *Skin:* impaired wound healing, thin fragile skin, petechia, ecchymosis, acne, facial erythema, increased sweating, may mask infections; Topical: burning, itching, irritation, dryness, folliculitis, hypertrichosis, hypopigmentation, allergic contact dermatitis, maceration of the skin, secondary infection, **skin atrophy, striae, miliaria.** *Hemic:* **thrombocytopenia.** *Endocrine:* **HPA-axis suppression,** menstrual irregularities, Cushing's states, **secondary adrenocortical, pituitary unresponsiveness.** *Musculoskeletal:* **suppression bone growth, osteoporosis,** muscle weakness, **aseptic necrosis of femoral and humeral heads.** *Sensory:* ENT: hoarseness, dry, irritated throat, dry mouth, infection nose and pharynx by *Candida albicans*, ulceration, bloody mucus, epistaxis, nasal septum perforation, **shortness of breath, tightness in chest, wheezing;** Ophthalmic: **posterior subcapsular cataracts, increased intraocular pressure.** *Other:* Hypersensitivity (ENT): urticaria, angioedema, rash, **bronchospasm; negative nitrogen balance, hypokalemia, hyperglycemia,** susceptibility to infections; Withdrawal symptoms: rebound inflammation, fatigue, weaknesa, arthralgia, fever, dizziness, lethargy, depression, fainting, orthostatic hypotension, dyspnea, anorexia, hypoglycemia, nausea and vomiting, shortness of breath, unusual weight loss

**Nursing Implications:**
*Assess:* Obtain baseline weight, height; before long-term therapy: ECG, chest and spinal x-rays, glucose tolerance test, evaluation of HPA-axis function, and BP. Oral Inhalation: drug should not be given during acute asthma attack.

Topical: observe and record appearance of involved area for baseline information.

**_Administer:_** Best to calculate drug dosage on mg/m$^2$; reduces overdosage possibilities in very short or heavy children. **_PO:_** Take with food or milk to reduce GI irritation. Best to give daily dosage before 9 AM. It suppress adrenal cortex activity less, which may reduce risk of HPA-axis suppression. Alternate-day therapy recommended to reduce growth retarding effects. Tablet can be crushed, mixed with small amount of food or fluid. **_IM:_** Shake well before withdrawal. Drug causes subcutaneous tissues to abscess and atrophy. Burning and pain may occur with injection. INTRALESIONAL or INTRABURSAL: Do not use 40 mg/ml for intralesional injection. Drug should not be mixed with parenteral local anesthetic formulation containing preservatives such as parabens and phenol, because flocculation of the adrenocorticoid could occur. First, withdraw the adrenocorticoid suspension into a syringe, then add the local anesthetic. This prevents introduction of local anesthetic into triamcinolone vial. **_Oral Inhalation:_** If bronchodilation inhaler prescribed, use it 5 to 15 minutes before triamcinolone so steroid's penetration will be augmented into peripheral airways. To use aerosol inhaler, see Part I. Shake well prior to usage. If second inhalation prescribed, wait about 1 minute between inhalations. Rinse mouth after use of inhaler to prevent further drug absorption. **_Topical:_** Cleanse with water before application or as physician prescribes. Cleaning prevents cumulative deposit effect, which may increase systemic absorption, duration of drug's action and side effects. Apply thin coat, gently rubbing into area, avoiding eye area and mucous membranes. Do not cover with occlusive dressing unless directed by physician. If occlusive dressing is used it should not remain in place for more than 16 hours; it increases incidence of side effects. Disposable diapers or plastic pants act as an occlusive dressing if covering medicated groin area. Aerosol: carefully spray only affected area for no more than 2 seconds and from distance of no less than 6 inches. Keep spray from being inhaled and away for the eye area.

**_Monitor:_** Carefully assessment of child's respond to drug, necessary for dosage adjustments. Observe for side effects, especially hypocalcemia, signs of adrenal insufficiency, symptoms of infections, or worsening of condition. Children more prone to muscular skeletal side effects; note any pain or gait changes immediately to physician. Monitor BP and daily weights, report any sudden weight gain to the physician. With long-term usage, monitor serum electrolytes and height. Encourage well-balanced diet low in sodium and encourage good hygiene and dental care (possible oral fungal infections). Tonometry (eye) examinations every 6 weeks. Discontinuing of drug dosage should be reduced gradually, especially after long-term usage so it does not cause acute life-threatening adrenal insufficiency. After discontinuation of short-term therapy (up to 5 days) with high dosage, adrenal recovery may occur within 1 week. After prolonged high-dose therapy, complete recovery of adrenal function may require up to 1 year. Topical: assess wound site with every new application of medication and record. Notify physician of any variations. If infection occurs, discontinue drug and inform physician. If child is on long-term therapy (over 2 weeks) or medicated over large body surface area (15% of body surface), the following laboratory tests may be helpful in evaluating the HPA-axis suppression: urinary free cortisol test and ACTH stimulation test. Itching can lead to scratching and introduction of infections. Younger children may need restraining especially during naps or at night. Keep the nails short and clean. Contact physician if itching persists. ORAL INHALATIONS: fungal infections of the oropharyngeal area are common; inspect mouth frequently.

***Patient Teaching:*** Do not alter dosage or stop drug abruptly, it could cause very serious side effects, even death. Gradual tapering of dosage is necessary. Increasing amount of medication will not hasten healing process. Demonstrate how to use medication form perscribed. Monitor for side effects of medication, symptoms of adrenal insufficiency or worsening of condition and report to physician. Obtain daily weights; report any sudden weight gains to physician. Importance of close medical supervision and follow-up. Regular ophthalmic examinations if on long-term therapy. Caution about receiving skin tests, vaccinations, or other immunizations, or coming in contact with persons receiving oral polio virus vaccine. Inform any health-care provider, including dentists, surgeons, or emergency care personal that child is on this medication. Child should carry a medical identification card. Observe for symptoms of infections. Do not use OTC medications without contacting health-care provider. Topical: Do not use medication on other than those prescribed by physican. Do not use oral inhaler during acute asthma attack.

**Drug Interactions:** This drug in combination with high dosage of acetaminophen may increase risk of hepatotoxicity. With analgesics and antiinflammatory drugs it may increase the risk of gastric ulceration. Amphotericin B and potassium-depleting diuretics increase risk of hypokalemia. Use with anabolic steroids may increase the risk of edema and acne. Drug in combination with anticoagulants may decrease anticoagulant effect. This drug used with anticonvulsants (phenytoin) may lower seizure threshold. Use with vaccines, live virus, or other immunizations may potentiate replication of the vaccine virus, increasing chance for developing the viral disease.

**Laboratory Test Interferences:** May increase serum cholesterol, sodium, and blood glucose. May decrease serum calcium, potassium, $T_4$, and reduce thyroid I-131 uptake, urine 17-hydroxysteroid and 17-ketosteroids. Tends to suppress skin tests; may give a false-negative result with nitrobluetetrazolium for bacterial infection. Adrenal function assessed by ACTH stimulation or plasma cortisol may be decreased.

**Storage Requirements:** Store at 15 to 30°C (59 to 86°F). Protect from light and freezing. Do not puncture or dispose of aerosol preparations into fire or incinerator.

---

# ☐ TRIAMTERENE                    (trye-am′ter-een)

(Dyrenium)

**Combination Products:** Dyazide, Matazine, Triamterene, and Hydrochlorothiazide

**Classification:** potassium-sparing diuretic

**Available Preparations:** 50, 100-mg capsules
Also available in tablets and capsules with hydrochlorothiazide

**Action and Use:** Blocks exchange of sodium and potassium in distal tubule, leading to excretion of sodium and water and retention of potassium. Increased excretion of calcium, magnesium, chloride, and bicarbonate also occurs. Does not block excretion of uric acid. Used in treatment of edema during congestive heart failure, nephrosis, cirrhosis.

**Routes and Dosages:**
*PO:* 4 mg/kg/day or 115 mg/m$^2$/day in two daily doses initially; maintenance dose may be increased up to 6 mg/kg/day (not to exceed 300 mg/day)

**Absorption and Fate:** Rapidly and variably (30 to 70%) absorbed from GI tract. Widely distributed in body tissues; approximately 70% protein bound. Partially metabolized by the liver and excreted in bile and urine. Onset of action: 2 to 4 hours; peak level: 2 to 4 hours; peak effect: 1 to 2 days; decreased activity: 7 to 9 hours after one dose; and duration of action: up to 24 hours. Half-life is 90 to 150 minutes.

**Contraindications and Precautions:** Pregnancy category B. Unknown if present in breast milk. Safety in children is not established. Contraindicated in lactation, renal failure, severe hepatic dysfunction, hyperkalemia, hypersensitivity. Cautious use in those with history of renal calculi, patients with elevated BUN, renal dysfunction, diabetes, hyponatremia, metabolic or respiratory acidosis.

**Side Effects:**
*CNS:* lethargy, confusion, fatigue, dizziness, headache. *CV:* **arrhythmia** (resulting from hyperkalemia). *GI:* nausea, vomiting, anorexia, abdominal cramps, diarrhea, dry mouth, thirst. *Hepatic:* elevated BUN. *Hemic:* megaloblastic anemia with cirrhosis, granulocytopenia, eosinophilia. *Metabolic:* **hyperkalemia** if renal failure develops or if on potassium supplements, **metabolic acidosis**, hyponatremia (especially with cirrhosis patients), hypomagnesemia, increased serum chloride, decreased serum bicarbonate. *Skin:* rash, urticaria, sweating

**Nursing Implications:**
*Assess:* Obtain baseline CBC, BUN, creatinine, EKG, serum electrolytes, weight, and vital signs, especially blood pressure.
*Administer:* Give with food to enhance absorption and decrease GI upset.
*Monitor:* Continue to monitor serum potassium and sodium, vital signs espe-

cially blood pressure, I & O, and daily weight. Watch for signs of hyperkalemia (paresthesias, confusion, weakness, cardiac irregularities). If giving combination product with hydrochlorothiazide, hypokalemia may occur. BUN, creatinine, EKG are monitored periodically. If given to diabetic, monitor blood glucose carefully as hyperglycemia may result.

*Patient Teaching:* Avoid excess intake of potassium such as potassium supplements and sodium-free salt unless also taking a potassium-depleting diuretic. Teach the signs of hyperkalemia (paresthesia, confusion, weakness) and teach to report. Report sore throat, fever, malaise, bleeding, or bruising.

**Drug Interactions:** Increases uric acid, therefore, allopurinol dose may need adjustment if on that drug concomitantly. Increased blood glucose in those on insulin. Hyperkalemia may result if potassium supplement is given; note that whole blood also contains potassium. Increased hyperkalemia may occur with captopril, therefore, that drug should be used with caution. May reduce excretion of digoxin; may inhibit inotropic effect of digitalis. Diuretic effect may decrease if salicylates are also given. Increased potassium excretion may occur with corticosteroids. Nonsteroidal antiinflammatories, estrogen, sympathomimetics can decrease the antihypertensive effect. Increased diuresis with other diuretics. Decreased blood pressure with other antihypertensives. Lithium will have reduced renal clearance and is not recommended for use with potassium-sparing diuretics. Do not use with other potassium-sparing drugs.

**Laboratory Test Interferences:** Interferes with fluorescent measurement of quinidine and lactic dehydrogenase. May elevate BUN, creatinine, plasma renin activity, magnesium, potassium, uric acid. Falsely elevates plasma digitalis level. May increase blood glucose in diabetics. Increases urinary calcium and decreases serum sodium. Causes inaccurate plasma and urinary 17-hydroxycorticosteroids.

**Storage Requirements:** Store at 15 to 30°C (59 to 86°F). Protect from light.

---

## □ TRIFLUOPERAZINE       (trye-floo-oh-per'a-zeen)

(Stelazine)

**Classification:** antipsychotic, antiemetic, phenothiazine

## Available Preparations:
- 10 mg/ml solution
- 1, 2, 5, 10-mg tablets
- 1, 2, 5, 10-mg film-coated tablets
- 2 mg/ml vials for parenteral use

**Action and Use:** This phenothiazine derivative may act on the CNS by blocking dopamine transmission, increasing adrenergic activity, and other effects. As compared to chlorpromazine, this drug has weak anticholinergic and sedative effects, and strong extrapyramidal and antiemetic effects. Used for treatment of psychosis.

## Routes and Dosages:
*PO:* Psychosis: 6 to 12 years: 1 mg QD or BID, increase PRN; not to exceed 15 mg/day
*IM:* Psychosis: 6 to 12 years: 1 mg QD or BID; IM doses given at least 4 hours apart

**Absorption and Fate:** Well absorbed from GI tract and injection. Widely distributed in the body and crosses blood-brain barrier; present in high concentrations in brain. Highly bound to plasma proteins. Extensively metabolized by the liver and excreted principally in urine. Rapid onset of action; peak level: 2 to 3 hours; duration about 12 hours.

**Contraindications and Precautions:** Pregnancy category C. Contraindicated in children under 6 years, those with prior hypersensitivity to phenothiazines, often manifested as jaundice; those with CNS depression, comatose, subcortical damage, bone marrow suppression; parenteral solution with sulfite used as a preservative is not to be used in those with hypersensitivity to sulfites. Cautious use in cardiovascular disease, seizure disorders, hepatic or renal disease, glaucoma, children with acute illness or dehydration, hypocalcemia, previous reaction to insulin, and in those taking drugs, such as antineoplastics, with which nausea and vomiting may signal toxic effects.

## Side Effects:
*CNS:* Dystonic reactions especially in children with acute illness or dehydration, manifested by neck spasm, torticollis, rigid back, opisthotonos, tics, TMJ dysfunction, tongue spasm, difficult swallowing, sweating, fever; effects in 24 to 48 hours of dose and relief obtained with anticholinergics. Dystonia, akathisia, extrapyramidal effects more common with this drug than chlorpromazine. Motor restlessness especially in children with acute illness or dehydration, manifested by foot tapping, excess movement, insomnia; effects generally in 2 to 3 days after therapy begins. Other CNS effects include tardive dyskinesia, **neuroleptic malignant syndrome**, drowsiness, restlessness, insomnia, depression, weakness, headache, **seizures**, hyperthermia or hypothermia. *CV:* **hypotension, tachycardia**, syncope, **EKG changes**; effects usually end in 30 to 120 minutes. *GI:* anorexia, constipation, dry mouth, diarrhea, paralytic ileus. *Respiratory:* **laryngospasm, bronchospasm, anaphylaxis** (rare). *Hepatic:* cholestatic jaundice after 2 to 4 weeks of therapy; effect seen in some newborns whose mothers received phenothiazines in pregnancy. Elevated bilirubin, alkaline phosphatase, transaminases. *Skin:* pruritus, photosensitivity, urticaria, dermatitis, hyperpigmentation; contact dermatitis upon skin contact with solutions. *Hemic:* **agranulocytosis, leukopenia, eosinophilia, thrombocytopenia,**

aplastic anemia; all rare but potentially fatal. *Endocrine:* glycosuria, gynecomastia. *Sensory:* ocular changes

## Nursing Implications:
*Assess:* CBC, liver function studies are done before therapy. Establish baseline vital signs. Physical assessment to rule out acute illness and dehydration.
*Administer:* Avoid contact of solutions with skin. Give with food or fluid to decrease gastric upset. Tablet may be crushed and added to small amount of food.
*Monitor:* Vital sign checks, especially during initial therapy. CBC periodically during long-term therapy. Monitor I & O. Weekly urine bilirubin during first month and serum bilirubin, alkaline phosphatase, transaminase regularly. Take temperature. Monitor urine glucose. Periodic eye examinations if on long-term therapy. Monitor hearing if patient is also on ototoxic drugs; monitor toxic effects of antineoplastic drugs if patient is on concurrent therapy with drugs whose toxicity is manifested by nausea and vomiting, as these effects may be masked by phenothiazines.
*Patient Teaching:* Take drug as directed. Avoid driving and operating hazardous machinery. Report continued insomnia or other side effects as they usually decrease with time. Good oral hygiene and nutritious food can decrease some side effects. Urine may turn red in color. Use a sunscreen during exposure to sunlight.

**Drug Interactions:** Additive effects with other CNS depressants. It can decrease phenytoin metabolism, has additive hypotensive effects with β blockers, additive effects with tricyclic antidepressants. Phenothiazines reverse effects of epinephrine and lower blood pressure; these two drugs should not be given together; effect not seen with norepinephrine or phenylephrine. Phenobarbital increases excretion of the drug. Acute encephalopathy possible when given with lithium.

**Laboratory Test Interferences:** False-positive urobilinogen, amylase, uroporphrins, porphobilinogens, 5-hydroxyindolacetic acid, phenylketonuria, pregnancy tests. May elevate serum bilirubin, alkaline phosphatase, transaminase, PBI, other liver function tests.

**Storage Requirements:** Store in tightly covered, light-resistant containers at 15 to 30°C (59 to 86°F). Avoid freezing. Slight yellow color of solution does not affect potency but marked discoloration or precipitates necessitate discarding solution.

---

## ☐ TRIFLUPROMAZINE     (trye-floo-pro′ma-zeen)

(Vesprin)

**Classification:** antipsychotic, antiemetic, phenothiazine

**Available Preparations:** 10, 20 mg/ml vials for parenteral use

**Action and Use:** This phenothiazine derivative may act on the CNS by blocking dopamine transmission, increasing adrenergic activity, and other effects. As compared to chlorpromazine, this drug has strong anticholinergic, sedative, antiemetic, and pyramidal effects.

**Routes and Dosages:** IV route only for adults
*IM:*
- Psychosis: over 2 1/2 years: 0.2–0.25 mg/kg/day; not to exceed 10 mg/day
- Nausea and Vomiting: over 2 1/2 years: 0.2 to 0.25 mg/kg/day in divided doses

**Absorption and Fate:** Well absorbed after IM injection. Widely distributed in the body and crosses blood-brain barrier. Highly bound to plasma proteins. Extensively metabolized by the liver and excreted principally in urine.

**Contraindications and Precautions:** Pregnancy category C. Contraindicated in children under 6 years; those with prior hypersensitivity to phenothiazines, often manifested as jaundice; those with CNS depression, comatose, subcortical damage, bone marrow suppression, Reye syndrome. Cautious use in cardiovascular disease, seizure disorders, hepatic or renal disease, glaucoma, children with acute illness or dehydration, hypocalcemia, previous reaction to insulin, and in those taking drugs, such as antineoplastics, with which nausea and vomiting may signal toxic effects.

**Side Effects:**
*CNS:* Dystonic reactions especially in children with acute illness or dehydration, manifested by neck spasm, torticollis, rigid back, opisthotonos, tics, TMJ dysfunction, tongue spasm, difficult swallowing, sweating, fever; effects in 24 to 48 hours of dose and relief obtained with anticholinergics. Motor restlessness especially in children with acute illness or dehydration, manifested by foot tapping, excess movement, insomnia; effects generally in 2 to 3 days after therapy begins. Other CNS effects include tardive dyskinesia, **neuroleptic malignant syndrome**, drowsiness, restlessness, insomnia, depression, weakness, headache, **seizures**, hyperthermia or hypothermia. *CV:* **hypotension, tachycardia**, syncope, **EKG changes**; effects usually end in 30 to 120 minutes. *GI:* anorexia, constipation, dry mouth, diarrhea, paralytic ileus. *Respiratory:* **laryngospasm, bronchospasm, anaphylaxis** (rare). *Hepatic:* cholestatic jaundice after 2 to 4 weeks of therapy; effect seen in some newborns whose mothers received phenothiazines in pregnancy. Elevated bilirubin, alkaline phosphatase, transaminases. *Skin:* pruritus, photosensitivity, urticaria, dermatitis, hyperpigmentation; contact dermatitis upon skin contact with solutions. *Hemic:* **agranulocytosis, leukopenia, eosinophilia, thrombocytopenia, aplastic anemia**; all rare but potentially fatal. *Endocrine:* glycosuria, gynecomastia. *Sensory:* ocular changes

## Nursing Implications:

**Assess:** CBC, liver function studies are done before therapy. Establish baseline vital signs. Physical assessment to rule out acute illness and dehydration.

**Administer:** Avoid contact of solution with skin. Give deep IM.

**Monitor:** Vital sign checks especially during initial therapy. CBC periodically during long-term therapy. Monitor I & O. Weekly urine bilirubin during first month and serum bilirubin, alkaline phosphatase, transaminase regularly. Take temperature. Monitor urine glucose. Periodic eye examinations if on long-term therapy. Monitor hearing if patient also is on ototoxic drugs; monitor toxic effects of antineoplastic drugs if patient is on concurrent therapy with drugs whose toxicity is manifested by nausea and vomiting, as above effects may be masked by phenothiazines.

**Drug Interactions:** Additive effects with other CNS depressants. It can decrease phenytoin metabolism, has additive hypotensive effects with β blockers, additive effects with tricyclic antidepressants. Phenothiazines reverse effects of epinephrine and lower blood pressure; these two drugs should not be given together; effect not seen with norepinephrine or phenylephrine. Phenobarbital increases excretion of the drug. Acute encephalopathy possible when given with lithium.

**Laboratory Test Interferences:** False-positive urobilinogen, amylase, uroporphrins, porphobilinogens, 5-hydroxyindolacetic acid, phenylketonuria, pregnancy tests. May elevate serum bilirubin, alkaline phosphatase, transaminase, PBI, other liver function tests.

**Storage Requirements:** Store in tightly covered, light-resistant containers at 15 to 30°C (59 to 86°F). Avoid freezing. Slight yellow color of solution does not affect potency but marked discoloration or precipitates necessitate discarding solution.

---

## □ TRIFLURIDINE                            (trye-flure'i-deen)

(Viroptic)

**Classification:** antiviral ophthalmic

**Available Preparations:** 1% solution for ophthalmic administration

**Action and Use:** Drug closely resembles thymidine (metabolite essential for DNA synthesis). During viral replication drug is used in place of thymidine, resulting in faulty viral DNA that is unable to infect, destroy tissue, or reproduce itself. Treats keratitis and keratoconjunctivitis caused by herpes simplex virus types 1 and 2, and some adenovirus strains.

## Routes and Dosage:

*Ophthalmic:* Drops: instill 1 drop 1% solution in conjunctival sac every 2 hours during day until reepithelialization. (Maximum dosage 9 drops per day); then 1 drop every 4 hours during day for 7 days. (Maximum dosage 5 drops per day)

## Absorption and Fate:
Absorbed through cornea and drug is found in aqueous humor. Corneal, stromal, or uveal inflammation increases absorption but this does not cause systemic absorption.

## Contraindications and Precautions:
Pregnancy category C and safe usage during lactation not established. Contraindicated in hypersensitivity to drug or its components.

## Side Effects:

*Sensory:* transient burning or stinging, mild edema of eyelid or cornea, (most common); lacrimation, photosensitivity, superficial punctate keratopathy, keratitis sicca, increased intraocular pressure

## Nursing Implications:

*Assess:* Note and record appearance of eye and surrounding tissue.

*Administer: Ophthalmic:* See Part I for instillation.

*Monitor:* Improvement of affective tissue can be evaluated by loss of fluorescein staining. If no sign of improvement in 7 days or if reepithelialization does not occur in 14 days, evaluation of therapy is required. Therapy is usually continued for 7 days after reepithelialization and medication should be used for no longer than 21 days.

*Patient Teaching:* Proper instillation of ointment. Use no more frequently than prescribed. Stress importance of close ophthalmic supervision. If side effects occur, contact ophthalmologist. Use sunglasses if photosensitivity occurs. Use good hand washing techniques to prevent spread of infection (liquid soap preferred). Child should have separate towels and washcloths. Do not share eye make-up. Encourage child to keep hands away from eyes. Do not use OTC eye preparations.

## Storage Requirements:
Store at 2 to 8°C (36 to 46°F) in light-resistant container.

---

☐ **TRIMETHOBENZAMIDE HYDROCHLORIDE**    (trye-meth-oh-ben′za-mide)

(Tegamide, Ticon, Tigan, Spengan)

**Classification:** antiemetic

## Available Preparations:
- 100, 250-mg capsules
- 100, 200-mg rectal suppositories

**Action and Use:** Structurally related to ethanolamine antihistamines. It appears to have depressant effect on chemoreceptor trigger zone of the medulla. Used primarily as an antiemetic and has only weak antihistaminic activity. It should not be used for control of severe vomiting.

## Routes and Dosage:
*PO:*
- weighing 13.6 to 45 kg: 100 to 200 mg 3 to 4 times per day; or 20 mg/ kg/day; or 500 mg/m²/day in 3 or 4 divided doses
- adults: 250 mg 3 or 4 times per day

*IM:* Not recommended for use in children.

*PR:* Do not use in prematures and neonates
- less than 13.6 kg: 100 mg 3 to 4 times per day
- 13.6 to 45 kg: 100 to 200 mg 3 to 4 times per day; or 15 mg/kg or 400 mg/m² daily in 3 to 4 divided doses
- adults: 200 mg 3 to 4 times per day

**Absorption and Fate:** Onset of action: PO, 10 to 40 minutes and duration is 3 to 4 hours. Metabolic fate unknown, excreted in urine and feces.

**Contraindications and Precautions:** Pregnancy category C and safety during lactation not established. Contraindicated parenterally in children, rectally in premature and neonates, hypersensitivity to drug, rectal form if sensitive to benzocaine or similar local anesthetics, acute viral illness (risk of developing Reye syndrome). Use with caution in treatment of vomiting in children, high fevers, dehydration, electrolyte imbalance, those receiving other CNS depressants.

## Side Effects:
*CNS:* Parkinson-like symptoms, blurred vision, depression, seizures, disorientation, vertigo, dizziness, drowsiness, headache, **coma, opisthotonos**. *CV:* hypotension. *GI:* diarrhea, exaggeration of preexisting nausea. *Hepatic:* jaundice. *Skin:* allergic skin reactions

## Nursing Implications:
*Administer: PO:* May be taken without regard to food. Capsules may be taken apart, mixed with small amounts of food or fluid. *Rectal:* For instillation, see Part I. Suppository form contains 2% benzocaine, do not use if hypersensitivity exists. After unwrapping, do not expose to direct sunlight.
*Monitor:* Report any side effects or symptoms of hypersensitivity to physician. Drug may masks symptoms of other illness such as appendicitis. Observe stools for passage of suppository.
*Patient Teaching:* Inform child and parents of side effect. Use only as prescribed; do not use as emetic with other illness without consulting physician. Store suppository in refrigerator in opaque container.

**Drug Interactions:** May potentiate depressive effects of alcohol, barbiturates, or tranquilizers. Drug may increase anticholinergic side effects of belladonna alkaloids. Do not give with aminoglycosides or other ototoxic drugs, may mask symptoms of ototoxicity.

**Storage Requirements:** Store at 15 to 30°C (59 to 86°F), in tightly closed containers. Refrigerate suppositories.

---

## □ TROPICAMIDE                                    (troe-pik'a-mide)

(l-Picamide, Minims Tropicamide, Mydriacyl, Mydriafair, Tropicacyl)

**Classification:** cycloplegic, mydriatics

**Available Preparations:** 0.5%, 1% drops for ophthalmic administration

**Action and Use:** Anticholinergic that blocks the response caused by acetylcholine. This causes sphincter muscle of the iris to dilate (mydriasis) and paralysis of accommodation of ciliary body (cycloplegia). Used in refraction, diagnostic ophthalmic procedures, and treatment of uveitis.

### Routes and Dosage:
*Ophthalmic:*
- Cycloplegic Refraction: instill 1 drop of 0.5 or 1% solution repeated in 5 minutes
- Fundus Examination: instill 1 drop of 0.5% solution 15 to 20 minutes before procedure

**Absorption and Fate:** Rapid acting. Peak effects: mydriasis, 20 to 40 minutes; cycloplegia, 20 to 35 minutes. Duration: mydriasis, 6 to 7 hours; cyclopegia, 50 minutes to 6 hours.

**Contraindications and Precautions:** Pregnancy category C. Use caution in infants and younger children because of increased susceptibility to drug's systemic effects. Contraindicated in hypersensitivity to this drug, its components, and in narrow-angle glaucoma. Use caution in infants and young children with spastic paralysis or brain damage, Down's syndrome, or blond, blue eyed children.

### Side Effects:
*Sensory:* stinging upon instillation, blurred vision, photophobia, increased intraocular pressure (less due to short duration of action). *Other:* Systemic Effects: clumsiness or unsteadiness, confusion, disorientation and unusual behavior, failure to recognize people, drowsiness, weakness, tachycardia, fever, urinary retention, flushing of face, dry mouth and skin, slurred speech, distended abdomen in infants, hallucinations

## Nursing Implications:

*Assess:* Tonometric examinations are recommended before drug usage.

*Administer: Ophthalmic:* Wash hands before and after administration; drug may cause contact dermatitis. Do not touch the dropper tip to the eye or any adjacent structures. *Drops:* Warn child that drug causes stinging just before giving. Apply finger on lacrimal sac using light pressure for 1 to 2 minutes after instillation to minimize systemic absorption. Very carefully blot excess eye drops from around the eye with a clean tissue. Brown or hazel eyes may require more medication because dark eyes seem to be less responsive to this drug. 0.5% drop form is inadequate for cycloplegia.

*Monitor:* Observe for symptoms of CNS systemic effects; these occur more frequently in children on long-term therapy. If blurring of vision or photosensitivity lasts longer than 72 hours, contact physician. Physostigmine is antidote for systemic toxicity.

*Patient Teaching:* Instruct child not to rub eyes. Wear sunglasses to decrease photophobic discomfort. Do not perform hazardous tasks until drug has worn off.

**Storage Requirement:** Store at 15 to 30°C (59 to 86°F) in tightly closed container. Do not refrigerate.

---

## □ TUBERCULIN                                    (too-ber′cue-lin)

(Aplisol, Aplitest, Mono-Vacc, PPD, SclavoTest, Tuberculin Old Tine Test, Tuberculin Purified Protein Derivative Tine Test, Tubersol)

**Classification:** skin test

## Available Preparations:
- 1 TU/0.1 ml, 5 TU/0.1 ml, 250 TU/0.1 ml vials for parenteral use
- disposable multiple puncture device

Also available in multiple puncture test with antigens for *Candida*, diphtheria, group C *Streptococcus, Proteus*, tetanus, trichophyton to assess cell-mediated immunity.

**Action and Use:** There are two types of preparations available. Old tuberculin is a filtrate obtained from cultures of tuberculosis, and purified protein derivative is a purified protein fraction of old tuberculin. The preparations stimulate the body's T cells if they have been previously sensitized by infection with tuberculosis, thereby demonstrating a hypersensitivity response at the injection site. Used to test persons to determine presence of tuberculosis infection.

## Routes and Dosages:
*ID:*
- Multiple Puncture Device: firmly applied to forearm and held for 1 second

■ Mantoux: 0.1 ml of 5 TU/0.1 ml solution of PPD (formerly intermediate strength PPD)

Old tuberculin is available only in multiple puncture devices with the active substance dried into tines or solution surrounding the tines. Purified protein derivative is available dried into tines of multiple puncture devices and as a solution to be give intradermally. The latter is called the Mantoux test.

**Absorption and Fate:** The presence of the tuberculin causes a local hypersensitivity reaction in those previously infected with *Mycobacterium tuberculosis* or immunized with BCG, a live strain of *Mycobacterium bovis*.

**Contraindications and Precautions:** Used during pregnancy only if clearly needed. It may be advisable to test a pregnant woman at high risk of tuberculosis as there has been no evidence of fetal harm from the test. Contraindicated in those with known prior tuberculosis and generally not used in those with prior immunization with BCG. The tine tests use acacia as a stabilizer and should not be used in those hypersensitive to this substance.

**Side Effects:**

**Skin:** Immediate hypersensitivity to some substance in the preparation manifested by wheal or flare for up to 24 hours. Persons with prior tuberculosis infection may have pruritus, necrosis, ulceration, pain at the site. **Other:** fever, lymphadenopathy, **anaphylaxis** (all extremely rare)

**Nursing Implications:**

**Assess:** Inquire about known history of tuberculosis or immunization with BCG. These will necessitate omitting the test and substituting a chest x-ray, physical examination, and sputum studies for diagnosis.

**Administer:** Tuberculin skin tests are to be given annually to children at high risk of tuberculosis, such as those with a family member with the disease or in areas with significant numbers of cases, and in immigrants from areas where the disease is prevalent. HIV-infected children should be screened regularly with the Mantoux test. If reaction is negative but potential symptoms of tuberculosis are present, a chest x-ray and physical examination should also be done. Other children should be screened at about 1 year, 4 to 6 years, and 14 to 16 years. Have epinephrine 1:1000 and resuscitative equipment readily available. **ID:** Multiple puncture devices are most commonly used due to convenience. The most accurate test is the Mantoux or direct intradermal injection of PPD, therefore, this is used if tuberculosis exposure has occurred or if a multiple puncture test results in a positive or questionable reaction. **Multiple puncture test:** Clean the forearm with alcohol or other antiseptic, dry the skin, stretch skin tightly over area to be used, select an area free of visible surface blood vessels, and firmly place the device on the skin for at least 1 second. The puncture sites and imprint from base of device indicates correct amount of pressure is used. Discard puncture device with care. **Mantoux test:** Clean the forearm with alcohol or other antiseptic, dry the skin, stretch skin tightly over area to be used, select area free of surface blood vessels, and inject 0.1 ml of 5 TU/0.1 ml PPD solution intradermally with a 26 to 27-gauge tuberculin syringe. A 6 to 10-mm bleb indicates correct technique; this absorbs within a few minutes. *Note:* Care should be taken to use only 5 TU/0.1 ml strength as a 250 TU/0.1 ml solution also exists and must not be used for screening.

*Monitor:* Observe patient for 20 minutes after administration for signs of anaphylaxis. *Multiple puncture test:* Examine site in 48 to 72 hours for induration and vesiculation; errythema without either of these is nonsignificant. A positive reaction is indicated by vesiculation or by induration of 2 mm or greater. Other tests are read as negative. Positive reactions must be followed by a Mantoux test. *Mantoux test:* Examine in 48 to 72 hours. If not suspected of contact with tuberculosis, induration of under 10 mm is insignificant. Some practitioners consider reactions of 5 to 9 mm questionable and require a second Mantoux test. For those who are suspected of the disease or contact with a case of tuberculosis, induration of under 5 mm is insignificant. All other results are significant and warrant follow-up with a second test and then physical examination and chest x-ray if positive or questionable.

*Patient Teaching:* Inform patient when and where to return for reading of results. Inform them of results and record on a medical record for them to keep. Positive reaction does not necessarily indicate active disease and must be followed by a repeat Mantoux test, physical examination, chest x-ray, and attempts to isolate the bacillus from the body (generally sputum). If the patient has positive reaction, provide teaching for follow-up care such as chest x-ray and medication treatment if needed. Teach positive patient never to have repeat tuberculin skin tests.

**Drug Interactions:** Tuberculin skin test reaction may be suppressed if given within 4 to 6 weeks after immunization with such agents as measles, mumps, rubella, polio, influenza. Tuberculin test should be given before, concomitantly with, or 6 weeks after these vaccines; generally tuberculin test is given at 12 months of age, MMR at 15 months. BCG vaccination frequently causes a falsely positive tuberculin reaction. Tuberculin skin test reaction may be suppressed if given with corticosteroids or aminocaproic acid. False-negative reactions may occur in patients with HIV infection, cancers of lymphoid system, some viral, bacterial, and fungal infections, those with dehydration, or renal disease. Those administered to areas with dermatitis or with exposure to ultraviolet treatments or excessive sun may be falsely negative. If tuberculosis is suspected in spite of a negative skin test, follow-up examination is needed.

**Storage Requirements:** Store multiple puncture devices at room temperature not to exceed 30°C (86°F). Solutions should be refrigerated at 2 to 8°C (35 to 46°F).

---

□ **VALPROIC ACID**                                    (val-proe'ic)

(Depakene, Depakote, Myproic Acid)

**Classification:** anticonvulsant

## Available Preparations:
- Valproate Sodium: 250 mg/5 ml oral solution
- Divalproex Sodium: 125, 250, 500-mg enteric-coated tablets
- Valproic Acid: 250-mg capsules

**Action and Use:** Exact mechanism of action unknown but may increase levels of the brain inhibitory neurotransmitter gamma aminobutyric acid. Used solo or in combination therapy for simple and complex absence (petit mal) seizures. Used without FDA approval in some other types of seizures.

## Routes and Dosages:
**PO:** 15 mg/kg/day initially; increase by 5 to 10 mg/kg/day at weekly intervals PRN; not to exceed 60 mg/kg/day; generally given in 2 divided doses

**Absorption and Fate:** Rapid GI absorption; delayed with food intake and with enteric-coated preparation. Highly protein bound. Distributed into plasma and extracellular fluid; crosses placenta. Metabolized in the liver and metabolites excreted in urine. Peak level for tablets 3 to 4 hours, for capsules 1 to 4 hours, for syrup 15 minutes to 1 hour. Onset of therapeutic effects in several days to a week. Half-life: 5 to 20 hours, with average of 10.6 hours; prolonged in children under 18 months. Therapeutic level is 50 to 100 $\mu$g/ml.

**Contraindications and Precautions:** Pregnancy category D. Fetal abnormalities in laboratory animals. An association with drug use in first trimester and neural tube defects in humans may occur, therefore, used during pregnancy only if essential to seizure control. Not recommended for use in lactation as drug is present in breast milk. Contraindicated in those hypersensitive to the drug, hepatic dysfunction, coagulation dysfunction. Cautious use in children under 2 years especially if on other medications as hepatic injury risk is increased. Caution with renal dysfunction, metabolic disorders, organic brain disease.

## Side Effects:
**CNS:** drowsiness, headache, tremor, anxiety, confusion, paresthesia, dizziness, incoordination, hyperactivity and behavior change may be more common in children. **GI:** nausea, vomiting, indigestion (common); hypersalivation, anorexia, weight loss, diarrhea, constipation, cramps. **Hepatic:** **hepatotoxicity** with increased liver enzymes, most common in children under 2 years who are receiving other drugs, have metabolic disease or mental retardation. **GU:** enuresis. **Skin:** rash, hair loss or changes, facial swelling. **Hemic:** decreased platelet aggregation and prolonged bleeding time; bruising, **thrombocytopenia, leukopenia, eosinophilia**, anemia, decreased fibrinogen

## Nursing Implications:
**Assess:** Baseline renal and hepatic function tests, CBC with coagulation stud-

ies, serum ammonia. Drug not given if hepatic function or coagulation studies are abnormal or with hyperammonemia.

***Administer:*** Tablets or capsules should be swallowed whole; may be taken with food to decrease GI upset.

***Monitor:*** Frequent hepatic studies, especially in first 6 months when risk of hepatotoxicity is greatest. Coagulation studies, such as bleeding time and platelets, are done periodically and before surgery. Periodic renal function and serum ammonia. Record seizure activity. Be alert for petechiae and ecchymosis. Serum valproic acid levels are routinely measured.

***Patient Teaching:*** Take drug as directed and do not change dosage. Report seizures. Return for scheduled health-care visits. Avoid other drugs such as OTC products and alcohol. Drug can alter mental alertness; therefore, avoid driving and adjust activities accordingly. Report this drug before having surgery or dental work performed. Wear identification stating person has seizures and is on valproic acid.

**Drug Interactions:** Increased CNS depression with other CNS depressants. Increases phenobarbital and primidone levels. Not recommended with clonazepam due to possible seizure activity. May alter phenytoin binding and action. Can potentiate MAO inhibitors and antidepressants. Use cautiously in those on anticoagulants. Can increase folic acid need. Increased risk of hepatotoxicity in young children on other anticonvulsants or with other hepatotoxic medications.

**Laboratory Test Interferences:** False-positive urinary ketones. Increases glycine, lactic dehydrogenase, alkaline phosphatase, SGOT, SGPT, bilirubin. Alters thyroid function test. Prolongs bleeding time.

**Storage Requirements:** Store tightly covered in light-resistant container between 15 to 30°C (59 to 86°F). Protect syrup from freezing.

---

## □ VANCOMYCIN HYDROCHLORIDE

(van-koe-mye′sin)

(Vancocin, Vancoled)

**Classification:** antibacterial

## Available Preparations:
- 250 mg/5 ml, 500 mg/6 ml solution
- 125, 250-mg capsules
- 500 mg, 1 g for parenteral administration

**Action and Use:** Interferes with phospholipid cycle of cell-wall synthesis, alters plasma membrane function, and inhibits RNA synthesis. It is effective against a variety of infections caused by gram-positive bacteria, notably staphylococci and enterococci. Not effective against gram-negative bacteria.

## Routes and Dosage:
**PO:** 40 mg/kg/day in 3 or 4 equally divided doses. (Maximum dosage 2 g/day)
**IV:**

- neonates, under 7 days, less than 1000 g: 10 mg/kg every 24 hours; 1000 to 2000 g: 10 mg/kg every 18 hours; over 2000 g: 10 mg/kg every 12 hours
- neonates, over 7 days, over 1000 g: 10 mg/kg every 18 hours; 1000 to 2000 g: 10 mg/kg every 12 hours; over 2000 g: 10 mg/kg every 8 hours
- infants and children: 30 to 40 mg/kg/day in equally divided doses every 8 hours or 1.2 g/m²/day in divided doses

**Absorption and Fate:** Poorly adsorbed from GI tract. After IV infusion, well distributed into body tissues with minimal amounts in CSF even if meninges inflamed. 52 to 60% bound to plasma proteins. Half-life: under 1 year, 4.1 hours; over 1 year, 2.2 to 3 hours; adults, 4 to 8 hours. Excreted in urine. Therapeutic level: 12 to 25 µg/ml; toxicity at 40 mg/L.

**Contraindications and Precautions:** Pregnancy category C and use with caution during lactation. Use with caution in premature and neonates due to renal immaturity. Contraindicated in hypersensitivity to drug, and those with hearing losses. Use with caution in impaired renal function, allergies to other antibiotics.

## Side Effects:
**CV:** rapid IV infusion causing **hypotension**, erythematous or maculopapular rash on face, neck, and upper body (red-neck syndrome), throbbing pain back and neck, **wheezing, dyspnea**, pruritus, **cardiac arrest** (rare). **GI:** nausea. **GU:** transient elevations in BUN and serum creatinine, hyaline and granular casts, albumin in urine, **nephrotoxicity, fatal uremia**. **Hemic:** leukopenia, eosinophilia, neutropenia. **Sensory: ototoxicity, permanent deafness** due to auditory branch of eighth cranial nerve damage, tinnitus. **Other:** Local: tissue necrosis, pain, thrombophlebitis; Hypersensitivity: chills, fever, **anaphylaxis, vascular collapse**

## Nursing Implications:
**Assess:** Obtain baseline renal, hematological, auditory function tests, and obtain cultures before therapy. Obtain baseline BP before IV therapy.
**Administer: PO:**Capsules taken apart, mixed with small amount of food or fluid. Parenteral form may be given orally by mixing vial contents with 30 ml water; has very bitter taste. Can give this parenteral mixture through nasogastric tube. **IV:** Reconstitute according to package insert directions with sterile water for injection. Do not give IM or IV push. Dilute with compatible IV solution to minimum dilution of 2.5 to 5 ml and infuse over 60 minutes. Make certain vein is patent; causes tissue necrosis with extravasation. Rapid infusion cause hypotension and red-neck syndrome. Compatible with $D_5W$, $D_5W/NS$, $D_{10}W$, NS, LR, Dextran 6%/NS. Many incompatibilities, avoid mixing with other drugs.

*Monitor:* IV can cause thrombophlebitis and avoid extravasation; change sites every 48 to 72 hours. Monitor BP frequently for hypotension during infusion. If red-neck syndrome occurs, stop infusion, notify physician. Report symptoms of tinnitus or any signs hearing loss to physician. Assess renal function: I & O, urinalysis, BUN, serum creatinine, and visual inspection of urine for casts. Assess hearing and hematologic function periodically. Long-term therapy: assess serum drug levels. Assess for side effects and report immediately to physician. Ototoxicity and nephrotoxicity more likely to occur with IV administration. Superinfections may occur. Maintain fluid intake for age group.

*Patient Teaching:* Inform physician of tinnitus or symptoms of hearing loss. Observe for side effects and report any symptoms ototoxicity and nephrotoxicity immediately. Maintain good oral hygiene, and inspect mouth daily for signs of superinfections. Importance of following dosage schedule and taking for entire duration even if symptoms dissipate. Do not take OTC medications without consulting physician.

**Drug Interactions:** Vancomycin and anesthetic agents have caused erythema and histamine-like flushing. Drugs with ototoxic and nephrotoxic side effects, such as aminoglycosides, amphotericin B, bacitracin, cisplatin, colistin, polymyxin B, viomycin, may cause increase of these effects if used with this drug.

**Storage Requirements:** Store at 15 to 30°C (59–86°F) in tight containers. Reconstituted oral solution stable for 14 days, if refrigerated. Reconstituted IV stable for 96 hours if refrigerated.

---

# ☐ VERAPAMIL                                    (ver-ap′a-mill)

(Calan, Isoptin)

**Classification:** calcium-channel blocking agent, antianginal, antiarrhythmic (class IV), antihypertensive

## Available Preparations:
- 40, 80, 120-mg film-coated tablets
- 240-mg extended-release film-coated tablets
- 2.5 mg/ml vials for parenteral use

**Action and Use:** Inhibits calcium ion transfer across myocardial and smooth muscle cells, thereby inhibiting contraction. Coronary and systemic arteries are thus dilated, which decreases peripheral resistance, decreases blood pressure, and lowers cardiac afterload. May decrease heart rate, cause sinoatrial block, prolong the PR interval, slow conduction, and prolong refractory period. Has local anesthetic action. Used to treat supraventricular tachyarrhythmias, angina, hypertension. Uses that are not approved by the FDA include treatment of hypertrophic cardiomyopathy and bipolar disorder.

## Routes and Dosages:
*PO:* dosage for children not established
*IV:* Supraventricular Tachyarrhythmia:
- under 1 year: 100 to 200 μg/kg given in 2 minutes with usual range from 0.75 to 2 mg. May repeat in 30 minutes PRN.
- 1 to 15 years: 100 to 300 μg/kg given in 2 minutes with usual range from 2 to 5 mg; not to exceed 5 mg. May repeat in 30 minutes PRN; not to exceed 10 mg total dose.

**Absorption and Fate:** Rapidly absorbed even from PO form; PO form is rapidly metabolized. 90% bound to plasma proteins. Metabolized by the liver and metabolites excreted mainly in urine with small amounts in feces. Onset of action after IV administration is 1 to 5 minutes. Peak action: 3 to 5 minutes after IV dose and duration of antiarrhythmic effect 2 hours. Half-life is 4 minutes initially, and 2 to 5 hours in terminal phase. Therapeutic level of over 100 mg/ml is needed for antiarrhythmic effect.

**Contraindications and Precautions:** Pregnancy category C. Rapid IV injection may cause maternal hypotension and resultant fetal distress. May be excreted in breast milk, therefore, not generally recommended during lactation. Controlled studies with children have not been done but the IV form has been used with children with results similar to those in adults. Marked hemodynamic effects have occasionally occurred in infants and newborns, therefore, caution must be used with these age groups. Oral forms have not been used with children. Contraindicated in those hypersensitive to the drug, those with severe hypotension, cardiogenic shock, atrial flutter or fibrillation of Wolff-Parkinson-White syndrome, ventricular tachycardia, second or third degree AV block, sick sinus syndrome, moderate or severe cardiac failure, severe left ventricular dysfunction. Only to be used in a hospital with facilities and personnel for constant monitoring. Cautious use in ventricular dysfunction, heart failure, hepatic or renal dysfunction, Duchenne type muscular dystrophy, bradycardia, aortic stenosis, cardiogenic shock, mild or moderate hypotension. Dosage may be reduced in congestive failure or conduction disturbance.

## Side Effects:
*CNS:* blurred vision, weakness, tiredness, dizziness, fainting, headache. *CV:* **tachycardia**, pounding heart, **bradycardia, hypotension, AV block, congestive heart failure**, peripheral edema, chest pain. *GI:* constipation nausea, dry mouth, gingival hyperplasia, GI discomfort. *Respiratory:* dyspnea, coughing, wheezing, pulmonary edema. *Hepatic:* increased SGOT, SGPT, alkaline phosphatase, bilirubin; hepatotoxicity. *GU:* gynecomastia, urinary frequency, impotence, disturbed menstruation. *Skin:* rash, hair loss. *Other:* rare **hypersensitivity** with bronchospasm, pruritus, urticaria; diaphoresis

## Nursing Implications:
*Assess:* Take baseline vital signs and EKG.
*Administer:* Given only in hospital with facilities and personnel for constant monitoring. *IV:* Given over 2 minutes with constant EKG, BP, and pulse

monitoring. Initial dose may be repeated in 30 minutes PRN. Stable in most infusion solutions for 24 hours at 25°C (77°F) if protected from light. Do not mix with human albumin, amphotericin B, hydralazine, co-trimoxazole.

***Monitor:*** Constant EKG, BP, and pulse monitoring are needed. I & O measures and daily weight are recommended. Hepatic and renal function are monitored.

## Drug Interactions: Increased incidence of congestive heart failure, arrhythmia, hypotension with β-adrenergic blockers such as propranolol. Additive effects with antihypertensives. Reduced antihypertensive effect if given with nonsteroidal antiinflammatories, estrogens, sympathomimetics. Calcium supplements may decrease the therapeutic response to verapamil. Carbamazepine, cyclosporine, prazosin, quinidine, theophylline, valproate may have increased concentration and toxicity as verapamil interferes with their metabolism. Although uncertain, cimetidine may inhibit verapamil metabolism, leading to toxic effects; close monitoring is needed. Increased serum digoxin levels may result when given concurrently. Other highly protein-bound drugs may compete with binding sites, resulting in high serum levels of verapamil or the other drugs; examples include coumarin, hydantoins, quinidine, antiinflammatory analgesics, salicylates, sulfonamides. May decrease serum levels of lithium and potentiate toxic effects of that drug. May potentiate effects of neuromuscular blocking agents.

## Laboratory Test Interferences: Elevated liver enzymes.

## Storage Requirements: Store in light-resistant containers at 15 to 30°C (59 to 86°F).

---

## □ VIDARABINE  (vye-dare′a-been)

(ARA-A, Vira-A)

## Classification: antiinfective, antiviral

## Available Preparations:
- 200 mg/ml for parenteral administration
- 3% ointment for ophthalmic administration

## Action and Use: Purine nucleoside whose action is not fully understood but appears to stop DNA synthesis through DNA polymerase. Major clinical use is in treatment of herpes simplex type 1 encephalitis (HSE) and neonatal herpes simplex infections. Ophthalmic form used to treat herpes simplex (HSV-1, HSV-2), keratitis, and keratoconjunctivitis.

## Routes and Dosage: (Dosage adjustment necessary with renal impairment)

*IV:* 15 mg/kg/day given over 12 hours for 10 days
*Ophthalmic:* instill 1 cm strip of ointment in conjunctival sac every 3 hours
5 times per day

**Absorption and Fate:** Minimal absorption into aqueous humor from ophthalmic form; IV rapidly deaminated to ara-hypoxanthine. Half-life: 3.3 hour.
Widely distributed to body fluids and tissues including CSF. Excreted in urine.

**Contraindications and Precautions:** Pregnancy category C. Contraindicated during lactation, in hypersensitivity to drug, herpes zoster-immunosuppressed child. Use caution in renal or hepatic impairment, susceptibility
to fluid overloads, cerebral edema.

**Side Effects:**
*CNS:* tremors, dizziness, malaise, insomnia, confusion, hallucinations **psychosis, ataxia**. *GI:* nausea, vomiting, diarrhea, anorexia, weight loss, **hateme-
sis** (rare). *Hepatic:* transient rise in SGOT, total bilirubin. *Skin:* rash,
pruritus. *Hemic:* **thrombocytopenia, leukopenia, anemia, neutropenia, decrease in hemoglobin, platelets, hematocrit; depression of bone marrow**
(doses 20 mg/kg/day). *Sensory:* blurring of vision, burning, itching, lacrimation, photophobia. *Other:* Local: IV pain, thrombophlebitis

**Nursing Implications:**
*Assess:* Confirm diagnosis by cultures before therapy; EEG and CT scan also
aid in diagnosis. Drug most effective for encephalitis if given before child
becomes semicomatose. Obtain baseline SGOT, WBC, RBC, hemoglobin, hematocrit, and platelet counts.
*Administer:* This drug is poorly absorbed from SC or IM sites. *IV:* Do not
give IV push. Vidarabine is a milky suspension and is poorly soluble in IV
solution (each 1 mg of drug requires 2.22 ml of IV fluid to dissolve). Compatible with most IV solutions but incompatible with biological or colloidal fluids.
Shake drug before withdrawal of dose. Warm diluting solution to between 35
and 40°C to further aid in dissolving solution. Visually inspect solution; when
completely clear no further agitation is required. Drug is slowly infused over
12 to 24 hours through an in-line filter (0.45 μm). This dilution is stable for
48 hours at room temperature; do not refrigerate. *Ophthalmic:* Used under
supervision of ophthalmologist. See Part I for instillation.
*Monitor:* Assess for cerebral edema and fluid overload. Monitor SGOT, RBC,
WBC, hemoglobin, hematocrit, platelet counts periodically. Assess for side
effects. Observe IV site for thrombophlebitis.
*Patient Teaching:* Proper instillation of ointment. Not to use more frequently
than prescribed; importance of close medical supervision. Warn child that drug
will blur vision for several minutes after instillation. If no signs of improvement in 7 days, drug is usually discontinued. Usually treatment continues for 5
to 7 days after reepithelialization to prevent reinfection. Dosage may be reduced to 2 times per day during this period. Use sunglasses if photosensitivity
occurs. Use good hand washing techniques to prevent virus spread (liquid soap
preferred). Child should have separate towels and washcloths. Do not share eye

make-up. Encourage child to keep hands away from eyes. Do not use OTC eye preparations.

**Drug Interactions:** Allopurinol and this drug appear to increase CNS effects.

**Storage Requirements:** Store at 15 to 30°C (59 to 86°F) in light-resistant containers.

---

## □ VINBLASTINE                                    (vin′blast′een)

(Alkaban-AQ, Velban)

**Classification:** antineoplastic, plant alkaloid

**Available Preparations:** 1 mg/ml and 10 mg vials for parenteral use

**Action and Use:** This salt from the periwinkle plant or *Cantharanthus roseus* is a vinca alkaloid. It binds proteins of the mitotic spindle, arresting cell division in metaphase. It is cell specific for the M phase of cell division. Used in stage III and IV Hodgkin's disease and non-Hodgkin's lymphoma, as well as some solid tumors such as neuroblastoma in children and histiocytosis X (Letterer-Siwe disease).

### Routes and Dosages:
*IV:* initially 2.5 to 6.5 mg/m$^2$ in one dose. Repeated in intervals of no less than 7 days if myelosuppression is not a problem with increases of 1.25 mg/m$^2$ weekly until WBC is 3000/mm$^3$ or tumor is reduced. Then, 1.25 mg/m$^2$ less than that maximum dose is given weekly.
Maximum weekly dose for children is 12.5 mg/m$^2$. Doses given for 4 to 12 weeks.

**Absorption and Fate:** Distributed widely in body tissues but does not cross the blood-brain barrier in amounts sufficient to achieve therapeutic levels in CNS. Metabolized by the liver and excreted in urine and feces. Half-life is biphasic with initial half-life of 4.5 minutes and terminally, about 25 hours.

**Contraindications and Precautions:** Pregnancy category D. Used in pregnancy only if the woman's life is in danger. Contraindicated in severe leukopenia, untreated infection, chicken pox or herpes zoster, persons with skin ulcers. Cautious use in hepatic disease, infections.

### Side Effects:
*CNS:* numbness, paresthesia, depression, ptosis, headache, autonomic nervous system dysfunction; neurotoxicity is less common than with vincristine but may

occur during prolonged therapy or with high dose. *GI:* nausea, vomiting begin in 4 to 6 hours after dose is administered and last under 24 hours, anorexia, constipation, diarrhea, stomatitis, GI pain. *Respiratory:* dyspnea, **broncho-spasm** especially if given with mitomycin. *GU:* hyperuricemia. *Skin:* phlebitis, necrosis, and tissue sloughing at IV site, especially if extravasation occurs, alopecia, dermatitis, phototoxicity, alopecia. *Hemic:* **leukopenia** with lowest WBC count at 4 to 10 days and return to normal at 7 to 21 days; **thrombocy-topenia** especially in those with prior radiation or chemotherapy; anemia. *Other:* fever

## Nursing Implications:

*Assess:* Establish baseline CBC. Obtain serum bilirubin. Gather history of previous radiation or chemotherapy.

*Administer:* This drug has potentially severe toxic effects and should be given only under the supervision of a physician with training and experience in cancer chemotherapy. The drug's potential for toxic effects on health-care personnel as well as patients necessitates careful handling during preparation and administration. Generally during preparation of antineoplastics, latex gloves, a mask, and a solid front gown are worn, and a laminar flow hood is used. Gloves and gown may also be recommended for administration. Contaminated equipment, such as needles, syringes, vials, and unused medication, is disposed of properly. Clean-up of spills is carefully performed and accidental contact by patient or personnel receives prompt flushing and cleaning. *IV:* Give IV only, as drug is irritating to tissues. Powder is reconstituted with saline. Given into tubing of running IV or into vein over 1 minutes. Not given in large amounts of fluid over prolonged time period due to danger of extravasation. Do not use extremities for infusion that have impaired circulation. After administration the syringe and needle can be rinsed with venous blood to minimize contact of the drug with tissues. If extravasation does occur, the infusion should be stopped and finished at another site; the area may be infused with hyaluronidase and heat applied or infused with saline and hydrocortisone and cold applied. Solutions reconstituted with normal saline are stable for 30 days if refrigerated. Avoid contact with eyes as corneal damage can occur. Rinse eyes copiously if contact occurs.

*Monitor:* CBC with total and differential WBC is done weekly or before each dose of drug. Dose is established so WBC remains just above 3000/mm³. Bilirubin levels are monitored and dose is decreased by half if bilirubin is above 3 mg/dl. BUN, SGPT, SGOT, creatinine, LDH, uric acid may be monitored. Close observation for signs of infection, such as fever and respiratory infections, as well as GI bleeding must be done. Observe for nausea and vomiting; antiemetics are usually helpful. Observe oral mucosa for signs of infection. Monitor I & O to ensure adequate hydration and prevent hyperuricemia. Carefully observe IV site before, during, and after injection to prevent tissue damage.

*Patient Teaching:* Return for future visits so course of therapy can be continued. Increase fluid intake. Avoid contact with persons with infections such as colds, influenza, chicken pox. Report drooping eyelids, jaw pain, depression, headache, pain in fingers and toes, difficulty walking. Report signs of infection and bleeding such as fever, sore throat, malaise, bruising. Avoid exposure to sunlight.

**Drug Interactions:** Suppresses immune response to immunizations. Live virus vaccines must not be given, nor oral polio vaccine to close contacts with the patient due to the chance of infection with a virus; these vaccines are delayed for at least 3 months after therapy when the patient is in remission.

**Storage Requirements:** Refrigerate at 2 to 8°C (35 to 46°F) and protect from light. Solutions reconstituted with saline are stable for 30 days if refrigerated.

---

# □ VINCRISTINE                                              (vin-kris'teen)

(Oncovin, Vincasar)

**Classification:** antineoplastic, plant alkaloid

**Available Preparations:** 1 mg/ml vial for parenteral use

**Action and Use:** This salt from the periwinkle plant or *Cantharanthus roseus* is a plant alkaloid. It binds proteins on the mitotic spindle, thus arresting cell division in metaphase. It is cell-cycle specific for the M phase of cell division. Interferes with protein synthesis; causes some immunosuppression. Used for treatment of acute leukemia, Hodgkin's disease, lymphomas, neuroblastoma, rhabdomyosarcoma, Ewing's tumor, and Wilm's tumor. Is used experimentally for some other tumors, such as osteogenic sarcoma and brain tumors, although not approved for these uses at present by the FDA.

**Routes and Dosages:**
*IV:* 1.5 to 2 mg/m² weekly
If child weighs 10 kg or less or is under 1 m² body surface area, dose is 0.05 mg/kg weekly.

**Absorption and Fate:** Absorbed quickly after IV administration and widely distributed in body tissues. Does not cross blood-brain barrier in amounts great enough to reach therapeutic levels in CNS. Highly protein bound (75%). Metabolized at least partly by the liver. Excreted mainly in feces by bile, lesser amount excreted in urine. Peak level is 0.19 to 0.89 μm and reached immediately after IV. Half-life is triphasic with 3 to 4 minutes initially, then 2 hours, and terminally 10.5 to 155 hours, average 85 hours.

**Contraindications and Precautions:** Pregnancy category B. Not used in pregnancy unless woman's life is in danger as drug is teratogenic. Not recommended during lactation. Contraindicated during chicken pox or herpes zoster infection. Use with caution and decrease dosage in persons with hepatic disease. Cautious use in those with leukopenia, neuromuscular disease, drugs with CNS side effects.

## Side Effects:

*CNS:* neurotoxicity is common and dose-limiting side effect; manifested by depressed Achilles reflex, loss of deep tendon reflexes, peripheral neuropathy, wrist and foot drop, changes in gait or difficulty walking, cranial nerve palsy, jaw pain, ptosis, disturbed vision, depression, seizures; will improve when drug is stopped. *CV:* orthostatic hypotension. *GI:* constipation (common), **paralytic ileus** common in young children, nausea, vomiting, diarrhea, abdominal distention, stomatitis. *Respiratory:* dyspnea, **bronchospasm** especially when given with mitomycin. *GU:* hyperuricemia, inappropriate secretion of antidiuretic hormone. *Skin:* phlebitis, necrosis upon extravasation; alopecia, rash. *Hemic:* less hemic toxicity than with vinblastine or many other antineoplastics; mild **leukopenia**, anemia, or **thrombocytopenia**; leukopenia improves within 1 week. *Other:* hyponatremia when inappropriate secretion of antidiuretic hormone occurs, fever, weight loss

## Nursing Implications:

*Assess:* Obtain baseline CBC and bilirubin. Take history of prior radiation or chemotherapy treatment, neuromuscular disease, or simultaneous use of neurotoxic drugs.

*Administer:* This drug has potentially severe toxic effects and should be given only under the supervision of a physician with training and experience in cancer chemotherapy. The drug's potential for toxic effects on health-care personnel, as well as patients, necessitates careful handling during preparation and administration. Generally, during preparation of antineoplastics, latex gloves, a mask, and a solid front gown are worn, and a laminar flow hood is used. Gloves and gown may also be recommended for administration. Contaminated equipment, such as needles, syringes, vials, and unused medication, is disposed of properly. Clean-up of spills is carefully performed and accidental contact by patient or personnel receives prompt flushing and cleaning. *IV:* Give into a running IV or directly into a vein over 1 minute. Avoid extravasation as the drug is toxic to tissues. If extravasation occurs, discontinue infusion and complete at another site. Extravasation may be treated by injecting area with hyaluronidase and applying heat, or injecting saline and hydrocortisone and applying cold. Overdosage can be lethal and should be treated with phenobarbital, fluid restriction, enemas, CV monitoring, daily CBC, and possibly leukovorin. Fluid intake is generally increased except in cases of inappropriate secretion of antidiuretic hormone when it is decreased.

*Monitor:* CBC and serum bilirubin are done before each dosage. Dosage is reduced by half if bilirubin is 3 mg/dl or greater. Monitor I & O, weight, and nutritional status. Perform neurological examination, especially including Achilles and other deep tendon reflexes and gait before and after each dose or daily if hospitalized. Monitor vital signs. Be alert for fever and other signs of infection.

*Patient Teaching:* Return for scheduled appointments so doses can be administered. Avoid persons with infections such as colds, influenza, chicken pox. Report signs of infection such as fever, sore throat, malaise, and signs of bleeding or bruising. Increase fluid intake (unless inappropriate secretion of antidiuretic hormone has occurred). Encourage nutritious foods. Report drooping eyelids, jaw pain, depression, headache, pain in fingers and toes, difficulty walking. If acetaminophen with codeine is ordered for jaw pain, instruct in proper use (generally needed 3 to 4 days after drug administration). Educate about possibility of constipation; stool softeners and enemas may be necessary.

**Drug Interactions:** Increased neutotoxicity may occur if given with other neurotoxic drugs. Bronchospasm can occur with mitomycin. Suppresses immune response to immunizations. Live virus vaccines must not be given, nor oral polio vaccine to those in close contact with the patient on this drug due to the chance of infection with a virus; these vaccines are delayed at least 3 months after chemotherapy when the patient is in remission.

**Storage Requirements:** Refrigerate at 2 to 8°C (35 to 46°F) and protect from light. Do not use if particulates or discoloration are noted.

---

## □ VITAMIN A

(Alphalin, Aquasol A)

**Classification:** nutritional supplement

## Available Preparations:
- 10,000, 50,000-unit tablets
- 10,000, 25,000, 50,000-unit capsules
- 5000 units/0.1 ml oral solution
- 50,000 units/ml vials for parenteral use

**Action and Use:** A fat-soluble vitamin with the biologic activity of retinol. It is necessary for stability of cellular membranes; important for normal visual adaptation to light, for growth, and integrity of mucosal and epithelial surfaces. Enters the body as preformed vitamin A in animal sources and as the precursor carotene in plant sources. Used in treatment of vitamin A deficiency such as in children with malabsorption syndromes, in certain GI and liver diseases, in those with dietary restrictions (persons on total parenteral nutrition), and when taking certain medications (see Drug Interactions section).

## Routes and Dosages:
*PO:*
- Dietary Supplement: 0 to 6 months: 1500 U/day (450 RE); 6 months to 3 years: 1500 to 2000 U/day (450-600 RE); 4 to 6 years: 2500 U/day (750 RE); 7 to 10 years: 3300 to 3500 U/day (990-1050 RE)

- Deficiency with Corneal Changes: over 8 years: 500,000 U/day (150,000 RE) for 3 days, then 50,000 U/day (15,000 RE) for 2 weeks, then 10,000 to 20,000 U/day (3000-6000 RE) for 2 months

Alternatively, 5000 U/kg/day for 5 days or until recovered

*IM:* Deficiency with Xerophthalmia: 5000 to 15,000 U/day (1500-4500 RE) for 10 days

Note: Vitamin A is calculated in international units or retinol equivalents (RE) as indicated above.

**Absorption and Fate:** Completely and rapidly absorbed from GI tract in healthy persons. Delayed and incomplete absorption with conditions such as cystic fibrosis, disease of liver or pancreas. Poorly bound to plasma proteins (5%). Stored in body organs, primarily the liver, with smaller amounts in kidneys, lungs, retina; body stores can supply need for 6 to 12 months. Metabolized by the liver and excreted mainly in urine with lesser amounts in stool; larger amounts in stool of those with GI disease.

**Contraindications and Precautions:** Pregnancy category X. Normal supplemental amounts during pregnancy are recommended with minimal crossing of placenta. Overdosage is to be avoided as urinary deformities, growth retardation, and possibly CNS problems can result in the fetus. Present in breast milk. Contraindicated in those with excess vitamin A levels, and in those allergic to the product. Caution in children as symptoms of overdosage can be severe, and in renal dysfunction.

**Side Effects:**
*CNS:* irritability, drowsiness, headache, weakness, fatigue, fever, sweating; **increased intracranial pressure**, bulging fontanels in infants. *CV:* gum bleeding. *GI:* stomach pain, anorexia, nausea, vomiting. *Hepatic:* hepatomegaly, **elevated liver enzymes**, jaundice, cirrhosis. *GU:* urinary frequency. *Skin:* pruritus, dry cracking skin, yellowed palms and soles of feet, desquamation, alopecia, hyperpigmentation. *Musculoskeletal:* epiphyseal closure, growth retardation, arthralgia. *Sensory:* papilledema, visual changes. *Other:* hypercalcemia

**Nursing Implications:**
*Assess:* Evaluate presence of GI disease. Obtain diet history. RDAs for vitamin A are:
- 0 to 12 months: 1500 U
- 1 to 4 years: 2500 U
- over 4 years: 5000 U
- pregnancy: 5000 U
- lactation: 6000 U

*Administer: PO:* Special water-miscible preparations are available for those with malabsorption syndrome such as cystic fibrosis. High doses may be needed for those with malabsorption syndrome. *IM:* Be certain to aspirate; not to be given IV.

*Monitor:* Monitor for side effects; most of them indicate overdosage. Be aware of side effects during all health-care visits; many people overdose with OTC products. The serious side effect of growth retardation and epiphyseal closure necessitates careful and frequent measurements in children on this vitamin. Periodic eye examinations are done. Serum levels of the vitamin done to establish deficiency but not to regulate dosage in therapy.

***Patient Teaching:*** Take vitamins only as directed. Overdosage can have serious side effects. Dietary teaching may be needed with information on vitamin A foods (dark yellow and green leafy vegetables, milk, egg, meat, fish). Report changes such as skin, vision alterations, GI complaints, fatigue, headache.

**Drug Interactions:** Decreased vitamin A absorption when given with mineral oil. Decreased vitamin A absorption during cholestyramine and neomycin therapy, therefore, vitamin A supplement may be needed. Can increase warfarin effects. Oral contraceptives may increase serum vitamin A. Increased storage and utilization when given with vitamin E.

**Laboratory Test Interferences:** False increased BUN. Increased SGOT, SGPT with hepatic side effects. Increased serum triglyceride and cholesterol. Lowered WBC, RBC, platelets. Increased PT and erythrocyte sedimentation rate.

**Storage Requirements:** Store at 15 to 30°C (59 to 86°F) in tightly covered, light-resistant containers. Protect solutions from freezing.

---

## □ VITAMIN B12
### or
### CYANOCOBALAMIN
### or
### HYDROXOCOBALAMIN

(Alphamin, alphaREDISOL, Berubigen, Betalin, Codroxomin, Crysti-12, Cyanoject, Cyomin, Droxomin, Hydrobexan, Hydro-Cobex, Kaybovite, LA-12, Redisol, Rubesol-1000, Rubramin, Sytobex)

**Classification:** nutritional supplement

## Available Preparations:
***Cyanocobalamin:***
- 25, 50, 100, 250, 500, 1000-μg tablets
- 30, 100, 1000-μg/ml vials for parenteral use

***Hydroxocobalamin:*** 1000 μg/ml vials for parenteral use
Also available in a liver extract formula, with intrinsic factor, and in combination with other vitamins and minerals.

**Action and Use:** This water-soluble vitamin is a coenzyme in DNA synthesis and protein synthesis. Essential for hematopoietic and neurologic metabolism and function. Rapidly dividing cells require large amounts. Deficiency causes megaloblastic anemia, decreased myelin and other nerve damage, and GI lesions. Used in treatment of vitamin $B_{12}$ deficiency such as pernicious anemia. Children with malabsorption syndrome may require therapy (e.g., gluten enteropathy, GI resection). Those on strict vegetarian diets may have vitamin $B_{12}$ deficiency. The vitamin has been used for a variety of other problems such as trigeminal neuralgia, delayed growth, multiple sclerosis, allergies, viral hepatitis, skin ailments, all without FDA approval.

## Routes and Dosages:
*PO:* Nutritional Supplement: 0 to 1 year: 0.3 μg/day; over 1 year: 1 μg/day
*IM:*
- Nutritional Supplement: 30 to 50 μg/day for 2 weeks; total dose 1 to 5 mg; then 60 to 100 μg/month PRN
- Familial Selective Vitamin $B_{12}$ Malabsorption: neonate: 1000 μg/day for 11 days

## Absorption and Fate: 
Well absorbed from GI tract (mainly ileus) in normal absorptive states when intrinsic factor is present to facilitate absorption. Distributed into liver and bone marrow and crosses placenta. Highly bound to plasma proteins. Stores are depleted slowly, therefore, it may take even a few years for deficiency to manifest. Metabolized by the liver and excreted in urine and stool. Peak level in 8 to 12 hours after PO administration. Half-life: 6 days.

## Contraindications and Precautions: 
Pregnancy category C. Contraindicated in those allergic to the drug or to cobalt; preparation with intrinsic factor contains hog protein and should not be given to those who might manifest this allergy. Contraindicated in those with hereditary optic nerve atrophy.

## Side Effects:
*GI:* diarrhea. *Respiratory:* wheezing in **anaphylactic reaction**. *Skin:* itching, urticaria, swelling. *Other:* rare anaphylaxis, most often to additives to the preparation

## Nursing Implications:
*Assess:* Serum folic acid, reticulocyte count, and vitamin $B_{12}$ levels are done before therapy to rule out folic acid deficiency, which may have same symptoms as vitamin $B_{12}$ deficiency.
RDAs for vitamin $B_{12}$ are:
- 1 to 3 years: 2 μg
- 4 to 6 years: 2.5 μg
- over 7 years: 3 μg
- pregnancy: 4 μg
- lactation: 4 μg

*Administer:* **PO:** Low doses and PO route are used in those with normal GI tract who need the vitamin as a nutritional supplement due to strict vegetarian diet. **IM:** Higher doses and IM administration are used in those with malabsorption states. The preparation is occasionally given SC but must be given deep SC if this route is chosen; IM is preferred. Not to be given IV, so careful aspiration must be done. Incompatible with chlorpromazine, prochlorperazine, warfarin, ascorbic acid, dextrose, alkaline and strong acidic solutions. Small amounts are sometimes added to total parenteral nutrition feedings.

**Monitor:** Repeat serum folic acid, reticulocyte count, and vitamin $B_{12}$ levels on day 5 to 7 after beginning therapy. Serum potassium within 48 hours of beginning treatment as hypokalemia may lead to sudden death. Record dietary intake. Side effects are generally not serious or life threatening in persons with normal kidney function as this water-soluble vitamin is readily excreted.

**Patient Teaching:** Take as directed; megadoses are not useful. Foods high in vitamin $B_{12}$ include meats, fish, eggs, milk, cheese.

**Drug Interactions:** Reduced absorption of vitamin $B_{12}$ with excess alcohol, aminoglycosides, anticonvulsants, cholestyramine, neomycin, extended-release potassium, cobalt bowel treatment. Vitamin C may destroy vitamin $B_{12}$, therefore, should not be given within 1 hour of each other. Folic acid lowers vitamin $B_{12}$ levels. Chloramphenicol can alter hematopoietic response to vitamin $B_{12}$.

**Laboratory Test Interferences:** Most antibiotics interfere with serum measurements of vitamin $B_{12}$. False-positive intrinsic factor antibodies.

**Storage Requirements:** Store at 15 to 30°C (59 to 86°F) in tightly covered, light-resistant container.

---

## □ VITAMIN C

(Ascorbicap, Cebid, Cecon, Cee-1000, Cemill, Cenolate, Cetane, Cevalin, Cevi-Bid, Ce-Vi-Sol, Cevita, C-Span, Flavorcee, Sunkist)

**Classification:** nutritional supplement

### Available Preparations:
- 50, 100, 250, 500 mg, 1 g tablets
- 100, 250, 500 mg, 1 g chewable tablets
- 500 mg, 1, 1.5 g extended-release tablets
- 1 g effervescent tablets
- 500 mg extended-release capsules
- 60, 100 mg/ml oral solution
- 100, 250, 500 mg/ml ampules for parenteral use

**Action and Use:** This water-soluble vitamin is used in oxidation–reduction reactions and is essential for cell repair and collagen formation. It plays a role

in utilization of carbohydrate, fats, and protein; in production of phenylalanine, in biosynthesis of steroid hormones, in preventing oxidation of folic
acid, and facilitating absorption of iron. Deficiency results in scurvy manifested
by tissue injury, lesions, and blood vessel damage. Needs increase with need
for tissue repair and in infection. Used in treatment of vitamin deficiency.
Unapproved uses for which data does not support use include the common
cold, cancer, hematuria, depression, adjunct to deferoxamine in iron overdose,
tyrosinemia in prematures on high protein diet, and numerous other disorders.

## Routes and Dosages: PO, IM, SQ. IV
*PO:*
  - Nutritional Supplement: under 4 years: 20 to 50 mg/day
  - Deficiency: 100 to 300 mg/day in divided doses

*IM, IV:* Deficiency: 100 to 300 mg/day in divided doses

## Absorption and Fate: Well absorbed from GI tract, principally in jeju-
num. Absorption of high doses is not appreciably increased as active transport
is required. Distributed throughout body with higher amounts in glandular
tissue, liver, and white blood cells. Crosses placenta and present in breast milk.
Metabolized in the liver and excreted in the urine. Normal levels are 10 to 20
$\mu$g/ml; in serum with scurvy observed below 1 $\mu$g/ml.

## Contraindications and Precautions: Pregnancy category C. Mega-
doses in pregnancy can lead to increased requirements and deficiency in the
newborn. Cautious use in G-6-PD deficiency as hemolysis can occur; in diabetes, thalassemia, sickle cell anemia, and with history of renal stones. Sodium
ascorbate used cautiously in those on salt restriction.

## Side Effects:
*CNS:* dizziness and fainting with IV administration, headache, flushing with
high doses, insomnia. *GI:* diarrhea with high doses; nausea, vomiting, cramping. *GU:* polyuria, acidic urine. *Skin:* pain at IM or SC site

## Nursing Implications:
*Assess:* Obtain diet history. The RDAs for ascorbic acid are:
  - 0 to 12 months: 35 mg
  - 1 to 10 years: 45 mg
  - 11 to 14 years: 50 mg
  - 15 to 18 years: 60 mg
  - pregnancy: 80 mg
  - lactation: 100 mg

*Administer: PO:* Give as directed. For example, chewable tablets should be
chewed, extended-release tablets should be swallowed whole, effervescent tablets should be dissolved in a glass of water. *IV:* Protect solution from air and
light; do not add to alkaline solution.
*Monitor:* Urinary pH is measured if drug is given to acidify urine. Observe
for improvement of deficiency state.
*Patient Teaching:* Use of megadoses is discouraged. Dietary sources of as-

corbic acid should be discussed as the vitamin must be replenished through daily diet as the body cannot synthesize it. These include citrus fruits, tomatoes, strawberries, cantalope, leafy vegetables, broccoli, green peppers. Cooking and aging destroy large amounts of ascorbic acid. Increased need in smokers.

**Drug Interactions:** Barbiturates, primidone, and salicylates may increase the need for ascorbic acid. May increase absorption of oral iron when given together. May increase effect of warfarin. Acidifies urine which may influence excretion of some drugs.

**Laboratory Test Interferences:** False high or low urine glucose depending on test used. Can decrease urine pH, serum bilirubin. May increase urine oxylate. Interferes with LDH and transaminase.

**Storage Requirements:** Store tightly closed in light-resistant container at 15 to 30°C (59 to 86°F). Avoid freezing solutions.

---

## □ VITAMIN D, CALCIFEDIOL

(Calderol);

## □ CALCITRIOL

(Calcijex, Rocaltrol);

## □ DIHYDROTACHYSTEROL

(DHT, Hytakerol);

## □ ERGOCALCIFEROL

(Calciferol, Deltalin, Drisdol)

**Classification:** nutritional supplement

**Available Preparations:**
*Calcifediol:* 20, 50-μg capsules
*Calcitriol:*
- 0.25, 0.5-μg capsules
- 1, 2 μg/ml ampules for parenteral use

*Dihydrotachysterol:*
- 0.125, 0.2, 0.4-mg tablets
- 0.125-mg capsules
- 0.2, 0.25 mg/ml oral concentrated solution

### *Ergocalciferol:*

- 1.25-mg tablets
- 1.25-mg capsules
- 200 µg/ml oral solution
- 12.5 mg/ml ampules for parenteral use

**Action and Use:** These products are all analogs of fat soluble vitamin D, which facilitates absorption of calcium and phosphate, thereby promoting bone calcification. Some forms are found in milk and the body synthesizes the form cholecalciferol upon exposure to sunlight. Deficiency results in rickets and osteomalacia. Used in treatment of vitamin D deficiency such as that caused by malabsorption, familial hypophosphatemia, vitamin D-dependent rickets, prolonged anticonvulsant use, chronic renal failure, and hypocalcemic tetany in prematures.

**Routes and Dosages:** PO, IM (ergocalciferol), IV (calcitriol)
*PO:*
Calcifediol: under 2 years: 20 to 50 µg/day; 2 to 10 years: 50 µg/day; over 10 years: 50 to 100 µg/day
Calcitriol: 0.25 µg/day; increase by 0.25 µg q2–4wk; not to exceed 1 µg/day for vitamin D-dependent rickets, or 2 µg for hypocalcemia in dialysis, or 0.08 µg/kg/day for hypoparathyroidism, or 0.041 µg/kg/day for renal osteodystrophy
Dihydrotachysterol:

- Hypoparathyroidism: 1 to 5 mg/day for 4 days; Maintenance: 0.5 to 1.5 mg/day
- Familial Hypophosphatemia: 500 µg to 2 mg/day initially; Maintenance 200 µg to 1.5 mg/day

*IM:* Ergocalciferol:

- Nutritional Supplement: 1000 to 4000 U/day initially; 400 U/day maintenance
- Vitamin D–dependent Rickets: 3000 to 10,000 U/day
- Prolonged Anticonvulsants: 1000 U/day
- Hypoparathyroidism: 50,000 to 200,000 U/day
- Renal Osteodystrophy: 4000 to 40,000 U/day

*IV:* Calcitriol: Hypocalcemic Tetany in Premature: 0.05 µg/kg/day for 5 to 12 days; dosage established by clinicians rather than manufacturers

**Absorption and Fate:** Well absorbed from small intestine when fat absorption is achieved; bile necessary for ergocalciferol absorption. Stored in body fat and liver. Metabolized in liver and kidneys and excreted through bile in feces and in urine. Onset of calcitriol action in 2 to 6 hours and for ergocalciferol 10 to 24 hours. Peak level of calcifediol in 4 hours and calcitriol in 2 hours. Duration of calcitriol action is 3 to 5 days; of ergocalciferol is 2 months; of calcifediol is 15 to 20 days; and dihydrotachysterol is 9 weeks.

**Contraindications and Precautions:** Pregnancy category C. Cautious use in children as some infants are hyperreactive to the drug and some children may have slowed growth. Safety of calcifediol and IV calcitriol has not been demonstrated for children, nor has PO calcitriol for children on dialysis. Contraindicated in hypercalcemia, excess vitamin D levels, renal osteodystrophy with hyperphosphatemia. Cautious use in cardiovascular disease, hyperphosphatemia, renal dysfunction, sarcoidosis.

## Side Effects:
*CNS:* headache, fatigue, mood changes, seizures. *CV:* hypertension. *GI:* constipation, diarrhea, nausea, vomiting, abdominal pain. *GU:* kidney stones. *Skin:* pruritus, calcification of soft tissue. *Other:* hypercalcemia, nephrocalcinosis especially in infants

## Nursing Implications:
*Assess:* Obtain diet history. Serum phosphate is measured and must be at normal levels. Take baseline height and weight. RDAs are:
- birth to 18 years: 10 μg
- pregnancy: 10 μg
- lactation: 10 mg

*Administer:* Can be mixed with small amount of food or fluid.

*Monitor:* BUN, creatinine clearance, creatinine, alkaline phosphatase, phosphorus, and calcium levels are measured regularly. Urine calcium, phosphate, albumin also monitored. Monitor for signs of hypervitaminosis D such as constipation, nausea, vomiting, fatigue, hypotonia, light sensitivity, hypertension, mood changes, pruritis, and report. There is a narrow therapeutic range, or small difference between therapeutic and toxic doses.

*Patient Teaching:* Take as directed and do not overdose. Dietary teaching about sources of vitamin D may be needed. These include yeast, fish liver oils, fortified milk. Ask health-care provider before taking OTC medication as some contain calcium or phosphates and regulation of these substances will be difficult. Ensure generous fluid intake unless contraindicated.

## Drug Interactions:
Absorption decreased by cholestyramine and mineral oil. Hypercalcemia with thiazide diuretics. Decreased serum levels of vitamin D analogs in those on chronic phenobarbital and phenytoin. Increased arrhythmias with digitalis.

## Laboratory Test Interferences:
Decreased alkaline phosphatase. Increased serum calcium, cholesterol, magnesium, and phosphate. Increased urinary calcium, phosphate, albumin. Increased SGOT, SGPT.

## Storage Requirements:
Store tightly covered in light-resistant container at 15 to 30°C (59 to 86°F).

---

## □ VITAMIN E

(Aquasol E, Chew-E, Eprolin, Epsilan-M, Pheryl-E, Viterra E)

**Classification:** nutritional supplement

## Available Preparations:

- 100, 200, 400, 500, 600, 1000-unit tablets
- 100, 200, 400-unit chewable tablets
- 100, 200, 400, 600, 1000-unit capsules
- 100, 200, 400-unit water-miscible capsules
- 50 units/ml water-miscible oil

**Action and Use:** This fat-soluble vitamin is an antioxidant that likely protects other necessary metabolic substances from oxidation. It may serve to promote some enzyme action and prevents red blood cell hemolysis. Deficiency is rare but can occur in infants, particularly if premature or small for gestational age and are not fed a fortified formula. Deficiency is manifested by anemia, edema, thrombosis, and irritability. Used in treatment and prevention of deficiency such as with malabsorption (cystic fibrosis) and with total parenteral nutrition. Used in prematures to prevent hemolytic anemia, retrolental fibroplasia, and bronchopulmonary dysplasia.

## Routes and Dosages:

*PO:*

- Nutritional Supplement: premature: 5 U/day; full-term neonate: 5 U/L of formula
- Retinopathy Prevention: premature: 15 to 30 U/kg/day; dose established by clinicians rather than manufacturers
- Deficiency Treatment: 4 to 5 times RDA or 1 U/kg/day

One unit equals 1 mg of *dl*-alpha-tocopherol acetate, 1.12 mg of *dl*-alpha-tocopherol acid succinate, and 0.6 mg of *d*-alpha tocopherol.

**Absorption and Fate:** Variable (20 to 80%) absorption based on age, form of medication, presence of bile. Absorbed mainly in duodenum. Bound to plasma proteins and stored in fat tissue. Some transfer across placenta and present in breast milk. Metabolized in the liver and excreted in urine. Serum vitamin E (tocopherol) levels range from 6 to 14 µg/ml. Serum levels of newborns are about 30% of normal; lower in prematures.

**Contraindications and Precautions:** Pregnancy category A. IV form has caused a fatal syndrome in prematures and is no longer available.

## Side Effects:

Generally no side effects. Overdose can cause nausea, diarrhea, fatigue, weakness, increased CPK, and necrotizing enterocolitis. The IV form that is no longer available was shown to cause **thrombocytopenia, hepatospenomegaly, renal and hepatic dysfunction, and even led to death**.

## Nursing Implications:

*Assess:* Assess normal intake and presence of malabsorption disease. RDAs are:

- 0 to 12 months: 4 to 6 units
- 1 to 10 years: 7 to 10 units
- pregnancy: 15 units
- lactation: 16 units

*Administer:* Can be mixed with food or fluid for administration. Water miscible form for those with decreased fat absorption.

*Monitor:* Dietary intake and general assessments are done periodically.

*Patient Teaching:* Take drug as directed; overdose is not recommended and can be harmful. Dietary teaching regarding sources of vitamin E may be performed; these include vegetable oils, whole grains, wheat germ, eggs, milk, muscle meats, fish, cereals.

**Drug Interactions:** Cholestyramine and mineral oil may decrease vitamin E levels; antacids decrease its absorption. Possible increased absorption and usage of vitamin A. May decrease response to iron supplements in iron deficiency. Increased potential for hemorrhage in those on anticoagulants due to interference with vitamin K activity.

**Laboratory Test Interferences:** Increased serum cholesterol and triglyceride.

**Storage Requirements:** Store tightly closed in light-resistant container at 15 to 30°C (59 to 86°F). Protect solution from freezing.

---

## □ VITAMIN K, MENADIOL

(Synkayvite)

## □ PHYTONADIONE

(AquaMEPHYTON, Konakion, Mephyton)

**Classification:** nutritional supplement

## Available Preparations:
*Menadiol:*
- 5-mg tablets
- 5, 10, 37.5 mg/ml vials for parenteral use

*Phytonadione:*
- 5-mg tablets
- 2, 10 mg/ml vials for parenteral use

**Action and Use:** This fat-soluble vitamin facilitates the liver's production of several factors necessary for coagulation. Deficiency is rare but can occur in GI absorption problems. Used for deficiency states such as in malabsorption syndromes (cystic fibrosis and sprue). Phytonadione is used for overdose of coumarin and for hypoprothrombinemia caused by other drugs, and to prevent and treat neonatal hemorrhage.

## Routes and Dosages: PO, SQ, IM, IV
### PO:
Menadiol: Hypoprothrombinemia: 5 to 10 mg/day
Phytonadione: Hypoprothrombinemia and Nutritional Supplement: 5 to 10 mg/day
### SC, IM:
Menadiol: Hypoprothrombinemia: 5 to 10 mg QD or BID
Phytonadione:
- Nutritional Supplement: infant: 1 mg/month
- Hypoprothrombinemia: infant; 1 to 2 mg; child: 5 to 10 mg
- Hemorrhagic Disease of Newborn: 0.5 to 1 mg after birth.

## Absorption and Fate: Well absorbed from GI tract; phytonadione requires bile presence. Some amounts do cross placenta and appear in breast milk. Metabolized by liver and excreted by urine and bile. Onset of coagulation activity after IM or SC injection in 1 to 2 hours for manadiol with normal prothrombin in 8 to 24 hours. Onset of action after PO phytonadione in 6 to 12 hours; after IM or SC in 1 to 2 hours. Normal prothrombin in 12 to 14 hours after IM or SC injection of phytonadione.

## Contraindications and Precautions: Pregnancy category C. Has sometimes been given to women just before delivery to prevent bleeding in newborn but such use is not recommended. Manadiol is not recommended for newborns as it can cause hepatotoxicity, hyperbilirubinemia, kernicterus, anemia, and death; phytonadione is used. Contraindicated in those hypersensitive to the drug. Menadiol may contain sulfite and should not be given to those with an allergy to this substance. Cautious use in hepatic dysfunction and G-6-PD deficiency.

## Side Effects:
**CNS:** headache. **Other:** hypersensitivity reaction with **anaphylaxis** (rash, urticaria, dyspnea, cardiac changes, dyspnea, shock) particularly with IV administration; neonates, especially prematures, may react to menadiol with **hyperbilirubinemia**, anemia, kernicterus; such reactions to phytonadione are rare and after doses of 10 to 20 mg; the benzyl alcohol preservative may be the causative factor in the latter case

## Nursing Implications:
**Assess:** Prothrombin time is measured when drug given for hypoprothrombinemia. RDAs for vitamin K are not established but MDRs are 1 to 5 $\mu$g/kg for children.
**Administer: IM, SC:** IV dose is not recommended except in emergency due to possibility of hypersensitivity reaction. Medadiol incompatible with protein hydrolysate and phytonadione with phenytoin. Injection solution with benzyl

alcohol not given to neonates due to possibility of CNS depression, acidosis, hypotension, intracranial hemorrhage. Only phytonadione is given to neonates to prevent bleeding after birth. This is due to their inability to synthesize vitamin K in the GI tract related to inadequate intake and intestinal flora. Normal flora is reached within first week after birth with usual intake. Neonates of mothers on anticonvulsants during pregnancy may require higher doses of vitamin K.

***Monitor:*** Monitor prothrombin time for those on the drug for hypoprothrombinemia.

***Patient Teaching:*** Vitamin K is normally synthesized by the intestinal flora. Dietary sources include green leafy vegetables, tomatoes, cheese, egg, liver.

**Drug Interactions:** Decreased vitamin K with antibiotic, quinidine, salicylate intake. Decreased effect of anticoagulants when given with vitamin K. Decreased absorption of vitamin K with antacids, cholestyramine, mineral oil.

**Laboratory Test Interferences:** Falsely elevated 17-hydroxycorticosteroids.

**Storage Requirements:** Store in tightly closed, light-resistant container at 15 to 30°C (59 to 86°F). Protect solution from freezing.

---

## □ WARFARIN                                        (war'far-in)

(Coumadin, Panwarfin, Sofarin)

**Classification:** anticoagulant

**Action and Use:** Inhibits the action of vitamin K, thereby blocking hepatic formation of clotting factors II, VII, IX, and X. Effective to prevent extension of existing thrombi and to avoid additional thrombus formation. Used to treat deep vein thrombosis and pulmonary emboli. Potassium and sodium preparations of warfarin are available.

### Available Preparations:
- 2, 2.5, 5, 7.5, 10-mg tablets
- 50-mg vials for parenteral use

**Absorption and Fate:** Well absorbed from GI tract; varies among different tablets, absorption slowed by food. 97% bound to plasma proteins. Crosses placenta but not present in breast milk. Peak level in 1 to 12 hours; peak PT change in 12 hours to 3 days with duration of action 2 to 5 days. Half-life is 12 hours to 3 days.

### Routes and Dosages:
***PO:*** Dose is individualized. Started with lowest dose and adjusted upward to achieve desired PTT. Common initial dose is 2 mg daily.

**Contraindications and Precautions:** Pregnancy category D. Contraindicated in pregnancy, in patients who are bleeding or have a tendency to bleed (such as hemophilia), in abortion, recent surgery or other open wounds, GI ulcers, stroke, aneurysm, pericardial effusion, pericarditis, subacute bacterial endocarditis, eye, brain or spinal cord surgery, regional or lumbar anesthesia, vitamin C or K deficiency. Cautious use in hepatic dysfunction, diabetes, disorders that may affect prothrombin time, during menstruation, in tuberculosis, during radiation therapy, when IUD is in place. Dental procedures are performed cautiously with PT at 2 times control.

**Side Effects:**
*CV:* bleeding. *GI:* anorexia, nausea, vomiting, diarrhea, cramps, stomatitis. *Hepatic:* jaundice. *GU:* hematuria, dysuria, renal damage. *Skin:* blue and painful toes 3 to 8 weeks after therapy begins; dermatitis, hives, pruritus. *Hemic:* leukopenia, agranulocytosis. *Other:* hypersensitivity manifested by pruritus, dermatitis, hair loss, **anaphylaxis**, edema, chills, fever, weakness

**Nursing Implications:**
*Assess:* PT is measured. Consult PT before administering each dose. It should be between 1 1/2 to 2 1/2 times control. The Panwarfin brand 7.5-mg tablets contain tartrazine (yellow dye #5) that has been noted to cause allergy, particularly those with ASA sensitivity. Histories should be taken to identify patients with asthma or other allergy, especially to ASA.
*Administer:* Drug is often used as maintenance therapy after initial treatment with parenteral heparin. The two drugs may be used together for several days before heparin is withdrawn. Patients should not switch brands when desired PTT time has been reached due to potential change in clinical response. Vitamin K or fresh-frozen plasma may be administered before surgery to the patient on this drug. *IM, IV:* 2 ml sterile water is added to the 50-mg vial and a solution of 25 mg/ml is obtained. Use immediately and discard unused portions.
*Monitor:* Consult PT before administering each dose. PT is measured before therapy and daily until stabilized; then 1 to 2 times weekly for 3 to 4 weeks; then at 1 to 4-week intervals. Watch potential bleeding areas such as urine and stool; perform stool for guaiac.
*Patient Teaching:* Teach parent and child to recognize and report signs of bleeding such as blood in mouth, nose bleed, black stools, blood in urine. Urine may turn reddish orange from the medication. Infants are at highest risk of hemorrhage due to low vitamin K levels, therefore, need closest monitoring. Teach to avoid all medications, especially OTC medications such as aspirin unless contacting the prescribing physician first. Warn that many OTC products contain aspirin. Teach that illness and diet can affect PT. Tell physician before going to the dentist when on this drug. No contact sports may be played. Avoid alcohol. Eat a normal diet and call physician if child is ill and cannot eat. Child should wear a medication alert tag noting warfarin is being taken. Many rodent killers contain warfarin. These products need to be kept out of reach of all children.

**Drug Interactions:** Many drugs alter the activity of warfarin. Aspirin enhances anticoagulation and should never be given with warfarin. Broad-spectrum antibiotics alter the normal GI flora and inhibit synthesis of vitamin K, increasing the anticoagulant effect. Vitamin K will decrease warfarin's activity. Barbiturates increase metabolism of warfarin and increase PT while griseofulvin inhibits its absorption. Examples of other drugs that increase warfarin action include high dose acetaminophen, allopurinol, inhalation anesthetics, chloral hydrate, chlorampenicol, cimetidine, diazoxide, disulfiram, erythromycin, ethcyric acid, heparin, ibuprofen, indomethacin, MAO inhibitors, methotrexate, neomycin, phenothiazines, propoxyphene, quinidine, sulfonamides, tetracycline, thiazide diuretics, thyroid hormones, tricyclic antidepressants, valproic acid, verapamil, vitamins A and E. Drugs that may decrease warfarin activity include antacids, barbiturates, carbamazepine, corticosteroids, cyclophosphamide, estrogen, griseofulvin, laxatives, mercaptopurine, rifampin, smoking, spironolactone, vitamin K, high-dose vitamin C. Although close monitoring is recommended when any of these drugs is given with warfarin, concomitant administration of some should be avoided. Examples are chloral hydrate, chloramphenicol, disulfiram, phenylbutazone, aspirin, barbiturates, estrogen.

**Laboratory Test Interferences:** Increased SGOT, SGPT, alkaline phosphatase; increased bilirubin is rare. False decreased serum theophylline. Interferes with spectrophotometric urinary tests.

**Storage Requirements:** Protect from light and moisture. Store between 15 and 30°C (59 to 86°F).

# Appendices

## SCHEDULE OF CONTROLLED SUBSTANCES

- Schedule I: no accepted medical use; high-abuse potential (Examples: heroin, LSD)
- Schedule II: accepted for medical use; high-abuse potential (Examples: meperidine, amphetamine, morphine, secobarbital)
- Schedule III: accepted for medical use; lower abuse potential (Examples: paregoric)
- Schedule IV: accepted for medical use; low-abuse potential (Examples: diazepam, chloral hydrate, phenobarbital)
- Schedule V: accepted for medical use; low-abuse potential; small amounts of narcotics in combination with other products; available without prescription when certain requirements of packaging and sale are followed (Example: expectorants with codeine)

# Appendix B

## PREGNANCY CATEGORIES

- Category A: No demonstrated risk for fetal harm in controlled studies
- Category B: No demonstrated risk for fetal harm in controlled studies on women, although harm has been shown in laboratory animals; or no demonstrated risk for fetal harm in controlled studies on laboratory animals, although no controlled studies on women have been carried out
- Category C: Demonstrated risk of fetal harm in laboratory animals, although there are no controlled studies in women; or no controlled studies in animals or humans; given only if potential benefit outweighs potential harm
- Category D: Demonstrated risk of fetal harm in women; given only when serious disease is present in the pregnant woman
- Category X: Demonstrated risk of fetal harm in laboratory animals or women; potential benefit cannot outweigh risk; contraindicated in pregnancy

# Appendix C

## LAXATIVES

**Action and Use:** Laxatives in clinical use act by different mechanisms. They are categorized as follows:

1. Bulk-forming laxatives, which absorb fluid and swell in the intestine, thereby promoting peristalsis by mechanical distention and facilitating passage of stool. Cannot be given dry.
2. Stimulant laxatives, which promote peristalsis by local irritation of the mucosa.
3. Saline laxatives, which stimulate small-bowel activity, inhibit absorption of fluid and electrolytes from jejunum and ileum, attract fluid into the intestinal lumen, and increase peristalsis by osmotic force.
4. Lubricant laxatives, which soften fecal contents by coating them and preventing colonic absorption of fecal water.
5. Surfactant laxatives, which have detergent activity; they lower surface tension at the interface of oil and water, therby facilitating the mixture of water and fatty substance with fecal material to soften it.

**Considerations for Administration:** Onset of action should be considered when establishing the time of drug administration, so that the bowel movement will occur when the patient is awake and near a bathroom.

The table on the following pages shows classes of laxatives and their pharmacologic properties.

## CLASSES OF LAXATIVES AND THEIR PHARMACOLOGIC PROPERTIES

| Class | Examples | Brand Names (and Form) | Dose/Day | Onset of Action | Site of Action | Administration and Side Effects |
|-------|----------|------------------------|----------|-----------------|----------------|-------------------------------|
| Bulk-forming | Psyllium | Metamucil, Modane Bulk Mucilose, Plain Hydrocil and others | 6–11 y, 1.25–15 grams each dose prn over 12, 2.5–30 grams prn | 12–24 h up to 3 days | small and large intestine | When taken in the dry form, it may cause intestinal obstruction; take with large amount of fluid. Should be mixed immediately prior to administration; if allowed to sit, the solution will thicken. |
| | Malt soup extract | Maltsupex | infants under 2 yr, 2.5–10 ml once or twice a day older children, 5–10 ml once or twice a day | 12–24 h up to 3 days | small and large intestine | Can be given to infants under 2 months. Can be added to 1–2 oz formula, water, or fruit juice for flavoring purpose. Follow with fluids; tablet cannot be chewed or crushed. |
| Stimulant | Senna extract | Black Draught, Gentlax Senokot Senna-Gen, X-prep | 1 month to 1 y, 2.5 ml b.i.d. 1–5 yr, 5 ml b.i.d. 5–15 yr, 10 ml b.i.d. | 6–10 h | Colon | Rare. Give on empty stomach and follow with full glass fluid. May discolor urine (alkaline: pink to red) (acid: yellow to brown) |
| | Bisacodyl | Bisco-Lax, Dulcolax, tablet, 5 mg suppository, 10 mg | over 3 y, 5 mg q.d. Do not use under 2y, 1/2 to 1 prn | 6–10 h 0.25–1 h | colon colon | Wait at least 1 hour after taking milk or antacid. Swallow whole, since the enteric coating prevents the drug from causing abdominal cramps or diarrhea. Suppository may cause burning sensation. |

| Drug | Trade name | Dose | Onset | Site of action | Comments |
|------|-----------|------|-------|----------------|----------|
| Phenolph-thalein | Ex-Lax | not recommended for children under 2 y, 2–6 y, 15–20 mg; over 6 y, 30–60 mg | 6–8 h | colon | Bile must be present for phenolphthalein to be effective. About 15% is absorbed and undergoes enterohepatic circulation; hence, effect may last up to 3–4 days.<br><br>Prolonged use of phenophthalein can impair absorption of vitamin D and calcium. May impart a pink-to-red color to akaline but not to acidic urine. This drug has been known to cause skin eruptions; overdose results in excessive diarrhea, colic, cardiac and respiratory collapse. |
| Castor oil | Alphamul, Necloid, Purge | Before colonic procedure, 10–60 ml single dose (Neoloid dose); under 2y, 1–5 ml; 2–11 y, 5–15 ml; over 12 y, 15–60 ml (all given as single dose) | 2–6 h | small intestine | Not recommended for treatment of constipation; prolonged use may result in excessive loss of fluid, electrolytes, or nutrients; has been shown to cause damage to intestinal villi. Neoloid is a castor-oil emulsion and the dose is twice that of castor oil (e.g., when 30 ml of castor oil is ordered, 60 ml of Neoloid is to be given.) oil preparation unpleasant taste—chill to improve palpability, mix with minimal amounts fluid |

**(Continued)**

## CLASSES OF LAXATIVES AND THEIR PHARMACOLOGIC PROPERTIES *(Cont.)*

| Class | Examples | Brand Names (and Form) | Dose/Day | Onset of Action | Site of Action | Administration and Side Effects |
|-------|----------|------------------------|----------|-----------------|----------------|--------------------------------|
| Saline cathartics | Mg citrate | Mg citrate, Citroma, Evac-Q-Mag | 2–5 y, 60–90 ml<br>6 y and older, 90–180 ml | 0.5–3 h | small intestine and colon | Should be kept refrigerated to retain potency and palatability. |
| | Mg hydroxide | Milk of magnesia, Magnesia | 2–5 year, 5–15 ml<br>6–12 years, 15–30 ml<br>over 12 years, 30–60 ml | 0.5–3 h | small intestine and colon | Twenty percent of the magnesium is absorbed systemically; patients in renal failure who are not able to excrete the magnesium ion may suffer from adverse effects of hypermagnesemia. Give on empty stomach. |
| | Sodium phosphate Sodium biphosphate | Phospho-Soda, Sal-Hepatica | 6–9 y, 5 ml/dose; 10 y or older, 10 ml/dose | 0.5–3 h | small and large intestine | Ten to 30% of the sodium and phosphate may be absorbed systemically and may result in hypernatremia, hypokalemia, hypocalcemia, hyperphosphatemia, dehydration, hypotension, tetany, and coma. Dilute solution c̄ at least 30 ml of fluid. |
| | | Fleets Enema | pediatric size per dose | 5–15 minutes | colon | The only indications for the enema are preparation for barium enema and fecal impaction. Its use is contraindicated in patients with renal failure, appendicitis, |

| Lubricant | Liquid petrolatum | Mineral oil, oral enema, Agoral, Kondremul Neo-Cultol | under 6 y, not recommended; 6 to 12 y, PO, 5–15 ml PR, 60 ml over 12 y, PO 15–45 ml/day P.R. 60–120 ml/day | 6–8 h | colon | megacolon, imperforate anus, or congestive heart failure (because of sodium load.) Side-effects are associated with chronic use: (1) systemic absorption may elicit a foreign-body reaction characterized by the presence of inflammatory cells; (2) it may impair the absorption of fat-soluble vitamins (A, D, E, and K); (3) it should not be taken with meals because it may delay stomach emptying; (4) more palatable if given cold c̄ 30 ml fruit juice or carbonated beverage; (5) it may leak through the anal sphincter and produce anal pruritis and other perianal discomfort; (6) when taken with dioctyl sodium sulfosuccinate, absorption of mineral oil is enhanced; (7) it should not be given to comatose, combative patients or patients with impaired pharyngeal reflex because aspiration can cause lipid pneumonitis. |
| Surfactant | Docusate sodium Docusate potassium | Colace, Surfak, Diactose and others | 5 mg/kg/d in 1–2 doses | 12–72 h | small and large intestine | Useful in keeping stool soft; not used in treating existing constipation or fecal impaction. Produce a |

(Continued)

## CLASSES OF LAXATIVES AND THEIR PHARMACOLOGIC PROPERTIES (Cont.)

| Class | Examples | Brand Names (and Form) | Dose/Day | Onset of Action | Site of Action | Administration and Side Effects |
|---|---|---|---|---|---|---|
| | Docusate calcium | | | | | temporary change in intestinal permeability lasting a few hours, which may enhance GI or hepatic uptake of other drugs given at the same time (e.g., greater mucosal damage is seen when aspirin and a surfactant are taken concomitantly). Liquid has bitter taste; do not crush or chew tablets. |
| Miscellaneous | Glycerin | Glycerin (PR) Babylax Sanisupp | suppository, 1–1.7 g or 2–5 ml as enema for children under 6 y, double the dose for older children | 0.25–1 h | colon | May produce rectal irritation; oral form of glycerin is used as an osmotic diuretic to reduce intraocular or intracranial pressure. |

**Patient Teaching:** Give laxatives to children only if ordered by physician. Teach parent about child's bowel patterns and how overusage can result in loss of bowel tone. Monitor bowel pattern.

# Appendix D

**CLASSES OF ANTIARHYTHMICS**

| Class | Examples | Characteristics |
|-------|----------|-----------------|
| IA | Quinidine<br>Procainimide<br>Disopyramide | Depresses sodium conduction<br>Suppresses automaticity<br>Prolongs refractory period<br>Decreases conduction velocity<br>Prolongs action potential duration |
| IB | Lidocaine<br>Phenytoin<br>Tocainide | Increases potassium conduction<br>Decreases action potential duration<br>Prolongs refractory period |
| II | Beta blockers<br>Propranolol<br>Nadolol<br>Metoprolol | Antagonizes catecholamine<br>Suppresses automaticity<br>Decreases conduction rate |
| III | Bretylium | Prolongs action potential duration<br>Prolongs refractory period |
| IV | Calcium-channel blockers<br>Verapamil<br>Nifedipine<br>Diltiazem | Slows impulse conduction<br>Prolongs refractory period |

**RESUSCITATION MEDICATIONS, BY WEIGHT AND AGE, FOR INFANTS AND CHILDREN 0–10 YEARS**

| Age | 50th Percentile Weight (kg) | Epinephrine | | Atropine | | Bicarbonate[a] | |
|---|---|---|---|---|---|---|---|
| | | *mg* | *ml* | *mg* | *ml* | *mEq* | *ml* |
| Newborn | 3.0 | 0.03 | 0.3 | 0.1 | 1.0 | 3.0 | 6.0 |
| 1 Month | 4.0 | 0.04 | 0.4 | 0.1 | 1.0 | 4.0 | 8.0 |
| 3 Months | 5.5 | 0.055 | 0.55 | 0.11 | 1.1 | 5.5 | 11.0 |
| 6 Months | 7.0 | 0.07 | 0.7 | 0.14 | 1.4 | 7.0 | 7.0 |
| 1 Year | 10.0 | 0.10 | 1.0 | 0.20 | 2.0 | 10.0 | 10.0 |
| 2 Years | 12.0 | 0.12 | 1.2 | 0.24 | 2.4 | 12.0 | 12.0 |
| 3 Years | 14.0 | 0.14 | 1.4 | 0.28 | 2.8 | 14.0 | 14.0 |
| 4 Years | 16.0 | 0.16 | 1.6 | 0.32 | 3.2 | 16.0 | 16.0 |
| 5 Years | 18.0 | 0.18 | 1.8 | 0.36 | 3.6 | 18.0 | 18.0 |
| 6 Years | 20.0 | 0.20 | 2.0 | 0.40 | 4.0 | 20.0 | 20.0 |
| 7 Years | 22.0 | 0.22 | 2.2 | 0.44 | 4.4 | 22.0 | 22.0 |
| 8 Years | 25.0 | 0.25 | 2.5 | 0.50 | 5.0 | 25.0 | 25.0 |
| 9 Years | 28.0 | 0.28 | 2.8 | 0.56 | 5.6 | 28.0 | 28.0 |
| 10 Years | 34.0 | 0.34 | 3.4 | 0.68 | 6.8 | 34.0 | 34.0 |

Volume (ml) is based on the following concentrations:
  Epinephrine: 1:10,000 (0.1 mg/ml)
  Atropine: 0.1 mg/ml
  Bicarbonate: ≤ 3 months = 4.2% solution (0.5 mEq/ml)
        > 3 months = 8.4% solution (1 mEq/ml)
[a]The use of bicarbonate in cardiac arrest is controversial (see text). Good ventilation must be established before bicarbonate is used.
*From Chameides Leon (1988) Textbook of Pediatric Advanced Life Support, Dallas TX: Amer Heart Association; by permission of the American Heart Association*

## EMERGENCY MEDICATIONS, BY WEIGHT AND AGE, FOR INFANTS AND CHILDREN 0–10 YEARS

**ADD**   0.6 mg (3 ml)[a] of **isoproterenol**
0.6 mg (0.6 ml)[a] of **epinephrine**
60.0 mg (1.5 ml)[a] of **dopamine**      **TO** 100 ml of diluent
60.0 mg (2.4 ml)[a] of **dobutamine**

**INFUSE**  at 1 ml/kg/hr or according to following table in order

**TO GIVE**   0.1 μg/kg/min isoproterenol
0.1 μg/kg/min epinephrine
10 μg/kg/min dopamine
10 μg/kg/min dobutamine

| Age | 50th Percentile Weight (kg) | Infusion Rate (ml/hr) |
|---|---|---|
| Newborn | 3 | 3 |
| 1 month | 4 | 4 |
| 3 months | 5.5 | 5.5 |
| 6 months | 7.0 | 7.0 |
| 1 year | 10.0 | 10.0 |
| 2 years | 12.0 | 12.0 |
| 3 years | 14.0 | 14.0 |
| 4 years | 16.0 | 16.0 |
| 5 years | 18.0 | 18.0 |
| 6 years | 20.0 | 20.0 |
| 7 years | 22.0 | 22.0 |
| 8 years | 25.0 | 25.0 |
| 9 years | 28.0 | 28.0 |
| 10 years | 34.0 | 34.0 |

These are starting doses. Adjust concentration to dose and fluid tolerance.
[a]Based on the following concentrations.
  Isoproterenol = 0.2 mg/ml
  Epinephrine = 1:1000 (1 mg/ml)
  Dopamine = 40 mg/ml
  Dobutamine = 25 mg/ml
*From Chameides Leon (1988) Textbook of Pediatric Advanced Life Support, Dallas TX: Amer Heart Association; by permission of the American Heart Association*

**COMMON TOXIC EFFECTS OF ANTINEOPLASTICS**

| Drug | Common Toxic Effects |
|------|---------------------|
| ARA-C | Myelosuppression: megaloblastosis, reticulocytosis, leukopenia, thrombocytopenia, anemia<br>High-dose:<br>  Neurological: cerebral and cerebellar dysfunction<br>  GI: severe ulceration<br>  Pulmonary: respiratory distress, pulmonary edema |
| Asparaginase | Hypersensitivity: rash, urticaria, hypotension, dyspnea, arthralgia, anaphylaxis<br>Hyperglycemia |
| Bleomycin | Pulmonary: interstitial pneumonitis, pulmonary fibrosis |
| Cisplatin | Renal: increased serum creatinine, BUN, uric acid; decreased creatinine clearance, glomerular filtration rate<br>Electrolyte imbalance: hypomagnesemia, hypocalcemia, hypokalemia, hypophosphatemia, hyponatremia<br>GI: severe nausea and vomiting<br>Ototoxicity: tinnitus, hearing loss<br>Myelosuppression: less severe than with other agents |
| Cyclophosphamide | Myelosuppression: leukopenia, thrombocytopenia, anemia<br>Hypothrombinemia<br>GU: hemorrhagic cystitis, hematuria |
| Dacarbazine | Myelosuppression: leukopenia, thrombocytopenia |
| Dactinomycin | Myelosuppression: leukopenia, thrombocytopenia; less often anemia, pancytopenia, reticulopenia, agranulocytosis, aplastic anemia<br>GI: stomatitis, diarrhea |
| Daunorubicin | Myelosuppression: leukopenia, thrombocytopenia, anemia<br>Cardiac: congestive heart failure |
| Doxorubicin | Myelosuppression: leukopenia, thrombocytopenia, anemia<br>Cardiac: congestive heart failure, cardiorespiratory decompensation |
| Etoposide | Myelosuppression: leukopenia, granulocytopenia, thrombocytopenia, anemia, pancytopenia<br>Cardiac: delayed hypotension |
| Fluorouracil | GI: stomatitis (day 5 to 8 of therapy), GI hemorrhage<br>Myelosuppression: leukopenia, granulocytopenia, thrombocytopenia, anemia |
| Hydroxyurea | Myelosuppression: leukopenia, thrombocytopenia, anemia<br>GI: severe nausea and vomiting |
| Lomustine | Delayed myelosuppression: leukopenia (6 weeks after ther- |

apy), thrombocytopenia (4 weeks after therapy), anemia (4 to 7 weeks after therapy), pancytopenia

| | |
|---|---|
| Mechlorethamine | Myelosuppression: leukopenia, anemia, thrombocytopenia, delayed hemorrhage<br>GI: severe nausea and vomiting |
| Mercaptopurine | Myelosuppression: leukopenia, anemia, thrombocytopenia, agranulocytosis, pancytopenia, hypoplastic bone marrow<br>Hepatic: jaundice, ascites, elevated liver enzymes, cholestasis |
| Methotrexate | GI: oral ulcers<br>Myelosuppression: leukopenia, thrombocytopenia, anemia, hemorrhage |
| Procarbazine | Myelosuppression: leukopenia, reticulocytopenia, thrombocytopenia, eosinophilia, anemia, blood cell hemolysis<br>Neurological: neuropathy, paresthesia, depression, tremors, confusion, seizures<br>GI: stomatitis, diarrhea |
| Thioguanine | Myelosuppression: leukopenia, thrombocytopenia, anemia<br>Hepatic: jaundice, elevated liver enzymes<br>GI: stomatitis, diarrhea |
| Vinblastine | Myelosuppression: leukopenia, granulocytopenia, thrombocytopenia, anemia<br>Neurological: numbness, paresthesia, peripheral neuropathy, depression |
| Vincristine | Neurological: peripheral neuropathy with Achilles tendon reflex, depression, then loss of other deep tendon reflexes<br>Myelosuppression: less severe than with other agents |

Note: Drugs cause various responses in the body. Antineoplastic agents are expected to cause toxicity due to their potency and desired action on abnormal body cells. The symptoms listed here are the most common and earliest toxic effects. They require dosage lowering or temporary cessation of the drug. Generally, the highest dose possible is given that allows for absence of toxic effects but maximum therapeutic effects in the body. Toxic effects can lead to serious, life threatening, and sometimes permanent damage in the body. They, therefore, require dosage adjustment, in contrast to other less threatening side effects. Each drug has unique toxic effects that indicate need for dosage adjustment.

These drugs have potentially severe toxic effects and should be given only under the supervision of a physician with training and experience in cancer chemotherapy. The drug's potential for toxic effects on health care personnel, as well as patients, necessitates careful handling during preparation and administration. Generally, during preparation of antineoplastics, latex gloves, a mask, and a solid front gown are worn, and a laminar flow hood is used. Gloves and gown may also be recommended for administration. Contaminated equipment, such as needles, syringes, vials, and unused medication, is disposed of properly. Cleanup of spills is carefully performed and accidental contact by patient or personnel receives prompt flushing and cleaning.

## EXAMPLES OF ANTINEOPLASTIC DRUG COMBINATIONS

- A-COPP = doxorubicin + cyclophosphamide + vincristine + procarbazine + prednisone
- ABVD = doxorubicin + bleomycin + vinblastine + dacarbazine
- ACE = cyclophosphamide + doxorubicin
- APE = doxorubicin + procarbazine + etoposide
- CAF = cyclophosphamide + doxorubicin + fluorouracil
- CAMP = cyclophosphamide + doxorubin + methotrexate + procarbazine
- CAVe = lomustine + doxorubicin + vinblastine
- CAVE or ECHO or CAPO or EVAC or VOCA = etoposide + cyclophosphamide + doxorubicin + vincristine
- CHOP = cyclophosphamide + doxorubicin + vincristine + prednisone
- CHOR = cyclophosphamide + doxorubicin + vincristine
- CISCA = cyclophosphamide + cisplatin
- CMF = cyclophosphamide + methotrexate + fluorouracil
- COPP = cyclophosphamide + vincristine + procarbazine + prednisone
- CVP = cyclophosphamide + vincristine + prednisone
- CY-VA-DIC = cyclophosphamide + vincristine + doxorubicin + dacarbazine
- FAC = fluorouracil + doxorubicin + cyclophosphamide
- MACC = methotrexate + doxorubicin + cyclophosphamide + lomustine
- MOPP = mechlorethamine + vincristine + procarbazine + prednisone
- MTX + MP + CTX = methotrexate + mercaptopurine + cyclophosphamide
- PVB or VBP = vinblastine + bleomycin + cisplatin
- T-2 = dactinomycin + doxorubicin + vincristine + cyclophosphamide
- VAP = vincristine + dactinomycin + cyclophosphamide
- VP-L = Asparaginase vincristine + prednisone + asparaginase

**REPORTABLE EVENTS FOLLOWING VACCINATION**

| Vaccine/Toxoid | Event | Interval from Vaccination |
|---|---|---|
| DTP, P, DTP/polio combined | A. Anaphylaxis or anaphylactic shock | 24 h |
| | B. Encephalopathy (or encephalitis)a | 7 days |
| | C. Shock-collapse or hypotonic-hyporesponsive collapsea | 7 days |
| | D. Residual seizure disordera | (See Aids to Interpretationa) |
| | E. Any acute complication or sequela (including death) of above events | No limit |
| | F. Events in vaccinees described in manufacturer's package insert as contraindications to additional doses of vaccinea (such as convulsions) | (See package insert) |
| Measles, mumps, and rubella; DT, td, tetanus toxoid | A. Anaphylaxis or anaphylactic shock | 24 h |
| | B. Encephalopathy (or encephalitis)a | 15 days for measles, mumps, and rubella vaccines; 7 days for DT, Td, and T toxoids |
| | C. Residual seizure disordera | (See Aids to Interpretationa) |
| | D. Any acute complication or sequela (including death) of above events | No limit |
| | E. Events in vaccinees described in manufacturer's package insert as contraindications to additional doses of vaccineb | (See package insert) |
| Oral polio vaccine | A. Paralytic poliomyelitis | |
| | - in a nonimmunodeficient recipient | 30 days |
| | - in an immunodeficient recipient | 6 mo |
| | - in a vaccine-associated community case | No limit |
| | B. Any acute complication or sequela (including death) of above events | No limit |

| | | |
|---|---|---|
| | C. Events in vaccinees described in manufacturer's package insert as contraindications to additional doses of vaccine[b] | (See package insert) |
| Inactivated polio vaccine | A. Anaphylaxis or anaphylactic shock | 24 h |
| | B. Any acute complication or sequela (including death) of above event | No limit |
| | C. Events in vaccinees described in manufacturer's package insert as contraindications to additional doses of vaccine[b] | (See package insert) |

---

[a]**Aids to Interpretation:**

Shock-collapse or hypotonic-hyporesponsive collapse may be evidenced by signs or symptoms such as decrease in or loss of muscle tone, paralysis (partial or complete), hemiplegia, hemiparesis, loss of color or turning pale white or blue, unresponsiveness to environmental stimuli, depression of or loss of consciousness, prolonged sleeping with difficulty arousing, or cardiovascular or respiratory arrest.

Residual seizure disorder may be considered to have occurred if no other seizure or convulsion unaccompanied by fever or accompanied by a fever of less than 102°F occurred before the first seizure or convulsion after the administration of the vaccine involved.

*And*, if in the case of measles-, mumps-, or rubella-containing vaccines, the first seizure or convulsion occurred within 15 days after vaccination *or* in the case of any other vaccine, the first seizure or convulsion occurred within 3 days after vaccination,

*And*, if two or more seizures or convulsions unaccompanied by fever or accompanied by a fever of less than 102°F occurred within 1 year after vaccination.

The terms seizure and convulsion include grand mal, petit mal, absence, myoclonic, tonic-clonic, and focal motor seizures and signs. Encephalopathy means any significant acquired abnormality of, injury to, or impairment of function of the brain. Among the frequent manifestations of encephalopathy are focal and diffuse neurologic signs, increased intracranial pressure, or changes lasting at least 6 hours in level of consciousness, with or without convulsions. The neurologic signs and symptoms of encephalopathy may be temporary with complete recovery, or they may result in various degrees of permanent impairment. Signs and symptoms such as high-pitched and unusual screaming, persistent unconsolable crying, and bulging fontanel are compatible with an encephalopathy, but in and of themselves are not conclusive evidence of encephalopathy. Encephalopathy usually can be documented by slow wave activity on an electroencephalogram.

[b]The health-care provider must refer to the *Contraindication* section of the manufacturer's package insert for each vaccine.

*From "National childhood vaccine injury act: Requirements for permanent records and for reporting of selected events after vaccination," 1988,* Morbidity and Mortality Weekly Report 37(13), 198.

## REPORTING OF EVENTS OCCURRING AFTER VACCINATION

| | Vaccine Purchased with Public Money | Vaccine Purchased with Private Money |
|---|---|---|
| Who Reports: | Health-care provider who administered the vaccine | Health-care provider who administered the vaccine |
| What Products To Report: | DTP, P, Measles, Mumps, Rubella, DT, Td, T, OPV, IPV, and DTP/Polio Combined | DTP, P, Measles, Mumps, Rubella, DT, Td, T, OPV, IPV, and DTP/Polio Combined |
| What Reactions To Report: | Events listed in Appendix I including contraindicating reactions specified in manufacturers' package inserts | Events listed in Appendix I including contraindicating reactions specified in manufacturers' package inserts |
| How To Report: | Initial report taken by local, county, or state health department. State health department completes CDC form 71.19 | Health-care provider completes Adverse Reaction Report-FDA form 1639 (include interval from vaccination, manufacturer, and lot number on form) |
| Where To Report: | State health departments send CDC form 71.19 to: MSAEFI/IM (E05) Centers for Disease Control Atlanta, GA 30333 | Completed FDA form 1639 is sent to: Food and Drug Administration (HFN-730) Rockville, MD 20857 |
| Where To Obtain Forms: | State health departments | FDA and publications such as *FDA Drug Bulletin* |

From *"National childhood vaccine injury act: Requirements for permanent records and for reporting of selected events after vaccination," 1988,* Morbidity and Mortality Weekly Report *37(13),* 199.

# References

Abhyanker S, Rao, SP, Pollio, L, Miller ST, et al. (1988). Anaphylactic shock due to dacarbazine. *Am J Dis Child, 142*, 918.

American Society of Hospital Pharmacists. (1990). *American hospital formulary service: drug information*. Bethesda, Md: American Society of Hospital Pharmacists.

Arnon S. (1979). Honey and other environmental risk factors for infant botulism. *J Pediatr, 92*, 331–338.

Babson SG, Pernoll ML, Benda GI, Simpson K. (1980). *Diagnosis and management of the fetus and neonate at risk* (4th ed.). St. Louis: Mosby.

Becker T. (1981). *Cancer chemotherapy: a manual for nurses*. Boston: Little, Brown.

Behrman R, Vaughan V. (1987). *Nelson textbook of pediatrics* (13th ed.). Philadelphia: Saunders.

Benitz W, Tatro D. (1988). *The pediatric drug handbook*. Chicago: Yearbook Medical Publishers.

Bernstein JG. (1988). *Handbook of drug therapy in psychiatry* (2nd ed.). Littleton, Mass: PSG Publishing.

Bindler R, Tso Y, Howry L. (1986). *The parents' guide to pediatric drugs*. New York: Harper & Row.

Breitzer GM. (1988). Practical approach to the treatment of otitis media in infants and children. *Pediatric Basics, 51*, 11–16.

Buchanan G. (1980). Hemophilia. *PCNA, 27*(2), 309–326.

Carlson B. (1983). [Guidelines for administration of intravenous medications to pediatric patients (17 years and under)]. *Deaconess Medical Center—Spokane, WA*. Unpublished data.

Chameides L. (1988). *Textbook of pediatric advanced life support*. Dallas, Tex: American Heart Association.

The choice of antimicrobial drugs. (1988, March). *Med Lett Drugs Ther, 30*, 33–40.

Cleary J. (1988). Two inotropic agents: dopamine and dobutamine. *Pediatric Nursing, 14*(5), 414.

Colley R, Wilson J. (1979). Meeting patient's nutritional needs with hyperalimentation: providing hyperalimentation for infants and children. *Nursing 79, 9*(7), 50–53.

Committee on Infectious Diseases. (1988). *Report of the Committee on Infectious Diseases* (21st ed.). Elk Grove Village, Ill: American Academy of Pediatrics.

Cox NH, Moss C, Forsyth A. (1988). Cutaneous reactions to aluminum in vaccines: an avoidable problem. *Lancet, 2*, 43.

Davis N, Sweeney L. (1989). Infantile apnea monitoring and SIDS. *J Pediatr Health Care, 3*(2), 67–75.

Deglin JH, Vallerand AH. (1988). *Davis's drug guide for nurses*. Philadelphia: Davis.

Dorr R, Fritz W. (1980). *Cancer chemotherapy handbook*. New York: Elsevier.

*Drug information for the health care professional (USPDI)* (9th ed.) (1989). Rockville, Md: U.S. Pharmacopeial Convention.

Drugs for parasitic infections. (1988, February). *Med Lett Drugs Ther, 30*, 15–24.

Drugs for tuberculosis. (1988, April). *Med Lett Drugs Ther, 30*, 43–44.

Evans W, Schentag J, Jusko W. (1980). *Applied pharmacokinetics: principles of therapeutic drug monitoring*. San Francisco: Applied Therapeutics.

Few B. (1987). Digoxin immune Fab. *MCN, 12*(6), 431.

Fitzgerald JJ, Shamy PG. (1987, July). Let your patient control his analgesia. *Nursing 87, 17*(7), 48–51.

Ford DC, Leist WR, Phelps SJ. (1988). *Guidelines for administration of intravenous medications to pediatric patients* (3rd ed.). Bethesda, Md: American Society of Hospital Pharmacists.

Foster R, Hunsberger M, Anderson J. (1989). *Family centered nursing care of children.* Philadelphia: Saunders.

Friedman WF, George BL. (1984). New concepts and drugs in the treatment of congestive heart failure, *PCNA, 31*(6), 1197–1227.

Gadow K. (1986). *Children on medication, Vols. I & II.* Boston: Little, Brown.

Gahart B. (1990). *Intravenous Medications* (6th ed.). St. Louis: Mosby.

Gibaldi M. (1984). *Biopharmaceutics and clinical pharmacokinetics* (3rd ed.). Philadelphia: Lea & Febiger.

Gibson G, Skett P. (1986). *Introduction to drug metabolism.* New York: Chapman & Hall.

Gilman AG, Goodman LS, Rall TW, Murad F. (eds.). (1985). *The pharmacological basis of therapeutics* (7th ed.). New York: Macmillan.

Govoni L, Hayes J. (1988). *Drugs and nursing implications* (6th ed.). Norwalk, Conn: Appleton & Lange.

Graef JW (ed.). (1988). *Manual of pediatric therapeutics* (4th ed.). Boston: Little, Brown.

Grinder D, Guastella C., Pellegrino M. (1988). Soft tissue damage and intravenous phenytoin. *Drug Intell Clin Pharm, 22,* 725–726.

*Handbook of nonprescription drugs* (8th ed.). (1986). Washington, D.C.: American Pharmaceutical Association.

Haskell CM. (1980). *Cancer treatment.* Philadelphia: Saunders.

Hazinski MF. (1984). *Nursing care of the critically ill child.* St. Louis: Mosby.

Howry L, Bindler R, Tso Y. (1981). *Pediatric medications.* Philadelphia: Lippincott.

Jacobson N. (1979). How to administer those tricky lipid emulsions. *RN, 42,* 63–67.

Kelley SJ. (1988). *Pediatric emergency nursing.* Norwalk, Conn: Appleton & Lange.

Klaus MH, Fanaroff AA. (1986). *Care of the high-risk neonate* (3rd ed.). Philadelphia: Saunders.

Landier WC, Barrell ML, Styffe EJ. (1987). How to administer blood components to children. *MCN, 12,* 178–184.

Leopold I, Burns R. (eds.). (1977). *Symposium on ocular therapy (Vol. 10).* New York: Wiley.

Levin, DL, Morriss FC, Moore GC. (eds.). (1979). *A practical guide to pediatric intensive care.* St. Louis: Mosby.

Lowrey GH. (1986). *Growth and development of children* (8th ed). Chicago: Yearbook Medical Publishers.

McEvoy GK. (ed.). (1989). *AHFS drug information 89.* Bethesda, Md: American Society of Hospital Pharmacists.

The Medical Letter. (1989). Drugs for epilepsy. *The Medical Letter, 31*(783), 1–4.

Mungall D. (1983). *Applied clinical pharmacokinetics.* New York: Raven Press.

National Cancer Institute. (1985). *Chemotherapy and you.* Bethesda, Md: U. S. Department of Health and Human Services.

National Childhood Vaccine Injury Act. (1988). *Morbidity and Mortality Weekly Report, 37*(13), 198.

Nelson JD. (1987). *1987–1988 pocketbook of pediatric antimicrobial therapy* (7th ed.). Baltimore: Williams & Wilkins.

Nice FJ. (1989). Can a breast-feeding mother take medication without harming her infant? *MCN, 14*(1), 27–31.

O'Hara WJ, Weidel RM. (1989). Therapy of childhood asthma. *J Pharm Pract, 2*(1), 45–54.

Pagliaro LA, Pagliaro AM. (1987). *Problems in pediatric drug therapy* (2nd ed.). Hamilton, Ill: Drug Intelligence Publications.

Penatzer M, Fissell G, Groover MC, Heim D, Emerson-Krolman ME. (1988). Pediatric drug information. *Pediatr Nursing, 14*, 56–57.

Penatzer M, Fissell G, Groover MC, Heim D. (1989). *Physician's desk reference* (43rd ed.). Oradell, N.J.: Medical Economics Co.

Pipes P. (1985). *Nutrition in infancy and childhood* (3rd ed.). St. Louis: Mosby.

Protocol for the use of ribavirin in the care of the patient with respiratory syncytial virus. *Deaconess Medical Center—Spokane, WA*. Unpublished data.

Rimar JM. (1987). Guidelines for the intravenous administration of medications used in pediatrics. *MCN, 12*, 322–340.

Rocchini AP. (1984). Childhood hypertension: Etiology, diagnosis, and treatment, *PCNA, 31*(6), 1259–1273.

Rowe PC. (1987). *The Harriet Lane handbook* (11th ed.). Chicago: Year Book Medical.

Rudolph AM. (ed.). (1987). *Pediatrics* (18th ed.). Norwalk, Conn: Appleton & Lange.

Schneeweiss A. (1986). *Drug therapy in infants and children with cardiovascular diseases*. Philadelphia: Lea & Febiger.

See-Lasley K, Ignoffo R. (1981). *Manual of oncology therapeutics*. St. Louis: Mosby.

Skidmore-Roth L. (1988). *Mosby's nursing drug reference*. St. Louis: Mosby.

Speck WT, Blumer JL. (1983). Anti-infective therapy. I. *Pediatr Clin North Am, 30*(1).

Speck, WT, Blumer JL. (1983). Anti-infective therapy. II. *Pediatr Clin North Am, 30*(2).

Stewart C, Stewart L. (1984). *Pediatric medications*. Rockville, Md: Aspen Systems Corp.

Traver GA, Martinez M. (1988). Asthma update. Part II: treatment. *Journal of Pediatric Health Care, 2*(5), 227–233.

Weinberger M, Lindgren S, Bender B, Lerner JA, Szefler S. (1987). Effects of theophylline on learning and behavior: reason for concern or concern without reason? *J Pediatr, 3*(3), 471–474.

Weintraub M, Evans P. (1986). Fab: an immunologic treatment for severe digoxin overdose. *Hospital Forum, 21*(12), 196–197.

Whaley LF, Wong DL. (1987). *Nursing care of infants and children*. St. Louis: Mosby.

Worthington-Roberts B, Vermeersch J, Williams S. (1985). *Nutrition in pregnancy and lactation* (3rd ed.). St. Louis: Mosby.

Zimmerman DR. (1983). *The essential guide to nonprescription drugs*. New York: Harper & Row.

Zimmerman SS, Gildea JH. (1985). *Critical care pediatrics*. Philadelphia: Saunders.

# Index

Generic names are *italic*; trade names are capitalized and in regular type. Page numbers followed by a *t* refer to tables.